DERMONICS

A MNEMONICS-DENSE REVIEW BOOK FOR THE UPDATED DERMATOLOGY BOARD EXAM

Dr. Jeffrey Morris, DO, FAAD

First Edition

NEWMAN SPRINGS PUBLISHING
320 Broad Street
Red Bank, NJ 07701

First originally published by Newman Springs Publishing 2025

This review book is for educational and boards review purposes only. It is not meant to substitute for independent medical judgement of the treating physician. The information in this review book has been gathered from other review books (Alikhan), textbooks (Bolognia), journal articles (particularly JAAD CMEs), VisualDX, conferences, and question banks, and I cannot guarantee the accuracy, reliability, completeness, or timeliness of the information presented. I am not responsible for any actions taken in reliance on this book by a medical professional.

ISBN 979-8-89308-448-1 (Paperback)
ISBN 979-8-89308-449-8 (Digital)

Printed in the United States of America

To my wife, Sara

Contents

Chapter 4: Pediatric dermatology

How to use this book

This book is intended to provide the reader with the most up-to-date review on the topics most likely to be tested for the updated in-service exams and dermatology board exam. In addition to being the most complete and up-to-date review book, it also contains mnemonics to help you remember many important facts and concepts. It is known that having a mnemonic not only helps you remember facts and details, but it allows you to retain them for longer periods of time. Example: there are some "superhuman geniuses" that can remember thousands of numbers consecutively. They don't actually have superhuman abilities, they are regular people who just use mnemonics, which convert these random numbers into elements in a story which can be easily memorized. With these mnemonics, I have provided you with an easier way to memorize the thousands of facts we commonly get tested on (bolded items get tested more commonly). You'll notice I color certain letters and words the same color when I want to draw your attention to an association between them. Not all mnemonics will work for all people; if you do not like one, just strike a line through it and move on. The information is still all here, and it is all important, and if you have a better way of memorizing it, then write it down instead (and please email me so I can include it in version 2). Happy studies everyone!

Trigger warning

Some mnemonics you are about to read may come off as immature or sexually charged, but just as sex sells in business, it also produces an emotional response that greatly facilitates the process of memorization. The purpose of this book is not to offend anyone but to help dermatology residents remember the most board-relevant details of dermatology. With PC culture only picking up steam, I understand these are hypersensitive times, and if you believe the value provided by any mnemonic is outweighed by the negative emotions they may cause my readers, then please let me know via email, TikTok, or Instagram, and I will remove them from any future copies.

Last thing I'll say

Kodachromes are a big part of the dermatology boards, and this book does not have any pictures. I highly recommend looking at clinical and dermpath pictures of every disease you read about in this book, as well as clinical "signs" (e.g., fringe sign in traction alopecia) on VisualDX or google. I can promise you, if you know this book cold and you know what every entity looks like, you will absolutely ace your applied exam.

Chapter 1: Basic science, billing and statistics in dermatology

1.1 Structure and Function of the Skin

Structure of the epidermis

- Epidermis is composed of squamous epithelium comprised of keratinocytes connected by Desmosomes, Adherens junctions, Tight junctions and Gap junctions ("**DAT Gap**")
  - o Desmosomes connect keratinocytes by anchoring to **keratin tonofilaments**
    - ▪ Mediates **slow but strong** cellular adhesions ("Desmo-slowms")
    - ▪ Consist of **intercellular desmoglein/desmocollin** that binds cytoplasmic **plakoglobin** that binds desmoplakin/plakophilin that binds **keratin**
  - o Adherens junctions connect keratinocytes by anchoring to **actin** filaments
    - ▪ Mediates **fast but weak** cellular adhesions
    - ▪ Consist of intercellular classic cadherins (P-, E-, N-cadherins) that binds cytoplasmic β-catenin/plakoglobin that binds α-catenin that binds actin
      - Notice plako-globin is present in both ("present globally")
  - o Tight junctions are composed of claudins and occludins which form a tight seal
  - o Gap junctions allows for intercellular communication and transfer of small molecules between

cells; gap junction defects are the MCC of genetic deafness

DAT gap

Desmosome proteins (Cadherin family)

- Desmocollins (associated condition when defected is listed)
    - Desmocollin 1: Subcorneal pustular type of IgA pemphigus
- Desmogleins: **PISS ARV Vulgar ALARM** ("Piss off vulgar alarm")
    - Desmoglein 1 (PISS): Pemphigus foliaceus, Impetigo (bullous), SSSS, Striate PPK
        - Expressed in all levels of epidermis in skin (superficial > deep)
    - Desmoglein 2 (ARV): Arrhythmogenic Right Ventricular dysplasia
    - Desmoglein 3 (Vulgar): P. Vulgaris (oral PV only Dsg3; mucocutaneus PV is 1 & 3)
        - Expressed in just deep epidermis and all levels of mucosa and fetal skin
    - Desmoglein 4 (ALARM): AR Localized hypotrichosis, AR Monilethrix
        - Expressed in hair follicles

Desmosome proteins (Armadillo family): Armadillo family always **starts** with "plako"

- Plakoglobin (PG): Naxos syndrome ("The movie is not PG if it's X-rated")
    - Present in both desmosomes and adherans junctions ("present globally")
- Plakophillin (PP): ectodermal dysplasia with skin fragility ("your PP is fragile")

Desmosome proteins (Plakin family): "Plakin family usually **ends** with plakin"

- Desmoplakin 1 (250 kDa) and 2 (210 kDa) ("Plays at his desk in the principle's CLASSS")
    - Paraneoplastic pemphigus (antibodies to DSG 1, 3 and entire plakin family)
    - Carvahal syndrome
    - Lethal Acantholytic EB
    - Striate PPK (mutation in desmoplakin 1, DSG 1 and keratin 1: "straight like #1")
    - Skin fragility/wooly hair syndrome
    - SJS/EM Major (anti-desmoplakin antibodies)
- Remember Plakins and their molecular weight with **PEB DP** mnemonic
    - Periplakin (190 kDa)
    - Envoplakin and Desmoplakin 2 (210 kDa)
    - BPAg1 (230 kDa)
    - Desmoplakin 1 (250 kDa)
    - Plectin (500 kDa)

Adherans junction proteins of importance

- Classic cadherans (E-, P- and N- cadherin) attach to either plakoglobin or β-catenin (armadillo family) which attach to α-catenin which attaches to actin filaments
    - Plakoglobin mutated in Naxos disease
    - β-catenin mutations are seen in pilomatricomas (which are common in Myotonic dystrophy, garners syndrome (APC gene), Turners and Rubinstein-Taybi

Tight junctions have no important disease associations

Gap junction mutations: "**KEV & Deaf Bart** go **HOMe**"

- KEV & Deaf Bart are all **Connexin 26 (GJB2) mutations except** Erythrokeratoderma variabilis which is

Connexin 30.3 and 31 (GJB4 and GJB3; "variable/multiple connexins")
  - o KID (Keratitis-ichthyosis-deafness) syndrome
  - o Erythrokeratoderma variabilis
  - o Vohwinkel syndrome
  - o PPK with deafness
  - o Bart-Pumphrey syndrome
- HOMe ("say BAC HOM to keep the GJs straight")
  - o Hidrotic ectodermal dysplasia, aka Clouston's: Connexin 30 (GJB6)
  - o Oculo-dental-digital dysplasia: Connexin 43 (GJA1)
  - o Milroys disease (MC mutation is FLT4): Connexin 47 (GJC2) is 2nd MC

Epidermal layers

Stratum basale

- Keratins 5 and 14 are produced here
- About 10% of cells in the basal layer are stem cells and about 10% are melanocytes
- Expresses ornithine decarboxylase (a/w proliferative states) and catalase
  - o Increased by factors such as trauma (Blunt force trauma) and UVB
  - o Inhibited by Vitamin D3, Corticosteroids, Retinoids
    "It's OD (Ornithine Decarboxylase) that the VCR in the basement (basal layer) is not working (inhibited)"

Stratum spinosum: "spines look like a 1 or an l → lame land, lys lip, leg leq, link"

- Keratins 1 and 10 are produced here
- Lamellar granules (Odland bodies) are produced by Golgi bodies in the spinous layer
  - o Specialized lysosomes which discharge lipids (most important is **Ceramide**) that extrude their

  - contents to form the intercellular lipids in the stratum corneum
  - Flegel's disease and Harlequin ichthyosis are due to ↓ lamellar granules
  - X-linked ichthyosis occurs due to absent steroid sulfatase in lamellar granules

Stratum granulosum: "KLIP your basophilic keratohyalin granules"

- Keratin intermediate filaments: binds filaggrin
- Loricrin: Largest component of CCE (mutated in Vohwinkel variant/PSEK; ↓ in psoriasis)
- Involucrin: cross-links with loricrin by transglutaminase (↑ in psoriasis)
- Profillagrin: becomes fillagrin (↑ in lamellar ichthyosis; ↓ in ichthyosis vulgaris and AD)
- Cornified cell envelope (CCE) production primarily takes place in the s. granulosum
- Cross-linking of CCE occurs via Transglutaminase 1 (TG mnemonic is "I'D Peel")
  - Icthyosis (Lamellar/CIE): Transglutaminase 1 is mutated
  - Dermatitis herpetiformis: Transglutaminase 3 is antigenic
  - Acral peeling skin syndrome: Transglutaminase 5 is mutated

Stratum corneum

- Serves as a water-impermeable mechanical barrier between the epi and environment
- Made of corneocytes which are terminally differentiated keratinocytes that contain a cornified envelope composed of cross-linked proteins (**loricrin**, involucrin, periplakin)
- **Urocanic acid** ("uro-corneum acid") is a filaggrin biproduct found in the cornified layer

- **Absorbs UVR** and forms natural moisturizing factor which hydrates s. corneum
- **Major protein component is loricrin; major lipid component is ceramide**

Epidermal cells

Keratinocytes and keratin

- Keratinocytes produce keratin filaments which form the cell's cytoskeletal network
  - Desmin, vimentin, neurofilaments ("neurofinaments"), nuclear lamins and nestin are types of keratin intermediate filaments
- Class 1 keratins: low molecular weight; acidic; K9- 28
  - "1st class girls with low body weights and nice ass get higher ratings (9-28)"
- Class 2 keratins: high molecular weight; basic; K1-8
  - "2nd class girls with high body weights are basic and get lower ratings (1-8)"
- There are > 50 epithelial/hair keratins expressed as either type I (acidic), type II (basic), or type I/II coexpressed together as heterodimers (e.g., K5/14) aka **double helix structure** which are bonded together with disulfide bonds utilizing the many cysteine amino acids
- **Basic structure is an α-helical rod consisting of heptad (7) amino acid repeats** ("keratino-sevens") vs collagen which is a triple helix w/ triple repeat sequence (Gly-X-Y)
  - "Keratino-sevens" also helps you remember that collagen 7 and 17 are produced by keratinocytes, all other collagens (except 8/18) are produced by fibroblasts
- Release and respond to various cytokines most notably **TNF-α** ("keraTiNoFytes")

Keritin filament expression pattern Some Girls Can Make Boys Have Nice Puberties	Some Girls Can Make Boys Have Nice Sex
K1: Spinous layer → Ichthyosis Hystrix, Unna thost (non-epidermolytic) PPK, Greithers, EHK (HUGE)	K10: Spinous layer→ Epidermolytic hyperkeratosis (EKH/bullous CIE) and Ichthyosis en confetti
K2: Granular layer → Ichthyosis bullosa of Siemens	K11: Granular layer → Nothing
K3: Cornea → Meesmans corneal dystrophy	K12: Cornea → Meesmans corneal dystrophy
K4: Mucosal epithelium → White sponge nevus	K13: Mucosal epithelium → White sponge nevus
K5: Basal layer → EBS, Dowling-Degos disease	K14: Basal layer → EBS, NFJ, DPR
K6a: Hair, nail, palmoplantar skin → PC type 1	K16: Hair, nails, mouth, palmoplantar skin → PC type 1 and **non-epidermolytic Unna thost PPK**
K6b: Nail, hair follicle, palmoplantar skin → PC type 2	K17: Nails, hair follicles, sebaceous glands → PC type 2
K9: Palmoplantar skin→ Vörner PPK (epidermolytic; "the umlaut in ö looks like keratin clumps lysing")	K19: Stem cells → Nothing

***K5/K14 is the epidermal target proteins for haptens** as this is the heterodimer expressed in basal keratinocytes
*K1/K9 is the keratin heterodimer expressed **exclusively in palmoplantar skin**
*K8/K18 is not in this mnemonic because they are only expressed in epithelial tissues like the liver
***K6/K17 and K7/17 are found in hair/adnexal structures and are upregulated in wound healing**

Melanocytes

- Neural crest-derived melanin-producing dendritic cells found in the stratum basale
    - 1:10 ratio of melanocytes to keratinocytes when viewed in 2-dimensional plane

  - Each melanocyte interfaces with 36 keratinocytes in 3-dimensions
  - Ratio is 1:5 in hair (graying caused by gradual ↓ in # of follicular melanocytes)
- Connected to keratinocytes via **E-cadherin** receptors not desmosomes
- Melanin is produced in melanosomes (lysosome-like organelles) from its precursor tyrosine w/ the **copper-dependent enzyme tyrosinase** ("PHARCK I inhibited tyrosinase")
  - Phenylalanine, Hydroquinone, Azelaic acid, Retinoids, Cysteamine, vitamin C and Kojic acid are competitive inhibitors of tyrosinase
- Melanin absorbs UVR and protects against UV-induced mutations
- Racial variation: melanosomes in darker skinned individuals are larger, more abundant, have more melanin, are more stable and are transferred as individual organelles (vs smaller, less melanin, less stable and transferred in membrane-bound clusters of 3-6 melanosomes in lighter skin individuals); **# of melanocytes is the same between races**
  - "Small white unstable melanosomes must stick together in groups of 3-6"
- Chronic sun exposure causes melanosomes to get larger over time
- Pheomelanin: red color with spherical shape, a microvesicular ("microphesicular") internal structure and increased sulfur ("sulphur") content which is made from cysteine
- Eumelanin: black color w/ oval shape and lamellar structure → You (Eu) are overly lame
- Melanin production is stimulated by melanocyte-stimulating hormone (**product of proopiomelanocortin gene**) on melanocortin 1 receptor (MC1-R) on melanocytes

- **MC1-R loss of function mutations → ↑ pheomelanin:eumelanin ratio** (phenotype = red hair/fair skin with ↑ risk of melanoma)
  - "MC1-R defect p/w My Color Red"
- **Promotion of Agouti protein** also causes red phenotype

- Autoimmune destruction of melanocytes: vitiligo
- Defect in **melanocyte migration** (C-Kit): piebaldism ("here kitty makes cat move")
  - C-kit is also mutated in acral/mucosal melanoma and mastocytosis
- Defects in **melanin synthesis** enzymes: oculocutaneous albinism ("white like TP")
  - OCA1A/1B (Tyrosinase), OCA2 (P gene), OCA3 (TYRP), OCA4 (MATP/SLC45A2)
- Defects in **melanosome synthesis** >> transfer: Hermansky-Pudlak syndrome
- Defects in **melanosome trafficking/transfer** → Griscelli and Chediak-Higashi syndrome
  - "Greasy Hash drug traffickers"

Langerhan Cells (LC)

- BM-derived dendritic cell of monocyte-macrophage lineage ($CD34^+$) in s. spinosum
- Recognize and present foreign antigens (haptens) to specific T lymphocytes
  - After APCs like LCs take up antigen, they activate **and drain to nearby LNs**
- Like melanocytes, they are connected to keratinocytes via **E-cadherin** receptors
- During inflammatory states **MMP-9** is secreted which Makes LCs Move out of epidermis
- During non-inflammatory states **BRAK/CXCL14** is expressed homing LCs to the epidermis
  - "BRAK makes Langerhan cell stay BACK in the epidermis"

- Kidney or coffee-bean shaped on H&E (due to folded nucleus)
- Distinct intracytoplasmic organelles (Birbeck granules) w/ tennis racquet-shape on EM
- Positive immunostains: **CD207 (langerin)**, CD1a, S100, CD34, vimentin and actin
- Downregulated by UV, upregulated by TIM (TGF-β, IL-34, MCSF)
    - "TIM lends a hand to Langerhan's cells"
- Langerhan Cell Histiocytosis: Say "Letter Hand Cell" (this terminology may be obsolete)
    - Letter-Siwe: acute disseminated form occurring before 2 years old (yo)
    - Hand-Schuller-Christian: DI, osteolytic bone lesions, exophthalmos; 2–6 yo
    - Congenital self-healing (Hashimoto Pritzker): skin-limited, rapid resolution; birth
    - Eosinophilic granuloma: bone lesions (cranium); 6–12 yo

Merkel Cells

- Ectoderm-derived mechanoreceptor found among basal keratinocytes in areas with high tactile sensitivity (lips, fingers, ORS, oral mucosa) which communicates with neurons
- Markers: "Merkel will Merk a Very Important Person's CNS"
    - MAP-2 (most sensitive and specific neuroendocrine marker)
    - Vasoactive intestinal peptide (VIP)
    - **CK20**, Calcitonin gene-related peptide, Chromogranin A, NSE, Synaptophysin

Basement membrane zone

- Semipermeable barrier b/w epidermis and dermis w/ distinct layers (from superficial to deep):
    - Basal keratinocytes (keratin intermediate filaments)
        - K5 (EBS, Dowling-Degos)
        - K14 (EBS, Naegeli-Franceschetti, dermatopathia pigmentosa reticularis)
    - Hemidesmosome-anchoring filament complex: ("Peanut Butter BIL"): **PB** (hemidesmosomal plaque; **connects keratin intermediate filaments to the hemidesmosome**), BI (**lamina lucida;** anchoring filaments), L (**lamina densa**; connects hemidesmosome-anchoring filament complex to anchoring fibrils in lamina densa); because "L" is below lamina lucida it stains blister floor on SSS
        - Plectin: EBS with muscular dystrophy (only EBS that's AR) and PNP
        - BPAg1: BP, PNP (remember paraneoplastic pemphigus affects all plakins)
        - BPAg2 (Coll 17): "Called 17 times w/ no answer, what a Judgmental BICH"
            - Genetic Disease: Junctional EB (milder phenotype than Herlitz)
            - Autoimmune disease: BP, linear IgA bullous dermatosis/CBDC, Cicatricial pemphigoid, (Carboxy terminus: all others in this mnemonic are N16A terminus of BPAg2), Herpes gestationis
                - N-terminus of BPAg2 is iNtracellular
                - C-terminus of BPAg2 is eCxtracellular
        - Integrin α6β4
            - Genetic disease: junctional EB w/ pyloric atresia has crumpled skinny ears, skinny gastric pylora, ureteral stenosis → renal failure

- "I is a skinny letter so think skinny stenoses"
- Autoimmune disease: ocular cicatricial pemphigoid (β4 integrin)
  - "The β looks like glasses for your eyes"
- Laminin 332 (Laminin 5 or anti-epiligrin): **stains floor on SSS** starting now
  - Genetic disease: Junctional EB (severe version of JEB, aka Herlitz)
  - Autoimmune disease: anti-epiligrin cicatricial pemphigoid (a/w malignancy so it is the severe version of cicatricial pemphigoid)
- Lamina densa: "lamina FEHNsa
  - **Laminin 5** (lamina densa/hemidesmosome-anchoring filament complex)
  - **Type Four collagen**: mutated in Goodpasture and Alport syndrome
  - Entactin/nidogen: connects laminin 1 to collagen 4 (**unique to skin BMZ**)
  - Heparan sulfate proteoglycan (perlecan): gives the BM a negative charge
  - Nidogen: connects laminin 1 to collagen 4 (**unique to skin BMZ**)
- Sublamina densa: **Type 7 coll** (anchoring fibrils) hook to dermal type 1/3 collagen
  - "Type VII collagen fibers anchor up my BED" (Bullous SLE, EBA, DEB)

Dermis

- Dermal cells: "the Five Massive Giant Mononuclear Dermal cells"
  - Fibroblasts: create extracellular matrix and play a role in wound healing
  - Mast cells: discussed in section 1.5

- Glomus cells: smooth muscle cells which allow for shunting of blood
  - Derived from Sucquet-Hoyer canals on palms and soles ("Suck yer nailes")
- Mononulcear phagocytes: discussed in section 1.5
- Dermal dendritic cells: highly phagocytic APC in the dermis

Extracellular matrix (ECM)

- Synthesized by dermal fibroblasts and composed of "CLEFT PIG"
  - **Collagens**, Laminins, **Elastins,** Fibulins, Three modifying enzymes
  - Proteoglycans, Integrins, Glycoproteins
- Collagen
  - **Triple helix** configuration composed of 3 amino acids on repeat (**Glycine**-x-y where x is usually proline and y is often hydroxylysine or hydroxyproline)
  - MC component of skin and accounts for 75% of dry weight of the dermis
  - Biosynthesis of collagen
    - Intracellular: lysyl hydroxylase (mutated in kyphoscoliotic EDS and inhibited by minoxidil) and proline hydroxylase catalyze hydroxylation to procollagen; **vitamin C-dependent** process (deficiency → scurvy)
      - Mnemonic "Hy-C"
    - Extracellular: procollagen N-proteinase/ ADAMTS2 (mutated in dermatospraxis EDS) cleaves the N-propeptide of procollagen and then lysyl oxidase (mutated in Menkes and occipital horn syndrome; **copper dependent**) catalyzes cross-linking between collagen molecules
  - Collagen (types 1, 2 and 3) is degraded by matrix metalloproteinases (MMPs)

- Collagen synthesis is ↑ by retinoic acid and doxycycline (inhibits MMPs)
- Collagen synthesis is ↓ by The Ugly PIIG
  - TNF-α
  - UV irradiation
  - Penicillamine (inhibits lysyl oxidase which crosslinks collagen and elastin)
  - IL-1 (↑ MMP expression)
  - IFN-γ
  - Glucocorticoids
- Types of collagen: location → disease state
  - Coll 1 (one): #1 most abundant collagen and is found in dermis, scars, tendons, teeth, ligaments and Bone → EDS (arthrochalasic form) and Osteogenesis imperfecta
  - Coll 2: cartilage ("car-2-lage") → Relapsing polychondritis and MAGIC syndrome
  - Coll 3 ("Big Gross Stinky Feet"): Blood vessels (arterial walls), GI tract and Granulation tissue, Scars, Fetal skin → EDS (vascular form)
  - Coll 4: **basement membrane** (of epidermis/BVs) → Alport, Goodpasture
  - Coll 5: skin EDS (classic form)
  - Coll 6: aorta, placenta → Ullrich Scleroatonic muscular dystrophy
  - Coll 7: anchoring fibrils (attach BM to ECM; BED) → Bullous SLE, EBA, DEB
  - Coll 17 (BPAg2): anchoring filaments of hemidesmosome → JEB, BP, IgA linear, Cicatricial pemphigoid, Herpes gestationis ("Judgmental BICH")
  - Coll 8 (eight) and 18 (eighteen): endothelial basement membrane
- **All collagens are produced by dermal fibroblasts except coll 7/17 (produced by keratino-**

cytes; "keritino-sevens") and Coll eight and eighteen (endothelial cells)

- Elastin
  - Elastic fibers are highly cross-linked proteins which provide resilience from stretching and account for 4% of dry weight of the dermis
  - 90% elastin (core) and 10% fibrillin (surrounds elastin)
  - Elastin contains **desmosine** and **isodesmosine** which crosslink with fibrillin via lysyl oxidase (same copper dependent enzyme which crosslinks collagen)
    - Enzymes that require copper ("never TALC to cops")
      - Tyrosinase (mutated in OCA type 1)
      - ATP7α (Menkes and XLR cutis laxa, aka occipital horn syndrome)
      - Lysyl oxidase (LMNOP): Lysyl oxidase is ↓ by Lathyrism from sweet Pea ingestion and Penicillamine; mutated in Menkes/Occip horn)
      - Cystathione β-synthase (homocystinuria)
  - Elaunin fibers run horizontal in reticular dermis and oxytalan fibers run vertical
    - "Stand up straight (vertical), high (high in dermis) and tall with oxytalan"
  - UV radiation damages elastic fibers (dermal elastosis hallmark of photodamage)
- Microfibrils
  - Connects perlecan in the BMZ to horizontal elaunin fibers in the reticular dermis
  - Consists mainly of fibrillins ("Do not be a fibber and tell on me to MS. C")
    - Fibrillin 1: linear Morphea (autoAbs), Marfans, Stiff skin syndrome

        - Fibrillin 2: mutated in Congenital Contractural arachnodactyly
    - Also consist of fibulins: fibulin 4 and 5: mutated in AR cutis laxa
    - Loss of function of the microfibril-associated glycoprotein (MFAP) Latent-TGF-β binding protein 4 (LTBP4) also causes AR cutis laxa and activating mutations in TGF-β receptors 1 and 2 cause Loeys-Dietz syndrome
- Extrafibrillar matrix
    - Amorphous material that the dermal fibril network and cells are embedded into
    - Consists of proteoglycans/GAGs, glycoproteins, hyaluronic acid and water
    - Glycosaminoglycans (GAGs) are negatively charged sugars that bind water
        - GAGs bind proteins via serine hydroxyl groups forming proteoglycans
        - The most ubiquitous protein-free GAG (non-sulfated) is hyaluronic acid
        - Chondroitin/dermatan/keratan/heparan sulfate are protein-bound GAGs
    - Glycoproteins: fibronectin, vitronectin, matrilins, tenascins and ECM proteins
        - Tenascin X deficiency: classic EDS and hypermobile EDS
        - ECM-1: lipoid proteinosis (gene mutation), LS&A (auto-antibody)
- Integrins
    - Mediates attachment to either ECM or to other cells
    - "JIL" has an integrin mutation
        - JEB with pyloric atresia: α6β4 integrin (MMP has autoAbs to β4 integrin)
        - Juvenile hyaline fibromatosis: CMG-2 gene (encodes an integrin receptor)

    - Infantile systemic hyalinosis: CMG-2 gene ("Can't Move Good")
    - Leukocyte adhesion deficiency: $\beta 2$ integrin
    - Lupus erythematosus: integrin α_M

Cutaneous vasculature

- **VEGF** is the primary mediator of vasculogenesis
- Lymphatic markers include VEGFR-3, Prox1, D2-40 (Podoplanin), LYVE-1
    - "Vegan Proxies are Down 2 Live in lymph"
- Anatomy
    - Veins, arteries and arterioles are composed of smooth muscle and elastic tissue surrounding the basement membrane (BM) and endothelial cells
        - The smooth muscle layer is just much thicker in arteries
    - Venules and capillaries are made of endothelial cells surrounded by **pericytes**
        - "The venue has a cap of 100 persons"
    - Lymphatics: endothelial cells and BM w/o pericytes or smooth muscle

Cutaneous neurology

- Sensory nerves are divided into free nerve endings and corpuscular nerve endings
    - Free nerve endings include small unmyelinated C-type fibers (dull pain) and larger myelinated Aδ fibers (sharp pain and temperature)
        - "The δ sign is a sharp symbol"
    - Specialized nerve receptors (corpuscular nerve endings; be able to recognize!)
        - Krause end bulbs: found on genitalia, perianal region, and vermillion lips
            - "Krazy Krause ends on erotic areas"
        - Meissner corpuscle: **on dermal papillae of digits** for pressure/light touch

        - "Well-Mannered Meissner lightly touches fingers"
    - Pacinian corpuscle: onion shaped mechanoreceptor of palmoplantar skin, nipples and genital region; suited for vibration located in deep dermis/fat
        - "Women always pack their vibrators deep in their suitcases"
    - Ruffini corpuscle: on fingernails in deep fat; suited for sustained pressure
        - Ruff sex = fingernails deep in your back with a sustained pressure
    - Merkel nerve endings: found on fingertips, lips, and external genitalia in the basal epidermis (superficial); suited for pressure

Adnexal structures

- Eccrine glands
    - Secretory gland of merocrine secretion (exocytosis) w/ thermoregulatory effects
    - They produce a clear, odorless substance consisting mostly of **sodium** and water
    - Eccrine Everywhere Except External auditory canal and Euphoric areas (lips, glans penis, clitoris and labia minora)
    - Most numerous on palms and soles "sweaty palms"
    - No relationship to pilosebaceous follicle
    - Innervated by sympathetic fibers that have Ach (not NE) as the neurotransmitter
        - Neurotoxins (botox) blocks Ach release and treats hyperhidrosis
    - Delivers hypotonic sweat to skin, but the faster you sweat, the more isotonic it is
        - "Your skin gets salty when you exercise intensely"

  - ECCrine Gland Stains: EMA, CEA, Cytokeratin, GCDFP-15 (apocrine>eccrine), S100
- Apocrine glands (ABCDE)
  - Secretory gland of apocrine/**decapitation (part of cell) secretion** located on…
    - **Anogenital area, Axilla**
    - Breast (areola/nipple), **Belly button**
    - Canal of external ear, Dividing line of lip, Eyelid margin
      - C, D, and E are all the facial orifices except nose
  - **Connect to infundibulum of hair follicles** except 3 named ectopic apocrine glands which empty directly onto surface (mammary glands of breast, Moll's gland of eyelid margin and ceruminous glands of external auditory canal)
  - Innervated by β-adrenergic receptors stimulated by circulating catecholamines
  - Secretory products include cholesterol, cholesterol esthers and fatty acids
  - Bromhidrosis: smelly sweat from apocrine secretions mixing w/ surface bacteria
  - Chromhidrosis: pigmented sweat due to its rich lipofuscin content
  - Stains for CEA, keratins (same stains as eccrine glands)
- Sebaceous glands
  - Secretory gland of holocrine (whole cell lyses off) secretion located mainly on the scalp, face and chest ("seborrheic areas") but NOT on palms and soles
  - Associated with terminal hair follicles except the ectopic sebaceous glands
    - Ectopic seb-eye-ceous glands all have the "eye" sounds

        - Zeis glands on eyelid margin next to Molls glands ("Z-eye-s")
        - Meibomian glands on eyelid tarsal plate ("M-eye-bomian")
            - More deep (more letters) in eyelid than Zeis and Molls
        - Fordyce spots on vermillion lip/penis ("Ford-eye-ce")
        - Montgomery tubercles on areola/nipples ("Montgom-eye-ry")
        - Tysons glands on labia minora/prepuce ("T-eye-sons")
            - "Mike Tyson beats up the genitals"
    - Composition of secretions is "Three Wacky Sebaceous Contents"
        - **Triglycerides** (#1 component; makes up > 50% of sebaceous secretion)
            - Of importance, in acne vulgaris, resident microorganisms like P. acnes secrete lipases which split triglycerides into free fatty acids which alter the pattern of keratinization in the infundibulum (comedones) and which attracts neutrophils (inflammatory acne); pubertal androgens stimulate sebaceous glands which produce more free fatty acids from triglycerides in the presence of P. acnes
        - **Wax esters** (2nd MC), **Squalene** (3rd MC), Cholesterol/Cholesterol esters

Hair anatomy

- Infundibulum: from epidermis to opening of sebaceous gland duct (**apocrine gland connects to the follicle above the sebaceous gland in the infundibulum**)

  - No IRS but contains an **ORS with normal epidermal keratinization** (has **keratohyalin** granules (KHG)/granular layer)
- Isthmus: from sebaceous gland duct to arrector pili insertion (bulge)
  - No IRS but contains an **ORS with trichilemmal keratinization** (no granular layer)
    - "Pilar cysts are also called trichilemmal cysts and isthmus-catagen cysts"
  - **Bulge**: part of ORS at level of arrector pili (**major site of hair follicle stem cells**)
- Lower hair follicle: from arrector pili insertion to hair bulb
  - **Contains an IRS** and a **non-keratinized ORS**
    - IRS is not present in telogen hairs ("The IRS won't rest until you pay tax")
    - IRS only present in lower hair follicle ("The IRS stoops so low")
    - IRS has **trichohyalin** granules found in Huxley's layer ("The IRS is tricky")
  - Critical line of Auber is the widest area where most mitotic activity occurs
    - "Auber is pronounced like Ober which sounds like Obese (widest part)"
  - Hair bulb is the lowest part of follicle which contains melanocytes for hair color
    - 1 melanocyte: 5 keratinocytes (melanocytes only produce pigment in anagen phase because melanocytes in matrix apoptose in catagen phase)
- Hair anatomy in cross section
  - Layers (inner to outer): hair shaft (medulla, cortex and cuticle), IRS (cuticle, Huxley's layer and Henle's, layer), ORS, glassy membrane
    - Just remember that the Huxley layer hugs the cuticle, and from there it's easy to remember

that the Henley's layer is next followed by the ORS
        - Cuticle from IRS and hair shaft fuse → split ends (trichoptilosis)
- Hair growth (ACT)
    - Anagen: **hair grows 0.4mm/day or 1cm/month**; lasts **3 years** (89% of scalp hair)
        - Hair (1cm/month), toenails (1mm/month), fingernails (2–3mm/month)
        - **Hairs look like a hockey stick** (anagen effluvium hairs will be surrounded by a clear sheath whereas loose anagen hair syndrome hairs lack this)
    - Catagen: regression phase where IRS of lower hair follicle is lost and melanocytes in matrix apoptose; lasts **3 weeks** (1% of scalp hair at any given time)
        - Can be identified by a very **thick vitreous sheath** (just outside the ORS)
    - **T**elegen: Rest (**T**ired phase); **Club-shaped**; high in dermis; lasts **3 months** (10%)
        - "Night Clubs give you a high but then get you tired and need a rest"
- ShApe of follicle (oval → curly; round → straight) and Disulfide Bonding via Cysteine residues determines Curliness of hair (these bonds brake when hair is straightened)

Nails

- Nail anatomy
    - Proximal nail fold is contiguous with/in proximity to both skin and the matrix
    - Eponychium, aka cuticle ("Every pony is cute") which is b/w the plate and matrix
    - Nail matrix: proximal matrix forms Dorsal nail plate; Distal matrix forms ventral nail plate ("just remember that the Ds are opposite")

        - Nail Matrix has Melanocytes and **lacks a granular layer**
            - Proximal matrix: forms 80% of nail Plate (biopsy → nail dystrophy)
            - Distal matrix (lanula is visible distal portion): 90% of melanocytes
        - Nail thickness is determined by the length of the nail matrix
    - Lunula (distal nail matrix) → nail bed → nail plate
        - Nail bed extends from the lunula to the onychodermal band (reddish pink transverse band) and has minimal contribution to nail plate synthesis
        - Nail bed **lacks a granular layer** (like isthmus of hair follicle)
- Nail growth
    - Fingernails: 2–3 mm/month (0.1 mm daily; 6 months to grow out)
        - Beau's lines 1/3rd up the fingernail plate → insult occurred 2 months ago
    - Toenails: 1 mm/month (12–18 months to grow out)

1.2 Embryology

- Skin structures all derived from 2 of 3 primary germ layers (ectoderm or mesoderm)
    - Ectoderm ("stays"): epidermis, adnexa, nerves, Merkel cells, and melanocytes
    - Mesoderm ("Moves"): dermal fibroblasts, LCs, vessels, and inflammatory cells
- Epidermal layers
    - 5 weeks (2 layers): periderm (transient **glycogen-rich** layer) and inner basal layer
        - Periderm becomes the vernix caseosa (a layer that coats the newborn)

  - 8 weeks (3 layers): **periderm (studded w/ microvilli by week 8)**, intermediate layer (start of "epidermal stratific-8-tion") and inner basal epidermal layer
    - **p63 gene** is required for the process of epidermal stratification
  - **24 weeks (4 layers): intact epidermis** (corneal layer) is found in the 3rd trimester
    - Although skin does not have full barrier function until **4 weeks after birth**
- Skin layers/zones
  - 9 weeks: distinction b/w the epidermis and dermis (DEJ) and b/w dermis and SQ
    - "Nine rhymes with line (between zones)"
  - 12–15 weeks: distinction b/w the papillary and reticular dermis
- Epidermal and dermal cells (cells appear in alphabetical order)
  - 6–8 weeks: Fibroblasts appear beneath epidermis ("Fibroblasts First")
  - 9–12 weeks: LCs, Melanocytes and Merkel cells migrate into epidermis
    - Melanocytes migrate 2° to KIT (Piebaldism has anterior depigmentation)
    - Melanocytes produce melanin at **16 weeks** and they become fully functional (transfer melanosomes to keratinocytes) at 16–20 weeks
      - Melanin production at 16 weeks ("Melanie had her sweet 16")
- Other components of dermis and the subcutis
  - 9–12 weeks (eleven): primordial vessels form
  - 17 weeks: fat forms in the SQ ("seventeen is a big fat word")
- Hair (sebaceous gland development parallels hair follicle development)

- o 9–12 weeks: primordial follicles 1st form on the eyebrows, scalp, upper lip, chin
- o Hair canal fully formed at 18–20 weeks and starts cycling (A → C → T) at 24–28
    - ▪ "Hair follicle development reminds me of men's genitals → it starts growing at age 9–12 and is fully developed by 18–20 (hair keratinization at 15); then he starts cycling it amongst various women at 24–28 years old"
- o Developing follicle has 2 bulges which become certain structures (in apocrine skin, there are 3 bulges, and the superficial bulge becomes the apocrine gland)
    - ▪ **Superficial bulge → Sebaceous gland**
    - ▪ **Deep bulge →** insertion of arrector pili muscle; **follicular stem cells**
        - • "The deep bulge in his pants are where his stem cells (sperm) are"

- Nails (**fingernails: start at 10 weeks**; **toenails: 14 weeks**): structures form in alph order
    - o 9–12 weeks: nail Bed demarcation (beginning w/ the **hyponychium** which marks the transition between the nail bed and the epidermis of the digits)
    - o 12 weeks: proximal nail Folds form
    - o 17 weeks: nail Plate forms and completely covers the nail bed by 20 weeks
- Keratinization: 1st in **nail bed** (11 wks), hair canal (15 wks), interfollicular skin (24 wks)
- Adnexal glands
    - o Eccrine glands begin to form on palms/soles at 10 weeks and mature at 20
        - ▪ Whorls of mature eccrine glands result in dermatoglyphics at 20 weeks
    - o Truncal eccrine glands and apocrine glands develop later (22 weeks)

- **Notice that vessels, hair, sebaceous glands, nails, palmar eccrine glands and melanocytes all start to develop around 9–12 weeks and are fully formed by 20 weeks**

1.3 Wound Healing

Phases of wound healing (IPR: in alphabetical order)

- Inflammatory phase (hours to days): vascular response (**1st**) → cellular response
    - Vascular response: vessels initially constrict then vasodilate (due to histamine release), **platelets** come to wound first (**thrombin** is 1st substance released) and release various factors (PDGF, TGF-α, TGF-β → recruits WBCs); **fibrin** (first ECM component deposited) and **fibronectin serves as a scaffold for cell adhesion**
    - Cellular response: neutrophils are the 1st nucleated cell to arrive but **macrophages** (2nd to arrive) are the most important cell in wound healing
    - Macrophages release various growth factors (VEGF, TGF, TGF-α, **TGF-β**, PDGF)
- Proliferative phase (days to weeks): "prolife-FAR-ative" (from latest to earliest)
    - Re-epitheliazation (within hours): keratinocytes leapfrog over each other from the **sides** adjacent to the wound; stimulated by **KGF, EGF, TGF-β**
        - Matrix metalloproteinases and collagenases also exhibit ↑ expression in wound healing and help keratinocytes migrate
- Angiogenesis (within days): ↑ by VEGF and ↓ by **thrombospondin**

- Fibroplasia (within weeks): fibroblasts synthesize collagen and GAGs
    - **PDGF: stimulates fibroblasts** (you would think FGF would stimulate fibroblasts, but like VEGF, FGF actually stimulates endothelial cells)
    - **TGF-β**: transforms fibroblasts into myofibroblasts which helps w/ wound contraction (max at **2 weeks;** "Your max is too weak")
        - Persistence of myofibroblasts → hypertrophic scar/keloid
    - Vitronectin and tenascin: facilitates cell adhesion/migration
    - Fibronectin: needed for granulation tissue formation and is **replaced by collagen 3** (peaks in 5–7 days) and is ultimately replaced by Collagen 1
        - Collagen 3 upregulated (1:1 vs 1:5 with collagen 1 normally)
    - Hyaluronic acid (non-sulfated GAG): #1 GAG in 1st week of wound healing
    - Chondroitin/dermatan sulfate (sulfated GAGs): MC GAGs > 1 week
- Remodeling (weeks to months): apoptosis of granulation tissue (endothelial cells die first, macrophages last); collagen remodeling (normal 5:1 collagen 1 to collagen 3 ratio)
    - Hypertrophic scars have ↑ collagen 1 (20:1 ratio of collagen 1 to collagen 3)

Other testable wound healing facts

- Scar strength: week 1 (5%), week 2 (10%), week 3 (20%), week 4 (40%), >3 months (80%)
    - Notice how scar strength doubles q weekly for the 1st 4 weeks
- Select drugs and their effect on wound healing ("WHOOPS, I impaired wound healing")

    - Warfarin/Heparin, ↓ Oxygen (O_2; OO), Penicillin (↓ collagen cross-link), Steroids
    - Zinc, vitamin A or C improve epithelial repair (but a deficiency would impair it)
- Differences in adult vs fetal wound healing
    - Fetal wound healing has no inflammatory phase and does not heal w/ scars
- **K6/K17 and K7/17 are found in hair and are upregulated in wound healing**

Predominant cell in wounds ("Please, No More Lies Fauci")

- Immediately after injury: Platelets
- Day 1 and 2: Neutrophils ("Two-trophils")
- Day 3: Macrophages
- Day 4: Lymphocytes
- Day 5 and on: Fibroblasts ("Five-roblasts")

1.4 Ultraviolet Light

- UV light spectrum
    - UVC (200–290 nm)
    - UVB (290–310 nm): excimer laser (308 nm) falls in here ("8-xcimer")
    - UVAII (310–340 nm)
    - UVAI (340–400 nm): woods lamp (365 nm)
        - "Only AI could get wood 365 days a year"
    - "I just remember that UVB is 10 away from 300 so 290–310 (B and three rhyme). Then UVA is 90 above 310 (310–400) and UVC is 90 less than 290 (200–290)"
- Longer wavelength **UVA** causes **free-radicals (oxidative DNA damage)** → photo-Aging
    - UVA causes immediate pigment darkening in Mins d/t melanin Redistribution
        - "An immediate MR (mister)"

  - UVA causes **persistent pigment darkening** within **Hours** d/t **melanin Oxidation**
    - "A persistent HO"
- **UVB** is more erythemogenic (sun-Burn; 12 hours after exposure), involved in delayed tanning response (2–31 days after exposure) and **activates photosynthesis of vitamin D**
  - **UVB** light causes **Delayed pigmentation** (tanning) **Days** after exposure to light which is due to **↑ Synthesis of Melanin** ("Keep straight w/ mnemonic BDSM")
  - Nitric Oxide and Prostaglandins are ↑ in sunburnt skin and are early mediators involved in sunburns ("NO prostitutes get sunburns b/c they work night shifts")
- UVB was thought to drive carcinogenesis but since UVA can penetrate windows and is more abundant on Earth, we now know both play a crucial role
  - 300 nm (UVB) is the most effective wavelength for inducing DNA photoproducts
    - **Cyclobutane-pyrimidine (specifically T-T) dimers** is the MC photoproduct
    - UV signature mutations (**C → T is MC**; CC → TT is 2nd MC) results from failure of nucleotide excision repair to remove these DNA photoproducts
- UVA is Always present from sunrise to sunset while UVB Bumps up highest at noon
- **"FIT": Dose, aka Fluence (J/cm^2) = Irradiance (J/s cm^2 aka W/cm^2) × exposure Time (s)**
- Effects of UV light on the immune system
  - Proinflammatory: skin cells secrete IL-1, IL-6, IL-18, and TNF-α
  - Anti-inflammatory: **skin cells secrete IL-10** and α-MSH, depletion of Langerhans cells (inhibits

antigen presentation) and induction of regulatory T cells

- Erythema from UVB exposure appears at 4 hours and peaks at 1 day
- Erythema from PUVA exposure appears at 1 day and peaks at 4 days

Know your D's
Ergocalciferol (vitamin D2): derived from irradiated ergosterol in **plants** Cholecalciferol (vitamin D3): produced in animals (and humans) **7-dehydrocholesterol (provitamin D3): absorbs UVB** Calcidiol (25-Hydroxyvitamin D3): circulating form which is hydroxylated in the **liver** Calcitriol (1,25- Hydroxyvitamin D3): hormonally active form hydroxylated in the **kidneys** Calcipotriene: 1,25- Hydroxyvitamin D3 derivative used topically to treat psoriasis

1.5 Immunology

Innate immunity

- Initial defense w/ no memory ("innept"); only recognizes foreign ("invader") antigens
- Toll-like receptors ("toll-line receptors") bind to unique patterns on pathogens (PAMPS)
- Compliment ("complimint") cascade plays an important role in innate immunity
- Cathelicidins and defensins are antimicrobial peptides of the innate immune system
- Cells of significance: granulocytes, macrophages, dendritic-cells, and NK cells

Adaptive immunity

- Occurs After innate immunity when antigen-specific T- and B-cells are created via gene rearrangement in response to an antigen

- The T- and B-cell receptors recognize foreign AND self-antigens (Autoimmune disease)
- Cells of significance: dendritic cells, T- and B-cells (Antibodies)

Cytokines

- Greek lesson: "cyto" means cell, and "kinos" means movement, so cytokines move cells
- First aid mnemonic for IL-1 through IL-6 is Hot T- Bone stEAK
    - IL-1: fever ("hot"), ↑acute phase reactants, triggers innate immune response
    - IL-2: T-cell stimulator
    - IL-3: Bone marrow stimulator (GM-CSF-like)
    - IL-4: IgE isotype switching (a more specific mnemonic for the "1 percenters" out there is "BEG 4 iT"→ B cell growth, IgE switching, IgG switching, Th2 response)
    - IL-5: IgA isotype switching and **eosinophil activator ("eosino-five")**
    - IL-6: stimulates aKute phase protein production; stimulated by adipocytes
- IL-8: neutrophil chemotaxis ("clean up on aisle 8")
    - Neut chemotactic factors: ("LICK my pus") → Leukotriene B4, IL-8, C5a, Kallikrein
- IL-10: inhibition of the inflammatory response (↓IL-12 expression, **↓Th1 response**)
    - "When you see a 10 (hot girl) walk by, you get nervous and inhibited"
- IL-12: ↑ Th1 response/cell mediated immunity; composed of p40 and p35 subunits
- **IL-23: ↑ Th17 response** (key role in psoriasis); composed of p40 and p19 subunits
    - Ustekinumab inhibits the common p40 subunit on both IL-12 and IL-23

  - All other IL-23 blockers bind to the p19 subunit of IL-23
  - Major cytokines in psoriasis
  - IL-22 and **IL-23 stimulate Th17 cells** to release IL-17, IL-22, TNF-α
    - IL-17, IL-22 and IL-23 have a key role in psoriasis
  - Th1 cells release IFN-γ, IL-2, IL-8, IL-12, IL-18
- **IL-18: ↑IFN-γ** → ↑ macrophage activation, ↑ Th1 pathway, ↓Th2 pathway
  - All interferons (IFN-α, -β, -γ) interfere with viral replication
- TNF-α: secreted by macrophages to cause ↑ proinflammatory cytokines
  - TNF-α is a/w the **Jarisch Herxheimer reaction**
- TGF-β: acts via MAP kinase pathway as a key regulator in cell proliferation and apoptosis

Toll-like receptors (TLR)

- Proteins in the innate immune response that recognize PAMPS expressed on APCs → activation of APCs → presentation of antigen to T-cells (forms a link between the innate and adaptive immune system) → phagocytosis of pathogen → proinflammatory state
- Various types exist: all use the **myd88 signaling pathway** upon activation except TLR3
  - TLR1: recognizes gram-negative bacteria and mycobacteria
  - **TLR2**: recognizes gram-positive bacteria like **P. acnes** ("acne has 2 syllables")
  - TLR3: recognizes viral DsRNA ("3D") and does not use myd88 signaling pathway
  - TLR4: recognizes **LPS** of gram-negative bacteria ("4 lips touch when people kiss")
  - TLR5: recognizes bacterial flagellin ("five-gellin")
  - TLR6: recognizes mycobacteria

- o TLR7/TLR8: recognizes viral **ssRNA**; imiquimod is a synthetic TRL7 and -8 agonist
  - ▪ **Imiquimod uses the myd88 signaling pathway**
- o TLR9: recognizes hypomethylated bacterial DNA

Antimicrobial peptides (AMPs)

- Have a wide range of inhibitory effects against bacteria, fungi, parasites and viruses
- **IL-17 activates AMPs** ("when you are 17 you get AMP'd about going to college")
- Many AMPs are ↑ in psoriasis ("psoriatic plaques look like A CHIP")
  - o Antileukoprotease
  - o Cathelicidin (LL-37)
  - o Human β-Defensins (HBD-2, -3, -4): HBD-2 is ↓ in atopic dermatitis
  - o Involucrin: actually not an AMP but it is an epidermal component ↑ in psoriasis
  - o Psoriasin
- Dermicidin (and HBD-2) is an AMP that is ↓ in atopic dermatitis

Complement pathways

- Small plasma proteins that circulate in the blood in an inactive state known as zymogens
- Upon activation they are cleaved, activating the next protein in the cascade
- Functions of compliment: "The best complement you can get is you're such A COOL kid"
  - o Anaphylaxis, Chemotaxis, Clears immune complexes, Opsonizes/Lyses bacteria
- There are 3 complement pathways all leading to formation of MAC (C5b to C9)
  - o Classical pathway

- Activated by immune Complexes (C1q binding to Fc portion of Ig**M** or Ig**G**)
  - **IgG3** > IgG1 > IgG2; IgG4 does not activate the classical pathway
    - Best is IgG3 ("C is the #3 letter of the alphabet")
- Forms C3 convertase (C4b/C2a) which cleaves C3 into C3a (anaphylatoxin) and C3b (IgG and C3b are the opsonins → phagocytosis)
- C3b joins to C4b2b to form C5 convertase which cleaves C5 into **C5a (mast cell/neutrophil chemotactic facto**r and anaphylatoxin) and C5b
- C5b, C6, C7, C8, C9 join to form the Membrane Attack Complex (MAC)

- Lectin pathway
  - Activated by mannose-binding lectin protein (without Ag-Ab complexes)
  - Subsequent pathway is similar to the classical pathway
- Alternative pathway ("ABCD")
  - Activated by **IgA** or Bacteria (without Ag-Ab complexes)
  - Factor B, **C3 (most abundant compliment protein)** and factor D are required to generate the C3 convertase which is stabilized by properidin ("propels alt. pathway") and inhibited by factor H ("Halts alt. pathway")

Cells

- Main cells include lymphocytes (T-cells, B-cells, NK-cells), monocytes (dendritic cells, Langerhans cells, macrophages), and granulocytes (mast cells, eosinophils, neutrophils)

T-cells

- Formed in the BM, mature in the thymus, reside in the LN where naïve T cells meet APCs
- T-cell receptors recognize antigens on MHC class I/II molecules (1° stimulation)
- Also, costimulatory signals between T-cells and APCs are needed (costimulation)
    - CD28 on T-cell binds B7-1 or B7-2 (CD80 or CD86) on APC ("8 looks like B")
        - Abatacept: blocks B7-1 (CD80) → **blocks T-cell activation**
        - If CTLA-4 on T-cell binds B7-1 on APC, T-cells are ↓ (ipilimumab blocks CTLA-4 and stops this inhibition → ↑T-cells → treats melanoma)
    - CD2 on T-cells binds LFA-3 ("#2 in CD2 is close to #3 in LFA-3")
        - Alefacept blocks this → **blocks T-cell activation** (was used in psoriasis)
    - LFA-1 on T-cells binds to ICAM-1 on APCs ("#1 and #1")
        - Efalizumab (off-market) is an Ab to CD11a which is a part of LFA-1
- Markers include CD2, -3, -4 (on helper T-cells) and CD8 (cytotoxic T-cells)
- T-cells include CD4 T-helper cells (Th1, Th2, Th17, Treg) and CD8 cytotoxic T-cells
    - Th1 T-helper cells
        - Activated by **intracellular pathogens** and used in cell-mediated immunity
        - Activates macrophages and cytotoxic T-cells
        - Transcription factors are T-bet, STAT1, and STAT4
        - Th1 differentiation requires stimulation by IL-12 and IFN-γ
        - Th1 cells produce IL-2, IL-12, TNF-α, and IFN-γ
    - Th2 T-helper cells

        - Activated by **extracellular pathogens** and important in humoral immunity
        - Activates eosinophils for parasite defense and ↑ IgE by B-cells
        - Transcription factors are STAT6 and GATA-3
        - Th2 differentiation requires stimulation by IL-4
        - Th2 cells produce IL-4, -5, -6, -10, and -13
    - Th17 T-helper cells
        - Activates neutrophils and important in chronic inflammation (psoriasis)
        - Transcription factors are RORγT, STAT3, and TGF-β
        - Th2 differentiation requires stimulation by IL-6 and TGF-β
        - Th17 cells produce IL-6, -17, -22, -23, -36, and TNF-α
    - Treg T-helper cells
        - Express CD25; transcription factor is FOXP3; downregulates immune response ("Treacy is a 25-year-old fox who is always down")
    - CD8 T-cells
        - Become cytotoxic T-cells or memory T-cells
        - **Recognize intracellular antigens when bound to MHC class 1**
            - **All other T-cells (e.g., helper T-cells) recognize MHC class 2**
        - Kills viruses or tumor cells via perforin/granzyme pathway or binding of Fas ligand on $CD8^+$ T-cells to Fas on target cells
- Disease associations of T-helper cells ("PAT C CAL'D")
    - Th1 (PAT C): Psoriasis, ACD, Tuberculoid leprosy, Cutaneous leishmania
    - Th2 (CAL'D): CTCL (Sézary), Atopic dermatitis, Lepromatous leprosy, Disseminated leishmania; also think autoimmune diseases (scleroderma, SLE)
    - Th17 and Th22: psoriasis

B-cells

- Formed in the bone marrow and reside mainly in the LNs
- B-cells isotype switch (IgM to IgA, IgG, IgE) if they interact with T-helper cells
- Whereas T-cells are activated by fragments of proteins degraded in APCs and act short range, B-cells recognize intact antigens and secrete antibodies which can act far away
- Initial exposure results in low Ab production (mainly IgM) while subsequent exposures to the same antigen results in rapid development of IgA, IgG, IgE (↑ isotype switching)
- B-cell markers include CD19, CD20 and CD79a
- Main function is antibody production
    - Antibodies have heavy and light chains connected by disulfide bonds
        - One end binds to specific bacterial antigens (variable region/Fab) while the other end has a constant region (Fc) which interacts with human cells
    - IgM: pentomer; activates complement; 1st Ab in 1° immune response
        - IgG,-M activate compliment (classic pathway)
            - "I go to the GyM to get compliments classically"
    - IgA: dimer; present on mucosal surfaces (IgA can activate Alternative pathway)
    - IgG: monomer; activates complement (except IgG4); only Ab that crosses placenta ("G mom, thanks"); opsonize (except IgG2, IgG4; "Odds Opsonize")
        - **Half-life of IgG is about a month**, the others are about a week
    - IgE: monomer; binds to mast cells/basophils; response to helminths

Natural killer cells

- Key cell in the Innate immune system
- Main cell surface markers are CD56, CD2, and CD16
- **FasL on NK-cell surface** bind to Fas on target cells → apoptosis via caspases
- **Granzymes and perforins are in cytosolic granules** and released causing apoptosis of infected viral or tumor cells w/ ↓ MHC I expression
- Activated by IL-12, IL-15 and type I interferons; secretes **IFN-γ**

Monocytes

- Macrophages and dermal dendrocytes are types of monocytes in the skin
- They are derived from a common CD34+ progenitor cell in the bone marrow
- Cell markers include **CD11c** ("11 letters in macrophages"), **CD6** ("6 letters in phages"), Fc receptor for IgG and MHC II (for antigen presentation)
- Functions of macrophages: "MAC-rophages, more like WAC-rophages"
    - o Wound healing/tissue remodeling
    - o Antigen presentation, Angiogenesis
    - o Cytokine production, Coagulation

Eosinophils

- Important role in fighting against parasites/helminths and in allergic disease
- Activated by IL-5; secrete Th2 cytokines (IL-4, -5) → ↑ IgE which coats helminths
- **Contain cytoplasmic granules composed of Major Basic protein** causing the degranulation of Mast cells and Basophils

Mast cells

- Important role in immediate-type hypersensitivity (urticaria, anaphylaxis)
- Present in urticaria pigmentosa, mastocytosis, urticaria, and **neural tumors**
- Express CD34, CD13, c-kit, c-kit receptor (CD117), and its ligand stem cell factor
    - Mast cell progenitor cell is $CD34^+$
- Compliment protein C5a triggers chemotaxis of cutaneous mast cells
- Anaphylatoxins (C3a, C4a and particularly **C5a) triggers mast cell degranulation**
- **Prostaglandin D2** is a marker for mast cell activation ("Degranulates mast cells")
- **Prostaglandin E2 inhibits mast cell degranulation ("Ends degranulation")**
    - Mast cell degranulation contains pro-inflammatory mediators
        - Preformed (no #s): histamine, tryptase, heparin, chymase, cathepsin G
        - Newly formed (#s): prostaglandin D2, leukotrienes C4/D4/E4, IL-1, -4, -5
- Mast cell stains: Kit (CD117), tryptase, Leder, toluidine blue, Giemsa
    - "Master Kit led them on a trip to the tall-blue gems"
    - Kit and Leder are the stains still reliable in recently degranulated (rubbed) skin
        - Leder is commonly used and will function even after rubbing skin/recent degranulation ("rub me and take me to your leader")
    - Toluidine blue and Giemsa are the metachromatic stains
- Degranulation triggers can be divided into immunologic and nonimmunologic mechanisms: ("When you go to CAMP Everyone Pack your DARN SOCKS")

  - Immunologic: autoAbs against FcεRI due to Cephalopsorin, AutoAbs, Asparaginase, Minocycline/Medical devices (latex gloves), PNC
  - Non-immunologic: **Epinephrine**, Polymyxin B, Dietary pseudoallergens, ASA, ACE inhibitors, Radiocontrast media, Nettle stings/NSAIDS, Substance P (and other neuropeptides), Opiates, C5a anaphylatoxin, KIT ligand (Stem cell factor)
    - Use lidocaine w/o epinephrine (unless staining with Kit or Leder as these still stain mast cells even after recent degranulation)

Neutrophils

- First cell to arrive in the inflammatory cascade
- Neutrophil chemotactic factors: "LICK my pus" → LTB4, IL-8, c5a, Kallikrein
- Kills microbial pathogens by phagocytosis and release of ROS
- Neutrophilic granules
  - Primary granules (LMNoP) aka azurophilic granules: contain Lysozyme, Myeloperoxidase, Neutral serine proteases, Proteinase-3, Proteoglycans
  - Secondary granules: contain lactoferrin, alkaline phosphatase, phospholipase A2

Langerhans cells (LCs)

- Dendritic APCs which reside in the epidermis which are activated by "TIM"
  - **TGF-β1**, IL-34, M-CSF ("TIM lends a hand to Langerhans cells")
- Adhere to keratinocytes via E-cadherin
- Following antigen uptake, LCs move to the LNs where they present MHC-bound antigen to T-cells resulting in their activation
- Markers: Langerin (CD207) is the most sensitive and specific marker as it stains Birbeck granules (rod-

shaped organelles visible on EM); CD1a, S100, vimentin also stain

Major histocompatibility complex (MHC)

- Human leukocyte antigens (HLA) are part of the MHC that **presents peptides to T-cells**
- MHC locus is on chromosome 6 ("six and Major histocompatibility complex end in x")
- Divided into two main classes
    - MHC class I: presents endogenous antigens (e.g., viral, tumor) to $CD8^+$ T-cells
        - Expressed on all nucleated cells (e.g., keratinocytes)
        - Three main MHC I genes: HLA-A, HLA-B, HLA-C
    - MHC class II: presents exogenous proteins (bacterial proteins) to T-helper cells
        - Expressed on APCs (macrophages, dendritic cells, B-cells)
        - Three main MHC II genes: HLA-DP, HLA-DQ, HLA-DR
- High-yield MHC-associated diseases
    - HLA-DR2: Bullous SLE, EBA ("2nd letter of the alphabet is B")
    - HLA-DR3: SCLE, Childhood/juvenile DM and Herpes gestationis (CHERPES G is my mnemonic in section 3.24) → "3rd letter of the alphabet is C"
    - HLA-DR4: Vitiligo (and A33, B13, B44, DRB1), pemphigus Vulgaris (and DRw6), RA (and DR1), Relapsing polychondritis (and DR6), chronic Urticaria, Mixed CTD
        - "The 4th DR drives in his fast car which goes VVRRUM"
    - HLA-B27: sacroiliitis (reactive arthritis, PsA, ankylosing spondylitis, IBD, SAPHO)
    - HLA-Cw6: psoriasis ("Cw6 aka C-why-a-six sounds like psoriasis")

- HLA-B13 and HLA-B17: erythrodermic and guttate psoriasis
  - "Ery (every) gutt B 13 to 17 inches too wide in America"
- HLA-B51: Behçet's disease ("5+1=6 and there are 6 letters in Behçet")
- HLA-B57, -B8, -DR1 and -DR10 are a/w lichen planus
- HLA-A1, -B8, -**DQ2** a/w dermatitis herpetiformis ("celiacs can't go 2 Dairy Queen")
- HLA-DQ7: LS&A ("a 7 rotated 180° looks like an L")

1.6 Genetics and Laboratory Techniques

Genetics

- AR: both parents are carriers and offspring have 1 in 4 chance of being affected
- AD: one parent is affected, and **offspring have a 1 in 2 chance of being affected**
- XLR: mother is a carrier and sons have a 1 in 2 chance of being affected while daughters have a 1 in 2 chance of being carriers (no male-to-male transmission)
- XLD: mother is affected and sons either die in utero or are born unaffected while daughters have a 1 in 2 chance of being affected

Laboratory techniques

- Polymerase chain reaction (PCR)
  - Amplifies a specific piece of DNA by these steps: DA ER (sounds like "the ER")
    - Denaturation → Annealing/hybridization→ primer Extension→ Repeat

    - Quantitative PCR can measure gene rearrangements in cancer ("Quancer")
    - An alternative method to measure DNA is by Southern blot
        - **First aid mnemonic was SNoW DRoP**
            - Southern blot: DNA detected with a DNA probe (PCR-like)
            - Northern blot: RNA detected with a DNA probe (RT-PCR-like)
            - Western blot: Protein detected with an antibody probe (ELISA, immunoprecipitation and immunohistochemistry-like)
- Reverse transcriptase PCR (RT-PCR)
    - Amplifies a piece of mRNA by first converting it to DNA via reverse transcriptase
    - Like PCR, it is very sensitive for detecting mutations, but RNA is more fragile
    - A modification is quantitative RT-PCR (allows quantification of RNA transcripts)
    - An alternative method to measure RNA is by Northern blot
- Western blot
    - Can detect, quantify, and determine the molecular weight of specific **proteins** and identify antibody activity to a known antigen
    - Requires Abs specific for proteins of interest (can't cross react w/ other proteins)
    - A modification is the dot blot and alternatives include ELISA, IP and IHC
        - ELISA: used to detect specific immunoglobins (anti-Mi-2) in blood but can be modified to detect specific proteins in tissue (immunohistochemistry)
- Gene expression profiling detects abnormal gene expression through expression of RNA

  - The technology used to assess the expression of these genes is qRT-PCR
- Comparative Genomic hybridization: detects chromosomal Gain/loss in tissue samples
  - Advantage: genome-wide screening of chromosomal gains/losses
  - Disadvantage: low % of neoplastic cells in the sample leads to false negatives
- Fluorescence in situ hybridization (FISH): detects Translocations, Amplifications and Deletions ("TAD pole = FISH") by using dyes to attach to specific parts of chromosomes
  - Each nucleus is evaluated individually so no risk of false negatives
  - Can detect cancers, predict outcomes and whether they will respond to chemo
    - Ex: detects t(17;22) translocation in DFSP, n-MYC in neuroblastoma and c-MYC amplifications in radiation-induced angiosarcoma
  - Can detect polyploidy in melanoma and if (+) would predict a more aggressive melanoma (but does not prove malignancy as polyploidy can be seen in Spitz)
  - Can also detect inherited genetic mutations and identify microorganisms
- Flow cytometry: separates cells through a narrow stream of liquid and uses lasers to detect fluorescent antibodies and proteins bound to the cells
  - Commonly used for analyzing T-cells in CTCL
- Single nucleotide polymorphism (SNP) arrays: assesses DNA sequence variation that occurs when a single nucleotide (e.g., adenine) in the genome sequence is altered

1.7 High Yield Dermatology Billing and Coding

E/M (evaluation and management) codes (992xx)

- 99211: office visit that may not require presence of a doctor (e.g., biologic injection)
    - Only add a J code (J3590) if the drug was supplied by the physician
- 99212: straightforward medical decision making (e.g., evaluation of nevi)
- 99213: low medical decision making (e.g., acute uncomplicated issue w/ OTC treatment)
- 99214: moderate decision making (e.g., chronic illness w/ exacerbating w/ prescription)

CPT (current procedural terminology) Codes

Skin biopsy (11102-11107)

- Physician's intent is to sample tissue for the purpose of histopathologic diagnosis
- 11102: tangential biopsy of one lesion +/- 11103 for any additional shave biopsies
- 11104: punch biopsy of one lesion +/- 11105 for any additional punch biopsies
- 11106: incisional biopsy of one lesion +/- 11107 for any additional incisional biopsies

Excisions (114xx to 116xx)

- Physician's intent is to remove the lesion
- Must document medical necessity for excision (and destruction) of benign lesions
- Requires that a lesion be excised through the dermis **(down to SQ)** and include margins
- The surgeon must specify the size of the lesion and the margins

- Simple suturing is included in the code (intermediate/ complex suture coded separately)

Repairs

- Simple (12001-18): only epidermal sutures (or staples or tissue adhesives) are used
- Intermediate (12031-57): epidermal and dermal sutures are used
- Complex (13100-53): in addition to the requirements for intermediate repair, it requires at least one of the following ("RUDE af")
  - Placement of Retention sutures
  - Extensive Undermining (defined as a distance equal to or greater than the max width of the defect along at least one entire edge of the defect)
  - Debridement of wound edges (e.g., traumatic lacerations or avulsions)
  - Exposure of bone, cartilage, tendon, or named vascular structure
  - Involvement of a free margin (e.g., helical rim, nostril rim or vermillion border)

Destruction of actinic keratoses (AK)

- 17000: 1 AK
- 17000 (x1) and 17003 (x1 to x13): 2 to 14 AKs
- 17004: 15 or more AKs

Modifiers

- 24 modifier: separate E/M in the post-op global period
  - Ex: pt underwent excision and develops unrelated rash 1 week later
  - "Twenty-four, they're back for more"
- 25 modifier: separate E/M on the same day as a procedure
  - Ex: they also show you a rash during a MOHs procedure

- 50 modifier: identifies the service as being performed on both sides of the body
    - Ex: application of an unna boot
    - "50/50 is the most bilateral number"
- 51 modifier: multiple procedures on the same day (subsequent procedure is paid less)
    - Ex: you are doing MOHs and you also perform a biopsy
    - "51 is near 50 (half) which reminds me that every extra procedure bills at half"
- 57 modifier: allows physician to bill for an E/M pre-op code the day of or the day before a major surgery with a 90-day global period (e.g., grafts/flaps but NOT MOHs)
- 58 modifier: related/staged procedure within the post-op global period (not same day)
    - Ex: re-excision of incompletely excised lesion or slow MOHs
    - "Fifty-eight finishes same procedure late"
- 59 modifier: unrelated procedure performed on same day as an E/M encounter
    - Ex: they are in for a rash and you do an unrelated biopsy

More modifiers with mnemonics

- 76 modifier: same procedure performed again on the same day (e.g., double-site MOHs)
    - "76-year-old is younger and wants both his MOHs done the same day"
- 78 modifier: unplanned return to OR for related procedure in the post-op period
    - "Poor old 78-year-old had a complication after MOHs and had to come back"
- 79 modifier: unrelated procedure performed in the global period (not same day)

- "79-year-old is too old to have more than one MOHs w/ repair on the same day so he does his 2nd MOHs later (but within the repair post-op period)"

Global period

- A period of time starting w/ a surgical procedure and ending some period of time after in which normal post-op charges are bundled into the global surgery fee (coded 99024)
- No global period: biopsies, shaves, injections and MOHs
- **10-day global period: benign/malignant excisions and destruction codes**, repair, I&D
- 90-day global period includes flaps, grafts, soft-tissue tumor excisions, dermabrasion

1.8 Statistics and Studies

Construct your diagram/plot ("disease always ends up on top")...

	Positive Disease	Negative disease
Positive test	True Positive (TP)	False Positive (FP) Type I error
Negative test	False Negative (FN) Type II error	True Negative (TN)

- Sensitivity = TP / (TP + FN)
  - SNOUT (high sensitivity rules out): high sensitivity means if the test is negative, we can confidently rule out disease due to few false negatives (screening test)
- Specificity = TN / (TN + FP)
  - SPIN (high specificity rules in): high specificity means if test is positive then disease is likely due to very few false positives (confirmatory test)

- Positive predictive value (PPV) = TP / TP + FP
  - PPV is the probability of having a disease given a positive test result
  - Affected by prevalence (positive relationship)
- Negative predictive value (NPV) = TN / TN + FN
  - NPV is the probability of not having the disease given a negative test result
  - Affected by prevalence (negative relationship)
- Null hypothesis: assumption that there is no difference between 2 groups being studied
  - Type I error (FP): incorrect rejection of a true null (type I error rate is the alpha)
    - "If I was doing a study, I would probably make a type I error because I am an alpha male that is overly confident that I will show a true difference"
  - Type II error (FN): incorrect acceptance of a null hypothesis (type II error rate is called the Beta which is related to power of a test → power = 1 – Beta)
    - Power is ↑ (and type II error is ↓) by increasing the # of test subjects

Statistical definitions

- Prevalence: proportion of the total population affected by a disease
- Incidence: **# of new cases** of a disease diagnosed over a set period of time
- Precision: how consistently repeated the results are (Reliability)
- Validity: how close the test assay comes to the truth (Accuracy)
  - Accuracy = TP + TN / TP + FP + TN + FN

Studies and bias

Observational studies

- Case control (all are retrospective): we know who has the disease (case) and the investigator does a chart review/questionnaire to see if they have the exposure
    - Odds ratio: confidence interval < 1 is protective, 1 is no effect, > 1 is ↑ risk
- Prospective cohort: we know who is exposed and follow to see if they get the disease
- Restrospective cohort: we know who is exposed and the investigator does a chart review and follows them back in time to see if they have the disease
    - Relative risk: confidence interval < 1 is protective, 1 is no effect, > 1 is ↑ risk
- Cross sectional: analyses data (using medical records) at one specific time (snapshot)

Randomized control trial (RCT)

- Interventional study where participants are randomly assigned to a Rx or control group
- Randomization reduces Selection bias and Blinding reduces Ascertainment bias
    - "R is next to S, and B is next to A in the alphabet"

Meta-analysis

- A statistical analysis that combines the results of multiple scientific studies

Bias

- Search satisfying bias: the predisposition to stop a search once something is found
- Attrition bias: subjects drop out of the clinical trial before it has completed
- Recall bias: subjects have distorted Recollection of events in a Retrospective study

- Sunk cost bias: when pt/doctor continues to invest resources in a plan that is suboptimal
- Availability bias: occurs when we overweigh evidence that comes easily to mind
- Lead time bias: when a pt w/ a disease found earlier in its course appears to live longer
- Ascertainment bias: results are distorted because researchers know if subjects are in the intervention or the control group (Blinding eliminates this; A next to B)
- Selection bias: subjects not randomly selected (Randomization fixes this)
- Confirmation bias: researcher uses respondents' info to confirm pre-held beliefs
- Publication bias: selective publication of results when a positive effect is shown
- Reporting bias: selective dissemination of findings based on the nature of results
- Response bias: tendencies for participants to respond inaccurately/falsely to questions
    - Acquiescence bias: tendency to agree w/ all questions or indicate positive results
    - Social desirability bias: tendency to give the perceived socially acceptable answer
    - Extreme responding: tendency to select the most extreme options available

Medical errors and safety events ("NP'S commit many medical errors")

- Near miss: error w/ potential to cause harm but was caught before reaching the patient
- Precursor safety event: safety event that reaches patient but causes minimal to no harm
- Sentinel event: error that results in serious harm to the patient

Chapter 2: Dermatopharmacology

2.1 Retinoids

- Retinoids bind to retinoid binding protein in the cytoplasm which is transported to the nucleus where they bind to nuclear receptor **RARs or RXRs (each which have 3 isotypes α, β and γ)** and where **dimers** of retinoid receptors (RAR/RXR or RXR/RXR) bind to retinoid hormone response elements (RAREs) to affect DNA transcription
  - **RAR-γ is the MC receptor in skin** (all retinoids except bexarotene hit this hard)
- Binding to RAR/RXR effects various genes and transcription factors (↓OK TAN, ↑TH1)
  - ↓Ornithine decarboxylase, Keratinization (**K6/K16**), Tumorigenesis (induces apoptosis), TH2 (Two) cytokines, **TLR2** (Toll-like receptor Two), AP1 and NF-IL-6
- SEs of systemic retinoids are "STOP Doing Retinoids"
  - **Staph aureus folliculitis**/colonization, **Sticky Sensation on palms and Soles**
    - Sticky DIK mnemonic (Doxorubicin, Isotretinoin and Ketoconazole)
  - Teratogenicity, Telogen effluvium, ↑ Triglycerides, **↓ TSH and T4 (Bexarotene)**
  - Ossification of bones (DISH), Ocular effects and Onychorrhexis/Onychoschizia
  - Pseudotumor cerebri, Palmoplantar Peeling, Photosensitivity, Pancreatitis, **Pyogenic granuloma-like lesions** and **Premature epiphyseal closure (SE in a kid)**

  - DISH, Diarrhea and Dry lips, eyes, nasal mucosa and skin
  - **Reduced night vision**
- CIs: more P words (Pregnancy/lactation and Paraben hypersensitivity)
- Monitor triglycerides (D/C if > 800), LFTs (D/C if > 3x upper limit of normal), urine/serum pregnancy test in females and TSH/T4 (bexarotene)
- Most isotretinoin-exposed pregnancies result in healthy-appearing births but ↓ mental function becomes apparent over time (majority have mild-moderate deficits): Get a CT (not actually just a mnemonic) to look for specific features of retinoid embryopathy
  - Craniofacial: ears (**microtia**) and eyes don't fully form, cleft palate, hypertelorism
  - CNS: microcephaly, hydrocephalus and Bell's palsy
  - CV: septal defects, Tetralogy of Fallot, TOGV and aortic arch hypoplasia
  - Thymic: thymic aplasia or ectopia
- Interactions (FAST: continuation on SE/CI mnemonic "STOP Doing Retinoids FAST")
  - Fatty meals ↑ bioavailability because retinoids are lipophilic
    - Absorbica is lidose coated isotretinoin and can be taken w/o a fatty meal
  - Alcohol ↑ hepatotoxicity and ↑ conversion of acitretin to etretinate
  - Vitamin A supplements ↑ risk of hypervitaminosis A
  - CYP3A4 drugs: gemfibrozil ↑ bexarotene levels, 3A4 inhibitors (macrolides, azoles, etc.) ↑ retinoid levels and retinoids ↑ cyclosporine levels
  - Simvastatin and gemfibrozil may not be used (use other statins to ↓ LDLs and **use fenofibrate to ↓ triglycerides**; "SimvaStatin Sucks, FenoFibrate is Fine")

    - Tetracycline coadministration ↑ risk of **pseudotumor cerebri**
- Topical retinoids for acne (adapalene, tazarotene, tretinoin and trifarotene)
    - All pregnancy category C except tazarotene (cat X)
    - All synthetic except all-trans-retinoic acid/tretinoin (naturally present in plasma)
        - "Liberals say that all trans athletes are natural girls"
    - All have hepatobiliary excretion except tazarotene (urine and feces)
    - **Adapalene and tazarotene effect RAR-**$\beta/\gamma > \alpha$, trifarotene is selective for the RAR-γ receptor, and tretinoin (all-trans-retinoic Acid) effects all RARs equally
    - All light stable and benzoyl peroxide stable except tretinoin, which is inactivated by UV light and oxidized by benzoyl peroxide
    - All used for acne and photoaging and cause irritation, erythema and pruritis
        - Tazarotene is also used in psoriasis
- Other topical retinoids that we do not commonly use
    - Alitretinoin (9-cis-retinoic acid) is an endogenous retinoid, pregnancy cat D, binds all nuclear receptors (RAR > RXR) and used in Kaposi sarcoma ("kap-all-si")
        - "Liberals say that All cis males can get Kaposi sarcoma too"
    - BeXarotene is preg category X, binds all RXR (**RXR-**$\beta/\gamma > \alpha$) and is used for CTCL
- Systemic retinoids (to remember half-lives remember order "TB, IAE"- this rhymes)
    - Tretinoin (1 hour): for promyelocytic leukemia but causes **scrotal/mouth ulcers**
    - Bexarotene (8 hours): for CTCL but causes **central hypothyroidism** and **↑ TGs**

    - Isotretinoin (1 day; 13-cis retinoic acid): for acne but SE are STOP Doing Retinoids
        - Requires contraception 1 month before to 1 month after stopping drug
    - Acitretin (2 days): for psoriasis but converts to etretinate upon alcohol consumption so patient **needs contraception for 3 years after cessation**
        - Similar SEs as isotretinoin: ↑ TGs, ↑ LFTs, alopecia, hepatitis
    - Etretinate (120-day half-life because it is 50 times more lipophilic than acitretin)
- iPLEDGE requirement for isotretinoin
    - Females of childbearing potential (anyone w/ a functional uterus)
        - Day 1: patient registers and has her first pregnancy test (done in office)
            - Must be on 2 forms of contraception for 30 days (**abstinence counts as both forms**) after registration in iPLEDGE
        - As early as day 31 pt can have office visit and doctor confirms counseling
            - The 2nd pregnancy test (in lab) must occur within 7 days after this office visit and during the first 5 days of the pt's menstrual cycle
            - If pt answers all iPLEDGE questions (in this 7-day window) and pregnancy test is negative the pt can fill the prescription
        - This process repeats and 2 forms of contraception is continued until 30 days after therapy (final pregnancy test occurs 30 days after therapy)
    - Males or females of non-childbearing potential (e.g., trans females)
        - Day 1: pt registers and office visit/counseling (no 30-day waiting period)
            - Pt has 1 week to fill prescription

        - All pts should not donate blood for at least 1 month off therapy

2.2 Corticosteroids (CS)

- Basic structure is three 6 sided rings and 1 five-sided ring
- Absorbed in jejunum ("steroid and jejunum have same # of letters")
- Desired effect in derm is through glucocorticoid not mineralocorticoid activity
    - Long-acting (dexamethasone and betamethasone) systemic CS have the Least (none) mineralocorticoid activity ☺ and are the Least allergic topical CS ☺
    - Prednisone/Prednisolone (intermediate) and Cortisol/Cortisone (short-acting) have 1+ and 2+ mineralocorticoid activity respectively (PC culture gives me HTN)
    - Methylprednisolone and triamcinolone are also intermediate-acting but have no mineralocorticoid activity so are **best in CHF**
- CS bind to glucocorticoid receptors in the cytoplasm and then translocate to nucleus
- When CS is bound to cortisol-binding globulin (CBG) it is inactive
    - Thyroid and estrogen ↑ CBG → ↓ active free fraction
        - "Hyperthyroid women need more exogenous steroid to have effect"
    - Liver disease, renal disease and obesity ↓ CBG → ↑ active free fraction
        - "Fat hypothyroid men with renal and liver disease don't need as much"

- 11-β-hydroxysteroid dehydrogenase (3-β…was defect in CHILD syndrome) in liver converts steroid to active form (cortisone → cortisol / prednisone → prednisolone)
    - "Liver disease ↓ this conversion so give active cortisol/prednisolone in old liver"
- MOA: retinoids ↓ OK TAN and ↑TH1 cytokines; steroids ↓ OC PAN and ↑IL-10
    - ↓"Ornithine decarboxylase", Cox-2, Prostaglandins, "AP-1", **NFKβ**
        - These changes have major effects on **cellular** >> humoral immunity
- Major SE from systemic CS is **HPA suppression** (Hypothalamus → Pituitary → Adrenal)
    - Adrenals get lazy and atrophied and stop making their own cortisol
        - Adrenals are last to get suppressed and slowest to recover
    - Only "PC culture" (Prednisone/prednisolone, Cortisone/-ol) suppresses mineralocorticoid axis (renin-angiotensin-aldosterone) → **HTN, ↑ Na, ↓ K**
    - Risk factors: course > **1-month**, abrupt cessation, major stressors, divided doses
    - Exogenous adrenal insufficiency has two clinical presentations
        - **Steroid Withdrawal syndrome (common)**: pt has flu-like symptoms with **no change in serum cortisol level ("Serum cortisol within avg limits")**
        - Adrenal crisis (uncommon): life-threatening hypotension from ↓ cortisol
- Other side effects can be remembered by the DIT mnemonic "BAM CUSHINGOID"
    - Buffalo hump
    - Amenorrhea
    - Moon faces, Myopathy
    - Crazy (psychosis), Cataracts, CHF, **↓Calcium**

- **Ulcers (peptic) → bowl perforation (prevent with H2 blockers in high-risk pts)**
- Skin changes: "A SHIT Prednisone Taper" → Atrophy, ACD, Acne, Striae, ↓wound Healing, Hirsutism, Infections (staph/HSV), Telangiectasias, Purpura, Perioral dermatitis, hypoPigmentation, Pustular Psoriasis (withdrawal), Telogen effluvium
- **HTN, Hypertriglyceridemia, Hypokalemia**
- Infection
- **Necrosis of femoral head (avoid trauma/alcohol/smoking; Dx MRI; Rx: referral)**
- Glaucoma, Growth impairment in kids
- **Osteoporosis (ppx calcium and vit D; Dx DEXA; Rx bisphosphonate)**
  - We even start bisphosphonates for osteopenia (A T score of -1 to -2.5)
- Immunosuppression
- **Diabetes**

- These SEs are a result of the catabolic effect that CS have, which pulls energy from the liver, SQ fat, connective tissue, muscles and bones to the brain in this fight or flight state
- Most complications are dose-related and their risks can therefore be ↓ w/ QOD dosing except **cataracts** ("Qataracts"), **Osteoporosis and Osteonecrosis of femoral head**
- BID (divided doses) are Better (more effective) but have Bigger (more) side effects
- Lab abnormality caused by steroids: **neutrophilia, ↓Ca, ↑ Na, ↓ K, ↑ glucose**
- Pregnancy cat C but likely safe for short courses (Prednisolone is safest in Pregnancy)
- Unique intramuscular CS side effects ("Ken 40 is a CHAMP")
  - **Cold abscesses, Crystal deposition**
  - **↑HPA axis suppression compared to PO**

- **Atrophy of SQ fat**
- Menstrual irregularities
- Purpura

- Intralesional CS SEs: fat atrophy and **streaky hypopigmentation, especially in dark skin**
- Pulse IV Steroids indicated for PG, Pemphigoid, Systemic vasculitis and SLE but it's not very "SAFE" (**Sudden cardiac death, Seizures, Anaphylaxis, A-Fib, Electrolyte shifts**)

2.3 Non-steroidal immunomodulatory agents

Apremilast

- PDE-4 inhibitor (like Crisaborole used in AD) used for Psoriasis and Psoriatic arthritis
    - PDE4 expression causes immune activation (Th1, Th2, Th22) so also treats AD
    - Sildenafil is a PDE5 inhibitor
- Side effects makes you Puke (**nausea**, diarrhea, headache, **depression**)
- In renal disease you half the dose
- **Roflumilast**: topical PDE4 inhibitor that can be used in AD, seb derm, inverse psoriasis

Janus Kinase inhibitors

- Normally JAK phosphorylates/activate STAT proteins which translocate to the nucleus to trigger downstream effects (these drugs **block this phosphorylation**/activation of STAT)

- Know your JAKs: "JAK U BRAT, that Russian Bartender wants To Fac Dude"
    - JAK1 ("U BRAT"): Upadacitinib, Baricitinib, Ruxolitinib, Abrocitinib, Tofactinib
        - Cytokines: γc family (IL-2, **-4**, -7, -9, -15), gp130 family (IL-6, -11), IFN$\alpha/\beta/\gamma$
    - JAK2 ("Russian Bartender"): Ruxolitinib, Baricitinib
        - Cytokines: gp130 family (IL-6, -11, OSM, LIF), βc family (IL-3, -5, GM-CSF), erythropoietin, thrombopoietin, IFNγ, **IL-12/IL-23**
    - JAK3 ("To fac"): Tofacitinib
        - Cytokines: γc family (IL-2, **-4**, -7, -9, -15)
    - TYK2 ("Dude"): Deucravacitinib
        - gp130 family (IL-6, -11, OSM, LIF), IFNα/β, **IL-12/IL-23**
- Only JAK2 can couple w/ itself ("it takes 2 to tango except with JAK2")
    - TYK2/JAK1 (IFN-α, -β) → B/T cell survival, antibody production, MHC expression
    - **TYK2/JAK2 (IL-12, -23) → Th1 and Th17 cell differentiation**
    - JAK1/JAK2 (IL-6, IFN-γ) → Th1 cell differentiation
    - JAK1/JAK3 (IL-2, **-4**, -7, -9, 15, -21) → T-cell and Treg survival, Th2 differentiation
    - **JAK2/JAK2** (erythropoietin, GH, leptin, thrombopoietin, prolactin, GM-CSF) → hematopoiesis, growth factor response, myelopoiesis)
- Upadacitinib (Rinvoq) and abrocitinib (Cibinqo): inhibits JAK1
    - FDA approved for AD (unique **SE is acne**)
- Ruxolitinib: inhibits JAK1/JAK2
    - Topical cream (Opzelura) is FDA approved for AD and vitiligo
    - Oral form (Jakafi) is FDA approved for AD, polycythemia vera and myelofibrosis

- Baricitinib (Olumiant): inhibits JAK1/JAK2
  - FDA approved for **alopecia areata**
- Tofacitinib (Xeljanz): JAK1/JAK3 > JAK2/TYK2 ("Three and One")
  - FDA approved for RA, PsA and UC but works well for alopecia areata and vitiligo
  - Like rituximab, there is a risk of intestinal perforation (ask about diverticulitis)
- Deucravacitinib (Sotyktu): selective TYK2 inhibitor
  - FDA approved for psoriasis
  - Does not have black box warning for clots and cancers like the other JAKs
- Ritlecitinib: selective JAK3 and TEC kinase inhibitor
  - Works well for alopecia areata
- Brepocitinib: TYK2 and JAK1 inhibitor
- SEs: GI perf, infections, **blood clots**, cancer (particularly lymphoma), **hypertriglyceridemia**, **cytopenias**, ↑ LFTs, acne, **shingles**
  - Deucravacitinib has different SE and may ↓ risk of cancers
- Get **CBC**, CMP, CK, **lipid** at baseline and q 3 months (hepatitis panel, TB just at baseline)
- Pregnancy test in females (do not want to get pregnant within 4 weeks of last dose)
- **JAK does not directly modulate IL-1, IL-17** (but indirectly via IL-23) **or TNF-α**

Cyclosporine

- MOA: **cyclosporine binds cyclophilin** (calcineurin inhibitors bind FK506-binding protein) which **inhibits Calcineurin** → ↓NFAT-1 → ↓ IL-2 → ↓ CD4 and CD8 T-cells
- Maximum dermatologic dose is 5 mg/kg/day; maximum length of treatment is 1–2 years
  - For obese patients, use ideal body weight to calculate starting dose

- Only FDA approved for psoriasis but used off-label in various inflammatory conditions
- SEs: **nephrotoxicity, progression of CTCL/SCCs/BCCs**, epidermal Cysts, palmoplantar dysesthesia w/ temperature change, acne, **↓ Mg and "hyper-KLUTS"**
  - o **Hyper... -Kalemia, -Lipids, -LFTs, -Uricemia (gout), -Tension, -Trichosis, -Teeth/gums (gingival hyperplasia), and Sebaceous hyperplasia**
    - ▪ Oral tacrolimus has same labs: ↓ Mg, ↑ lipids, K^+, uric acid
  - o **Nephrotoxicity and HTN are MC** and are dose and duration dependent
    - ▪ After 2 elevated BP readings, reduce dose by 25–50% and start a CCB
    - ▪ **CCB is prescription of choice for HTN** (does not alter drug levels or ↑K)
      - **Isradipine** is best CCB as it does not cause gingival hyperplasia
- "Remember the #5"
  - o Max derm dose is 5 mg/kg/day
  - o If two Cr levels ↑ to > 50% over baseline then discontinue cyclosporine
  - o If 2nd level ↑ to > 25% over baseline then ↓ dose by 1 mg/kg/day or by 25–50%
    - ▪ If Cr drops back down to < 25% over baseline you can continue therapy
- Baseline labs: 2 BP and Cr (1 day apart), BUN, CBC, LFTs, fasting lipids, Mg, K, uric acid

Anti-Malarial agents

- Incudes hydroxychloroquine (HCQ), chloroquine (CQ) and quinacrine
  - o HCQ has only 2/3rd the efficacy of CQ but is only half as toxic
- MOA: inhibition of UV-induced skin reactions by binding to DNA and ↓ superoxide production; raises intra-

cytoplasmic pH and stabilizes Microsomal Membranes → ↓ ability of Macrophages to express MHC complex antigens on cell surface (↓ lymphs)

- "Dapsone is for neutrophilic, anti-malarial drugs are for lymphocytic disorders"

- **Long half-life: takes 3–4 Months to achieve clinical benefit so be patient**
  - Mycophenolate mofetil and rituximab can also take up to 4 months for full effect
    - "I'm glad PCR (Plaquenil, Cellcept, Rituxan) tests don't take 4 months"
- FDA approved for malaria, SLE and RA but useful in many disorders w/ significant lymphocytic infiltrate (PMLE, lupus panniculitis, discoid lupus, Jessner's)
- CI (absolute): pts w/ retinopathy and those w/ hypersensitivity to the drug
- CI (relative): Myasthenia gravis, full dose in PCT (risk of hepatitis so we use low-dose here), hepatic dysfunction, severe blood dyscrasias, psoriasis, pregnancy/lactation
- Side effects (think eyes and Mucocutaneous drug reactions)
  - Ocular toxicity (not seen in quinacrine): corneal deposits/neuro-Muscular eye toxicity (reversible), retinopathy (irreversible; **p/w central scotoma/blind spot**)
    - Get baseline eye exam and then most recommend yearly thereafter
  - Mucocutaneous drug reactions (W is an upside-down M)
    - **Minocycline pigmentation-like darkening of shins, face, mouth and nails**
      - **Minocycline is more gray-blue, HCQ/CQ is more gray-brown**
    - **Mustard yellow skin pigmentation (only seen with quinacrine)**

        - **Morbilliform drug reactions in DM (30%) > SLE (3%)**
        - Worsens psoriasis and cause drug-induced LP and acute porphyria attacks
        - Whitening of the hair seen w/ all 3 drugs (in blonds and red heads)
    - **GI symptoms are MC SE** (can do BID dosing to lower risk)
    - Myositis, CNS, ↑ LFTs, cardiac toxicity (only w/ CQ), **AGEP** and hemolytic SEs are rare (even in G6PD deficient populations)
- ↓ dose in renal disease or you risk side effects such as pigmentation and retinal toxicity
- Baseline labs: ocular exam, CBC, CMP (LFTs)
- Boards factoids
    - HCQ can delay the time to fulfill criteria for SLE and delay dx of lupus nephritis
    - Low-dose HCQ can be used in PCT (100 mg/day vs 400 mg/day for lupus)
    - **Quinacrine added to HCQ or CQ ↑ efficacy** (never give HCQ and CQ together)
    - Preg category C but most suggest continuing treatment for SLE in pregnancy

Dapsone (HELP)

- MOA: **inhibits myeloperoxidase** (where have we seen myeloperoxidase before? HeLP)
    - Histiocytoid sweet's is MPO+
    - Leukemia cutis is MPO+ (chloromas in AML are green due to MPO activity)
    - P-ANCA is also known as anti-MPO
    - Primary granules of neutrophils use MPO to create reactive oxygen species hence why dapsone is effective in various neutrophilic dermatoses

- Important pharmacology points (HELP)
    - Hydroxylation leads to clinically relevant variability in metabolism b/w patients
    - **Hydroxylamine metabolite is responsible for Hematologic SEs like Hemolysis**
    - Hemolysis has been demonstrated in nursing infants of mothers taking dapsone
    - Enterohepatic recirculation → remains in circulation for 30 days after one dose
    - Low risk of *in utero* harmful developmental effects but still classified as…
    - Pregnancy category C
- FDA approved indications (Help): dermatitis Herpetiformis and leprosy
- Off label dermatologic uses (HELPS): various dermatoses including but not limited to Hypereosinophilic syndrome, **Erythema elevatum diutinum**, Lupus (bullous), LCV, **Linear IgA dermatosis**, Pemphigus/**Pemphigoid (especially mucosal predominate)**, Pyoderma gangrenosum, Sweet's syndrome, Subcorneal pustular dermatosis
- Side effects: "MAD HELP" → the SEs in green are predictable (pharmacologic) events and occur in 100% of individuals, the other SEs are idiosyncratic (dose-independent)
    - **Methemoglobinemia**: ↓ oxygen carrying capacity → exacerbates preexisting cardiopulmonary disease → give **oral methylene blue in emergencies**
        - Dx: get CBC and methemoglobin level (pulse ox doesn't show it)
        - **Rx: methylene blue (G6PD deficient pts cannot use this), blood transfusion, cimetidine** (vit B2, vit E, and vit C helps too)
    - **Agranulocytosis**: serious idiosyncratic reaction; **occurs at 7 weeks; p/w fever**

    - Dapsone hypersensitivity syndrome: DRESS-like syndrome (fever, rash, hepatitis)
    - **Hemolytic anemia**: Hydroxylamine metabolites are potent oxidants that deplete glutathione → Heinz body formation and splenic sequestration of RBCs
    - **Elevated liver enzymes**
    - **Leukopenia**
    - **Peripheral motor neuropathy**: may present with atrophy of hand muscles
- Labs: baseline **G6PD level**, CBC, CMP and **UA** (check compliance w/ reticulocyte count)
    - CBC weekly x 1 month, then every 2 weeks for 2 months then every 3–4 months
        - You will see signs of hemolytic anemia: ↑ retic count, ↑LDH, ↓ Hg
    - CMP every 2 weeks for first 3 months then every 3–6 months thereafter
- If dapsone can't be tolerated an alternative is sulfapyridine which has more mild SEs

Cytotoxic agents

- Antimetabolites mimic the natural building blocks of cells and are **active during the S-phase of the cell cycle** ("5-MATH"; S looks like 5)
    - **5-FU (pyrimidine analog that inhibits thymidylate synthetase)**
    - Methotrexate, Mycophenolate mofetil (both inhibit enzyme in **purine synthesis**)
    - Ara-C, aka cytarabine (pyrimadine analog)
    - Azathioprine (**purine analog** that inhibits purine synthesis)
    - Thioguanine (**purine analog** that inhibits purine synthesis)

    - Hydroxyurea (**inhibits ribonucleotide reductase** which is needed to produce purine and pyrimidine deoxyribonucleotides)
- Alkylating ("alCylating") agents directly damage DNA and are **cell-cycle non-specific**
    - Cyclophosphamide
    - Chlorambucil

Methotrexate (MTX)

- MOA: binds and irreversibly inhibits **dihydrofolate reductase** w/ greater affinity than folic acid → ↓ conversion of dihydrofolate to tetrahydrofolate (cofactor for thymidylate and purine nucleotides involved in DNA/RNA synthesis) → ↓ cell division
- This inhibition of dihydrofolate reductase can be bypassed by **leucovorin** (**folinic acid** not folate/folic acid) or **thymidine** (these inhibit the MTX toxin without ↓ MTX efficacy)
- FDA approved for severe psoriasis and Sezary syndrome but commonly used off-label
- Absolute CI: pregnancy (category X) and lactation
    - **3 months off drug for men and 1 month off for women** before conceiving
        - "Men need to go More time without sex than women w/ MTX"
- Relative CI: hepatic or renal disease, metabolic syndrome, hematologic abnormalities
- High yield side effects: "going to war with MTX is fought with Flags and HARPOONs"
    - **Flag sign**: hair w/ horizontal hyperpigmented bands alternating with normal hair
    - **Hepatotoxicity**/Hepatic fibrosis
    - Alopecia, Acral erythema
    - Radiation recall: inflammatory skin reaction at a previously irradiated field

  - **Pulmonary fibrosis**/Pneumonitis, **Pancytopenia** (occurs early), **Phototoxicity**
    - Pancytopenia RFs: old age, ↓ renal function, no folic acid supplements
  - **Oral and cutaneous ulcers** (commonly the presenting sign of MTX toxicity)
  - Opportunistic infections
  - Nausea/vomiting (GI SEs common), **Necrosis in preexisting psoriatic plaques**
    - MTX preferentially affects hyperproliferative skin (e.g., psoriatic plaques)
  - **Nodule development: classically on fingers** (similar to rheumatoid nodules)
  - **NMSC** (but also ↑ risk of melanoma, non-Hodgkin's lymphoma, breast cancer)
    - Data is weak that MTX given in doses used in psoriasis cause malignancy
- ↑ risk of myelosuppression/pancytopenia when coadministered w/... "STAND for MTX"
  - **Sulfonamides (TMP-SMX)**, Salicylates, Trimethoprim, **TCNs (doxy)**, ...Azines (phenothiazines), NSAIDS, Dapsone, Dipyridamole
    - Pancytopenia may p/w fatigue, easy bruising and epistaxis
  - Systemic retinoids and alcohol should be avoided due to synergistic liver damage
- **Leucovorin** (and thymidine) reverses MTX toxicity and **glucarpidase** is FDA approved to treat toxic levels of MTX caused by impaired kidney function
- Baselines labs: CBC, LFTs, Cr/BUN, hepatitis panel (repeat all except hepatitis panel weekly x 1 month then gradually decrease frequency to q 3 months)
- **Liver biopsy** is gold standard for checking hepatic fibrosis (cumulative doses > 1.5–4 g) but serial **pro-collagen 3** levels can also be used for psoriatic patients on long-term MTX

- No live vaccines while on MTX

Mycophenolate mofetil ("my cop")

- **Inhibits inosine monophosphate dehydrogenase**, a key enzyme in **de novo synthesis of purines** (Adenosine, Guanine; "Pure As Gold") which lymphocytes need for replication
- "Side effects are not my cop but HIS COP"
    - **Hematologic** (various cytopenias); Hematochezia
    - Infections (progressive multifocal leukoencephalopathy is controversial)
    - Stomach symptoms are most common side effect (N/V/D)
        - Gut bacteria secrete β-**glucuronidase** which **produces active mycophenolic acid (↑ GI SEs); vancomycin** eliminates β-glucuronidase-expressing bacteria and MMF-induced GI side effects
    - Carcinogenesis (NMSC and lymphoma controversial)
    - CNS symptoms (HA, tinnitus)
    - Occasional GU urgency/frequency/dysuria/sterile pyuria but no nephrotoxicity
    - Pseudo-Pelger-Huet anomaly (nuclear hypolobation)
- "Drug interactions are not my cop or his cop but A COP"
    - **Azathioprine** → myelosuppression
    - **Antacids**: requires gastric acidity for absorption → ↓ efficacy
    - Cholestyramine: ↓ enterohepatic recirculation → ↓ efficacy
    - **Calcium** → ↓ efficacy
    - OCPs are less effective
    - Phenytoin is more toxic
    - Polycarbophil → ↓ efficacy

Azathioprine ("6 SHOPPING SCAMs")

- **Onset of action is in 6 weeks**
- Azathioprine is converted to 6-MP (**purine analog**) and 6-TG (thioguanine) which are purine imposters and get incorporated into DNA/RNA → ↓ cell division of lymphocytes
- Xanthine oxidase (XO) and thiopurine methyltransferase (TPMT) convert azathioprine into **inactive** metabolites so ↓ XO from allopurinol or ↓ TPMT activity in certain populations can result in life-threatening myelosuppression by shunting more 6-MP through the anabolic hypoxanthine-guanine phosphoribosyltransferace (HGPRT) pathway leading to more active metabolites (**always test TPMT levels first**)
    - If TPMT is < 5 U then azathioprine is CI; if TPMT is 5–15 U just lower the dose
- Azathioprine SEs ("SHOPPING"; very similar to MTX SEs as both inhibit purines)
    - **SCCs**
    - Hypersensitivity syndrome, **Hepatotoxic**, Hepatosplenic T-cell lymphoma
    - Oral ulcers, Opportunistic infections
    - **Pancytopenia**
    - **Pancreatitis**
    - Infections (HSV, HPV, scabies), Immunosuppression
    - Non-Hodgkin's B-cell lymphoma
    - GI side effects like N/V **(MC side effect)**
- Azathioprine drug interactions (SCAMs)
    - **Sulfasalazine (TPMT inhibitor) → myelosuppression**
    - **Coumadin** (↓ anticoagulant effect); Contraceptive (IUD) failure
    - **Allopurinol and febuxostat (XO inhibitors) → myelosuppression**
    - **ACE inhibitors** (various mechanisms) → myelosuppression

    - Methotrexate → myelosuppression +/- hypersensitivity syndrome
    - Mycophenolate mofetil → myelosuppression

Hydroxyurea ("DUMP HER")

- MOA ("DUMP HER"): **anti-Metabolite** of Purine and Pyrimidine that Hypomethylates DNA (which inhibits/Ends DNA synthesis) and **inhibits Ribonucleotide Reductase**
- Uses: head/neck SCC, melanoma, erythromelalgia, Sweet's, Hypereosinophilic syndrome
- SEs ("DUMP HER"): **Drug-induced Dermatomyositis (MCC)**, **leg Ulcers**, Megaloblastic anemia/ **Myelosuppression (MC SE)**, Photosensitivity, **Hyperpigmentation of skin and nails**, lichenoid Eruption resembling GVHD or dermatomyositis, Radiation Recall

Cyclophosphamide

- Alcylatng agent that directly damages DNA by forming cross-links within DNA strands
- FDA approved for Mycosis fungoides but used off-label for ocular CP, vasculitis, AI-CTD
- **SE: hemorrhagic cystitis** (prevent w/ hydration) → ↑ risk of transitional cell carcinoma
    - **Monitor with periodic UA** w/ cytology
- Other SE: N/V (MC), **infertility**, hyperpigmentation of teeth/skin/nails, anagen effluvium

Chlorambucil

- Like cyclophosphamide it directly damages DNA by cross-linking, it is a nitrogen mustard derivative, and a common SE is infertility (azoospermia, amenorrhea) and N/V
- FDA approved for CLL but used off label for NXG, PG, Behçet's, and several AI-CTDs

- Other SEs: pulmonary fibrosis, hepatoxicity, bone marrow suppression, and oral ulcers

2.4 Biologics

- Drugs referred to as "biologics" are produced by cells or living organisms
- Bind/inhibit a specific arm of immune system
- Do not give live vaccines **1 month before**, during and **3 months after stopping biologics**
  - **Live vaccines**: MMR, varicella-zoster, yellow fever, rotavirus, oral polio, vaccinia
    - Zoster: Zostavax (no longer used in USA) is live, Shingrix is inactivated
    - The only live vaccines still used in USA are MMR and yellow fever (travel)
    - 2020 consensus recommends giving MMR 1 month before Dupilumab
    - No BCG vaccine 1 year before, during and 1 year after ustekinumab
- Biologics can be stopped 3 half-lives before and started 2 weeks after high-risk surgeries
  - Etanercept has shortest half-life (3.5 days); secukinumab has longest (27 days)
- Suffix of biologics
  - Ends in "omab": murine (0% human)
  - Ends in "ximab": chimeric (65% human; "Xi Jing Ping is half human half animal")
  - Ends in "zumab": humanized (> 90% human)
  - Ends in "umab": fully human
    - The more human the drug, the lower the potential for immunogenicity
  - Ends in "cept": receptor fusion protein
- Labs: CBC, CMP, PPD (if PPD+, can start biologic after 1–2 months of treatment w/ INH)

TNF-α inhibitors

- Adalimumab (SQ): fully human IgG mAb against transmembrane TNF receptor
- Etanercept (SQ): **soluble** human dimeric **fusion protein** that binds both TNF-α and TNF-β
    - o Approved down to 4 years old in psoriasis; weight based (great for obese pts)
- Infliximab (IV): **chimeric** (**mouse** + human) IgG monoclonal antibody binding only TNF-α
- Certolizumab (SQ): antigen-binding fragment of humanized monoclonal antibody coupled to polyethylene glycol (lacks Fc component → **cannot cross the placenta**)
- Golimumab (SQ): fully human monoclonal Ab to both soluble and transmembrane TNF-α
- FDA approved for plaque psoriasis and psoriatic arthritis (adalimumab also for HS)
- Pregnancy cat B
- CI: **active infections** (**can be safely used in active hep C infections**), **demyelinating disorders such as MS, class III or IV heart failure and recent malignancies**
- Black box warnings ("LGBTq")
    - o Malignancy: Lymphoma (hepatosplenic T-cell lymphoma)
    - o **Serious infections: Bacterial (Legionella, Listeria), invasive fun-gal, Hep B, TB**
- SEs: **injection site reactions (MC SE)**, demyelinating diseases, psoriasis/palmoplantar pustulosis, LCV, opportunistic infection, lupus-like syndrome, autoimmune hepatitis
- Avoid TNF inhibitors in demyelinating diseases, hepatitis B, history of latent TB and CHF
- Avoid live vaccines (this goes for all biologics) and concurrent use of IL-1 antagonists
- Infliximab-specific side effects: infusion reactions (p/w N/V, HA, flushing, dyspnea, taste perversion; prevent by

↓ infusion rate and premedicate), CHF, infliximab-associated-Anti-drug Antibodies (ADA; ↓ drug efficacy and ↑ SEs such as infusion reactions)

- Labs: CBC, CMB, quant gold and hep C at baseline and repeat PPD/quant gold annually

Ustekinumab

- Fully human monoclonal **IgG1 Ab against the common p40 subunit of IL-12 and IL-23**
- FDA approved for psoriasis (12 years and up) but also used in HS and PRP
- Approved in peds down to 6 years old
- Like etanercept, ustekinumab is weight based (great for obese patients)
- SEs: URI (MC), HA, back pain, fatigue, and other infections (TB, viral, fungal)
- Labs: quant gold at baseline and yearly thereafter

IL-23 inhibitors

- Guselkumab, tildrakizumab, risankizumab, mirikizumab (not used)
- Guselkumab and risankizumab also FDA approved for psoriatic arthritis
- SEs: infections (e.g., URI)

IL-17 inhibitors ("IBS")

- Ixekizumab (IL-17A inhibitor), Bimekizumab (**Both IL-17 A and F inhibitor**), Brodalumab (IL-17 **receptor** antagonist), Secukinumab (IL-17A inhibitor)
    - IL-17A is more potent but IL-17F is more abundant in psoriatic lesions
- Ixekizumab and secukinumab are approved in peds down to 6 years old
- Better than TNF-α inh for plaque psoriasis and similar efficacy for psoriatic arthritis

- SEs: nasopharyngitis (MC), IBS/IBD, **candida** (esp w/ bimekizumab), injection site reaction (esp w/ ixekizumab); brodalumab has a black box warning for suicidality
    - o Candidiasis is manageable and not a reason for discontinuation
- Avoid IL-17s if personal history of inflammatory bowel disease

IL-13 inhibitors ("Lets Treat Dermatitis and Pruritis")

- Lebrikizumab and Tralokinumab: monoclonal antibody which binds to IL-13 (treats AD)
    - o Do not get confused with tildrakizumab which is an IL-23 blocker
- Dupilumab: monoclonal Ab which **binds to the IL-4Rα subunit inhibiting IL-4 and IL-13**
    - o Treats AD, BP, alopecia areata, Grovers and chronic spontaneous urticaria
    - o SEs: MC is conjunctivitis (eye pain may indicate keratitis → send to ophtho) and enthesitis (Rx: NSAIDS; if severe send to rheum)
- Pitrakinra: inactive human recombinant protein that like Dupilumab, targets the IL-4Rα subunit to inhibit IL-4 and IL-13 (being studied for AD and pruritis)

IL-1 inhibitors ("1 CAR": Canakinumab, Anakinra, Rilonacept)

- MOA: recombinant IL-1 receptor antagonists
- FDA approved for RA but also used for HS, Schnitzler's and cryopyrin-associated periodic fever syndromes (Muckle-Wells, familial cold autoinflammatory syndrome, NOMID)
- SE: injection site reactions, flu-like symptoms, neutropenia, thrombocytopenia, infection
- CI: renal failure or active infections
- Monitor absolute neutrophil count and do not give w/ TNF-α inhibitors or live vaccines

Omalizumab

- Monoclonal IgE antibody → ↓ IgE levels and IgE receptors on mast cells and basophils
- FDA approved for allergic asthma and chronic idiopathic urticaria
- SE ("xo-LAIR"): Lethal cancers, Anaphylaxis (inject in office 1st 3 times), Injection site Rxn

Rituximab

- **Chimeric** (mouse) IgG monoclonal antibody targeting the B-cell surface antigen (**CD20**)
    - o CD20 is found on all types of B-cells (pre-Bs and mature Bs) but **not plasma cells**
- Takes 2–4 months for full effect
- FDA approved for **PV**, non-Hodgkin's lymphoma, GPA/MPA, CLL, RA but used off-label for severe skin diseases (BP, AI-CTD, chronic GVHD, LCV, and **cutaneous B-cell lymphoma**)
- **Depletes B-cells in weeks and last for 6 months** (normal B cell #s 1 year after starting)
- SEs: infusion reactions (occurs in everyone's 1st infusion), HTN, URIs, arthralgias, and pruritis
- Serious but rare SEs: **arrythmias**, **intestinal perforation**, HBV reactivation, SJS/TEN, serious infection, hepatic/BM failure, and progressive multifocal leukoencephalopathy
- Considered safe in pregnancy
- Get routine vaccines at least 4 weeks before starting Rituximab and wait 3–5 months to get vaccines after stopping (vaccines won't work if you don't wait)

Emerging biologics

- **Spesolimab: IL-36 inhibitor for generalized pustular psoriasis flares**
- Mogamulizumab: anti-CCR4 antibody FDA approved for refractory CTCL

    - SE: increased risk for GVHD
    - Compare to Maraviroc (CCR5 inhibitor) which treats visceral GVHD
- Tezepelumab: monoclonal antibody that targets thymic stromal lymphopoietin (TSL), FDA-approved for asthma but is showing promise for pruritis
- **Fezakinumab: monoclonal antibody against IL-22 showing promise in AD (eczema)**
    - "Fez was a 22ish-year-old character in *That '70s Show* who had eczema"
- Aprepitant, serlopitant and tradipitant: blocks substance P/neurokinin-1R
    - Uses: refractory pruritis in CTCL, Sézary, brachioradial pruritis and others
    - SEs: fatigue and diarrhea
- Nemolizumab: monoclonal antibody against IL-31 showing promise in pruritis

Tapinarof

- Small molecule **Topical Aryl hydrocarbon receptor modular for AD and psoriasis**
- SE: folliculitis

2.5 Oncologic Agents in Dermatology

Melanoma

Dacarbazine

- Cell cycle non-specific chemotherapeutic alkylating agent that halts DNA replication
- Use: metastatic melanoma but fallen out of favor w/ more tolerable and effective meds
- SE: GI (vomiting), pancytopenia, allergic reactions (anaphylaxis) liver injury, neuropathy

Interferon alpha

- Works as a cytokine that signals and modulates immune responses
- Uses: FDA approved for melanoma, hairy cell leukemia, and RCC
- SE: flu-like symptoms, injection site reactions, N/V/D, pancytopenia, liver injury, depression, and rare but fatal **rhabdomyolysis** w/ multiple organ failure

Taliomogene laherparepvec (T-VEC)

- Genetically engineered **herpes virus type 1** that selectively infects and replicates in tumor cells producing granulocyte-macrophage colony-stimulating (GM-CSF) which promotes anti-tumor immunity capable of destroying tumor at distant sites
- NCCN: intralesional T-VEC is used as a 2nd line agent in combo w/ an immune checkpoint inhibitor or targeted therapy in those that have progressed on initial 1st line therapy

Interleukin-2 (IL-2)

- MOA: activates immune response to kill tumor cells
- Initially used systemically in 1998, but now NCCN recommends intralesional IL-2 (due to severe toxicity of IV) and only as a 2nd line therapy for those who have progressed on targeted or immune checkpoint therapy and only when T-VEC is unavailable
- SEs (IV): **capillary leak syndrome** (oliguria, generalized edema, tachyarrhythmias, hypotension), fever, N/V/D, catheter-related sepsis and death
- SEs (IL): pyrexia, flu-like symptoms, GI symptoms, injection site pain/redness/swelling

BRAF inhibitors (VEmurafenib, dabrafenib, encorafenib)

- MOA: serine/threonine signal transduction kinase that inhibits BRAF (targets the V600E mutation of BRAF) in the MAPK pathway; given PO
    - Substitution of valine (V) for glutamic acid (E) at amino acid codon 600
- **MAPK pathway: BRAF is a phosphorylating serine/threonine kinase** that with the GTPase activity of NRAS, leads to the phosphorylation of MEK and ERK → phosphorylated ERK activates **nuclear cyclin D1** ("nucl-ERK cyclin D1") which complexes w/ CDK4 and phosphorylates Rb → phosphorylated Rb releases the transcription factor E2F, which leads to progression through the S phase of the cell-cycle
- **NCCN guidelines**: use in pts w/ stage 3 melanoma or higher and a known BRAF mutation
- **Quicker onset** of action vs immunotherapy (use BRAF/MEK combo over immunotherapy if pt has organ failure/symptoms); benefits are not as long lasting as w/ immunotherapy
    - "Use a BRAF to give Rapid relief"
- SEs: **Verrucous keratoses**/KP (MC skin lesions), **Eruptive KAs/SCCs/AKs** (blocking BRAF leads to new SCCs by paradoxical activation of RAF), Elevated temperature/pyrexia (MC SE), **Erythema nodosa (neutrophilic)**, palmoplantar Erythrodysesthesia, new BRAF wild-type melanomas/nevi (blocking BRAF pathway causes new melanomas by shunting to the MEK pathway), photosensitivity, dysgeusia, muscle aches, alopecia, **prolonged QT**, seb-derm-like rash, acneiform eruption, **KP-like rash,** photosensitivity, N/V/D, arthralgia

- **Resistance** develops after 6 months of therapy unless combined w/ MEK inhibitors
  - o There are currently 3 combinations: "Biden was Tested for COV-19"
    - Binimetinib/ encorafenib
    - **Trametinib/dabrafenib**
    - Cobimetinib/Vemurafenib
- Sorafenib also targets the BRAF V600E mutation (in addition to PDGFR, c-KIT, VEGFR)
  - o SEs: **hand-foot-skin reaction**, alopecia, rash/desquamation, facial erythema, nail changes, pruritis, mucositis, eruptive benign nevi, **KAs/SCCs**

MEK inhibitors ("MECK": trametinib, cobimetinib, binimetinib, selumetinib)

- Serine/threonine/tyrosine kinase that inhibits MEK1/2 of the MAPK pathway; given PO
- Uses: **neurofibromatosis (selumetinib)** and late-stage melanoma (commonly Combined w/ BRAF inhibitors which is more effective and ↓ risk of BRAF-induced KAs/SCCs)
  - o 2-year survival goes from 30% w/ BRAF monotherapy to over 50% w/ combo
- SEs: **MC SE is acneiform reactions** (Rx w/ doxycycline), photosensitivity, pruritis, alopecia, peripheral edema; Cardiomyopathy and retinal vein occlusion were reported

Ipilimumab and tremelimumab

- **Blocks CTLA4** (cytotoxic T-lymphocyte associated antigen 4) on cytotoxic T-cells; given IV
- Use: metastatic melanoma (commonly used in combination w/ PD-1 blockers)
  - o 2-year survival w/ ipilimumab is 30% and if combined w/ PD-1 inhibitors is 65%

- Unlike BRAF inhibitors, responses take long (3 months) to develop, but are more durable
- SEs: immune-related SEs → **Diarrhea, Dermatitis (MC)**, and **Deadly colitis (most severe)**
  - o Treat grade 3 or 4 colitis toxicity w/ high dose steroids (infliximab given if no improvement after 3 days) and pt should permanently discontinue ipilimumab
  - o Other SEs remind me of DRESS: rash, facial swelling, hypothyroidism, hepatitis
    - ▪ Treat these immune-related side effects w/ systemic steroids
  - o **SE of vitiligo-like leukoderma is correlated w/ improved clinical response**
- SE onset: rash/pruritis (4 weeks), diarrhea/colitis/liver toxicity/hypophysitis (6 weeks)

PD-1 (on T-cells) inhibitors (Cemiplimab, Nivolumab, Pembrolizumab, Pidilizumab; "Cem Nice Pembroke Pines PD"): PD-1L (on tumor cells) inhibitors (atezolizumab, durvalumab, avelumab)

- Checkpoint inhibitors that target the Programmed cell death-1 (PD-1) receptor; given IV
  - o PD-1 inhibit T-cells from attacking tumor cells (these meds stop this inhibition)
- Uses: late-stage melanoma, Merkel cell carcinoma and NMSC
  - o Avelumab/pembrolizumab are FDA-approved for locally advanced Merkel
  - o **Cemiplimab** is FDA-approved for unresectable NMSC (BCCs and SCCs)
- **NCCN guidelines**: preferred adjuvant treatment for stage 3 melanoma after primary treatment and pre-

ferred monotherapy in stage 4 (unresectable/metastatic) disease
  - o Pembrolizumab is approved adjunctly for stage 2B/2C melanoma after excision
- SEs: common SEs include fatigue, diarrhea, nausea, **pruritis, rash**, hypothyroidism
  - o Pruritis Rx ("PD"): Potent topical steroids (grade 1), Pregabalin/gabapentin (grade 2), Dupilumab/omalizumab (grade 3)
  - o Rash ("PD-1L"): the two MC reaction patterns are **Lichenoid (MC; 50%)** and maculo-Papular (spongiotic; 40%) but others include **bullous Pemphigoid**, Photo-distributed vitiligo, Psoriasiform, and vacuolar interface Dermatitis
    - ▪ SJS/TEN, sarcoid, AI-CTD like eosinophilic fasciitis are much less common
- Efficacy improved when combined w/ ipilimumab (pitfall is ↑ immune-related SEs)
- The combination of **Relatlimab (LAG-3 blocker)** and Nivolumab (PD-1 blocker) was FDA approved in 2022 for unresectable and metastatic melanoma
  - o SE: 5% get hepatitis and 5% get adrenal insufficiency
  - o "The RN Lagged 3 steps behind the PD (Program Director)"
- Management latter: if they fail a PD-1 add a CTLA-4, if they fail that try a PD-1 + LAG3
- Development of **vitiligo-like leukoderma** is correlated w/ **improved clinical response**
  - o And spongiotic (eczematous/psoriasiform), lichenoid and BP to a lesser degree
- Relative contraindication: **solid-organ transplant patients**

Immunotherapies for the treatment of skin cancer

- Class of treatments that use persons own immune system to help kill cancer cells
- "Immunotherapies make you itch" (PICA is itch in Spanish")
    - Pembrolizumab (PD-1 inhibitor): used in advanced Merkel, melanoma and NMSC
    - Poly ICLC (toll-like receptor 3 agonist): used in advanced SCC (not FDA approved)
    - Ipilimumab (CTLA-4 inhibitor): used in advanced melanoma
    - Imiquimod (toll-like receptor 7/8 agonist): used topically in subsets of BCC/SCCs
    - Cemiplimab (PD-1 inhibitor): used in unresectable NMSC
    - Avelumab (PD-1 inhibitor): used in metastatic Merkel cell carcinoma

Imatinib mesylate (Gleevac)

- Inhibits multiple tyrosine kinases (Bcr-Abl, c-Kit, platelet-derived growth factor receptor)
- Derm uses: CML (Bcr-Abl), DFSP (COL1A-PDGFR), Hypereosinophilic syndrome (FIP1L1-PDGFR), acral/mucosal Melanoma (C-Kit), Mastocytosis (C-Kit and FIP1L1-PDGFR)
    - "CBDC's are a Highway to Financial Prison and will Make the Masses Controlled"
- SE (GLEEvac): **Gingival/tooth/nail hyperpigmentation**, **Loss of pigment** (via inhibition of c-Kit), Lichenoid eruption (usually oral), **Eye edema (periorbital)**

BCC

Hedgehog pathway (Hp) inhibitors (vismodegib, sonidegib, taladegib, saridegib, patidegib)

- Pathway: in the normally functioning Hp, patched (PTCH) normally binds and inhibits smoothened (SMO); when this pathway is activated, Hp proteins bind to the transmembrane PTCH receptor which ↓ the inhibition of PTCH on SMO, allowing SMO to activate a downstream cascade (e.g., GLI) that results in cell proliferation
  - Even without smoothened, GLI is normally inhibited in the cytoplasm by SUFU
- MOA: acts as a cyclopamine-**competitive antagonist of smoothened (G-protein coupled receptor)** in the sonic hedgehog pathway → ↓ gene transcription of various cancers
  - "The 3 vegetarian PA's (Erivedge, PATCH, Pategedib gel, cyclopamine) always flirt w/ the smooth doctor and inhibit him (SMO) from doing his work in cancer"
  - Smoothened is a G-protein coupled receptor ("the smooth doctor is such a G")
- Uses: metastatic (vismodegib only), locally advanced BCCs and pts w/ Gorlin's syndrome
  - Vismodegib has a 30% response rate in pts w/ metastatic BCC and 45% in those w/ locally advanced inoperable BCC; medium duration of treatment is 10 months
  - Cemiplimab (PD1) is used if BCC got worse on Hp inhibitors or if can't tolerate SE
- SEs ("MAD side effects"): **Muscle spasms (68%) > Alopecia (63%), > Dysgeusia (51%)**
  - Sonidegib has less muscle spasms (taking w/ L-carnitine can lessen this SE)

  - Other SEs: teratogenicity (**cyclopia**), fatigue, **SCC**, amenorrhea/azoospermia, DVT
- Females and males need contraception x 24 months and 3 months off drug, respectively for Vismodegib and for 20 months (females) and 8 months (males) for sonidegib
- Females and males must avoid donating blood for **24 months** off drug (20 for sonidegib)

CTCL

Brentuximab vedotin ("Brent is 30 years old MALE Nurse Practitioner")

- Antibody-drug conjugate of monoclonal **anti-CD30** conjugated to an antimicrotubule
- Uses ("30-year-old MALE"): MF (large cell change), Anaplastic large cell lymphoma, LyP
  - Use is restricted to multifocal or refractory cases
- SE: **peripheral sensory Neuropathy (Numbness)**, N/V, Pneumonia, Pyrexia, Neutropenia
- Black box: JC virus infection resulting in Progressive multifocal leukoencephalopathy

Alemtuzumab

- Humanized monoclonal antibody **against CD52** surface Ag on T- and B-cells
  - "Its's not **all** (alemtuzumab), its actually just slightly more than half (52%)"
- Use: CTCL w/ peripheral blood disease (e.g., Sézary)
- Black box warning for cytopenias, infusion reactions and infections

Romidepsin, Remetinostat and Vorinostat

- Histone deacetylase inhibitors ("he was treated for CTCL in his RV")

- Use: FDA-approved for CTCL pts w/ recurrent disease refractory to 2 systemic therapies
  - o Vorinostat also shows promise for patients w/ advanced head and neck SCC
  - o Topical remetinostat may be effective in treating early localized cutaneous SCC
- SEs: GI SEs, fatigue, cytopenias, infections, and T-wave flattening

Denileukin diftitox

- Binds **IL-2α** or **CD25** and introduces diphtheria toxin into cells → cell death
  - o "Di means 2 which helps me remember it inhibits CD25 component of IL-2"
- Use: CTCL whose malignant cells express the **CD25 component of the IL-2 receptor**
- SEs: **capillary leak syndrome** (oliguria, generalized edema, arrhythmias, and hypotension)
- Black box: fatal infusion rxns, capillary leak syndrome, and loss of visual acuity/color vision

Lenalidomide

- **Thalidomide analog:** ↑ Th1-cytokines and enhances T and NK cell-mediated killing
- FDA approved for myelodysplastic syndrome, MM, mantle cell lymphoma, CTCL, Sézary
- SEs: cytopenias and fatigue/malaise

Mechlorethamine hydrochloride and Carmustine

- Nitrogen Mustard alkylating agents used for patch/ plaque stage MF
- SEs (mechlorethamine): contact dermatitis (MC), anaphylaxis and SCCs
- SEs (carmustine): local reactions (MC) and myelosuppression

Topical oncologic agents used in dermatology

- 5-fluorouracil ("PTSD"): **Pyrimidine analog which binds to Thymidylate Synthetase** (thus **Deoxyurine cannot convert to thymidine**) and results in ↓ DNA synthesis
  - Uses: AKs and superficial BCCs (SCCIS is not mentioned in label)
  - SEs: erythema, erosions, and blistering at application site
  - **Severe seborrheic dermatitis which p/w burning (simulates 5-FU reaction) can be seen weeks after 5-FU treatment (pearl: pretreat w/ topical ketoconazole)**
  - Do not use in patients w/ **dihydropyrimidine dehydrogenase** (DPD) deficiency → even topical application can cause severe toxicity → pancytopenia → death
  - Pregnancy category X
- Imiquimod: **activates TLR7** > TLR8 → activates **NFkB** transcription factor → ↑ cytokines (**TNF-α, IFN-γ**, IFN-α, IL-12) which trigger an antiviral and antitumoral T-cell mediated adaptive immune response (can only use in immunocompetent adults)
  - Uses: AKs on face/scalp (2x per week for 16 weeks), superficial BCC on trunk/extremities/neck (5x per week x 6 weeks), SCCIS/lentigo maligna (off label)
  - SEs: local reactions like 5-fluorouracil, flu-like symptoms, eruptive milia/cysts
  - **Topical steroids make imiquimod less effective but not 5-fluorouracil**
  - 10% of people have ↓ toll-like receptors in skin and don't respond to imiquimod
  - Pregnancy category C
- Diclofenac: ↓ cyclooxygenase enzymes → ↑ apoptosis
  - Uses: AKs (apply BID x 2–3 months)

    - SEs: more mild local reactions, photosensitivity, headache, ↑ LFTs
    - Pregnancy category B
- Tirbanibulin: inhibits microtubules (↓ tubulin polymerization) and **inhibits Src kinase**
    - Uses: AKs
    - SEs: local side effects
- Pategedib: inhibiting smoothened receptor in the sonic hedgehog pathway
    - Uses: BCCs
- Remetinostat: histone deacetylase inhibitor
    - Uses: superficial BCCs

Radiation therapy (RT)

- Ionizing electromagnetic radiation in the form of high energy photons produces **double-stranded breaks in DNA** when absorbed by tissues (esp in rapidly dividing cells)
- The MC form of cell death induced by RT is **mitotic catastrophe** (mitotic cell death)
- Main dermatologic indications ("MAD DUCKS"): Merkel cell, Angiosarcoma, Desmoid tumor, DFSP, Desmoplastic melanoma, UPS, CTCL, Keloids, Kaposi sarcoma, SCC/BCCs
    - Alternative treatment for skin cancers in nonsurgical candidates
    - Adjuvant treatment for aggressive tumors to decrease risk of recurrence
        - BCC/SCC: PNI of nerves ≥ 1mm, multiple nerves or cranial extension
    - Palliative treatment to provide symptomatic relief for incurable disease
- The unit of radiation dose is Gray (Gy): absorbed energy (J) per unit mass of tissue (kg)

- Malignant tumors: **50 Grey** ("50 shades of Grey") in 20 daily fractions is typical
- Success rate of keloids w/ surgical excision followed by RT is 75% (12 Gy in 3 fractions)
    - RT should be initiated within 24 hours post-op to induce apoptosis of fibroblasts
- CI: **genetic syndromes** predisposing patients to skin cancers (e.g., XP/Gorlin's syndrome)
    - Relative CI: **AI-CTD**, poorly vascularized tissue (**lower leg**, dorsum of hand), edematous tissue, trauma, thermal burn, ulcer, prior RT to site
        - "Don't hang out with Christian Grey if you have genetic conditions, connective tissue diseases or if your skin is already poorly vascularized, swollen, traumatized, or ulcerated"
- SEs
    - Early: erythema, epilation, desquamation, or ulceration
    - Late: telangiectasias, fibrosis, ulceration, necrosis, or secondary malignancies
- Forms done by dermatologists in the outpatient clinic for thinner tumors
    - Brachytherapy: radiation source is applied on the skin surface
    - Superficial x-ray therapy (SXRT): source applied at a distance and aimed at site
- Forms done by radiation oncologists for thicker tumors
    - Electron beam RT: source is an electron delivered through a linear accelerator

2.6 Antimicrobial Agents

Topical antimicrobial agents

Bacitracin

- MOA: binds **C55-prenol pyrophosphatase** (inhibits phospholipids) → disrupts **cell wall**
- Made from Bacillus subtilis; bactericidal against G+ and G- (Neisseria)
- Neisseria and gram-positive activity
- SE: ACD

Polymyxin B

- MOA: ↑ **cell membrane permeability** via detergent-like Phospholipid interaction
    - o "poly-mixin' the membrane"
- Made by B. subtilis and B. polymyxa; bactericidal against G- only (Pseudomonas)
    - o Cross reacts with bacitracin as both are made by Bacillus species
    - o Only agent in the triple antibiotic ointment (polymyxin B, bacitracin and neomycin) to cover pseudomonas and to not cover G+ (staph)
- Degranulates mast cells so do not use in mastocytosis
- Pregnancy category B

Topical antimicrobials safe in Pregnancy (category A or B; "My Really Sterile Pregancy CAME")
Mupirocin, Retapamulin, Silver sulfadiazine, Polymyxin B Clindamycin, Azelaic acid, Metronidazole, Erythromycin

Systemic antimicrobials safe in Pregnancy	Systemic antimicrobials unsafe in Pregnancy
"Pregancy CAME" Penicillins Clindamycin, Cephalosporins Aminopenicillins (Amoxicillin) Metronidazole Erythromycin	"SAFe Children Take Really Good Care" Sulfonamides (kernicterus) Aminoglycosides (ototoxicity) Fluoroquinolones (cartilage damage) Clarithromycin (embryotoxic) TCNs (discolored teeth, ↓ bone growth) Ribavirin (teratogenic antiviral) Griseofulvin (teratogenic antifungal) Chloramphenicol ("gray baby")

Neomycin

- MOA: **binds 30s subunit** of bacterial ribosome RNA (↓ protein synthesis) and may **inhibit bacterial DNA polymerase** (Neosporin: bacitracin, polymyxin B and neomycin)
- Aminoglycoside made from Streptomyces fradiae; bactericidal against **G+ and G-**
- SE: **ACD** and there are reports of neural deafness in neonates

Gentamycin ("Gentle People")

- MOA: binds 30s subunit of bacterial ribosome RNA → ↓ Protein synthesis
- Aminoglycoside made from M. Purpurea; bactericidal for G+ and G- (esp **Pseudomonas**)
- SE: Photosensitization

Ozenoxacin

- Topical quinolone which is FDA approved for impetigo

Mupirocin ("MuPIRocin")

- MOA: binds bacterial **Isoleucyl tRNA synthetase** → ↓ bacterial RNA/protein synthesis

- Made from **Pseudomonas** fluorescens; bactericidal against **G-Positives** (**MRSA**, strept)
- Use: 1st line topical therapy for impetigo
- SEs: Polyethylene glycol component can cause Nephrotoxicity in Neonates if applied over a large surface area (only approved for ages 3 months and up)

Retapamulin ("RetapamuLin")

- MOA: binds to **L3 protein on 50s subunit of bacterial ribosome** → ↓ protein synthesis
- Made from clitopilus schpoides; bactericidal against G+ (**MRSA**)

Iodoquinol

- High iodine concentration quinolone-derivative
- GP, GN, dermatophyte and yeast activity

Benzoyl peroxide

- Broad spectrum w/ strong oxidizing (P. acnes activity) and keratolytic properties
- Bacterial resistance NOT reported
- SEs: can Bleach hair/fabric and can oxidize (degrade) certain formulations of tretinoin; orange-Brown pigment on clothes when used w/ topical dapsone/ sodium sulfacetamide

Sodium sulfacetamide

- Inhibits bacterial Dihydropteroate Synthetase (prevents conversion of PABA to folic acid)
  - Dapsone, SMX (TMP-SMX) and Sodium sulfacetamide all have this same MOA
- P. acnes activity (used in acne, rosacea, perioral dermatitis and seborrheic dermatitis)

Silver sulfadiazine

- MOA: **Binds bacterial DNA** → ↓ DNA synthesis
    - Silver sulfadiazine, metronidazole and azelaic acid all ↓ DNA "Zynthesis"
- Bactericidal against G+ (MRSA) and G- (P. aeruginosa); used for burn wounds
- **SEs** (rare): "PURE silver" → Porphyria is Unmasked, Renal insufficiency, Eliminates blood cells (hemolysis in G6PD patients, methemoglobinemia and neutropenia), silver (argyria)
    - Neutropenia/leukopenia is enhanced when combined with cimetidine
    - Topical silver sulfadiazine may cause SJS/TEN in sulfa-allergic patients
- CI in neonates < 2 months due to hyperbilirubinemia/ kernicterus ("turns them silver")

Metronidazole

- MOA: nitroimidazole that disrupts DNA synthesis
- Protozoa and anaerobe activity
- Use: used for rosacea ("rozacea") primarily for anti-inflammatory properties
- SE of oral metronidazole is **disulfiram reaction**

Azelaic acid

- MOA: **Dicarboxylic acid** ("acid spelled backwards is dica") that disrupts mitochondrial respiration, ↓ DNA synthesis (esp. in melanocytes) and ↓ ROS production by PMNs
- MOA (ACID): And **Competitively Inhibits tyrosinase ("Dyrosinase") → ↓ pigmentation**
- Use: used to treat P. acnes (acne, rosacea) and hyperpigmentation (melasma, PIH)

Systemic antibacterial agents

Penicillins (PNCs)

- MOA: β-lactam ring in PNC binds bacterial DD-transpeptidase → ↓ cell wall synthesis
- Consists of natural penicillins (penicillin V/G/K), β-lactamase resistant penicillins (methicillin, nafcillin, oxacillin, dicloxacillin, cloxacillin), aminopenicillins (ampicillin, amoxicillin), carboxypenicillins (carbenicillin, ticarcillin), ureidopenicillins (piperacillin)
  - All patients with mononucleosis, ALL/CLL patients and patients taking Allopurinol who also take ampicillin will get a pruritic generalized morbilliform eruption
- β-lactamase inhibitors (clavulanate, sulbactam, tazobactam) HELPS for polymicrobial infections (Haemophilus, E. coli, Enterobacter, Listeria, Proteus, Salmonella, Shigella)
  - Amoxicillin-Clavulanate: TOC for Animal/human bites; ↑ risk of Cholestatic injury
  - Ticarcillin-clavulanate is great for diabetic foot ulcers
  - Ticarcillin-Piperacillin → ↑ Na, ↑ LFT, diarrhea ("TP makes me think diarrhea")
- Uses: streptococci skin infections (ABC pyogENES → peri-Anal strept, Blistering distal dactylitis, Cellulitis in adults, Ecthyma, Necrotizing fasciitis in kids, Erysipelas), erysipeloid, scarlet fever, SSSS, spirochete infections, MSSA skin infections (impetigo)
- SEs ("Penicillin HAG"): Probenecid ↓ renal clearance and ↑ drug levels), Photo-onycholysis(dicloxacillin), Hypersensitivity, AGEP, GI symptoms (common)

Cephalosporins

- MOA: same as penicillins (structure is β-lactam ring + 6-membered dihydrothiazine ring)

- Resistant to bacterial β-lactamases
- Generations
    - First: cefadroxil, cephalexin, cefazolin (1st AID mnemonics below)
        - Activity against gram positives and PEcK (Proteus, E. coli, Klebsiella)
        - **Cephalexin should be dosed at 500 TID to QID due to short half-life**
    - Second: cefaclor, cefuroxime, cefprozil, cephamycins (cefotetan, cefoxitin)
        - Activity against gram positives and HENS PEcK (H. influenza, Enterobacter, Neisseria, Serratia, Proteus, E. coli, Klebsiella)
    - Third: cefixime, cefdinir, cefotaxime ceftazidime, cefpodoxime, ceftriaxone
        - Good G- but poor G+ activity (diabetic foot ulcers, soft-tissue abscesses)
    - Fourth: cefepime (IV)
        - Broad coverage against MSSA, streptococci and G- (pseudomonas)
    - Fifth: ceftaroline (IV)
        - Good for acute bacterial skin infections (MRSA, VRSA)
- SEs ("SAD HAG"): **Serum sickness-like reaction (cefaclor)**, Aminoglycoside coadministration causes nephrotoxicity, hemolytic Anemia (cofotetan, ceftriaxone), Disulfiram-like reactions (cofotetan), Hypersensitivity reactions, AGEP, GI symptoms
- If no response, consider if it is being dosed correctly (e.g., **cephalexin should be QID)**

Vancomycin

- MAO: inhibits bacterial cell wall synthesis
- Activity against G+ including MRSA
- Resistance is plasmid-mediated
- IV administration except for C. difficile diarrhea (PO)

- SEs of vancomyin: **Linear IgA bullous dermatosis, Nephrotoxic (if given w/ aminoglycosides), Color red (red man syndrome; Rx: antihistamines), Ototoxic**

Antibiotics that bind to bacterial ribosomes (30s subunit vs 50s subunit)	
"Buy AT 30"	"Pam CELS at 50"
Aminoglycosides Tetracyclines	Retapamulin (L3 protein on 50s ribosome) Clindamycin, Chloramphenicol Erythromycin (all macrolides) Linezolid (23s portion of 50s ribosome) Synercid (Quinupristin and dalfopristin)

Macrolides

- MOA: binds to 50s subunit of bacterial ribosome → ↓ protein synthesis
- Activity against G+ (except MRSA and enterococcus) and some G-
- Indications: macrolides treat PUSS: Pneumonia (atypical), URIs, STDs, Strept/Staph
  - o Erythromycin
    - ▪ Other indications: acne, rosacea, pityriasis rosea, erythrasma, pitted keratolysis, erysipeloid, lyme disease, anthrax
    - ▪ Side effects (MACROlide)
      - Motility defects of GI tract (GI symptoms; Pyloric stenosis in baby)
      - Arrythmias (QT prolongation); potent CYP3A4 inhibitor
      - Cholestatic hepatitis in pregnant mothers
      - Rash (hypersensitivity reaction)
      - Ototoxicity

- Azithromycin (ABCD)
  - Other indications: 2nd line ppx in derm surgery for PCN/CSN-allergic patients, animal/human bites, atypical mycobacterium, acne, STDs
  - Drug interactions: Absorption ↓ with Antacids
  - SEs: Angioedema, Burns (photosensitivity), Contact dermatitis, Deafness
  - Does not inhibit the CYP3A4 system or have significant drug interactions
- Clarithromycin ("Clare is my Bitter HALF")
  - Other indications: atypical mycobacteria, T. pallidum
  - SEs: Bitter metallic taste, Hypersensitivity rxn, AKI/CKD is a CI, LCV, FDE

- Macrolides can cause increased serum levels and **toxicity of theophylline** (via CYP1A2)
- Tacrolimus, pimecrolimus, and sirolimus are functionally similar to cyclosporine but **structurally similar to macrolide antibiotics** (immunosuppressive macrolide antibiotics)

Fluoroquinolones

- MOA: inhibits DNA gyrase/bacterial topoisomerase II (G- target) +/- topoisomerase IV (G+ target) → DNA fragmentation
  - Keep your topoisomerases straight
    - Anti-topoisomerase I (anti-Scl-70) a/w diffuse systemic scleroderma (SSc)
    - Anti-topoisomerase II (anti-DNA gyrase) present in all forms of morphea
      - "Morphea has one more topoisomerase than SSc"
    - Topoisomerase II inhibited by 1st and 2nd generation quinolones (CON: Ciprofloxacin,

Ofloxacin Nalidixic acid) → only effective against G-

        - Topoisomerase IV > II is inhibited by 3rd and 4th generation quinolones (levofloxacin, moxifloxacin, sparfloxacin, gatifloxacin) → ↑ G+ coverage

- Indications: anthrax, pseudomonas and other gram-negative infections (chancroid, donovanosis, GN toe-web infections, diabetic foot ulcers, gram-negative folliculitis)
- Quinolones (& tetracyclines) are excreted renally except moxifloxacin (& doxycycline)
    - **Use these in renal failure ("Moxi and doxy are not renal toxy")**
- SEs (GRAPH)
    - GI symptoms (#1)
    - **Ruptured tendons**/tendonitis
    - Absorption ↓ with divalent cations (Ca, Mg, Al, zinc); CYP1A2 inhibitor
    - **Photosensitivity**/Photo-onycholysis: "SLE is most photosensitive"
        - Sparfloxacin (visible spectrum), Lomefloxacin (UVA spectrum), Enoxacin (UVA spectrum) > ciprofloxacin > norfloxacin > ofloxacin > levofloxacin
    - Hypersensitivity reaction; HA (and other CNS SEs)

Tetracyclines (saracycline, tetracycline, minocycline, doxycycline, omadacycline)

- MOA: **binds 30s subunit** (antibacterial); ↓ **matrix metalloproteinase** (antiinflammatory)
- Uses ("LARGE CRAMPS")
    - **LGV (doxycycline is TOC); Lyme disease (doxycycline is TOC)**
    - Acne (saracycline is a narrow-spectrum TCN developed for acne)

- **R**ickettsia/Rickettsia-like infections (RMSF, Q-fever, trench fever, rickettsialpox)
- Granulomatous diseases (sarcoidosis, silicone granuloma, Melkersson-Rosenthal)
- **EGFR inhibitor-induced acneiform eruption**
- **CARP (minocycline is TOC)**
- Rosacea (sub-antimicrobial doses effective and do not ↑ bacterial resistance)
- Acne keloidalis nuchae
- MRSA/**M. Marinum (minocycline)**
- PLEVA/PLC
- Syphilis including pinta/yaws (in PCN-allergic patients)

- The more lipophilic a tetracycline is (**minocycline** > doxycycline > tetracycline), the less the absorption is ↓ with divalent cations via chelation (Ca, iron, zinc, Mg, Al, bismuth)
- SEs (GP): G- folliculitis, GI symptoms (esp. doxy), esophageal erosion, vaginal candida, Photosensitivity and **distal** (vs proximal w/ taxanes) Photo-onycholysis ("DTM = Down To Melt": **Demeclocycline** > Doxycycline > Tetracycline > Minocycline; UVA spectrum)
  - "With Mino you can go outside Mid-day (least photosensitive) and you can drink Milk without it decreasing efficacy because it's the most lipophilic ("lipo-milic")
- TCN class strengthens bones and fights osteoporosis by inhibiting osteoclasts
- SEs more specific to minocycline ("PASS That DVD")
  - **Pseudotumor cerebri** (possible w/ all TCNs); **Pigmentation of skin**
  - **Autoimmune hepatitis**
  - **Sweets syndrome**
  - **Serum-sickness-like reaction:** p/w fever, itchy red "bruise-like" rash, arthritis

    - **SLE-like syndrome (ANA+):** p/w photosensitivity, morning joint pain, malaise
    - Tooth pigmentation (Mid-1/3rd in Mino vs gingival/Top 1/3rd in Tetracycline)
    - Thyroid pigmentation (black thyroid syndrome)
    - **Dizziness (vertigo)**
    - **Vasculitis/cutaneous PAN (p-ANCA+)**
    - **DRESS (important to differentiate from autoimmune hepatitis)**
- Minocycline hyperpigmentation types (after cumulative dose of > 70 g)
    - Type 1: blue-gray on facial scars ("1 face") → stains for iron and melanin
    - Type 2: blue-gray on shins ("2 shins") → stains for iron and melanin
    - Type 3: diffuse brown on sun-exposed skin ("3 letters in sun") → stains melanin
- Do not give to pregnant mothers or children < 8 years old → tooth/nail discoloration
    - If given in pregnancy to 6 months old, it will only stain primary teeth
    - If given from **6 months to 6 years old,** it will stain permanent teeth
- Doxycycline may cause brain swelling and ↑ ICP (evaluate optic disc; CI w/ isotretinoin)
- **Do not give TCN with lithium** as it decreases clearance and causes lithium toxicity
- All excreted renally except doxycycline ("Moxi and doxy are **not** renal toxy")
- Point mutation at 16s ribosome confers tetracycline resistance in G+ bacteria

Rifampin

- MOA: binds β-subunit of bacterial DNA-dependent RNA polymerase → ↓ RNA synthesis

- Uses: various mycobacteria, Bartonella infections, MRSA/MSSA, Rhinoscleroma
- Do not give as monotherapy because Rapid development of Resistance (**rpoB** mutation)
  - SEs: Red discoloration of body fluids, Red man syndrome (exfoliative erythroderma), **Reduces efficacy of OCPs**, **Ramps-up CYP3A4 (most potent inducer of CYP3A4)**, worsens porphyria and causes Red soft contact lenses

Contraceptive failure: "Your mom will be a GRANMA if you take these meds with your OCPs"

Griseofulvin/Rifampin (OCPs), Azathioprine/NSAIDs (IUDs), Mycophenolate mofetil (OCPs)

Trimethoprim-sulfamethoxazole (TMP-SMX)

- Dihydrofolate reductase inhibitor (TMP) + dihydropteroate synthetase inhibitor (SMX) → ↓ tetrahydrofolic acid → ↓ bacterial protein synthesis
  - Dapsone, SMX and Sodium sulfacetamide inhibit Dihydropteroate Synthetase
- BACTRIM uses: B. mallei (glanders), Acne/HS, Actinomycetoma (Nocardia), Cat-scratch, Traveler's diarrhea, Resistant bacteria (MRSA), granuloma Inguinale, Meliodosis
- SEs for TMP is "Treats Marrow Poorly": agranulocytosis, pancytopenia, megaloblastic anemia from folate deficiency, hemolytic anemia in G6PD deficiency
  - But can also treat skin poorly: SJS/TEN and hypersensitivity reactions esp. in HIV
  - Cross reacts w/ PABA → allergic reactions
- Pregnancy cat C: treats fetus' marrow poor → hemolytic anemia → jaundice/kernicterus
- Drug interactions from BATRIM ("DACTRIM"): Dapsone (↑ dapsone levels), ACE/ARBS (↑ K^+ levels), Amantadine (toxic delirium), Cyclosporine (↑ renal toxicity),

Coumadin (↑ risk of bleeding), **MTX (↑ hematologic toxicity as both ↓ tetrahydrofolic acid)**

Clindamycin (A-E)

- Lincosamide derived from Strept lincolnensis which binds to ribosomal **50s subunit**
- Activity against **Anaerobes** (Bacteroides, C. perfringens), **G+ Cocci** (GAS, MRSA), the G- organism Capnocytophaga Canimorsus and the protozoa T. gondii
- D-zone test: sometimes the lab will mistakenly say that CA-MRSA is Erythromycin- resistant and Clindamycin-sensitive but if D-zone test is performed next, a positive test will confirm inducible bacterial resistance to clindamycin (bacteria w/ **erm gene**)
    - MLSb: resistant phenotype (via erm gene) w/ dual resistance to clindamycin and erythromycin due to methylation of the shared ribosomal binding site
- Uses: MRSA, soft tissue infections including Deep soft tissue infections (strept myositis, C. perfringes, Diabetic foot ulcers), invasive GAS infections (toxic shock, SSSS)
- SEs: **C. Difficile Colitis** >> Cutaneous rashes, enhances neuromuscular Blocking agents
- Should be dosed TID

Bacteriostatic antibitoics: "ECSTaTIC"	-cidal: "Be Very Finely Proficient At Cell Mur-Der"*
Erythromycin Clindamycin (bactericidal at high dose) SMX TMP TCNs Chloramphenicol	Bacitracin Vancomycin Fluoroquinolones PCNs, Polymyxin B Aminoglycosides Carbapenems, Cephalosporins Metronidazole, Monobactams Daptomycin

*1st AID mnemonic

Linezolid

- MOA: binds **23s portion of 50s ribosomal subunit** of bacteria
- Uses: complicated G+ skin and soft tissue infections
- SEs of linezolid ("think of a line of SNOT"): **Serotonin Syndrome**, Neuropathy, Optic neuritis, **Thrombocytopenia (MC) > myelosuppression**, Tongue-discoloration

Quinupristin and dalfopristin combination (Synercid)

- MOA: binds 50s ribosomal subunit → ↓ protein synthesis
- Uses: complicated G+ skin and soft tissue infections
- SEs (ABC): Angioedema/Anaphylaxis, ↑ Bilirubin levels, potent CYP3A4 inhibitor

Daptomycin

- MOA: Depolarizes bacterial cell membrane → cell Death
- Uses: complicated G+ skin and soft tissue infections
- SEs ("Dapto-MENN"): Myopathy, Eosinophilic pneumonia, Neuropathy, Nephrotoxicity

Antiviral agents

Acyclovir and related drugs

- MOA: **Guanosine (purine) analog** that requires **phosphorylation by viral thymidine kinase** to acyclovir monophosphate, and then subsequent phosphorylation by human guanylate kinase to acyclovir triphosphate (here it competes w/ deoxyguanosine triphosphate to **inhibit viral DNA polymerase → terminates viral DNA elongation)**
- Uses: available topically (HSV), PO (HSV, VZV, EM 2° to HSV) and IV (disseminated HSV/VZV, eczema herpeticum and HSV infection in immunosuppressed patients)
- SEs: N/V/D/HA and **renal impairment w/ IV infusions 2° to crystalline nephropathy**
    - o **SE of Gancyclovir is granulocytopenia**
    - o **SE of valacyclovir is anemia/thrombocytopenia (TTP/HUS) in HIV patients**
- Drug interactions
    - o Probenecid ↓ renal clearance (↑ famciclovir, PNC, cephalosporin levels too)
    - o Combination of Acyclovir w/ Zidovudine → severe drowsiness
        - ▪ "Saying entire alphabet from A to Z causes severe drowsiness"
- **Viral resistance occurs via mutations in thymidine kinase (#1)** or DNA polymerase (#2)
    - o Switch to foscarnet (considered 1st line in acyclovir-resistant HSV) or cidofovir
- Famciclovir (PO) is the prodrug of penciclovir (topical; only treats herpes labialis)
- Use famciclovir or valacyclovir for VZV (better at ↓ VZV pain than acyclovir)

Foscarnet

- MOA: pyrophosphate analog that binds to **pyrophosphate-binding site on viral DNA polymerase** → ↓ pyrophosphate cleavage from deoxyadenosine → ↓ DNA elongation
- Uses (CAR): CMV skin infections in HIV, **Acyclovir-resistant HSV (TOC)**, CMV Retinitis
- SE (NET): Nephrotoxicity, **penile Erosions**, Thrombophlebitis
    - All-trans-retinoic acid and sunitinib cause scrotal ulcers

Cidofovir ("Have you tried Cid MOCH? NA CU!")

- MOA: IV nucleoside phosphate analog of deoxycytidine monophosphate that is phosphorylated to cidofovir diphosphate which inhibits viral DNA polymerase → ↓ DNA elongation (like foscarnet, it does not require viral thymidine kinase)
- Uses (MOCH): Molluscum, Orf, CMV retinitis, HSV/HPV
- SEs (NA CU): **Nephrotoxicity (MC),** Neutropenia, Alopecia, Cardiomyopathy, Uveitis/iritis

Bleomycin

- IL chemotherapeutic agent which **Binds DNA/RNA** to cause single strand Breaks
- Uses: warts, hemangiomas, cutaneous malignancies, condyloma acuminata, leishmania
- SEs ("When you inject bleo, make sure it doesn't DRIP"): Dystrophy of nails, Raynaud's phenomenon, Injection pain, flagellate Pigmentation (more a SE of systemic bleomycin)

Podophyllin and podofilox

- Antimitotic agents used for genital warts that bind tubulin and arrests cell in **metaphase**
  - Meds that bind to tubulin ("CRAP in the Tube"): Colchicine, griseofulvin, Albendazole, Podophyllin, Tirbanibulin (all work in M → G2 phase of cell cycle)
- Podophyllin is administered in office; podofilox administered at home by patient (safer)
- SEs: local reaction; do not use in pregnancy (teratogen)

Cantharidin (ABCDEF)

- Blistering Agent derived from the Blister Beetle/ **Spanish Fly**
- MOA: Disrupts Desmosomes → Acantholysis of Epidermis → Bullae
- Uses: applied topically in the office for warts and molluscum
- SEs: pain from blister; ring wart formation (center of wart is treated but not periphery)

Sinecatechins

- Green tea (Camellia sinensis)-derived polyphenol epigallocatechin gallate → apoptosis
- Use: condyloma acuminata (CA)
- SEs: local (ulceration, pain, itch, swelling)

5-FU and imiquimod discussed in section 2.5

Antifungal agents

Allylamines/benzylamines

- MOA: **inhibits squalene epoxidase** (converts squalene to lanosterol); **fungicidal**
  - Remember SLE: Squalene goes to Lanosterol via squalene epoxidase and then Lanosterol goes to

Ergosterol via 14α demethylase to form the cell membrane

Terbinafine (oral benzylamine)

- Use: Tinea infections (in tinea capitis it is great against endothrix organisms like T. Tonsurans but less effective than griseofulvin for ectothrix organisms like M. canis)
- Common SEs are GI, rash, HA and ↑ LFTs but rarer (more testable) SEs = THIRD
    - **Taste/smell disturbances** (**dysgeusia**)
    - Hepatobiliary dysfunction/Hepatitis/**Hepatic failure and Hematologic (penias)**
    - In-grown toenails
    - Rhabdomyolysis and Renal dysfunction (do not give if CrCl < 50)
    - **Drug-induced SCLE** and exacerbation of SLE, Depression and **CYP2D6 inhibitor**
        - Warfarin doesn't use CYP2D6 ("terbinafine is fine to use w/ warfarin")
        - Inhibiting CYP2D6 → toxicity of β-blockers, TCAs (doxepin), antipsychotics
- Terbinafine is Pregnancy category B ("fine in pregnancy")
- Lab monitoring: **obtain LFTs only at baseline only** (unless signs of liver damage arise)
    - Although neutropenia has been reported, all cases are reversible upon discontinuation and thus it is only advised to order a CBC for signs of infection

Naftifine and Butenafine (topical benzylamines)

- More effective than azoles against dermatophytes (tinea)

<u>Azoles</u>

- MOA: **inhibits 14α demethylase** (converts lanosterol to ergosterol); **fungistatic**
  - o "Terbinafine is closer to S (Squalene epoxidase) and Azole is closer to (14-Alpha)"
- Inhibits cytochrome P450 (mostly CYP3A4)→ increase P450 substrates such as PPIs
- Pregnancy category C (except high-dose fluconazole and voriconazole which are Cat D)

Itraconazole

- Metabolized mainly in the liver (inhibits CYP3A4)
- **Absorbed better in an Acidic environment (concurrent Antacids/PPIs ↓ effectiveness)**
  - o "Taking omeprazole/pantoprazole will make itraconazole not work"
  - o This was also the case in mycophenolate mofetil (mycophenolate mofetil, TCNs and fluoroquinolones had decreased absorption with divalent cations, e.g., Ca^{2+})
- Uses: onychomycosis, extensive TV, systemic and dimorphic mycoses
- CI: **Arrythmias/CHF**, Active liver disease and concurrent use of CYP3A4 drugs and ABCDE drugs: Atorvostatin, Benzos (midazolam), CCBs (nisoldipine), Dofetalide, Ergot alkaloids
- SEs (ABCDE): Abdominal pain (MC), Acute liver toxicity, Blood changes (↓WBCs, ↓K^+), Cold symptoms (rhinitis, fever), Cutaneous rash, CNS symptoms (HA, peripheral neuropathy), CV events (CHF), Deafness, Edema, pulmonary Edema
- **Black-box warning for congestive heart failure**
- **Inhibits sonic hedgehog pathway (Rx BCCs) by inhibiting accumulation of smoothened**

Fluconazole

- Uses: Candida infections, Cryptococcus, Coccidioidomycoses, TV, tinea, seb derm
- CI: pregnancy and concurrent use of CYP2C9 drugs
- SE are minor but similar to itraconazole w/ the addition of Cholestasis → hyperlipidemia
    - o While there is no black box warning for CHF, there is a precaution for QT ("Cutie") prolongation and is CI to combined w/ cisapride, pimozide, quinidine
- In addition to inhibiting CYP3A4 (like itraconazole), it also inhibits CYP2C9
- Unlike other azoles, fluconazole is not affected by food or gastric acidity
- Total dose > 300 mg is pregnancy category D but single dose use is category C

Ketoconazole

- Not used systemically due to hepatic toxicity (black box warning for hepatotoxicity)
- Topical uses: tinea/candida infections, tinea versicolor, seborrheic dermatitis
- CI: concurrent use of Cisapride, Astemizole, Terfenadine ↑ QT ("say QT-conazole CAT")
- SEs: similar azole SEs (GI/hepatic toxicity) w/ ↑ QT and **impotence/gynecomastia**
    - o "Long QT but short PP"

Voriconazole

- Use: **severe invasive fungal infections not responding to amphotericin**
- SEs: similar azole SEs (GI/hepatic toxicity/↑QT) w/ **severe photosensitivity** → pseudo-porphyria (acral blisters) and **xeroderma-pigmentosa-like changes (↑ risk of SCC)**
    - o "Long QT and sensitive to UV"

Miconazole, clotrimazole, econazole, luliconazole, efinaconazole (topical azoles)

- Uses: candida, tinea versicolor, seborrheic dermatitis, and tinea
- Topical azole creams in the groin/vagina **can interfere with condoms**

Griseofulvin

- MOA: interferes with tubulin → stops mitosis in metaphase
- Uses: tinea infections (better than terbinafine for tinea capitis caused by M. canis)
- **Like isotretinoin, griseofulvin is absorbed much better when taken w/ a fatty meal**
- SEs ("Greasy PHAT"): GI, **Photosensitivity** (CI in SLE/porphyria; drug induced SCLE), HA, CYP3A4 inducer, Teratogenic (Pregnancy cat X and harms sperm: women must use contraception during and 1 month after drug cessation and **men must wear condoms during treatment and at least 6 months after last dose)**
- **CYP3A4 inducer** → may ↓ effectiveness of OCPs (best to use 2 forms of contraception)
- Lab monitoring: LFT and CBC alterations are rare and thus lab monitoring is unnecessary

Ciclopirox olamine

- MOA: a hydroxypyridone which blocks fungal **cell membrane** transport
- Uses: tinea, Malessezia (TV, seb derm), candidiasis (non-inferior to azoles for candida)

Selenium sulfide

- MOA: antibacterial and antifungal; antimitotic action results in ↓ epidermal turnover
- Uses: tinea, psoriasis, tinea versicolor, seborrheic dermatitis, tinea capitus
- SEs ("CBDC"): Contact dermatitis, Brown discoloration of the distal nail Bed, **Discoloration** of the hair (usually orange to red-brown), Conjunctivitis
    - A selenium deficiency causes hypopigmentation which helps me remember that giving pts selenium sulfide shampoo can cause pigmentation

In-vitro potency comparison of select topical antifungals
Dermatophytes: butenafine > terbinafine > naftifine = ciclopirox > azoles >> nystatin Candidiasis: nystatin > azoles = ciclopirox > butenafine > naftifine > terbinafine

Nystatin

- MOA: topical **polyene** that **binds fungal cell membrane sterols** (e.g., **ergosterol**) and puts holes in the membranes (pore formation)
    - Amphotericin B is a systemic polyene which also Binds cell membrane sterols and is Pregnancy category B (considered safest systemic antifungal in pregnancy)
        - "Ampho-terrible (terrible side effects) but ampho-terrific in pregnancy"
- Best anti-fungal for mucocutaneous candidiasis; **worst anti-fungal for dermatophytes**

Caspofungin, micafungin and anidulafungin (echinocandins)

- MOA: **inhibits β-(1, 3)-D-glucan synthesis** → ↓ cell wall synthesis
- Uses: invasive candida infections

- SEs: **facial swelling (Fat Face)**, ↑ alk phos, hypokalemia, hematuria/proteinuria

Aluminum Acetate (borrows solution)

- MOA: astringent (shrinks body tissue when applied to skin)
- Use: OTC product used to temporarily relieve irritation (e.g., poison ivy)
- SEs: local skin irritation

Antifungal agents that are acceptable in Pregnancy (All are Category B)
Topicals (CON): Ciclopirox, Clotrimazole, Oxiconazole, Naftifine Orals: (AT): Amphotericin, Terbinifine

Antiparasitic agents

Systemic antiparasitic agents

- Ivermectin: binds glutamate-gated **Chloride** ion channels ("Ivermectin treats COVID?")
    - o Uses: onchocerciasis (give w/ doxy to prevent Mazzotti reaction), scabies, strongyloidiasis, cutaneous larva migrans, pediculosis; do not use for loiasis
    - o SEs (Ivermectin treats SARS?"): **Seizures**, Adenopathy, Rashes, face/limb Swelling
- Albendazole: inhibits tubulin polymerization ("Al bends the tube")
    - o Uses: various worms ("worms are bendy")
    - o SEs: Aplastic Anemia, Agranulocytosis, pancytopenia (↑ risk in liver failure)
- Thiabendazole: inhibits fumarate reductase ("t close to r in alphabet")
    - o Uses: worms ("worms are bendy")
    - o SEs: hepatotoxicity, GI/CNS side effects

Topical antiparasitic agents

- Permethrin ("that perm is So Curly"): inhibits **Sodium** channels; related to pyrethrins (insecticide in **Chrysanthemum** species/**Compositae** genus which causes airborne ACD)
    - Uses ("So Curly"): TOC for Scabies and pediculosis Capitis
    - SEs: local but avoid if pt has allergies to ragweed (chrysanthemum)
    - **TOC of scabies in pregnancy and in infants greater than 2 months**
- Lindane: organochlorine
    - Uses: scabies and pediculosis capitis
    - SEs: seizures (avoid if pt has history), neural tube defects, teratogenic
        - "Linda is LOST: Lindane, Organochlorine, Seizures, Teratogenic"
- Malathion ("Mal means bad in Spanish"): organophosphate (inhibits cholinesterase)
    - **Ovicidal** (kills live lice AND eggs → does not require repeat treatment)
        - vs permethrin/ivermectin which only kill live lice and require repeat Rx
    - Use: pediculosis capitis (not used in scabies)
    - SEs: **flammable**, malodorous and causes organophosphate poisoning if ingested
        - "Bad (mal) because it kills babies (lice eggs) and lights people on fire"
- Spinosad: used for pediculosis capitus and is ovicidal (works very fast)
    - Malathion (bad) and Spinosad: bad and sad both kill babies (ovicidal)
- Crotamiton: 10% cream or lotion is FDA approved for scabies but also helps w/ non-scabietic pruritis via unknown mechanism

- Precipitated sulfur (5–10%): used for scabies in pregnancy and **infants < 2 months**
- Benzoyl alcohol, benzyl benzoate and dimethicone are other anti-scabietic meds

2.7 Phototherapy

UVA modalities

- PUVA (Psoralen + UVA; "PUVA is not PC"): Photoactivated Psoralen (usually 8-methoxypsoralen) forms **DNA Crosslinks** → ↓ DNA synthesis (Cell Cycle Cessation)
  - Cyclophosphamide also forms Crosslinks between DNA strands
  - Uses: many dermatoses (psoriasis, vitiligo, CTCL, AD, GVHD, LP, scleroderma)
  - SEs (PC): Phototoxic reactions, Pruritis, Photoaging, skin Cancer (**SCC**), Cataracts
  - CI (PC): Pregnancy/lactation, Pemphigus/-oid and Photosensitive conditions (SLE)
- UVA-1 (340–400 nm): not widely performed
  - Uses: **scleroderma**/sclerodermoid conditions, AD, and MF
  - SEs: temporary erythema
- Instruct patients to stop all photosensitizing meds (which are in UVA range) such as doxycycline or St Johns wart (contains hypericin which is phototoxic to skin)

UVB

- MOA: multiple mechanisms including ↑ **p53** (cell-cell arrest), ↓ DNA synthesis (cell cycle arrest), ↓ proinflammatory cytokines and ↓ Langerhans cells in skin
- Narrowband UVB (311–313 nm)
  - Given 3x/week (start at 70% of minimal erythema dose and ↑ by 10% each time)

  - UV-opaque goggles covering eyes and genitals (**this is why periocular and genital vitiligo will be least effective w/ phototherapy**)
  - Uses: psoriasis (1st line for generalized psoriasis **w/o PsA**), vitiligo (TOC), AD, patch/plaque stage MF, photodermatoses (desensitization), LP, and pruritis
  - SEs: erythema, herpes simplex reactivation (unlike other forms of phototherapy, there is **no clear association between NBUVB and melanoma or NMSC**)
- Broadband UVB (280–320): largely replaced by NBUVB but still used for guttate psoriasis
- Excimer laser (308 nm; "Eight-cimer"): high-intensity treatment w/ higher efficacy than standard UVB for treating small/localized areas (< 2 cm^2 of psoriasis, AD, vitiligo)
  - "Limited wavelength range (308 nm) used for limited surface areas"
- Pts do not need to stop photosensitizing meds (e.g., doxy) as these sensitize in UVA range

Extra-Corporeal photo-Chemotherapy

- Catheter phereses blood from patient which is separated into WBCs and RBCs (RBCs are given back to patient while WBCs are exposed to 8-methoxypsoralen and irradiated before being given back) → results in a **net gain of 500 mL** (initial loss of 300 mL)
  - Immune effects include ↓ active T cells, ↓ Langerhans cells, ↑ regulatory T-cells
- Uses: **CTCL** (targets lymphoma cells), Chronic GVHD, NSF, pemphigus, scleroderma
- SEs: N/V, photosensitivity, hypotension, CHF, tachycardia
- CI in **CHF** (net addition of 500 mL); caution in those with low BP (initial loss of 300 mL)

Photodynamic therapy (PDT)

- Activation of topical photosensitizer by **visible light (peaks at 410 and 636 nm)** converts it to **Protoporphyrin 9** within cells → production of ROS → apoptosis of malignant cells
    - Aminolaevulinic acid (ALA; blue light) vs methyl-aminolevulinate (MAL; red light)
    - Hypericin: new photosensitizer w/ photosensitizing and **anti-tumor properties**
- Uses: AK, acne, skin-rejuvenation (PDT w/ IPL light source), CTCL (w/ hypericin)
- Technique: cleanse skin (Acetone for ALA and curette scale/crust for MAL), then apply photosensitizer (ALA vs MAL), then let photosensitizer incubate for 1–4 hours, then give light (10 J/cm^2 for 16 mins for ALA; 37 J/cm^2 for 8 mins for MAL)
- SEs: Photosensitivity (avoid sunlight for 48 hours), Pigmentary alterations

2.8 Miscellaneous Agents

Antihistamines

- MOA: H1 anti-H1stamines are H1nverse agonists and mediate urticaria/angioedema related itching by blocking H1 receptor (role less clear in eczema)
- First generation H1 antihistamines ("CBCD"): Cyproheptadine, Benadryl (Diphenhydramine), Chlorpheniramine; promethazine and hydroxyzine are others
    - SEs ("CBDC"): **anti-Cholinergic** (dry as a Bone, red as a Beat, Blind as a Bat), long term use is a/w **Dementia**, Crosses blood-brain barrier (drowsiness/sedation)
    - SEs in pregnancy ("CBDC"): premature uterine Contractions, **retrolental fibroplasia** of baby

(Blindness) if used peripartum (36–40 weeks), Preg Cat B

- Second-generation antihistamines are less sedating and lack anti-cholinergic effects
  - Includes fexofenadine, loratadine, **cetirizine (most sedating),** and levocetirizine
  - Loratadine, Levocetirizine and Cetirizine are preferred in pregnancy (Preg cat B)
    - "My LLC is about non-sedating antihistamines that are safe in pregnancy"
- Doxepin ("DOCS"): **blocks both H1 and H2**; used for urticaria and neurotic excoriations
  - MOA: Stronger affinity for histamine receptor than other antihistamines and lasts longer due to Slow half-life (qHS dosing)
  - SEs: **Sedation, Second-degree heart block, Seizures and Suicidality**
  - Pregnancy cat C: Congenital anomalies if used in 1st few weeks of pregnancy

Sunscreens

- Sun protection factor (SPF) is a measure of light filter efficacy
  - SPF = MED of protected skin divided by MED of unprotected skin
  - AAD recommends SPF > 30; FDA and USPSTF recommends SPF > 15
- Chemical sunscreens: aromatic compounds that absorb radiation and convert it to longer wavelengths (lower energy); must know if the sunscreen works for UVA or UVB
  - UVB ("he COPES w/ UVB"): Cinnamates (cross reacts w/ Balsam of Peru; ACD), "Oct" names (octisalate, octocrylene), Padimate O (PABA), Parasol SLX (dimethico-diethylbenzalmalonate), Ensulizole, Salicylates (trolamine salicylate)

        - Octocrylene and Ensulizole (vowels in COPES) stabilize photolabile agents
    - UVA: Avobenzone **(broadest UVA coverage** but **most photolabile),** ecamsule
    - UVA2 & UVB: **oxybenzone (MCC of contact derm; broadest chemical sunscreen)**
        - "Oxycontin is the chemical w/ contact to the broadest range of people"
- Physical blockers: chemically inert compounds (zinc/titanium) that reflect/scatter light
    - **Broadest spectrum** (covers UVB, UVA and some **visible light**)
    - No risk of contact dermatitis like the chemical sunscreens
    - Activity depends on particle size (large particles are cosmetically unappealing but offer protection well into UVA1 vs micronized particles which rub in much easier)
        - Tinted sunscreens w/ iron oxide and titanium dioxide offer better protection against visible light than micronized nanoparticles of zinc and titanium and should be recommended to POC w/ melasma
- Dihydroxyacetone (found in spray tan products): has SPF of 3 or 4
    - "Girls that do spray tans commonly have their ass tone"

Topical cosmetic agents

- Eflornithine (Vanique): **inhibits ornithine decarboxylase** which treats female hirsutism
- Hydroquinone: competes w/ tyrosine as a substrate for **tyrosinase** which lightens skin
    - SEs: dermatitis (MC) and **exogenous ochronosis** (paradoxical hyperpigmentation which has a grainy/textured appearance) w/ prolonged use

        - Resorsinol in the Jessner's peel can also cause exogenous ochronosis
- Bimatoprost (Latisse): **prostaglandin analog** which lengthens/thickens eyelashes
    - SEs: **iris and periorbital skin hyperpigmentation**

Topical calcineurin inhibitors (tacrolimus, pimecrolimus)

- MOA: **binds to FK506-binding protein** (**vs cyclophilin for cyclosporin**) → inhibits calcineurin (same as cyclosporin from here on) → ↓ activity of NFAT which normally transcribes cytokines → ↓ **IL-2** → T-cell proliferation
- Tacrolimus, pimecrolimus and sirolimus are functionally similar to cyclosporine but **structurally similar to macrolide antibiotics** (immunosuppressive macrolide antibiotics)
- Uses: various dermatoses (AD, LP, psoriasis, vitiligo, lupus, Zoon's balanitis
- SEs: **block box warning for cancer**; **high levels of absorption in Netherton's syndrome**

Psychiatric agents

- Pimozide: dopamine antagonist used for delusions of Parasitosis (DOP)
    - SEs: **extra-Pyramidal effects (Parkinsonism)**, arrythmias from **QT-Prolongation**, anti-cholinergic effects, weight gain, ↑ Prolactin
- Atypical (2nd generation) antipsychotics (**risperidone**, olanzapine, quetiapine): dopamine (D2) and serotonin receptor antagonists which are used for DOP
    - 1st line for DOP due to **less** extrapyramidal SEs, QT prolongation, drug interactions, anticholinergic effects and prolactin secretion than pimozide
    - Olanzapine is a/w weight gain; monitor fasting lipid panel

IVIG ("IVIG is a Dirty Lying SACK OF MEAT")

- Plasma from > 100 donors which primarily contains supraphysiologic IgG → ↓antibody production, blocks Fc receptor on autoantibodies, ↓ complement, ↓ TNF and other proinflammatory cytokines, ↓T-cells, ↑ regulatory T-cells, ↓ immune cell migration
- Uses ("Dirty Lying SACK"): **Dermatomyositis**, Livedoid vasculopathy, SLE, Scleroderma, **Scleromyxedema**, SJS/TEN, Serum Sickness, Autoimmune blistering disorders, Chronic autoimmune urticaria, **Kawasaki's disease**
- SEs ("OF MEAT")
  - "OF": **Overload of fluid, Fever/Flushing w/ Fast infusions, Forehead pain/HA**
  - Meningitis
  - **Dyshidrotic Eczema occurs 1-week post treatment → generalized Eczema**
  - Anaphylaxis: **only happens in those w/ IgA deficiency (screen Ig levels prior)**
  - AKI: occurs from osmotic effects of added stabilizers (sucrose, maltose, sorbitol)
  - **Thromboembolic events:** FDA issued a black box warning for this in 2013

Anti-androgens

- Spironolactone: **antiandrogen** w/ diuretic properties
  - Derm uses ("HAHA"): Hirsutism, Acne, HS, Androgenetic alopecia
    - Acne clearance in 80% of those on 100mg and 40% of those on 50mg QD
  - SEs: ("HAHAHA"): Hyperkalemia, Ataxia/dizziness, Huge breasts (gynecomastia), Agranulocytosis (rare), Headache, Anaphylactic reactions (rare)
  - CI in pregnancy (Category X) → feminizes male fetus
  - Avoid coadministration w/ meds that ↑ potassium: drospirenone (OCP w/ mineralocorticoid

activity), loop diuretics (furosemide), TMP-SMX, ACE inhibitors
  - **Labs: no need for baseline/routine potassium monitoring in healthy patients**
- Finasteride/dutasteride: 5-α-reductase inhibitors (finasteride = type 2; dutasteride = type 1&2)
  - Derm uses ("HAHA"): Hirsutism, Acne, HS, Androgenetic alopecia (and FFA)
  - SEs: sexual (impotence, gynecomastia, ↓ libido), depression, possible slight ↑ in high-grade prostate cancer (but ↓ risk of prostate cancer overall)
  - CI in pregnancy (Category X) → feminizes male fetus
- OCPs: **norgestimate**-ethinyl estradiol (Ortho Tri-Cyclen), **norethindrone** acetate-ethinyl estradiol (Estrostep), **drospirenone**-ethinyl estradiol (Yaz)
  - Only Yaz (drospirenone) has intrinsic anti-androgen effects
  - CI: **smoker > 35 y/o**, HTN of >160/100, active liver disease, severe headaches w/ neural symptoms, current breast cancer, pregnancy

Androgens (danazol and stanozolol)
- MOA: ↑ production of various proteins by the liver (clotting factors, C1 INH)
- Derm uses: **hereditary angioedema**, lipodermatosclerosis, livedoid vasculopathy
- SEs ("think guy on steroids after the gym"): deep voice, acne, myalgias/myopathy (esp if patient is on statins), HTN, CHF, HA, hepatic issues (jaundice/cancers)

Vitamin D analogs (Calcipotriene and Calcitriol)
- MOA: binds vitamin D receptors → this complex binds RXR-α to DNA → ↓ keratinocyte proliferation, ↓IL-2, -6, IFN-γ, GM-CSF, ↓ NK and Cytotoxic T-cell activ-

ity, ↑ involucrin and transglutaminase → enhanced Cornified envelope formation

- Derm uses: many dermatoses such as psoriasis, morphea, vitiligo, prurigo nodularis
- SEs: **hyper-Calcemia** (rare), Contact dermatitis/irritation (MC)
- Calcipotriene is inactivated by acid compounds (e.g., **salicylic acid** and steroids which require acid environment) but it is **compatible w/ halobetasol** (combination is more effective in psoriasis and there is less risk of contact dermatitis from the calcipotriene)

Agents for hyperhidrosis (glycopyrrolate, oxybutynin, sofpironium)

- Oral and topical (sofpironium, glycopyrrolate) anticholinergic agents for hyperhidrosis
  - Remember, eccrine glands are functionally cholinergic
- SEs: dry mouth, blurred vision, urinary retention, hyperthermia
- CI ("GUMP"): Glaucoma, Urine retention, toxic Megacolon, Myasthenia, Paralytic ileus

Clofazamine

- Riminophenazine dye used for multibacillary/lepromatous **leprosy** (in conjunction w/ Dapsone and Rifampin; "DR Clof") and **erythema dischromicum perstans**
- SEs: turns skin/body fluids orange (ceroid lipofuscin deposits), drug-induced ichthyosis and crystal deposition in organs → arrythmias, splenic infarct and eosinophilic enteritis

Colchicine

- MOA: **binds tubulin** in WBCs → mitotic arrest in **metaphase**

- Derm uses: familial Mediterranean fever, neutrophilic dermatoses, CSVV, AI-CTD, gout
- SEs: GI (cramping, abdominal pain, diarrhea), **BM suppression, neuropathy**
  - o "When riding coach (colchicine) on a plane, the terrible food gives you GI symptoms and the hard seats gives you neuropathy"

Nicotinamide (vitamin B_3): "take a NAP w/ nicotinamide"

- **MOA: inhibits PARP-1 and surtuins → ↓NFkB** transcription
  - o Remember, corticosteroids ↓NFkB and imiquimod ↑ NFkB transcription
- Uses: NMSC chemoprevention, Autoimmune bullous disorders (in a/w a TCN), Pellagra
- SEs: GI complaints and **drug-induced ichthyosis ("Nic rhymes w/ ich")**
  - o Unlike niacin, it does not cause flushing

Potassium iodide

- MOA: unknonwn
- Derm uses: sporotrichosis, erythema nodosum and erythema induratum
- SEs ("IODIDe"): Ioderma (acneiform eruption), **hypOthyroidism, DH exacerbation**, Iodism (metallic taste, burning mouth), Diarrhea, pregnancy category D
- Labs: check thyroid before starting medication

Thalidomide

- MOA: **inhibits TNF-α** and antigen presenting ability of epidermal LCs
  - o Due to its inhibition of TNF it was studied in SJS/TEN but caused ↑ mortality
- Derm uses: **erythema nodosum leprosum, prurigo nodularis, actinic prurigo,** neutrophilic dermatoses, GVHD, HIV-related pruritic disorders

- SEs: **Teratogenic** (results in phecomelia; **highest risk at 3–5 weeks gestation**; must be off drug for 1 month for men & women), motor and sensory neuropathy (**Tingling**), **venous Thrombosis, Tiredness** (MC SE; was sadly used as a sleeping aid for pregnant pts ☹)

Pentoxifylline

- **Phosphodiesterase inhibitor** (like apremilast) that ↓platelet aggregation and ↓**TNF-α**
- Derm uses: Raynaud's, livedoid vasculopathy, NLD, venous ulcers, lipodermatosclerosis
- SEs: mostly GI but there are reports of it causing **aseptic meningitis**

Capsaicin

- Derived from the hot pepper plant (Solanaceae family; Capsicum annuum)
- MOA: topical vanilloid that binds vanilloid receptor subtype 1 (TRPV1)
- Uses: neuropathic itch
- SEs: burning (keep away from eyes → capsaicin is the active ingredient in pepper spray)

Opioids in dermatology

- Oxycodone: mu, kappa and delta opioid agonist (inhibits adenylate cyclase → ↓cAMP) used for moderate to severe pain; significant addiction potential
  - o 2019 opioid prescribing guidelines published in JAAD recommend max dose of 10 tabs of oxycodone 5 mg for more complex repairs; add this to non-opioid regimen (1 g acetaminophen q 8 hrs and 400 mg ibuprofen q 4 hrs)
  - o 5mg of oxycodone is equivalent to 75 mg of tramadol, 50 mg of codeine, 7.5 mg of hydrocodone, 7.5 mg of morphine and 2.5 mg of oxymorphone

- Butorphanol: intranasal small molecule neuromodulating agent and mu/kappa opioid agonist used for pain and pruritis (prurigo nodularis)
- Tramadol: serotonin/NE reuptake-inhibitor and opioid agonist considered by some to be a lower risk opioid and in contrast to morphine, does not cause histamine release

Skin care products

- Moisturizers: more of a marketing term than a classification w/ scientific basis but they contain ingredients that attract water to the skin to restore barrier function
    - Contain ingredients that act as occlusives, emollients, humectants, preservatives
        - Occlusives: makes skin hydrophobic → ↓ transepidermal water loss
            - Best for super dry/damaged skin
            - Examples: cetyl alcohol, cocoa/shea butter, dimethicone, lanolin, petrolatum, silicone, oils (sesame seed, mineral, olive, soybean)
        - Emollients: makes skin feel soft/smooth ("molly makes skin feel so soft")
            - Best for dry skin
            - Example: overlaps w/ occlusives (oils, oatmeal, shea butter, etc.)
        - Humectants: draw water in from viable epidermis/dermis to skin surface
            - Best for oily skin
            - Examples: **Hyaluronic acid**, Hydrolyzed collagen, propylene Glycol and **Glycerin** ("G next to H in alphabet")
- Cleansers: remove dead skin cells, dirt, oil and other pollutants from the skin surface via complex physical and chemical interaction between a surfactant and the skin surface

2.9 Drug Interactions and Cytochrome P-450

Drug interactions that reduce efficacy of substrates

- Reduced GI Absorption: concomitant use of Antacids and Divalent Cations cause a **rapid ↓ in efficacy** of ABCD drugs (Azoles except fluconazole, Bisphosphonates, Cellcept, Ciprofloxacin and other fluoroquinolones, Dapsone, Doxycycline, and other TCNs)
    - o Avoid these interactions by taking drug 2 hours before and 6 hours after antacid
- Induction of CYP3A4: concomitant use of CYP3A4 drugs cause **slow ↓ in efficacy**

CYP3A4 Substrates	CYP3A4 Inducers	CYP3A4 Inhibitors
"I feel like a bullied substrate in this Lonely Sad Dull Boring PC TOWN"	"Neil DeGRASSE Tyson induces your interest in science (substrate works less)	"MISS C is a boring teacher and will inhibit your interest in science (aka she is toxic)"
Lidocaine Sirolimus/Simvastatin (lova) Digoxin/Dapsone Benzodiazepines Protease inh/Pimozide/ PPIs **Cyclosporine** Colchicine/ **Corticosteroids** Cyclophosphamide/ Cisapride Tacrolimus **OCPs** **Warfarin** Nifedipine (and other CCBs)	**Griseofulvin** **Rifampin (most potent)** Anticonvulsants (phenytoin) Antiretrovirals Steroids **St. Johns Wart** Ethanol (chronic use)	**Macrolides** (except azithro) Metronidazole **Itraconazole** Isotretinoin SSRIs **Sulfonamides** **Cimetidine**/CCBs **Ciprofloxacin** **Grapefruit juice**

Cytochrome P-450 system

- The CYP enzymes which metabolize drugs are located in the ER of hepatocytes
- CYP inhibitors result in toxicity of substrates while inducers result in ↓ efficacy
    - Example: itraconazole will ↑ cyclosporine levels while griseofulvin will ↓ levels

For the other CYP isoforms just know which main inhibitors will result in toxicity of substrates

- CYP1A2: Antibiotics (macrolides/fluoroquinolones) will ↑ warfarin/theophylline levels
- CYP2C9: fluconazole, Cimetidine and Clopidogrel will ↑ warfarin and phenytoin levels
- CYP2D6: **terbinafine**, Delavirdine, Diphenhydramine, Donepezil and **Doxepin** will ↑ anti-Depressants/psychotics/arrhythmics and **β-blocker levels (hypotension/bradycardia)**
- Notice, that of all systemic antifungals, only terbinafine has no effect on warfarin levels

High yield examples

- Terbinafine increases toxicity of β-blockers (bradycardia)
- Azole antifungals, macrolides and cimetidine can ↑ effect of warfarin (bleeding), and ↑ toxicity to lidocaine and cyclosporine ("hyper-KLUTS" mnemonic")
- St. John's wart can make OCPs less effective (warn your Accutane patients)

Chapter 3: General dermatology

3.1 Papulosquamous Dermatoses

Psoriasis

- Two distinct peaks (20–30 years old and 50–60 years old)
- Pathogenesis
  - HLA associations
    - HLA-Cw6 (PSORS1) is the strongest association ("C-Why-a-six")
      - (+) in 50% of cases, 75% of guttate, 90% of early-onset psoriasis
    - HLA-B13 and HLA-B17: a/w erythrodermic and guttate psoriasis
      - "In psoriatic patients, ery (every) gutt is 13 to 17 inches too wide"
    - HLA-B27: a/w sacroiliitis-associated psoriasis
    - HLA-DR3: a/w palmoplantar pustulosis
  - Immunologic factors
    - T-cell disorder with increased Th1 cytokines and ↓ IL-10
    - ↑ DCs in psoriatic skin → ↑ IL-23 Th17 cell stimulation → ↑ IL-17, -22 → ↑ keratinocytes which secrete antimicrobial factors ("A CHIP" is ↑)
      - Anti-leukoproteinase
      - Cathelicidin (LL-37): this is ↓ in atopic dermatitis
      - Human β-defensins (hBD1 and 2): this is ↓ in atopic dermatitis
      - Involucrin (not an antimicrobial factor, but it is ↑ in psoriasis)
      - Psoriasin

        - ↑CXCL8 → neutrophil chemotaxis
    - **K6 & K16** ("psoria-six") expression are ↑ in hyperproliferative psoriatic plaques
    - Triggers: "SICK TAN LIMBS" (TAN drugs have shorter latency periods; < 1 month)
        - Stress, Shots (alcohol), Infections (strept throat), ↓Ca, Köebnerization
        - Terbinafine, TNF-α inhibitors, ACE inhibitors, NSAIDS
        - **Lithium**, IFNs, Immune checkpoint inhibitors, anti-Malarials, Mesotherapy, **β-blockers**, Stopping Steroids, Smoking
- Clinical features
    - Plaque psoriasis: p/w symmetric well-defined red plaques with micaceous scale
        - Auspitz sign: plucking off psoriatic plaque → pinpoint bleeding
        - Woronoff ring (blanching around plaque): White oval ring on/off plaque
    - Guttate psoriasis: p/w symmetric well-defined drop-like lesions on the trunk and proximal extremities of kids (MC after perianal or oropharyngeal group A strept)
    - Erythrodermic psoriasis: generalized (> 90% BSA) erythema and scale MC due to abrupt withdrawal of systemic steroids or psoriatic medications
    - **Pustular psoriasis (↑ IL-36; "say 36 pustules")**: "Psoriatic Pustules are AALIVE"
        - Palmoplantar Pustulosis: pustules and yellow-brown macules on the palms/soles (chronic course); a/w inflammatory bone lesions (SAPHO)
        - Acrodermatitis continua of Hallopeau: purulent distal digits → nails shed
        - Annular pattern: pustules at advancing annular edge

      - Localized pattern: pustules at edge of existing psoriatic plaques
      - Impetigo herpetiformis: generalized pustular psoriasis in pregnancy which begins in the flexures (esp. groin); a/w hypocalcemia
        - Risk to fetus: placental insufficiency, still-birth, neonatal death
        - Rx: early delivery (systemic steroids if early delivery not possible)
      - Von Zumbusch: rapid and generalized pustules with painful skin and fever
        - Labs: ↑ WBCs, ↓ albumin, ↓ Calcium (risk factor)
      - Exanthematous type: presents like mild AGEP
- Site specific psoriatic sub-types
  - Scalp: overlaps with seborrheic dermatitis in this area ("sebo-psoriasis")
    - May present with **pityriasis amiantacea**
      - The Rx (10 Percent SAL aCid) also reminds you of the MC causes
        - Psoriasis > Seborrheic dermatitis > AD > Lice > T. Capitus
        - **Salicylic acid (t-sal) may cause tinnitus, N/V, acidosis, CRF**
  - Inverse psoriasis: red well-defined plaques without scale in intertriginous sites
  - Oral: annulus migrans (geographic tongue)
  - Nail psoriasis: fingers > toes (onychomycosis is opposite pattern)
    - Pitting: Parakeratosis in the Proximal matrix
    - Leukonychia, red spots in lanula ("colors"): distal matrix
    - Oil Spots (Salmon patches), Splinter hemorrhages, Subungual hyperkeratosis, onycholysis: nail bed affected ("Snail bed")

- Psoriatic arthritis
  - p/w morning joint stiffness that improves w/ activity
  - Highly a/w nail changes and tendon/ligament involvement (enthesitis)
  - Five distinct patterns in order of prevalence: "OD RAM"
    - Oligoarthritis (60%): DIP + PIP joints (sausage digits); spares MCP (vs RA)
    - DIP involvement only (16%): sausage digits
    - RA-like (15%): symmetric polyarthritis of small and medium joints
    - Anklyosing spondylitis (5%): Axial involvement; a/w HLA-B27, IBD, uveitis
    - Mutilating arthritis (4%): osteolysis of phalanges → "telescoping"
- Complications ("psoriatics CUM fast"): **CV disease**, Cancer, Uveitis, Metabolic syndrome
- Path: neutrophils above confluent parakeratosis in stratum corneum, alternating neutrophils and parakeratosis (sandwich sign), regular acanthosis, thin suprapapillary plates, hypogranulosis, clubbed rete ridges, neutrophils in stratum corneum (Munro microabscesses; "Marilyn Monro is always on top"), neutrophils in stratum spinosum (spongiform pustules of Kogoj), dilated capillaries in dermal papillae
  - Guttate: spongiosis and mounded parakeratosis w/ milder acanthosis
  - Pustular: large clusters of neutrophils in the upper epidermis
- Rx ("CBDC ATM")
  - Topicals/light/diet: Corticosteroids, UVB, vit D analogs, CNIs, Anthralin, Tapinarof, Tazarotene, Tar, low caloric Mediterranean diet (and roflumilast)
  - Systemic: Cyclosporine, Biologics, Deucravacitinib, oral Corticosteroids (only for impetigo her-

petiformis), Apremilast, Acitretin, Tofacitinib Methotrexate

- Biologics (all SC except infliximab which is IV)
  - TNF-α: adalimumab, etanercept, infliximab, certolizumab
  - IL-12 and -23 inhibitor: ustekinumab
  - IL-23: guselkumab, tildrakizumab, risankizumab, mirikizumab
  - IL-17 (IBS): Ixekizumab, Bimekizumab, Brodalumab, Secukinumab
  - IL-36 inh: **spesolimab** for generalized pustular psoriasis flares

- Before starting biologics or MTX, obtain a QuantiFERON (if quant + but CXR - pt must complete 9 months of isoniazid ppx but can start systemic drug after 1–2 months of ppx)
- Next best step for psoriatic subtypes: pustular (acitretin; "think retinoids for pustular acne"), psoriatic arthritis (biologics, MTX or **apremilast**), impetigo herpetiformis (early delivery), Guttate (**UVB +/- penicillin**), erythrodermic (cyclosporine or acitretin)

Conditions with two distinct peaks: "Some Lesions Have Distinct Peaks"
Sarcoidosis (25–35 years old; 45–65 years old)
Leprosy (10–15 years old; 30–60 years old)
Linear IgA bullous dermatosis (< 4 years old; > 60 years old)
LS&A (prepubertal; post-menopausal)
Herpetic whitlow (< 10 years old; 20–40 years old)
Dermatomyositis (5–15 years old; 45–65 years old)
Psoriasis (20–30 years old; 50–60 years old)
Pityriasis rubra pilaris (< 10 years old; 50–60 years old)

Pityriasis rubra pilaris (PRP)

- Unknown etiology; may be inherited (AD mutation in CARD14/PSOR2) which presents at very young age (CARD14-associated papulosquamous eruption → Rx: ustekinumab)

- Bimodal age distribution (1st and 6th decade)
- Classic presentation: follicular scaling papules on red base which begins on head/neck and progresses caudally (**keratotic "nutmeg grater" papules** on dorsal hands/fingers)
  - Papules coalesce into orange to salmon-colored plaques **w/ islands of sparing**
  - Orange waxy keratoderma on palms/soles; psoriatic nail changes (but no pitting)
- Six distinct subtypes (all except type 4 are generalized; all except 1 and 3 are chronic)
  - Type 1 (55%): classic presentation in an adult; resolves in 3 years
  - Type 2 (5%; "K sounds"): atypical adult form w/ Chronic course, ichthyotic legs, and Coarse Keratoderma
  - Type 3 (10%): classic juvenile form which mimics type 1
  - Type 4 (25%) **most common juvenile form** which p/w localized follicular papules on red base on the elbows, knees and distal extremities
  - Type 5 (5%): atypical juvenile form w/ sclerodermoid changes on the **hands/feet**
  - Type 6 (1%): similar to type 1 but a/w **HIV**, acne conglobate, HS, lichen spinulosa
    - Does not respond to classic therapies but may respond to HAART
- a/w solid organ malignancies (RCC, HCC and bronchogenic carcinoma)
- Overlap syndrome w/ dermatomyositis: Wong-type DM has overlap of DM and PRP
  - "There's nothing Wong with sliding in her DMs but People Recognize Players"
- Path: alternating orthohyper- and parakeratosis ("checkerboard pattern"), follicular plugging w/ parakeratosis (vs neuts in seb derm) next to follicular ostia

(corresponds w/ follicular prominence seen clinically), psoriasiform hyperplasia w/ **thick** suprapapillary plates (vs thin in psoriasis) and acanthosis w/ focal **acantholysis** (nice clue)
- Rx: psoriasis meds (MTX, acitretin, TNFs, IL-17s) except phototherapy (worsens PRP)

Seborrheic dermatitis

- M > F; infantile (Self-limited) and adult (chronic) forms
- Pathogenesis: link to Sebum overproduction by androgens and Malassezia overgrowth
- a/w Strokes, HIV, Parkinson disease, and mood disorders
- Clinical features
    - Infantile: begins 1 week after birth (vs AD which does not begin for months) with greasy Scale adherent to the vertex and anterior Scalp ("cradle cap") w/ acutely inflamed (but not pruritic) lesions in the folds (axillae, neck, groin: diaper ddx)
    - Adult: Symmetric, Sharply demarcated pink patches with greasy Scales on the Scalp, eyebrows, NL folds, ears, chest w/ pityriasis simplex capillitia (dandruff)
- Path: Spongiosis w/ Superficial PV/PF lymph infiltrate w/ parakeratosis and neutrophils on the Shoulder of follicular ostia
- Rx
    - Infantile: bathing, emollients, ketoconazole cream, keratolytics for thick scale
    - Adult: emollients, topical azoles, ciclopirox, low-potency topical steroids (2nd line treatments include zinc pyrithione, selenium sulfide, tar shampoos, and TCIs)

Pityriasis rosea (PR)

- Onset 10–35 y/o; F > M
- Likely viral etiology (**HHV-6, -7**)
- **PR p/w herald patch (large solitary Pink annular Plaque w/ trailing collarette of scale)** which heralds (by days) a generalized eruption of smaller oval scaly plaques which orient along Langer's lines/Relaxed skin tension lines ("**Christmas tree pattern**")
  - o Plaques are darker and more papular in darker skin tones
- Atypical variants: unilateral, inverse, vesicular, urticarial-like and EM-like
- Drug-induced PR ("alphabet drugs"): **ACE inhibitors (MC)**, Allopurinol, Accutane, β-blockers, Barbiturates, Bismuth, Clonidine, Diuretics (HCTZ), "ENSAIDS", Flagyl (metronidazole), Gold, HCTZ (notice there are many blood pressure meds)
  - o Typically appear more red-violet in color and do not p/w herald patch
- Path (PR): non-adherent thin mounds of Parakeratosis (guttate psoriasis has adherent thick-mounds), RBC extravasation, PV lymphocytic infiltrate and mild spongiosis
- Rx: self-resolves in 2 months; antihistamines and topical steroids if pruritic; if severe can hasten resolution w/ oral acyclovir or erythromycin; D/C any implicated drugs

Granular Parakeratosis

- Occurs mainly in adult women; likely due to anti-Perspirants or other skin care Products
- Defect processing Profilaggrin to filaggrin → retention of keratohyalin granules
- p/w Persistent Pruritic Purple Papules or Plaques in the folds (axillae is MC)

- **Path: thick stratum corneum w/ Prominent Parakeratosis w/ retained keratohyalin granules and a Paradoxically ↑/normal granular layer**
- Rx: largely unsuccessful; try topical Psoriasis drugs (steroids, vit D analogs, tazarotene)

Erythroderma

- p/w erythema and scale covering nearly the entire body (> 90% BSA)
- MC symptoms ("PADS"): Pruritis (MC; 90%); Adenopathy, Dehydration, Swelling
- Most severe complications: fluid and electrolyte abnormalities, high-output heart failure
- MC causes in order of frequency is "PADS"
    - Psoriasis (MC): usually due to drug withdrawal (MTX, steroid, cyclosporine)
    - Atopic dermatitis: p/w **severe pruritis**, lichenification and eosinophilia
    - **Drug reaction (MCC in HIV patients)**: allopurinol, antibiotics, antiepileptics, CCBs, opiates, gold, isoniazid, retinoids, lithium, thiazides, quinidine, thalidomide
    - Sézary syndrome: T-cell clone in blood plus one of the following: > 1000 Sézary cells/microliter, CD4:CD8 ratio > 10:1 or CD4+ cells w/ abnormal phenotype
    - Less common causes include PRP, GVHD, tinea, dermatomyositis
- Dx: KOH (tinea), biopsy (usually not diagnostic), flow cytometry (Sézary), ↑ eos (AD)
- Rx ("PADS"): Prednisone (1st rule out psoriasis → pustular psoriasis flare upon discontinuation), Admit to hospital (monitor fluids/electrolytes), D/C underlying meds and treat underlying condition, treat Secondary bacterial infections

Confluent and reticulated papillomatosis (CARP)

- Starts at puberty; MC in POC
- **p/w brown, rough, keratotic papules (acanthosis nigricans-like) MC on the Chest and back → papules coalesce into plaques in a reticulate pattern**
- Path: acanthosis nigricans-like (hyperkeratosis, acanthosis, papillomatosis)
- Rx: **minocycline** ("Carp is a type of fish which makes me think of minos")
- Pseudoatrophoderma Colli is a variant that appears on the neck (Rx minocycline)

Pityriasis rotunda

- Asymptomatic dermatosis seen in Mediterranean, African and far East ethnicities
- p/w large (>10 cm) annular hyperpigmented plaque w/ fine scale
- a/w malnutrition, mycobacterial infections and malignancy
- Dx: KOH is negative
- Path: looks like ichthyosis vulgaris (orthokeratosis w/ paradoxically ↓ granular layer)
- Rx: search for and treat underlying disorder; topical retinoids may be beneficial

3.2 Eczematous Dermatoses

Atopic dermatitis (AD; "Eczema")

- Part of the atopic march: "you can see atopics marching from AFAR"
    - o **AD and Food allergy (infants)**, Asthma (children), Rhinitis (adolescents)
- MC in high income/urban areas (↑ allergens/pollutants; poor skin microbiome)

- MC subset is Early onset (most pts with AD are affected by 1 year) which have allergen specific IgE autoAbs but late onset (after puberty) and senile onset (after 60) also occur
- A family history of atopic disease is the strongest known risk factor for AD
- Pathogenesis: Epidermal barrier dysfunction, IgE immune dysregulation, Environment
    - Barrier dysfunction: loss of function of filaggrin (strongest genetic risk factor; severe early onset AD), ↓ proteases (KLK5, KLK7) and abnormal lipids corneocyte dysfunction and ↑ trans-epidermal water loss (c/w disease severity)
    - Immune dysregulation: **Th2** (**thymic stromal lymphopoietin**, IL-4, **-13**, 31) and **Th22** (IL-22) cytokines → ↑ IgE production (chronic AD has Th1 predominance)
    - Environmental factors: scratching leads to penetration of environmental irritants and allergens → altered skin microbiome (↑ staph aureus)
- Mediators of itch: neuropeptides, proteases, kinins, cytokines (IL-31), TRPV1 (acts via afferent C fibers), Mas-related G protein-coupled receptor (chronic AD) >> histamine
- Clinical features based on lesion stage
    - Acute: Edematous, Erythematous papules and plaques +/- oozing, vesicles, crust
    - Chronic: thickened lichenified plaques +/- prurigo nodules
        - Perifollicular accentuation (papular eczema) is common in AA and Asians
- Clinical features based on age of patient
    - Infantile AD (**age < 2 years**): acute lesion morphology on the head/neck (esp. chEEks) and Extensor Extremities (**spares diaper area** vs seb derm)

        - The "Headlight sign" has been used to describe the typical sparing of the nose and medial cheek, even when there is extensive lateral involvement
    - Childhood/adolescent AD: chronic lesions on Ears (esp Earlobe and retroauricular), nipple ("ar-E-ola"), lips (cheilitis sicca: ICD > ACD > AD), flexures (antecubital fossa, neck), discoid lesions, hands/feet (dyshidrotic eczema, juvenile plantar dermatosis), frictional lichenoid eruption (Elbows > knees)
    - Adult/senile AD: marked xerosis, prurigo-like lesions, chronic hand eczema, Eyelids (involvement of periorbital skin vs other forms of eyelid dermatitis)
- Associated features: alopecia areata, Exaggerated skin markings (Dennie-Morgan folds on the lower lids, allergic salute on nasal crease, palmar/plantar hyperlinearity, anterior neck folds), white dermographism (central facial pallor, pityriasis alba, PIH), follicular prominence (AAs), periorbital darkening, KP, xerosis, ichthyosis, Hortoghe sign
    - Hortoghe sign is thinning of the LATeral eyebrow seen in Leprosy, AD, Thyroid
- Pruritis: worse with Exertion/stress/sweating and worse in the Evening → Excoriations
- Complications: bacterial (impetigo) and viral (eczema herpeticum) infections, **cardiac issues (Embolism/clot)**, **Eyes** (keratoconjunctivitis, corneal Elongation), alopecia areata
- Path
    - Acute: prominent spongiosis w/ PV lymphs and eos +/- epidermal vesiculation
    - Subacute: milder spongiosis w/ ↑ acanthosis
    - Chronic: marked irregular psoriasiform acanthosis with no spongiosis

- Dx: testing for aeroallergens (dust mites, pollen, fungi, animal dander) and **allergens in food ("White SPERM" is MC: Wheat, Soy, Peanuts, Eggs, Raw seafood, Milk)** with fluorescence enzyme immunoassays/ RAST testing (blood test that detects specific IgE antibodies), skin prick testing (detects immediate allergic reactions) and patch testing
  - Eggs is the food most often linked to Eczema flares
  - Consider limited food allergy testing in children < 5 y/o w/ mod-severe AD if…
    - They have persistent AD despite optimized management or…
    - Reliable history of immediate allergic reaction after eating a specific food
- Concomitant food allergy can cause treatment refractory dermatitis in infants (esp around the mouth like the chEEks) → **Rx: change diet**/switch to hypoallergenic formula
  - However, food allergens usually cause a type 1 hypersensitivity (e.g., urticaria) and elimination may not affect AD
- Rx: lukewarm showers, **moisturizers**, avoid fragrances, **avoid food/other allergens**
  - Topicals: steroids, crisaborole (PDE-4 inhibitor), TCIs, ruxolitinib (JAK), tapinarof
  - Phototherapy: induces T-cell apoptosis, ↓ dendritic cells, ↓Th2 cytokines
  - Systemic: cyclosporine, MTX, MMF, dupilumab (IL-4, -13), nemolizumab (IL-31), abrocitinib/baricitinib/upadacitinib (JAKs), tralokinumab/lebrikizumab (IL-13),
  - Adjunctive therapy: antimicrobials/antiseptics, antihistamines, omalizumab
  - ppx: moisturize baby and give vitamin D or **probiotics to pregnant mothers**

- Boards fact: natural infection w/ measles has been shown to mitigate atopic dermatitis
- Boards fact: **CCBs** are a known cause of drug-induced eczema

Asteatotic eczema

- Common in the elderly
- Pathogenesis: ↓ stratum corneum lipids, altered ratio of fatty acids esterified to ceramide-1, persistence of corneodesmosomes, premature expression of involucrin, ↓ natural moisturizing factor → ↓ water-binding capacity of stratum corneum → xerosis
- p/w xerosis of the shins (MC) w/ inflammation and white scales (pseudo-ichthyosis)
- Path: appears normal except for compact stratum corneum + spongiotic dermatitis
- Rx: topical corticosteroid ointment + emollients (petrolatum, urea, ceramide, lactic acid)

AuToSensitization (id reaction and disseminated eczema)

- Disseminated eczema develop after primary ACD/ICD, Tinea (pedis is MC) or Stasis derm
  - In children id reaction MC occurs after kerion/ severe **t. capitus** or ACD to nickel
- Pathogenesis: hematogenous dissemination of Allergens, circulating memory T cells, ↓ Sensitization threshold at distant sites
- p/w erythematous eczematous papulovesicles MC on upper extremities
  - In cases of t. pedis it p/w vesicles on lateral fingers (mimics dyshidrotic eczema)
  - **In cases of tinea capitis, it commonly presents on the face**
- Ddx (other widespread eczemas): AD, airborne/photo-ACD, eczematous drug rash, MF
- Path: Acute or Subacute Spongiotic dermatitis

- Rx: Antihistamines, **Treat underlying cause** and **topical Steroids** (if id reaction develops after starting antifungals for tinea, continue the antifungal and add topical steroids)

Nummular dermatitis

- Pathogenesis: unknown but a/w contact allergens (nickel, cobalt), venous HTN, atopy
- Can occur w/ AD, Asteatotic eczema, and Stasis dermatitis ("that ASS makes me numb")
- p/w pruritic round/discoid eczematous patches on the extremities (legs in M; arms in F)
- Path: subacute to chronic dermatitis
- Rx: high-potency topical steroid ointments

HTLV-associated infective dermatitis

- Affects children and adolescents (Toddlers to Teens) in Third world countries
- Pathogenesis: **Human T-cell lymphotropic virus type 1 (HTLV-1)** infects T-cells, B-cells and monocytes and causes immune system dysregulation → infection and eczema
- p/w crusty eczematous dermatosis affecting the **Head/neck and inter-Triginous sites**
    - Chronic watery rhinorrhea w/ crusts in the nasal cavity is a good clue
- Dx: HTLV-1 positivity on PCR or Western blot
- Rx: long term systemic antibiotic therapy (TMP-SMX is TOC) until puberty

Stasis dermatitis

- Pathogenesis: leaky leg valves → venous HTN and extravasation of venous contents into the interstitium → edema, fibrosis, inflammation and ulceration
    - "Legs in stasis dermatitis drain MILK"

  - **Medial ankle** is the first site effected (MC site for venous ulcers)
  - Inverted wine bottle appearance (Lipodermatosclerosis)
  - Kontact (contact) sensitization to topical antibiotics is common
- Contact sensitization commonly leads to secondary dissemination (id reaction)
- Path: spongiotic dermatitis with lobular ("cannon ball") capillary hyperplasia, fibrin cuffing, hemosiderin and dermal fibrosis
- Rx: **compression** socks/elevation + topical steroids
- Workup: consider patch testing for sudden worsening of symptoms

Dyshidrotic eczema

- Not an independent entity but a manifestation of other types of eczema (AD/ICD/ACD)
- a/w sweaty hands, hot climates, emotional stress, and **IVIG administration**
- **p/w symmetric, firm, Deep-seated vesicles on the palms/sides of Digits** (fingers > toes)
- Dyshidrosis lamellose sicca (keratolysis exfoliativa) is a mild variant which displays small annular collarettes of white scale but no vesicles
- Path: spongiotic dermatitis with micro- and macrovesicles within the epidermis
- Rx: keep hands Dry, potent topical steroids, PUVA, Dupilumab, Dysport/botox injections

Progesterone dermatitis

- p/w cyclic flares of dermatitis in the luteal phase of the menstrual cycle (flares 1 week before menses and resolves a few days after menses)
- Dx: intradermal injection of progesterone causes a skin reaction

- Rx: OCPs to inhibit ovulation

Topical steroid withdrawal (TSW) syndrome (from 2015 JAAD meta-analysis)

- Underrecognized disorder that presents shortly after topical steroid discontinuation
- MC occurs in adult women who use mid to high-potency topical steroids for > 1 year on the face (genitals is 2nd MC location) to treat their atopic dermatitis (cosmetic use for pigmentary disorders is 2nd MC condition being treated by steroids which causes TSW)
- Pathogenesis: largely unknown but vascular dilation, immune dysregulation and adrenal suppression following long-term use of topical steroids may be to blame
- Papulopustular and erythematoedematous types exist
    - Papulopustular: more likely to occur when steroids used for cosmetic purposes
        - p/w pustules, papules, erythema, burning/stinging > edema
    - Erythematoedematous: more likely to occur when steroids used for dermatitis
        - p/w intense erythema w/ sharp cutoff between affected cheeks and unaffected ears and nose ("headlight sign"; "reverse Rudolf sign"), burning, stinging, pain, pruritis, scaling, desquamation/peeling, crusting, swelling/edema, and diminished tolerance for emollients
- Path: thinned epidermis w/thinned/absent granular layer, spongiosis, numerous dilated dermal BVs w/ prominent sebaceous glands and degeneration of collagen fibers
- Workup: patch testing (rule out ACD to steroids/preservatives) and photo patch testing
- Rx: **D/C topical steroids**, antibiotics, pain management, and psychological support

- Consider TSW if burning is the prominent symptom, confluent erythema occurs days to weeks following topical steroid discontinuation and a history of frequent/prolonged topical steroid use on the face or genitals

Contact dermatitis

Irritant contact dermatitis (ICD)

- Four times more common than ACD
- Caused by direct damage of keratinocytes by irritant (most commonly by soaps)
    - Acids/bases cause acute ICD by direct cytotoxic damage to keratinocytes
    - Soap/water cause chronic ICD by removing lipids (↑ transepidermal water loss)
- Affects areas where soaps go (**hands** #1, face #2) and produce **burning** > itch
- Three types of irritant contact dermatitis: "Irritating APP"
    - Airborne ICD: rash includes upper eyelids, philtrum and submental region
    - Pustular ICD (LMNOP): Liquid metals, Metals, Naphthalenes, Oil (croton/mineral)
    - Phytophotodermatitis: furocoumarins + UVA light → erythema 1–3 days post-contact then hyperpigmentation 1–3 weeks post-contact
        - Berloque dermatitis: pigmentation from cologne (bergamot oil)
- Main types of specific contactants: "fiberglass AAPP"
    - Fiberglass dermatitis: p/w pruritic pink papules
    - Alkalis: worse reactions than acids (e.g., ammonia); Rx: weak acid (vinegar)
    - Acids: "This Nice SHHOP sells acid"
        - Nitric acid: burns skin yellow

- Sulfuric acid: burns skin brown (sulfur comes from dirt which is brown)
- Hydrofluoric acid: deep (bones) and delayed (1 day) burn
  - Hydro-FLOOR-ic acids burns deep down to the floor (painful)
  - Since their bones are burning treat with **Calcium Gluconate**
- Hydrochloric acid: superficial (blisters) and immediate burn
- Oxalic acid: hypocalcemia and gangrene of hands (ox has black hooves)
- Phenol: burns skin white (think frosting from Baker Gordon peel)
  - Systemic absorption causes arrythmias and glomerulonephritis
  - Neutralize with 65% ethyl or isopropyl alcohol

o Poop and other bodily fluids (saliva, urine); Rx: barrier protection (zinc paste)

o Plants: "This Nice CAMP has bad plants"

- Non-immunologic contact urticaria: stinging Nettle (urticaceae family)
  - A nettle HAS these toxins: Histamine, Acetylcholine and Serotonin
- Chemical ICD
  - Bromelain found in pineapples (Anas cosmosus)
    - o "Bros put pineapples in Anas cosmos"
  - Calcium oxalate found in Daffodils (Narcissus) and **Dumb Canes** (Dieffenbachia) and causes eczema in florists
    - o Dumb canes are common household plants; if eaten cause mucosal burn-

ing/edema/blistering/aphonia ("Can't talk")

- Capsaicin found in hot peppers (family Solanacea)
  - o Sol is sun in Spanish so makes you think "hot"
- Phorbol esters found in spurges, poinsettias and croton plants (family Euphorbiacea) → may cause temporary blindness
  - o "I phorbid ester from splurging on pointless Kratom tea. It produces euphoria but the tea can blind her from reality."
- Ranunculin found in buttercups produce linear vesicles
  - o "Ran straight (linear) to the buttercups"
- Thiocyanates found in garlic, black mustard and radish
  - o "All things that go on poisonous (cyanide) hotdogs"

▪ ACD (discussed in ACD section)

▪ Mechanical ICD: prickly pears (opuntia spp) produce glochid dermatitis

- Remove spines w/ tweezers and Rx for organisms that SAT on the spine (S. aureus, Sporotrichosis, Atypical mycobacteria, Tetanus)

▪ Phytophotodermatitis: phototoxic reaction (dermatitis within 24 hours; no prior sensitization required) due to plants that produce furocoumarins (psoralens) that are photosensitizing in the presence of UVA → "produces a pigment pattern on the ARM that looks Fabulous"

- **Apiacea/Umbelliferae (MCC) causes**
    - Parsley, parsnips, dill, **celery**, carrots
        - Hands of gardeners and grocery shop workers
    - Hogweeds, cow parsley and wild chervil
        - Linear vesicles on legs of weed wackers
    - "I imagine an Ape (apiacea) holding up an Umbrella (umbelliferae) because all these plants look like umbrellas"
- Rutaceae causes berloque dermatitis, dermatitis in bartenders (citrus fruits) and dermatitis from Hawaiian leis (flower necklace)
    - "I always Root (rut) for putting on cologne and going out for drinks with a Hawaiian lei around my neck"
- Moraceae: Mulberries and figs
    - "You always need More Mulberry-colored figs (scrubs)"
- Fabeaceae (legumes): Bavache pea and Balsam of Peru
    - "You see some fabulous legs in Bavache, Peru"
- Rx: topical steroids/cold compresses +/- hydroquinone (for PIH)
    - Plant extract takes 30 to 120 minutes to absorb so immediately wash skin after contact w/ plant

Allergic contact dermatitis (ACD)

- Most common cause is **Nickel (worldwide)** and **poison ivy (USA)**
- Caused by an immune mediated, delayed type hypersensitivity (sensitization required)

- Pathogenesis: upon re-exposure to allergen, LCs take up antigen and express **IL-1β** → migration of APCs to LNs to present antigen to native T-cells → T-cell activation
- Like all forms of spongiotic dermatitis, morphology depends on chronicity → p/w oozing and vesiculation (acute) vs acanthosis and crusting (subacute) vs lichenification (chronic)
- Distribution depends on exposure to allergen
  - **Linear streaks on extremities: rhus dermatitis (poison ivy/oak/sumac)**
  - Finger**tips** in florists: tul**ips** (tuliposide; α-methylene-β-hydroxy-γ-butyrolactone)
  - Hand dermatitis: **dorsal (ICD is MC)**, palmar (endogenous causes like dyshidrosis is MC) and **both palmar AND dorsal (ACD** from soaps, moisturizers and gloves)
    - Hand is MC location to result in negative patch test (generalized is 2nd)
  - Face: lateral face ("wash-off pattern") is due to shampoos and conditioners whereas central face is due to makeup (titanium dioxide, which is present in sunscreens and makeup, activates gold as an allergen and can cause facial ACD)
  - Eyelid: nail products like tosylamide ("toes makes you think of nails which you rub your eyes with"), **gold** rings ("eyes on gold") and shampoos and conditioners
    - **ICD is in eyelid creases** (intertriginous space when eyes are open → ↑ irritant absorption), **ACD involves eyelids AND beyond the boney orbit**
  - **Earlobe: nickel**
  - Waistline and where clothes fit tight (**spares axillary vault**): formaldehyde, formaldehyde releas-

ers, 106/124 **blue dyes**, carbamates (released by bleaching)
  - "Get in better form, like around 106 to 124 lbs by releasing carbs so you don't get an ACD when you wear tight clothes"
- Perianal: Wet Wipes (Methylisothiazolinone and Methylchloroisothiazolinone)
  - These chemicals have now been removed from leave-on products
- MCC of shoe dermatitis (spares webspace and instep) is **Mercaptobenzothiazole (rubber)** > Chromates like **potassium dichromate** (leather), Colophony (adhesive), Carbamix, Cobalt, p-tert-butylphenol formaldehyde resin (adhesive)
- Ulcers: Neomycin, Bacitracin, **Balsam of Peru** and Lanolin ("New Bottom Layer")
- Oral stomatitis (perioral erythema): Cinnamon/**cinnamates**, Gold, Amalgam and Mercury in dental fillings and Epoxy resins ("Cinnamon GAME")
- Airborne ACD: plants, most commonly **cOmpOsitae** (air is made up of O^2)
  - Involves areas normally shaded from photodermatitis like the eyelids, nasolabial folds and the submental region

High-yield ACD allergens

Metals: "A GNC Milkshake will make you strong like metal"

- Aluminum
  - 2022 American Contact Dermatitis Society allergen of the year
  - Produces reactions to vaccines and **patch test chambers (everything lights up)**
    - "All tested allergens react during a patch test in an Aluminum allergy"

- Gold
  - Found in jewelry and dental fillings and causes facial dermatitis (when combined w/ makeup/sunscreen), oral lichenoid reactions, and eyelid dermatitis (eyes on gold)
    - Titanium dioxide (found in sunscreens and makeup) activates gold as an allergen and causes ACD on face (switch from gold to platinum jewelry)
  - MCC of **persistently positive patch test reaction** and **delayed patch test reaction**
    - "It takes time and patience to acquire gold"
  - MCC of black dermographism: products such as those found in makeup and sunscreens (zinc oxide and **titanium dioxide**) abrade the metals off jewelry (gold, silver, copper, nickel, and iron) and cause this black skin discoloration
    - "The relentless pursuit of gold can turn your soul black"
  - Cross-reacts (immune system recognizes similar chemicals) w/ nickel and cobalt
    - "GNC cross reacts with each other"
- Nickel
  - **MCC of + patch test rxn** (poison ivy is MCC of ACD in US but is not in patch tests)
  - Found in jewelry, phones, zippers/buttons and foods like Nuts (peanuts, walnuts, almonds, hazelnuts) but also beans, lentils, spinach, licorice and cocoa/chocolate
  - Safe metals for pts w/ nickel allergy: sterling silver, stainless steel, platinum, titanium, rose gold, and yellow gold (**white gold** has nickel; "Nick is a white name")
    - **Dimethylglyoxime** ("di-Nethly…") **test** turns pink in presence of nickel

  - Baboon syndrome: symmetric eczematous eruption involving the elbows, axilla, eyelids, and sides of neck accompanied by bright red anogenital lesions
    - Pathogenesis: **allergic type IV reaction to systemically administered nickel > other allergens** (SDRIFE: drug-related type of Baboon syndrome)
- Chromates
  - Found in green felt on pool tables, cement, **leather**, **tattoo pigment**, matches
    - "Picture your mate Chris (chromate) as a guy playing pool on a cement floor with **leather shoes** and tattoos while lighting matches"
    - Chromates such as potassium dichromate are a common **occupational exposure in Cement workers**, bricklayers and Construction workers
- Cobalt (ABCDE)
  - 2016 American Contact Dermatitis Society allergen of the year
  - Found in Artificial joints, **vit B12** injections (vit B12 and cobalt may cross-react), Buttons, Cement, Ceramics, blue-green Dyes, glass potter-E (pottery)
  - Co-reacts (simultaneous exposure to two allergens w/o any immunologic basis) w/ nickel as these are commonly found together in various products
  - **Poral reaction**: ICD (toxic effect on acrosyringium) w/ brown pores (dermoscopy)
- Mercury
  - Found in amalgam (dentistry) and causes oral lichenoid reactions

Rubber and rubber additives: "Put on a rubber for some fun (phen) TLC MR"

- p-phenylenediamine (PPD)
  - Found in black **temporary tattoos**, black rubber, **dark hair dye**, and darkly colored cosmetics and

photograph development/photocopies/printer ink ("all dark ink")
        - "Temporary tattoos, rubber, hair dye and photographs are fun (phen)"
    - Presents as lichenoid hand dermatitis in rubber workers, hairdressers and photographers and presents as beard/scalp dermatitis in those who dye their hair or presents as dermatitis in the same pattern of a temporary tattoo
- Thiuram
    - Most common allergy in healthcare workers and **MCC of glove allergy**
        - Rx: switch from latex or nitrile to **vinyl gloves** (lacks rubber accelerators)
    - Bleach causes release from waistband and socks → eczema at waistline and feet
    - **Cross-reacts with disulfiram (Antabuse)**
        - "In the word Thiuram, the "TH" reminds me of health workers and the "RAM" reminds me that is cross-reacts with disulfiram
- Thioureas (neoprene; "Keanu Reeves plays Neo in the matrix")
    - Found in wet suits, goggles and knee braces/orthopedic supports
        - "Imagine Neo from The Matrix snorkeling with a knee brace"
    - Cross-reacts with **glutaraldehyde used in cold sterilization** procedures thus a surgeon/**dental assistant** who sterilizes would get this allergy
        - The "th" and "as" in thioureas reminds me of healthcare assistants"
- Latex
    - A pt w/ these qualities HAS (Healthcare workers, Atopic dermatitis, Spina bifida) ↑ risk of a latex-induced type 1 hypersensitivity immunologic contact urticaria

  - o Cross-reacts and cause oral/mucosal symptoms w/ ingestion of: "Eat fruit before latex sex to get Passion BACK" (Passion fruit, Banana, **Avocado**, Chestnut, **Kiwi**)
- Carba mix/Carbamates: released from bleached elastic; 2nd MCC of glove allergy; shoes
  - o Parts of the body where clothes are tight: waistband, hands (gloves), feet (shoes)
- Mercaptobenzothiazole (MBT)
  - o MCC of shoe dermatitis ("mecraptobenzothio-sole causes rash on the sole")
  - o Common cause of allergic diaper dermatitis
- Black Rubber mix: found in a variety of products (e.g., shoes, goggles)
  - o **Cross reacts with para-phenylenediamine (PPD)**

Adhesives: "the PRICE of Meth is that you'll get addicted to it and stick to it like glue"

- p-tert-butylphenol formaldehyde resin (PTBP)
  - o Adhesive used to glue leather (**shoes**, watches and purses) and rubber
  - o Can cause **a loss of pigmentation** ("occupational vitiligo")
- Rosin (colophony)
  - o Found in violins and other musical instruments, paint, chewing gum, de-epilation waxes, adhesives in shoes (shoe dermatitis) and hydro-colloid dressings
    - ▪ "Picture Rosi Cole who is playing the violin while also painting, chewing gum, waxing her leg hair and wearing shoes and hydrocolloid dressings"
- Isobornyl acrylate
  - o 2020 American Contact Dermatitis Society allergen of the year
  - o ACD related to **Insulin pumps/glucose monitors**

- Cyanoacrylates
  - Ethyl cyanoacrylate: used to glue on artificial nails ("ethyl has fake nails")
  - Butyl/octyl cyanoacrylate: closure of wounds without sutures
- Epoxy resin (bisphenol A)
  - Found in polyvinyl chloride (also causes scleroderma), plastic materials, and paint
- Methyl Methacrylate
  - Rigid plastic used in bone cement, artificial joints and in dental work
  - Diffuses through rubber and polyvinyl gloves to cause **parasthesias** and ACD on fingers of an **orthopedic surgeon or dentist**
    - "Surgeons/dentists shouldn't smoke meth or they'll get paresthesias"

Preservatives: "To preserve our friendship lets FaceTime in the PM"

- Formaldehyde
  - Found everywhere from meds to textiles to papers ("formaldehydes take many forms") but perhaps most notably in wrinkle free clothing
  - **Polyester has little to no formaldehyde (least of any clothing)**
    - "While playing tennis, Poly and Ester both have little to no form"
- Formaldehyde-releasing preservatives (chemicals that slowly release formaldehyde)
  - #2 cause of cosmetic (creams) related ACD behind fragrances
  - DMDM hydantoin, Diazolidinyl urea, Imidazolidinyl urea and Quaternium 15
    - "A DIQ releases various forms into the world that look like creams"

    - Quaternium-15 is found in soaps, shampoos and moisturizers ("skin Quare products") and is the #1 most "Quammon" preservative sensitizer in the USA
- Thimerosal (ethyl mercury)
    - Found in **hyaluronidase**, contact lenses and vaccines
        - "It's time ("thime") to say Hy to covid vaccines"
    - **MCC of clinically irrelevant patch test reactions** ("time is irrelevant")
    - Cross-reacts with Piroxicam and Mercury ("PM relates to time")
- Parabens
    - ACD society named it 2019 "non-allergen" of the year due to its low rate of ACD
    - Found in topical medications and cross-reacts with PPPASTA (Para-aminosalicylic acid, PABA (para-aminobenzoic acid), **PPD (p-paraphenylenediamine)**, Azo dyes, Sulfonamides, Thiazides, ester Anesthetics such as benzocaine)
- Methylchloroisothiazolinone/Methylisothiazolinone (kathon CG; MCI/MI)
    - Was found in Wet Wipes ("W is an upside-down M"); caused perianal dermatitis
    - Found in Water-based paints and may cause airborne ACD

Vehicles, emollients and emulsifiers

- Decyl glucoside
    - 2017 American Contact Dermatitis Society Allergan of the Year
    - **Foaming cleansers** ("Did you know Vin Diesel washes w/ foaming cleansers?")
    - Clue to rinse off products as the culprit is diffuse or poorly defined involvement

- Propylene glycol
    - Found in Antifreeze, Brake fluid, Creams, food Dyes, EKG jelly, Flavorings
    - **Both an irritant and an allergen** (ICD > ACD)
- Cocoamidopropyl betaine
    - Non-ionic surfactant found in shampoos/soaps and derived from coconut oil
- Ethylenediamine ("Ethyl's fun Baboon HAT")
    - Found in topical steroid and anti-fungal creams
    - Causes systemic ACD reaction (baboon syndrome); cross-reacts w/ **Hydroxyzine**, Aminophylline, Azines (piperazine), Theophylline to cause systemic ACD
        - Use **diphenhydramine** instead of hydroxyzine in ethylenediamine allergy
- Lanolin ("say lawnolin")
    - Allergy common in **Leg ulcer patients** ("New Bottom Layer")
    - Cross-reacts with **Aquaphor**
    - Allergan is a Wax-wool alcohol derived from **sheep** ("Baa like a sheep: Laanolin")
- Propolis ("say propolips")
    - Allergen found in lip balms and made by **bees**
    - Causes ACD of the **lips**

Fragrances: **MCC of cosmetic-related ACD** (**Finn chamber better than True-test for Fragrances**)

- Fragrance mix
    - Patch test has 8 fragrances including cinnamic alcohol and cinnamic aldehyde
    - **MCC of ACD in anogenital region**
    - Cross-reacts with propolis, colophony and turpentine
        - "Pro athletes, colons and turpins (fish) all smell bad and need fragrances"

- Balsam of Peru
  - Comes from Myroxylon pereirea tree
  - Key allergens are **cinnamic acid** and vanillin; cross-reacts w/ **tincture of Benzoin**
  - Common cause of ACD in venous ulcers ("New Bottom Layer")
  - Systemic contact dermatitis can occur w/ ingestion of citrus fruits, **tomatoes**, cinnamon, cloves, vanilla, curry, nutmeg, ginger, colas, wine, Beer, gin, and vermouth
- Lily of the valley
  - Found in perfumes, soaps, cosmetics, eye cream and aftershaves
  - Allergenic ingredient is hydroxycitronellal

Hair Products

- PPD (p-phenylenediamine): see above under "Rubber" heading for more info
  - Hand dermatitis in hairdressers and scalp dermatitis in those who use hair die
- Perms
  - Basic (home) perms contain **Ammonium Thioglycolate ("AT home")**
  - Acid (salon) perms contain Glyceryl monothioglycolate ("Go to salon")
- Hair bleach (contains ammonium persulfate and peroxides)
  - **Ammonium persulfate** causes a contact urticaria and generalized histamine rxn
    - "Bleaching your hair will make you let out a moan 2° to pruritis/urticaria"

Nail products

- Tosylamide, aka **toluene-sulfonamide** (know both names)

- Found in nail polish and causes **eyelid and peri-ungual dermatitis**
  - Nail polish goes on your toes and fingers which you rub your eye with
- Artificial nails are made of methacrylate and glued on w/ Ethyl cyanoacrylate

Medications

- Ester anesthetics
  - #1 sensitizer is benzocaine used for hemorrhoids (anesthetic for mucosa)
  - Cross-react with PPPASTA (PPD, PABA, PASA, Azo dyes, Sulfonamides, Thiazides)
- Antibiotics (neomycin, bacitracin, polymyxin)
  - Chronic leg ulcers are the main risk factor
  - **Neomycin co-reacts with bacitracin** and cross reacts with other aminoglycosides
- Corticosteroids ("AT BBs doing CBDH"): this classification may be outdated
  - Class A screening agent is Tixocortol pivalate (most allergenic class)
    - "People commonly react to the divisive topic of politix"
  - Class B screening agent is Budesonide (cross-reacts with agents in class D)
  - Class C screening agent is Betamethasone (least allergenic class)
    - "Beta Males don't react"
  - Class D screening agent is Hydrocortisone-17-butyrate (cross-reacts with class B)
  - Steroid being tested may suppress allergic reaction so delayed reading is critical
- Sunscreens
  - **Oxybenzone** is the MCC of allergic contact dermatitis from sunscreens

        - "All addicts want to get into contact with some oxy"
    - Cinnamates and PABA (cross react w/ Balsam of Peru and PPASTA, respectively)

Miscellaneous allergens

- Disperse blue dyes 106 and 124
    - Found on clothes so eczema **spares axillary vault**; seen on waistband area
- **Dimethylfumarate**
    - Antifungal agent used to prevent mold on Chinese **furniture** ("sofa dermatitis")
    - Dermatitis is usually seen on the posterior body and feet (touches couch)
- Acetophenone Azine
    - 2021 Allergen of the year
    - Found in Athletic wear (**footwear, goggles, athletic pads**) containing ethyl vinyl Acetate foam (not intentionally added but generated during manufacturing)

Patch testing

- T.R.U.E. test screens for 35 allergens and 1 control (use in adults)
- The Pediatric Baseline Series (PBS) contains 38 relevant pediatric allergens (use in kids)
- Apply allergens → patient **returns in 48 hours for 1st read** (remove patches and mark area w/ pen) → **2nd read is between 72 hours and 7 days after initial application**
- ICD tends to improve between initial reading and final reading, whereas ACD worsens
- Antihistamines do not affect results (no need to stop) but steroids do
    - Stop topical steroids for 1 week and PO/IM steroids for 2 weeks prior to test

ACD due to Plants

- Poison ivy (**Anacardiaceae** family/**Toxicodendron** species) contain **oleoresin,** aka **urushiol** (sensitizing agent is **pentadecyl catechol**) which cross react w/ **mango**, grinkgo, **cashew**, Japanese lacquer tree, Indian marking nut and the Brazilian pepper tree
    - "Go shew to Japan, India or Brazil so Ana's not so toxically pent up inside"
    - Systemic contact dermatitis w/ ingestion of mangoes and cashews
        - Mango actually contains resorcinol (similar to urushiol but not the same)
- The pine tree (Pinaceae) contains rosin (colophony/abietic acid) which also cross reacts with benzoin, turpentine, **Balsam of Peru** and wood tars
    - "Pine trees rose in Ben Turners Peruvian woods"
- **Asteraceae (compositae)** family causes **airborne ACD** via the sensitizer **sesquiterpene** ("ses-quiter sounds like sad camper") **lactone** and whose plants can be remembered by "SAD CAMPER" → Sunflower, Arnica, Dandelion, **Chrysanthemum**, Chamomile, Artichoke, Marigold, Mugwort, **Pyrethrum** (permethrin), Endive, **Ragwood**
    - Cross-reacts with **permethrin**, **turpentine, colophony** (rosin) and Balsam of Peru
- Onions, garlic and chive (Alliaceae) contains the sensitizer **diallyl disulfide** → ACD on thumb, index and middle fingertips of non-dominant hand
    - "All people that cry (these foods make you cry) are not dominant"
- Tulip bulb (Liliceae) and Peruvian lily (Alstromeria) both contain the sensitizer **tuliposide A (α-methylene-β-hydroxy-γ-butyrolactone)** and cause ACD on the dominant hand
    - "Lili wanted Tulips, but Alstrom wanted Peruvian lilies but since women always get their way, they

both walked out the store w/ Tulips in their dominant hand"

Contact urticaria (CU)

- Immunologic CU is mediated by allergen-specific IgE on mast cells → a/w anaphylaxis
  - "A worker at this contact urticaria LAB HAS a meat and potatoes diet"
    - Latex (cross-reacts with "passion BACK")
      - Healthcare workers
      - Atopic dermatitis patients
      - Aerosolized glove powder may induce anaphylaxis
      - Spina bifida patients
    - Ammonium persulfate (hair bleach)
    - Bacitracin (anaphylaxis when put on chronic leg ulcers)
    - Meat (raw meat, fish, and shellfish)
    - Potatoes are the MC raw vegetable, but celery can also cause anaphylaxis
- Non-immunologic CU
  - More common; occurs in any exposed person; low/No risk of anaphylaxis
  - MCC is stinging Nettles but another notable cause is dimethylsulfoxide (DMSO)
- p/w **urticaria within 1 hour (5 mins for stinging nettles)** of contact with food (meat/potatoes, "passion BACK"), topical or aeroallergens; **resolves in 24 hours**
- Dx (cOntact uRticaria): **Open patch testing** (wait 1 hour for wheal) and RAST testing
- Rx: avoidance and antihistamines (epinephrine if anaphylaxis)

3.3 Interface Dermatitis

Vacuolar interface dermatitis

- On path you see holes at the DEJ: "If you see holes, you DELVe G":
  - Drug eruption including FDE, EM/SJS/TEN, Lupus/DM, Viral exanthem, GVHD

Fixed drug eruption (FDE)

- MCC of FDE are PANTS ("If you can't keep it in your PANTS we'll get you fixed"): the drugs generally become more common as mnemonic progresses (P < A < N, T < S)
  - Phenolphthalein was previously in laxatives but has been removed; PPIs
  - Pseudoephedrine causes non-pigmented FDE ("causes a pseudo-FDE")
  - Aspirin, Acetaminophen, Azole antifungals
  - Antibiotics (macrolides, fluoroquinolones, and beta-lactams)
  - **NSAIDS especially Naproxen (predilection for the Lips**: N close to L in alphabet)
  - **Tetracyclines**
  - **Sulfonamides** like TMP-SMX (75% of cases, #1 cause on the genitals/Sex organs)
- p/w **well-demarcated round violaceous plaques with a central dusky hue, bulla or erosion which heal in 1–2 weeks with post-inflammatory hyperpigmentation**
  - "Dark PANTS" help me remember these lesions are dusky and heal with PIH
- **Genitals** ("PANTS") and oral mucosa > acral sites effected 1–2 weeks after drug intake
- Upon subsequent re-exposure lesion reoccurs at same exact site hours after drug intake

- Generalized FDE occurs if meds are continued (hard to distinguish from SJS/TEN)
- Non-pigmented FDE (commonly pseudoephedrine) show **large**, tender juicy red plaques
- Dx: patch testing of potential drugs in previously involved site can determine the drug
- Path: vacuolar interface w/ necrotic keratinocytes, **eosinophils,** and **dermal melanin**
- Rx: stop offending drug and treat symptomatically (topical steroids)
- Prognosis is good except in generalized bullous FDE (mortality similar to SJS/TEN)

Erythema multiforme (EM)

- Herpes-associated (HSV1 > HSV2) EM is the MCC of von Hebra's disease (EM minor)
- M. pneumoniae with severe Mucous Membrane involvement is MCC of EM Major
- Histoplasma capsulatum (EM with EN), Orf and drugs are less common causes
    - MC drugs are SJS drugs: **NSAIDS**, Anticonvulsants, Antibiotics (PCN, sulfa)
- p/w abrupt onset, symmetric macules → papules → targetoid lesions
    - Typical targets have three zones and favor acral sites (face and distal extremities)
    - Atypical targets have only 2 zones (helpful clue: atypical targets in **EM are Elevated papules**, while atypical targets in **SJS/TEN are Smooth macules**)
- EM Minor has target lesions, minor mucosal involvement and no systemic symptoms
- EM **Major** has targets, **major mucosal involvement** and systemic symptoms (**malaise**)

- Ddx includes other conditions that cause target lesions ("FES Up KEV, you're the target")
    - FDE, EM, SCLE, Urticaria, Kawasaki, EAC, Exanthematous drug eruption, Vasculitis
- Dx: positive HSV DNA by PCR
- Path: vacuolar interface w/ apoptotic keratinocytes (only EM/SJS, FDE, GVHD show this)
- Rx: **symptomatic treatment** (NSAIDS); if > 6 attacks/year consider long-term valacyclovir
- Prognosis: resolves in weeks without complications (except EM major → a/w eye issues)

Stevens-Johnson Syndrome and Toxic Epidermal Necrolysis: "GRAFI HAD A Bad Beer CHUG"

- Pathogenesis ("GRAFI")
    - Granulysin: cytotoxic molecule felt to be the major mediator of apoptosis
    - Granzyme B and perforin: pokes holes in target cells → apoptosis
    - RIP3 (receptor interacting protein kinase-3) is upregulated in skin of TEN pts
        - Dabrafenib inhibits RIP3 and represents a potential therapeutic target
    - Annexin A induces necroptosis of keratinocytes via binding to FPR1
    - Fas ligand (FasL, CD95L) is a member of the TNF family of cytokines that binds to its target on keratinocytes (FasL-Fas complex activates **caspases** → apoptosis)
        - "Fas rhymes with Cas"
    - IL-15 levels appear to be a/w the severity and mortality rate of SJS/TEN
        - IL-15 is also important in the pathogenesis of vitiligo and alopecia areata
- Epidemiology (H in "HAD")
    - Her (females > males)

- HIV infection (1000-fold ↑ risk due to loss of skin protective CD4+/CD25+ cells)
- HLA alleles
  - HLA-B*1502 (Asians and East Indians exposed to carbamazepine) and HLA-A*3101 (Europeans exposed to carbamazepine)
    - "Asians eat 1502 carbs/day while Europeans eat 3101 carbs/day"
  - HLA-B*5801 (Han Chinese exposed to allopurinol): DRESS and SJS/TEN
    - "The Han Chinese eat All things, about 5801 things"
  - HLA-B*5701 (abacavir): causes **DRESS** >> SJS/TEN
    - Abacavir is 100 back from the Han Chinese HLA (5801-100=5701)
  - HLA-DQB1*0601 (white patients with SJS and ocular complications)
    - "I have my white eyes on Dairy Queen"
    - HLA-DQB1*0301 is Caucasians with bullous pemphigoid, not SJS

- The precipitating factor in SJS are almost always drugs (A in HAD)
  - Acetaminophen
  - Allopurinol
  - Anticonvulsants (clobazam, carbamazepine, lamotrigine, phenytoin)
    - **Epoxide hydrolase deficiency** predisposes to anticonvulsant-related SJS
    - Lamotrigine is the most common anticonvulsant drug culprit
  - Antibiotics (**sulfonamides MC** > PNCs, cephalosporins, minocycline, quinolones)
    - 2018 JID article found TMP-SMX to be MC overall drug culprit in the US

- Anti-inflammatories, non-steroidal (NSAIDS) like piroxicam
- Antiretrovirals (**nevirapine** > abacavir, efavirenz, and etravirine)
  - ↑ risk of SJS in HIV patients due to an **acquired glutathione deficiency**

- Clinical features (D in "HAD")
  - After an initial prodrome, atypical (2 zones) targetoid macules ("SJS is Smooth") progress to atypical targets with Dusky center, Dusky macules and Dusky plaques
  - Detachment of the epidermis results in flaccid blisters from tangential pressure (Nikolsky sign) and vertical pressure (Asboe-Hanson sign)
  - **Distribution is opposite of EM (starts on the trunk and spares hands/feet)**
  - Mucosal involvement is severe and systemic symptoms present
- **SCORTEN criteria which predicts mortality** ("A Bad Beer CHUG")
  - Age > 40
  - Bicarbonate < 20 mEq/L (most important risk factor because its a/w septic shock)
  - Body surface area dusky/detached on day one > 10%
  - Cancer or hematologic malignancy
  - Heart rate > 120 bpm
  - Urea level > 10 mmol or BUN > 27 mg/dL
  - Glucose > 250 mg/dL
  - You want to know these values and the mnemonic makes it easier because "A" is > 40 y/o, half that for "Bad" (< 20 mEq/L of bicarb; careful this is the only "less than" value), half that for "Beer" (> 10% BSA on day 1) and "U" is also > 10 (mmol); now just remember to include hematologic cancer, HR > 120 and glucose > 250

  - Predicted mortality: 0–1 pt (3%), 2 pt (15%), 3 pt (30%), 4 pt (60%), ≥5 pt (90%)
    - Notice that 3% x **5** = 15%, 3% x **10** = 30%, 3% x **20** = 60%, 3% x **30** = 90%
- A 2017 JAAD article listed **renal failure** as the most important predictor of mortality
- Labs: CBC, BNP, Mg, bicarb, lactate, UA, ESR/CRP, urea, electrolytes, LFTs, coag studies
- Path: looks like EM but usually more keratinocyte necrosis and more eos (drug etiology)
- Rx (to finish the mnemonic, "GAFI HAD A Bad Beer CHUG because it had too much ICE")
  - high dose IVIG (2–4 gm/kg x 4 days) vs Cyclosporin 3–5 mg/kg/day x 7 days vs Corticosteroids (Dexamethasone 1.5 mg/kg/day x 3 days) vs **Etanercept 50 mg x1**
    - Etanercept is Bolognia's favorite one because of side effect profile
- Prognosis depends on how fast implicated drug is D/C'd (**drug timeline 1–3 weeks prior**)
  - 1%–5% mortality for SJS; 25%–35% mortality for TEN
- Ddx: TEC (skin sloughing involves skin folds, hands, foot, knees, elbows), SSSS (involves the folds and has perioral furrowing), generalized bullous fixed drug, PV, paraneoplastic pemphigus, vancomycin-induced LABD, **acute GVHD,** and **TEN-like acute cutaneous lupus**
- MC complication is ocular sequelae (like in EM major) and MCC of death is infection
  - "GAFI HAD A Bad Beer CHUG that got in his eyes and he died 2° to an infection"
- Workup: promptly D/C any offending drug, admit to ICU (burn unit), correct fluid/electrolyte abnormalities, caloric replacement, topical antibiotics, ophtho con-

sult, urology consult, periodic cultures, and biologic dressing, and consider Rx w/ "ICE" (above)

Graft versus host disease (GVHD): "GVHD is BS"

- **Pathogenesis**: immune competent donor WBCs target immunocompromised host tissue
- Occurs in most patients receiving **allogenic hematopoietic Stem cell transplants (HSCT)**
- Less common with Solid organ transplantation (Small intestine is MC), transfusion of non-irradiated blood to immunocompromised host and w/ maternal-fetal transmission
- **HLA incompatibility** is most important predictor of developing GVHD after HSCT
    - Risk of GVHD post HSCT in HLA-matched is 40% and HLA-mismatched is 60%–70%
- Other RFs: female donor to male recipient ("males usually put their DNA inside women not the other way around"), older age and collecting stem cells from the peripheral blood ("**Stem cells from Systemic circulation**") instead of directly from the BM
- Skin is the MC organ affected in acute and chronic GVHD (but GI and liver are common)
- Acute GVHD (aGVHD; traditionally occurring within 100 days of transplant)
    - GI tract involvement
    - Violaceous to red pruritic **acral** rash (face, hands, feet) **w/ follicular accentuation** assessed by % of BSA (stage 1: < 25%, 2 is 25–50%, 3 is > 50%, 4 is erythroderma)
        - Severe aGVHD can present like TEN w/ large areas of denuded skin
    - Hepatic dysfunction: accessed by degree of Bilirubin elevation
    - Diarrhea: accessed by volume (Bulk) of diarrhea

- Chronic GVHD (cGVHD; traditionally occurring 100 days after transplant)
    - Preceded by aGVHD (50%) or occurs de novo (50%) and can affect any organ
    - Classified as **Sclerodermoid cGVHD** (patchy-scleroderma or eosinophilic fasciitis-like) or non-sclerodermoid cGVHD (**lichenoid is MC non-sclerotic form**)
- aGVHD path
    - Vacuolar interface w/ **lymphs next to apoptotic cells (satellite cell necrosis)**
        - Generally less interface than FDE or EM due to poor immune function
    - **Hair follicles** also have dying keratinocytes (vs EM/FDE which are the other main conditions which show vacuolar interface w/ apoptotic keratinocytes)
        - Clinically, early lesions are centered around hair follicles
    - Dysmaturation of epidermis (resembles Bowenoid AK)
- cGVHD path: variable (the two MC patterns are sclerodermoid and lichenoid)
- Prophylaxis: Systemic Steroids, Sirolimus other immune inhibitors (MTX, cyclosporine)
- Rx: **JAK inhibitor (ruxolitinib)** and **Bruton tyrosine kinase inhibitor (ibrutinib)** are showing great promise in both acute and chronic GVHD
    - Acute GVHD: Systemic Steroids (if only limited to skin, topical steroids are fine)
        - **Maraviroc (CCR5 inhibitor)** can ↓ risk of visceral GVHD by blocking CCR5-mediated $CD8^+$ T-cell recruitment to liver and gut

- Chronic GVHD: prednisone + calcineurin inhibitor (cyclosporine or tacrolimus)
  - Low dose IL-2: expands T-regulatory cells to improve cGCHD
- Prognosis: 5-year survival is 70% (MCC of death is Bacterial infection)

Lichenoid interface dermatitis

Lichen planus (LP): "say lichen plaMus"

- Cutaneous LP affects 1% of adults but oral LP is 4X as common
- Pathogenesis: various triggers (e.g., viral, allergens, drugs) cause basal keratinocytes to express altered self-antigens on cell surface → T-cells target basal keratinocytes
  - MC viral, drug and contact allergen triggers ("ABCDEFGH")
    - Amalgam mercury (contact allergen), **ACE inhibitors, TNF-Alpha blockers**
    - **Beta Blockers**, Hep B vaccine
    - Chloroquine or hydroxy-Chloroquine, Copper (contact allergen), Hep C
    - Diuretics (especially HCTZ); D-Penicillamine
    - NSAIDS ("I say ENSAIDS")
    - Furosemide, Anti-Fungal medications (ketoconazole)
    - Gold (contact allergen)
    - **Hydroxyurea** (cause ulcerative LP-like dermatitis); **HCTZ; HSV6 (oral LP)**
- Inflammatory disease affecting skin, hair, nails, and mucosa with many clinical variants
- p/w pruritic purple polygonal flat-topped paps w/ Wickham striae and Köebnerization
- MC sites are oral **Mucosa (#1)** > ventral wrists/forearms, presacral area, **genitalia**, shins

- Labs: consider patch testing to contact allergens; consider **LFTs/hep C antibody**
- **Path**: orthohyperkeratosis, wedge-shaped hypergranulosis, "saw-toothed" rete, apoptotic keratinocytes confined to basal layer (Civatte bodies) and superficial dermis (Colloid bodies) and superficial dermal band-like lymphocytic infiltrate obscuring the DEJ
  - Lacks eosinophils (except in drug-induced LP and hypertrophic LP)
  - Lacks parakeratosis (except in drug-induced LP and oral LP)
  - Lacks apoptotic keratinocytes above basal layer except in drug-induced LP
- DIF: **shaggy fibrinogen along basement Membrane**; **Civatte bodies stain with IgM**
- Rx ("lichen PLAMUS"): withdrawal any potential offending medications or triggers
  - **Prednisone (also topical or IL steroids)**, Pimecrolimus, Protopic, Plaquenil (LPP)
  - **Low dose methotrexate**
  - Acitretin, Apremilast
  - Metronidazole, Mycophenylate mofetil
  - UV light
  - Sulfasalazine
- Prognosis: most forms resolve in 1 year but oral, hypertrophic and nail LP persist
  - ↑ risk of **SCC** in hypertrophic, oral (ulcerative type) and vulvovaginal LP

LP-variants (look up photos of these and be able to recognize Kodachromes)

- Hypertrophic LP: p/w pruritic **SCC-like** thick violaceous papules and plaques w/ white scale and Wickham striae on the dorsal lower legs/foot; may cause KAs/SCCs
  - Path is LP-like but w/ acanthosis +/- eosinophils

- Atrophic LP: p/w atrophic (morphea-like) hyperpigmented plaques on the lower legs
  - May represent a resolving phase of LP
- Actinic LP: Middle Eastern or Indian children (from Asian continent) w/ red-brown Annular plaques in sun-exposed skin and in intertriginous sites (Axilla)
- Annular LP: Asymptomatic Annular plaques (GA-like but scaly) in the Axilla > penis
- LP pigmentosa: round to reticulate hyperpigmented patches on **head/neck** in darker pts
- Ashy dermatosis: similar to LP pigmentosa but hyperpigmented macules are more oval, appear on the **trunk** and occur earlier in life (20s; vs 30s in LP pigmentosa)
- Inverse LP: clinically looks like LP pigmentosa, but it is in the folds (axilla)
- Bullous LP: blisters develop in previous LP sites due to expanded Max-Joseph spaces
- LP pemphigoids: blisters develop in locations away from previous LP sites due to circulating IgG antibodies to BPAG2 (type 17 collagen); patients are younger than in BP
- Drug-induced LP ("DEEP"): ABCDEFG drugs discussed above
  - Distribution is generalized; Delayed resolution after drug withdrawal (months)
  - Erased (absent) Wickham's striae; Empty mouth (spares mucous membranes)
  - Elderly people (60s vs 40s); Eczematous lesions
  - Photo-distributed lesions, Psoriasiform lesions, Prolonged latency period (**1 year**)
  - Path (vs normal LP): deeper lichenoid infiltrate, apoptotic keratinocytes in higher levels of the epidermis, eosinophils present

- Genital LP
  - Men: **annular** or **classic** LP lesions on glans/shaft (non-scarring; non-painful)
    - Ddx: bowenoid papulosis (more warty than lesions seen in classic LP)
    - Ddx: psoriasis (red and scaly vs more hyper-pigmented in annular LP)
  - Women: erosive lesions on vulva + oral lesions (vulvovaginal-gingival syndrome)
    - Lesions are painful and result in scarring; risk of malignant transformation
- Oral LP: oral lesions in 75% of LP cases; only 10% of those w/ oral LP develop skin lesions
  - Reticular LP: MC; p/w asymptomatic lacy white raised lines in B/L buccal mucosa
  - **Atrophic, erosive and bullous LP: painful; F > M; ↑ SCC risk; check genitals**
- Nail LP: seen in 10% of LP patients; affects multiple nails
  - Adults: trachyonychia (thinning), dorsal pterygium (adhesion of proximal nail fold to nail bed), onycholysis, nail thickening, yellow discoloration or red lunulae
  - Children: may present as 20 nail dystrophy
- Linear LP: lesions in a Blaschkoid distribution in young patients
- LP/LE overlap: pain, bullae, ulcers at acral sites; overlapping features of LP and lupus
- Palmoplantar LP: painful lesions (can be ulcerative esp on soles); refractory to treatment
- Lichen planopilaris (LPP): p/w perifollicular hyperkeratosis w/ erythematous rim; **pruritis**
  - Frontal fibrosing alopecia (FFA): variant effecting the **eyebrows** and frontal scalp
  - Graham-Little-Piccardi-Lasseur syndrome: variant w/ scarring alopecia on scalp, non-scarring pubic

and axillary hair loss, KP-like lesions and LP lesions on the skin

Erythema dyschromicum perstans (ashy dermatosis)

- p/w asymptomatic gray-brown oval macules/patches +/- erythematous rim symmetrically distributed on the neck, trunk, and proximal extremities
- More common in young adults w/ skin phototypes III and IV
- Path: subtle vacuolar interface with pigment incontinence (dermal melanophages)
- Rx: difficult to treat (steroids, hydroquinone, **clofazimine**, antimalarials, and dapsone)

Keratosis lichenoides chronica

- p/w erythematous to **violaceous keratotic papules forming linear or reticulate patterns on the limbs** (MC), buttocks and trunk w/ a greasy seb-derm-like centrofacial eruption
- Path: LP-like but epidermis has alternating areas of atrophy and acanthosis
- Rx: difficult to treat (systemic retinoids + UV light has been successful)

Lichen planus-like keratosis (benign lichenoid keratosis)

- Pathogenesis: inflammatory reaction to a preexisting solar lentigo, SK or AK
- p/w pink papule/plaque MC on the trunk (#1) or extremity (but can occur anywhere)
- Dermoscopy: diffuse gray dots and granules w/ sharp moth-eaten borders
- Path: looks like LP (may see a lentigo or SK at the periphery)

Pityriasis lichenoides

- PLEVA and PLC are on a spectrum; both have recurrent crops of lesions in kids
- PLEVA has more Vesicular, necrotic and crusted papules that heal with Varioliform scars
  - o Febrile ulceronecrotic Mucha-Haberman disease is a variant w/ severe skin involvement, high fevers, GI/pulmonary involvement and ↑TNF-α levels
    - Rx: **systemic steroids and transition to MTX**
- PLC has more scaly papules that heal with hypopigmentation (Color Changes)
- Path (PLEVA): **compact hyperkeratosis w/ Parakeratosis** (+/- neuts in the horn), Lichenoid to vacuolar infiltrate but w/ lymph in every whole, Extravasated RBCs, V (wedge)-shaped dermal lymph infiltrate w/ neuts but never any eosinophils, Apoptotic/dyskeratotic keratinocytes in a spongiotic epidermis w/ exocytosis of lymphs
  - o Path (PLC): very similar but infiltrate is less dense and more superficial
  - o CD8+ T cells predominate (PLEVA has 5 letters, PLC has 3 letters: 3+5=8)
- Rx (PLEVA/PLC): Phototherapy, Erythromycin/Azithromycin, topical Corticosteroids, MTX
- Prognosis: diffuse distribution of lesions resolves fastest (< 1 year) and then central distribution and then acral distribution resolves slowest (> 2 years)

Lichen nitidus ("ball and Claw")

- MC in Children
- p/w Clustered uniform pinpoint flesh-colored papules (hypopigmented in darker pts)
- Favored sites: **genitals**/lower abdomen/inner thighs ("ball") and hands ("claw")

- Path: classic "ball and claw" appearance
    - Ball: superficial dermal inflammatory nodule w/ lymphs, histiocytes, giant cells
    - Claw: hyperplastic rete ridges that surrounds and clasps the ball
- Ddx: lichen spinulosus and disseminate and recurrent infundibulofolliculitis (pruritic follicular-based eruption on trunk and proximal extremities in young AAs w/ AD)
- Rx: symptomatic with topical steroids, TCIs, and phototherapy
- Prognosis: majority resolve in 1 year

Lichen spinulosus

- p/w localized (often round) plaques of tiny discrete flat-topped papules
    - "Nutmeg-grater" texture has been described on palpation
- Rx: no treatment required as it is benign, asymptomatic, and resolves at puberty
    - May consider topical keratolytics (urea, ammonium lactate) and retinoids

Lichen Striatus

- Affects School-aged children (F > M), most of whom have AD
- ↑ incidence in Spring and Summer
- p/w Small, Scaly red papules in a linear (Blaschkoid) distribution on extremities (MC)
    - Erythema is more prominent in lighter skin tones and scale is more prominent in darker skin tones
    - Nail dystrophy may occur if digit is affected
- Ddx: ILVEN (presents earlier, more pruritic, red, psoriasiform and does not self-resolve)
- Path: Superficial (lichenoid) and deep (around the eccrine **Sweat glands**) lymph infiltrate

- Rx: Spontaneous resolution in 1–2 years but may consider topical Steroids or TCIs

Frictional lichenoid dermatitis

- Recurring cutaneous disorder affecting children between 4 and 12 years
- Half of pts have an atopic diathesis
- p/w aggregates of discrete tiny lichenoid papules on the elbows, knees and dorsal hands
- Rx: avoid frictional trauma, topical steroids, emollients

Lichen Sclerosis (LS&A)

- F >> M; bimodal peaks (post-menopausal females and prepubertal girls)
- Anogenital area involved in at least 85% of cases
    - Male penile involvement is called balanitis xerotica obliterans → phimosis
- a/w **autoimmune thyroid disease** (like in DH), other autoimmune diseases (celiacs, alopecia areata, vitiligo) and **HLA-DQ7** (Seven; DH had HLA-DQ2 > HLA-DQ8)
    - **IgG autoantibodies to ECM-1 in 80% (this gene is mutated in lipoid proteinosis)**
- Clinical features of genital LS&A
    - Sclerotic ivory white, fissured plaques
    - **"Figure-of-eight" pattern around vagina and perianal area in women**
    - Pruritus/Soreness → dysuria, dyspareunia and pain on defecation (constipation)
    - May see **purpura**/ecchymosis w/ hemorrhagic bullae (due to weakened BMZ)
        - Commonly confused w/ child abuse in young females
    - ↑ **SCC risk** (5% risk; 50% of all vulvar/penile SCCs occur in the setting of LS&A)

- Clinical features of extragenital LS&A (15% of cases)
  - **Shiny ivory Sclerotic wrinkled plaques**
    - **Ddx: morphea is not as shiny and wrinkled** (hypopigmented center w/ lilac border in active lesions and hyperpigmented throughout if inactive)
  - **MC site is upper trunk and neck** > proximal upper extremities
  - Lesions are asymptomatic (vs genital LS&A)
- Ddx: kids (sexual abuse); adults (morphea)
- Path (red/white/blue): orthohyperkeratosis w/ follicular plugging (red), papillary dermal edema w/ homogenization (white), underlying lichenoid lymphocytic infiltrate (blue)
- Rx: **ultra-potent topical Steroids** (kids and adults); circumcision in males with phimosis
- Prognosis: may resolve in children; relapsing course in adults

Annular lichenoid dermatitis of youth

- Occurs in children and adolescents w/ a travel history to the Mediterranean
- p/w annular plaques w/ red-brown border and central clearing MC on the flanks
- Path: lichenoid infiltrate localized to the tips of rete ridges
- Rx: topical/systemic steroids and phototherapy

3.4 Blistering Diseases

Preferred sites for obtaining biopsy specimens in autoimmune blistering diseases

- Routine H&E (affected skin; formalin): Rim of blister
- DIF (unaffected skin; Michel's or saline): Directly adjacent to blister (≤ 1cm away)

Pemphigus variants

Pemphigus foliaceous (PF)

- Autoantibodies to Dsg1
- Less common than PV but in **Brazil** it is 17x more common
  - o "There is a lot of foliage (P. foliaceous) in Brazil due to the Amazon"
- p/w subacute onset of transient impetigo-like crusted erosion on **seborrheic regions**
  - o Blisters are so superficial that you only see erosions (w/ a **"cornflake" scale**)
  - o No mucosal involvement (Dsg3 compensates) and there is a low mortality rate
- Fogo selvagem (endemic variant): found in rural Brazil effecting children ("shildren") living close to rivers rich in black flies (Simulium spp)
  - o "Selvagem, Shildren and Simulium all have 8 letters and start with S"
- **Pemphigus erythematosus (localized variant): overlap of lupus and PF with erythematous plaques and scale/crust and erosions on the malar face ("crusty SLE")**
- Pemphigus herpetiformis: mild variant of PF (**Dsg1** > Dsg3) which clinically resembles DH
  - o Path: eosinophilic spongiosis **without any acantholysis**
  - o Rx: responds well to dapsone +/- prednisone
- Path: subcorneal split (bullous impetigo has staph colonies and more neuts; SSS is DIF-)
- DIF (best test): shows "chicken wire" staining of IgG in upper epidermis
  - o Pemphigus erythematosus also shows granular to linear IgG and C3 along BMZ (this pattern of intraepidermal and linear BMZ staining is also seen in PNP)

- IIF and ELISA are not as sensitive as DIF but can be used to confirm diagnosis
- Rx: same treatment as pemphigus vulgaris (see below)

Pemphigus vulgaris (PV): "Vulgravis"

- Autoantibodies to Dsg3 (mucosal pemphigus) or Dsg1&3 (mucocutaneous pemphigus)
- MC form of pemphigus with a 10x increase rate in the Ashkenazi Jewish population
- a/w other autoimmune diseases (myasthenia gravis, thyroid disease) and thymoma
- In gravid mothers with PV, IgG against Dsg3 cross placenta → **transient blisters in baby**
    - o **Not seen in pemphigus foliaceous as fetal skin has sufficient Dsg 3 to compensate for a lack of Dsg 1 in these locations (similar to oral mucosa)**
- p/w gravely painful oral erosions (buccal and palatine MC sites) and 50% of patients also have skin involvement (flaccid blisters that rupture → painful erosions)
- PV can be fatal ("sends them to their grave") due to fluid imbalances and infections
- Path: suprabasal split ("tomb-stoning") w/ acantholysis down follicles (vs Hailey-Hailey)
- DIF (most sensitive): intracellular "chicken wire" staining of IgG in lower epidermis
- **ELISA and IIF Dsg Ab titers c/w disease activity** and can monitor response to treatment
    - o ELISA is a more sensitive test than IIF in PV and BP
- Rx: 1st line treatment for moderate-severe pemphigus is **rituximab** w/ prednisone PRN
    - o Tetracycline + nicotinamide + topical steroids for mild cases

Pemphigus vegetans

- Vegetative variant of pemphigus vulgaris

- Mild localized Hallopeau type and severe Neumann type exists
- p/w vegetating plaques in **mouth (cerebriform tongue), intertriginous areas, scalp**, face
- Ddx: Hailey-Hailey (will affect intertriginous sites but not mucosa) and pyoderma vegetans (rare vesiculo-pustular disease w/ vegetative plaques in intertriginous areas)
- Path: pseudoepitheliomatous hyperplasia (mimics SCC) **w/ eosinophilic pustules** and suprabasilar acantholysis that is more prominent in the hair follicles
- DIF and ELISA (same as PV): intraepidermal IgG on DIF and desmoglein 3 in ELISA
- Rx: same as PV (magic mouthwash or dapsone for oral lesions, surgery if localized)

Paraneoplastic pemphigus (PNP): "ParaneoPLASTIC pemphigus"

- Plakin family and Dsg1 and 3 are attacked by autoantibodies
- Polymorphous skin (PV-, lichenoid-, and EM-like)
- Polymorphous histology with an overalp of PV (**mild suprabasilar acantholysis**), EM (dyskeratotic keratinocytes) and LP (**lichenoid** infiltrate)
- **Palms and soles affected (rare in PV)**
- **PFTs to screen** for MCC of death (**bronchiolitis obliterans**) >> CT/chest X-ray
  - o Would show obstructive pattern on FPTs
- Poor prognosis (90% mortality)
- Lichenoid changes are the MC chronic presentation
- Autoantibodies to nearly all components of the desmosome
- **Severe Stomatitis (with extension onto lip) is the first, MC and most persistent sign**
- Thymoma is MC benign associated tumor in adults
- Immunoprecipitation/Immunoblotting + anti-Dsg IgG by ELISA is gold standard for Dx

- **Intercellular and linear (along DEJ) deposits of IgG and C3 on DIF**
    - Pemphigus erythematosus had this same pattern on DIF
- Corticosteroids and Corticosteroid sparing agent with **removal of Cancer is best Rx**
- Cancer (2nd MCC of death): **Non-Hodgkin Lymphoma** is #1, Castleman's is #1 in children
    - "Adults play for the NHL, children play and build sand Castles man"
    - **Refer them to hematology oncology** (treating cancer treats the disease)

Disorders with hemorrhagic crusts of the vermillion lips is "my lip chaps" (CHEPS)
Contact Cheilitis, Herpes (simplex and zoster), EM major, PV, PNP, SJS/TEN

Best IIF substrates for pemphigus variants
Pemphigus foliaceous: guinea pig esophagus ("Guinea pigs eat foliage") Pemphigus vulgaris: monkey esophagus ("Monkeys are vulgar") Paraneoplastic pemphigus: rat bladder ("rats, I have cancer")

*Pemphigoid variants do not have specific substrates (salt-split human skin can be used)

IgA pemphigus (intraepidermal neutrophilic type and subcorneal pustular dermatosis type)

- Both types have IgA Autoantibodies against the cell surface of keratinocytes
- p/w **fragile vesicles or pustules in an Annular pattern in the Axilla** most commonly (but also in the groin and other intertriginous zones); pruritis is a common feature
    - Rare mucosal involvement or significant morbidity ("patient is A OK")
- a/w Autoimmune diseases and **IgA gammopathy** (and other cancers)

- Path: neutrophilic mico-Abscesses in epidermis
- Rx: TOC is **dApsone** (Acitretin, colchicine or sulfapyridine if dapsone not tolerated)
- IEN type (unknown antibody but a small subset has antibodies to desmoglein 1 and 3)
    - Path: intra-epidermal neutrophilic infiltrate with minimal acantholysis
    - DIF: IgA intercellular staining throughout entire epidermis
- Subcorneal pustular dermatosis type (**antibodies to Desmocollin 1**)
    - Path: subcorneal pustule (looks like Sneddon-Wilkinson disease but w/ +DIF)
    - DIF: IgA intercellular staining in upper epidermis

Drug-induced pemphigus

- **PF** > PV presentation with the thiol (sulfhydryl) meds (**ACE inh and D-Penicillamine**)
    - DI-PF is more common than DI-PV, but ACE inh and D-Penicillamine are the MCC of both
- **For DI-PF/PV, LP and PR think of the "alphabet meds"** (many are blood pressure meds)
    - **ACE inhibitors**
    - β-lactams (PF/PV only), **β-blockers**
    - CCBs (PF/PV), Clonidine (PR), Chloroquine (LP)
    - **D-penicillamine**
    - "ENSAIDS"
    - Furosemide (LP and PR but not PV/PF)
    - **Gold**
    - Hydrochlorothiazide (LP and PR but not PV/PF)

Autoimmune subepidermal blistering diseases

- Subepidermal bullae result from damage to components of BMZ

- Must know location and disease associations of BMZ components ("Peanut Butter BIL")
  - Plectin and BPAG1 correspond to the **hemidesmosomal plaques**: EBS, BP
  - BPAG2 and Integrin correspond to anchoring filaments **(lamina lucida)**
    - BPAG2 is a "Judgmental BICH": Junctional EB (non-Herlitz type), BP, linear IgA/CBDC, Cicatricial pemphigoid, Herpes gestationis (+ LP pemphigoides)
    - Integrin is Junctional EB with atresias and ocular cicatricial pemphigoid
  - Laminin 332 corresponds to the **lamina densa**: Junctional EB (severe Herlitz type) and Laminin 332 cicatricial pemphigoid w/ malignancy

Bullous pemphigoid (BP)

- Pathogenesis: IgG attacks hemisdesmosomal target antigen NC16A domain of BP180 (BPAG2, type 17 collagen) which is the primary mediator but antibodies also arise to BP230 (BPAG1, Plakin family) as a secondary phenomenon ("epitope spreading")
  - a/w HLA-DQB1*0301 in whites (HLA-DQB1*0601 was SJS in whites w/ eye issues)
  - a/w DRB1*04, DRB1*1101 and DQB1*0302 in Japanese patients
- p/w fixed urticarial papules/plaques (early) and later evolves to figurate firm fluid-filled bullae on an urticarial base on the trunk, abdomen and flexural extremities
  - Oral involvement in 20% and peripheral eosinophilia in 50% of cases
- Path: sub-basal split with eosinophils in vessel cavity
- **DIF (best test)**: linear C3 and IgG along DEJ in an n-serrated pattern ("peNphigoid")
  - Vs U-serrated pattern in epidermoysis bUlossa aqUisita

- Salt-split skin stains the roof (epidermal) side
  - Only entity in "PB BIL" that stains floor is Laminin 332 cicatricial pemphigoid
- **ELISA** > IIF BP180 Ab titers c/w disease severity and can monitor response to treatment
  - ELISA is a more sensitive test than IIF in PV and BP
- Rx: prednisone +/- steroid spearing agent (cellcept)
  - TCN + nicotinamide (mild), dapsone (mucosal BP), or rituximab (recalcitrant BP)
- a/w dementia (Parkinson's) and bipolar depression which are risk factors for relapse

Pemphigoid variants ("LIVE GLAD")

- Lichen planus pemphigoides: LP/BP overlap with tense bulla on skin unaffected by LP
- Infantile/childhood BP: infants p/w acral bullae while children p/w face/genital bullae
  - "Infants play with their hands, kids play with their face and genitals"
- Vesicular pemphigoid: DH-like presentation with small grouped vesicles
- Pemphigoid Vegetans: vegetative plaques in intertriginous zones
- Erythrodermic pemphigoid: erythroderma along w/ blister formation (rare)
- Gestational pemphigoid (herpes gestationis): "CHERPES G"
  - Collagen 17 (BPAG2) antigen, C3 at DEJ on DIF, a/w Choriocarcinoma
  - HLA-DR3 (70%), DR4 (50%) or both; Herpetiform blisters in umbilicus → spreads
  - Exacerbation at birth or immediately after
  - Recurs in subsequent pregnancies
  - Premature infant
  - Exanthem (transient blisters) in 10% of infants

- Small for gestational age, Second or third trimester onset
- a/w Graves' disease

- Localized pemphigoid (RAP UP BP Variants locally): Radiotherapy sites, Amputated limb, Paralyzed limb, Umbilical, Peristomal, Brunsting-Perry (head/neck), Pretibial, Vulvar
- Anti-laminin γ1 pemphigoid (previously anti-p200): like classic BP but more likely to be on head and mucous membranes, more likely to have neutrophils (vs eos) on path, more likely a/w **psoriasis** and IgG binds to dermal side/floor on SSS (vs epidermal/roof)
- Anti-p105 pemphigoid: extensive blistering resembling TEN ("there is a ten in 105")
    - IgG binds to dermal side/floor of SSS
- Drug induced pemphigoid (< 60 yo): PF CHANGS → **Penicillamine**, Penicillins, Phototherapy, **Furosemide (#1)**, Cephalosporins, Checkpoint inhibitors (**Pembrolizumab**), ACE inhibitors, NSAIDS, Neuroleptics, Gliptins (**dipeptidyl peptidase-4 inhibitors** like vildagliptin), Gold, Sulfasalazine, SSKI, **Spironolactone**
- Dyshidrosiform pemphigoid: acral bulla resembling dyshidrotic eczema/pompholyx

Linear IgA bullous dermatosis (chronic bullous disease of childhood)

- Disease that usually affects children w/ linear IgA at the DEJ (instead of IgG/C3 in BP)
    - When adults effected it is usually drug induced (**vancomycin** > PF CHANGS)
- IgA autoantibodies against 2 components of BP180
    - LAD-1: **120 kD** portion of BP180
    - LABD97: **97 kD** portion of LAD-1
- p/w tense blisters and urticarial plaques in an **annular, polycyclic or herpetiform ("crown of jewels") pat-**

tern commonly on the face, thighs, lower abdomen, groin, butt

- Drug-induced cases resolve in about a month w/ drug withdrawal
- Path: superficial epidermal split w/ neuts lined up at DEJ (vs DH which has pockets of neuts at DEJ)
- DIF: linear IgA at DEJ (vs DH which has granular IgA in dermal papillae)
- Rx: **dapsone** (treats anything mucosal, IgA, or neutrophilic)

Cicatricial pemphigoid (CP; mucous membrane pemphigoid)

- "BIL in Peanut Butter BIL" corresponds to anchoring filament ("BIL rymes with fil") zone in which the forms of CP result from auto-Abs to all 3 portions of the anchoring filament
  - BP180 (C-terminus): head/neck skin and mucosal involvement (largest subgroup)
  - Integrin α6β4 (β4 subunit): exclusive ocular involvement ("β looks like glasses")
  - Laminin 332 (laminin5, epiligrin): strongly a/w underlying **solid organ malignancy**
- Chronic disease of elderly which effects **mucosa > head/neck skin** and has **scarring**
  - Mouth (#1 site): p/w stomatitis and **desquamative gingivitis (shallow erosions)**
  - Conjunctiva (#2 site, 40%): p/w symblepharon, trichiasis, ectropion and blindness
  - Skin involvement (25%): head/neck blisters/erosions that heal w/ atrophic scars
    - Brunsting-Perry variant: head/neck lesions with scarring alopecia
- Path: subepidermal split w/ lymphs > plasma cells and eos; **dermal fibrosis/scarring**

- DIF: linear IgA, IgG and C3 along the DEJ (n-serrated pattern except laminin 332)
    - o You cannot reliably differentiate cicatricial pemphigoid from BP based on path or DIF, you need salt split skin, IIF, immunomapping or genetics testing
- **SSS: stains roof (epidermal side), except anti-laminin 332 MMP which stains floor**
- Indirect immunofluorescence is only positive in 1 out of 5 cases
- Rx: **dapsone** and topical steroids
    - o Ocular disease: rituximab (1st line), cyclophosphamide (2nd line due to SE profile)

Bullous systemic lupus erythematosus (bullous SLE)

- IgG autoantibodies to NC1 and NC2 domain of type 7 collagen
- p/w vesicles/bulla on an urticarial background (like BP, linear IgA and DH)
- Path: **subepidermal split w/ neuts** (like linear IgA bullous dermatosis; DH looks similar)
- **DIF: full house (IgG, C3, IgA, IgM) in a granular pattern along the BMZ**
- Dermal (floor) staining on SSS since type 7 collagen is in the sublamina densa
- Rx: **dapsone**

Epidermolysis bullosa acquisita (EBA)

- IgG autoAbs to **NC1 domain of type 7 collagen** of sublamina densa anchoring fibrils
    - o "Type 7 collagen anchors up my BED" (Bullous SLE, EBA, Dystrophic EB)
- a/w MHC class II HLA-DR2 (Bullous lupus and EBA are HLA-DR2 as B is the 2nd letter of the alphabet)
- Most commonly presents like a mild dystrophic EB (mechanobullous form) with non-inflammatory bulla/

erosions on trauma-prone sites (**dorsal hands/feet, knees, elbows**) which heal w/ **atrophic scars**, milia, dyspigmentation +/- "mitten deformities" of hands

- May also present like BP (inflammatory form) without classic scarring or milia
- Mucous membrane involvement in 50% (vs 10–30% in BP)
- Strongly a/w **Crohn's** ("epidermolysis bullosa a-crohns-sica") but other associations are myeloma, SLE, RA, thyroiditis and diabetes
- Path: non-inflammatory subepidermal blister in **mechanobullous form (PCT-like)** vs inflammatory sub-epidermal split in the inflammatory form (BP-like) → need DIF serration pattern, SSS, IIF, ELISA to differentiate EBA from PCT/BP)
- DIF: linear **IgG** > C3 along DEJ in an **u-serrated pattern** ("epidermolysis bulossa aquisita")
    - o vs BP which shows C3 and IgG along DEJ in an n-serrated pattern ("penphigoid")
    - o vs PCT which shows Perivascular (Papillary dermis) staining of IgG and C3 on DIF
- DIF SSS: stains floor (dermal side) of blister cavity (vs stains roof/epidermal side in BP)
- ELISA and IIF autoantibody titers correlate with disease severity
- Rx: refractory to treatment ("EBA stands for Extremely Bad Antidotes") but systemic steroids, dapsone, IVIG, rituximab, and other immunosuppressants are used

Subepidermal autoimmune blistering disease (ABCDE)
Linear IgA bullous dermatosis (neutrophils along DEJ) Bullous pemphigoid (eosinophils along DEJ); Bullous lupus (neutrophils along DEJ) Cicatricial pemphigoid (mixed infiltrate with dermal fibrosis) Dermatitis herpetiformis (neutrophilic micro abscesses in dermal papillae) Epidermolysis bullosa acquisita (mechanobullous variant pauci-inflammatory like PCT but no festooning or caterpillar bodies) vs BP variant (looks like BP)

*We treat all of these w/ dapsone except BP (but we do treat mucosal BP w/ dapsone) and EBA

Dermatitis herpetiformis (DH)

- Pathogenesis: gluten breaks down into gliadin (antigenic) which complexes w/ transglutaminase-2 **(TTG2) in the gut**; this complex is recognized by HLA-DQ2 on APCs → production of IgA autoantibodies against TTG2 damages intestinal villi → epitope spreading (BP has this too) results in IgA autoantibodies against **epidermal TTG3** binding to TTG3 in the dermal papillae → neutrophilic subepidermal blister above papillae
  - TTG (I'D Peel): lamellar Ichthyosis (TTG1), DH (TTG3), acral peeling skin (TTG5)
- All have **HLA-DQ2** > HLA-DQ8 ("Celiacs can't go 2 Dairy Queen") and HLA-B8
- Autoimmune diseases a/w DH in order of frequency are "HIPAA": **Hashimoto's** > **Insulin dependent DM** > Pernicious anemia > Addison's disease, Alopecia areata
- a/w **MALT-type non-Hodgkin B-cell lymphoma** (as is Sjögren's syndrome)
- "The Wise Ruth Bater Ginsburg tells you what you can't eat. She only lets you eat ROCs"
  - Can't eat Wheat, Rye, Barley which contain Gluten
  - Can only eat Rice, Oats, Corn (4 letter words: "DH patients love 4 letter words")
- p/w **Herpetiform erosions** > vesicles on urticarial base distributed symmetrically on the **Hind (poste-**

rior) areas like extensor extremities, buttocks, back and posterior neck
  - o Vesicles may have Hemorrhagic crusts due to scratching from extreme pruritis
- Path: clusters of **neutrophils in Dermal papillae** w/ overlying sub-epidermal blister
- DIF (obtain from nearby Healthy appearing skin): granular IgA in the Dermal papillae
- **IIF: negative (DH and PCT do not have circulating antibodies that deposit in the skin)**
  - o But DH does have circulating antibodies that can be detected on ELISA → "GET these serologic tests": **anti-Gliadin, - Endomysial, aka TTG antibodies**
- Rx: **Dapsone** (clears DH quickly but no effect on GI disease or lymphoma risk)
  - o Gluten free diet treats skin disease, GI disease and lymphomas
- Avoid topical or systemic iodide → neutrophil infiltration into skin → DH exacerbation
- **DH is exacerbated by iodides (SSKI) and NSAIDS like indomethacin (ibuprofen is fine)**
- Workup: **IgA anti-TG2 Ab** (only if positive get IgA anti-endomysial Ab)
  - o These Abs can be monitored over time to assess compliance w/ gluten-free diet

Inherited blistering diseases

Epidermolysis bullosa (see section 4.4)

Darier's disease (keratosis follicularis)

- AD; peak age of onset is during puberty
- Mutation in **ATP2A2** (encodes **SERCA2** which is a Ca^{2+} ATPase of ER) → defective Ca^{2+} sequestration in ER (vs golgi in Hailey-Hailey) → keratinocyte acantholysis and apoptosis

- p/w malodorous, crusty, warty red/brown papules/ plaques in a seborrheic distribution
- Hands: **palmar pits** +/- acrokeratosis verruciformis (flat wart-like lesions on dorsal hand)
- Nails: red/white nail streaks ("candy cane nails") w/ v-shaped notches
- Mouth: oral cobblestoning
- ↑ risk for epilepsy, kaposis varicelliform eruption (eczema herpeticum), bipolar disorder
- Rx: systemic **retinoids** (very effective), high-dose vitamin A, JAK inhibitors are promising
- **Avoid lithium**: "Lit PAD" → lithium worsens Psoriasis, Acneiform eruptions, Darier's

Hailey-Hailey disease (familial benign chronic pemphigus)

- Compare to Darier's; both **AD** but Hailey-Hailey has a wider age of onset (teens-20s)
- Mutation in ATP2C1 ("Hailey's comet, 2C1 would be great") which encodes **hSPCA1**, a Ca^{2+} ATPase of the **Golgi** (G next to H in ABCs) apparatus → keratinocyte acantholysis
- Instead of warty plaques in seborrheic areas w/ oral lesions there are eroded plaques in **intertriginous zones** w/ moist malodorous vegetations and fissures **w/o oral lesions** (pemphigus vegetans has same distribution but more verrucous and has oral lesions)
    - BCCs, SCCs, and melanoma have all been reported to arise within affected skin
- Like Darier's, patients are prone to infections (e.g., Kaposi's varicelliform eruption)
- Unlike Darier's, retinoids are ineffective; try JAKs, dupixent, or **surgical** interventions (**CO2**)

Acral peeling skin syndrome

- Mutation in transglutaminase 5 → crosslinks proteins involved in cornification (loricrin)

- p/w superficial painless peeling skin on the hands and feet at birth

Other blistering disorders (A-F): all are cell poor except bullous arthropod (eos) and bullous CSVV (neuts); all are subepidermal blisters except bullous arthropod and friction blisters

- Bullous Arthropod assault ("BUG")
  - Blood malignancies (**CLL** in MC) are common causes
  - Bug bite-like reactions in lymphoma patients in absence of bug bite
  - Up in epidermis there is a split (**intraepidermal acantholysis**)
  - Grouped pruritic papules with central blistering clinically
- Bullous dermatitis Artifacta (self-inflicted injury)
  - Many etiologies (new fad among kids is salt and ice challenge)
  - Path: subepidermal blister with epidermal necrosis
- Bullous Bacterial infections (impetigo/cellulitis)
- Bullous Cutaneous small vessel vasculitis (CSVV)
  - Presents as LCV on lower extremities with hemorrhagic bulla
  - Path: LCV with massive subepidermal edema and epidermal necrosis
- Coma blisters
  - Tense blisters at sites of pressure 2–3 days after losing Consciousness
  - Path: cell poor subepidermal blister with **necrosis of eccrine glands**
- Bullous Diabeticorum
  - Sudden appearance of tense bulla seen in longstanding diabetics (feet MC)
  - Path: cell-poor subepidermal split
- Delayed postburn/postgraft blisters

  - o Blisters form about 1 month after wound has healed due to fragility of new DEJ
- Bullous Drug eruption (discussed below)
- Edema blisters
  - o Tense blisters in Edematous patients (MC on the lower Extremities)
  - o Path: marked epidermal spongiosis w/ dilated dermal BVs and mild infiltrate
- Friction blisters
  - o New pair of ill-Fitting shoes in young physically active patients → **painful intraepidermal blisters** with blood-tinged Fluid
  - o Path: blister is just below Granular layer (just like G is just below F in alphabet)
- Fracture blisters
  - o Tense bullae that develop within edematous skin that overlie bone fractures
- Suckling blisters is not an A-F letter but is seen on **hands and forearms of newborns**

Bullous drug eruptions (refer to individual sections for full mnemonics and more info)

- Fixed drug eruption ("dark PANTS"): clinically it is dark lesion which resolves with PIH
  - o Phenolphthalein < ASA, Acetaminophen < NSAIDS, TCNs < **Sulfonamides** (#1)
- SJS/TEN ("GAFI HAD A Bad Beer CHUG": The A in HAD referred to implicated drugs)
  - o Allopurinol, Anticonvulsants, Antibiotics (sulfonamides > β-lactams), Anti-inflammatories (NSAIDS), Antiretrovirals
- Drug induced autoimmune blistering diseases
  - o Linear IgA bullous dermatosis: **vancomycin** > β-lactams, captopril, NSAIDS
  - o Pemphigus (A-G): **ACE inhibitors** (captopril but not lisinopril), β-lactams, β-blockers, CCB,

D-penicillamine (MCC)**, "ENSAIDS", Furosemide, Gold
    - BP ("PF CHANGS"): Furosemide and dipeptidyl peptidase-4 inh (…gliptin) are MC
- Drug-induced pseudoporphyria: NSAIDS (esp **naproxen**), furosemide, TCNs, ciprofloxacin
    - Path identical to PCT but porphyrin studies are negative
    - More likely to be seen in **ESRF** ("bullous dermatosis of end-stage renal failure")
- AGEP (ABCs): Azithromycin, β-lactams, CCBs (diltiazem), Chloroquine
- Phototoxic drugs eruption ("my FAV TAN is a PhotoToxic Sunburn")
    - Flouroquinolones, Amiodarone, Voriconazole, TCNs, …Azines, NSAIDS, Psoralens, Thiazides, St. John's wort
- Bromoderma and iododerma: acneiform or vegetating lesions from bromides or iodide-containing drugs (SSKI, amiodarone) or radiographic contrast media
    - Path: pseudoepitheliomatous hyperplasia w/ neutrophilic abscess (no organisms)
- Palmoplantar erythrodysethesia (toxic erythema of chemotherapy): painful erythema on palms and soles after chemotherapy (esp cytarabine, aka "Cy-terrible")

Common blistering conditions and helpful clues to differentiate
- Contact dermatitis: blisters on a background of erythema
    - See if the erythema has square borders, suggesting extrinsic etiology
- Herpes: grouped vesicles on a red base which progresses to ulcers w/ a scalloped border
- Bullous impetigo: vesicles w/ yellowish crust
- Linear IgA bullous dermatosis: bullae will be in an annular configuration

3.5 Connective Tissue and Sclerosing Diseases

Ideal biopsy technique for connective tissue diseases

- For both H&E and DIF of lupus and DM: established lesional skin > 6 months
  - o Exception is the lupus band test where non-lesional skin is biopsied to see those at risk of renal disease (not commonly done as ds-DNA Abs also identifies this)

Antibodies in autoimmune connective tissue diseases

Antibodies in lupus

- Antinuclear antibodies (ANAs): most sensitive test for SLE (considered positive if > 1:40)
  - o ANAs also (+) in "ANA loves SPIRM ("I imagine Anasthesia Steele in 50 Shades of Grey") → SLE (99%), SCLE (70%), SSc (95%), Sjögren's, PNGD > IGDA (50%), Polymyositis/DM (40%), Idiopathic juvenile arthritis, RA, Morphea, MCTD
  - o ANAs may be detected via IIF utilizing Hep-2 tumor cells as substrate or via **ELISA**
    - ▪ SLE: rim pattern (IIF) or anti-dsDNA (ELISA/multiplex immunoassays)
    - ▪ SLE and drug-induced SLE: homogenous/diffuse pattern (IIF) or anti-dsDNA and anti-histone respectively (ELISA/multiplex immunoassays)
      - "SLE can be diffuse or rim but DI-SLE is always Diffuse pattern"
    - ▪ Non-specific but a/w Sjögren's, SCLE, NLE or MCTD: speckled pattern (IIF) or anti-Ro/SS-A,

La/SS-B, anti-U1RNP, anti-Smith, and anti-Scl-70 (ELISA)

- Systemic sclerosis and polymyositis (PM): nucleolar pattern (IIF) or RNA processing molecule fibrillarin, aka U3RNP (ELISA/multiplex immunoassay)
  - "You 3 (U3) fibbers lied and said you were going to systemically sclerose Panama with a nuclear bomb"
- CREST syndrome: Centromere pattern (IIF) or anti-Centromere (ELISA)

- Other antibodies (+) in lupus (prevalence in parentheses; "ABCD KRUSH")
  - ANA: discussed above
  - β2 glycoprotein (25%) and Cardiolipin (50%): antiphospholipid syndrome in SLE
  - C1q (60%): a/w renal dz in SLE and "hypoqomplementemic urtiqarial vasqulitis"
  - dsDNA (60%): very specific for lupus; monitors Disease Activity in **lupus Nephritis**
    - Crithidia IIF is used as a confirmatory test after positive anti-dsDNA ELISA
  - Ku (10%): overlap syndrome w/ SLE, DM/PM and systemic sclerosis
    - "When I Kiss u, our lips overlap"
  - rRNP (10%; 40% in Asians): specific for SLE; a/w neuropsychiatric LE
  - U1RNP (50%): overlapping features with other AI-CTDs (100% in MCTD)
  - SS-A/Ro (50%): MC in neonatal lupus (99%), SCLE (85%) and Sjögren's (70%)
  - Smith (20%): highly specific for lupus
    - Previous 4 Abs targeted ribonucleoproteins: "ribonucleoproteins R'USS"
  - ssDNA (70%): risk for developing SLE in DLE patients; also seen in linear morphea

- Histone (40%): drug-induced SLE

Antibodies in DM/PM ("MAPS")

- Mi-2 (helicase): a/w **classic** DM (myositis w/ classic skin findings); good prognosis
- MDA5 (CADM-140): a/w rapidly progressive ILD (adults and kids); amyopathic w/ unique skin findings (skin/oral ulcers, painful palmar papules, mechanics hands and panniculitis)
- Aminoacyl tRNA synthetase (Anti-**Jo**, -PL7, -PL12, -EJ/OJ): anti-synthetase syndrome (**rapidly progressive ILD**, **myositis**, mechanics hands, Raynaud's, arthritis)
  - "I imagine 2 guys named CAD ("MD") and Jo running a race so they are both SOB (ILD) but whereas CAD falls down early in the race onto his hands (skin ulcers, painful palmar papules), Jo finishes the race making his muscles very weak"
- ANA: MC IIF pattern is nucleolar; **most sensitive antibody in DM**
- **p155 (anti-TIF1γ): amyopathic DM a/w cancer** and psoriasiform lesions, **palmar hyperkeratosis** and verrucous papules in adults; MC antibody in juvenile DM (35%)
- p140 (NXP-2): a/w cancer (adults) and calcinosis cutis (kids)
- SRP: poor prognosis from severe cardiac involvement ("Severely Rapid Pulse")
- SAE: severe skin disease, cancer and myositis

Antibodies in systemic sclerosis ("Hard fibrotic CARS")

- Fibrillarin (U3RNP): a/w limited SSc which presents at a younger age
- Centromere: a/w limited SSc/**CREST** (a/w pulmonary HTN and digital ulcers) > SSc
- ANA: MC IIF pattern is **nucleolar**

- RNA polymerase (I and III): a/w diffuse SSc (**Renal** and severe skin disease) > CREST
- Scl-70 (DNA topoisomerase I): a/w diffuse SSc (**pulmonary fibrosis**) > CREST

Antibodies in morphea ("more hard HATS")

- Histones: linear and generalized morphea
- ANA
- Topoisomerase IIα
- ssDNA: linear morphea ("single stranded, aka linear"); also ↑ risk of SLE in DLE

Antibodies in rheumatoid arthritis

- RF (Fc portion of IgG): high levels c/w severe erosive RA and mixed cryoglobulinemia
- Cyclic citrullinated proteins: a/w severe RA

Sjögren's syndrome ("ASS": in order of decreasing sensitivity and specificity)

- **Anti-α-fodrin** (Actin-binding protein): most sensitive and specific
- ANA: speckled pattern on IIF
- SS-A/Ro (hyRNP): also important in neonatal lupus and SCLE
- SS-B/La (hyRNP): least sensitive and specific

Mixed connective tissue disease (MCTD)

- U1RNP shows high titers in MCTD and low titers in lupus

Lupus band test

- **Granular** continuous band of immunoglobin (**IgM** > IgG > IgA; "goes in reverse alphabetical order") and complement (C3) at the DEJ in patients w/ SLE seen on DIF

- Three different types of LBTs exist
  - Lesional LBT: high sensitivity for SLE, chilblains lupus and mucosal lupus (100%), fairly high sensitivity for DLE/SCLE (75%) and lupus profundus/ tumid lupus (50%)
    - May see false (+) in rosacea, telangiectasias, PMLE and dermatomyositis
    - The more immunoreactants present at the DEJ, the higher the specificity
  - Sun-exposed, non-lesional skin (e.g., forearm): fairly high sensitivity for SLE (75%)
    - Useful for making a diagnosis when no skin lesions are present
  - Sun-protected, non-lesional skin: positive in 50% of SLE
    - Useful for accessing disease activity/prognosis (poor prognosis if positive)
    - Although the sensitivity is lower, specificity is much higher if (+)
    - Correlates w/ anti-dsDNA Abs which c/w severe disease and Nephritis

Lupus erythematosus

Chronic cutaneous lupus (CCLE)

- MCC is discoid lupus (MC in African Americans)
  - Most pts w/ SLE will get discoid lupus; only 10% w/ discoid lupus will get SLE
- Subtypes
  - Discoid lupus erythematosus (DLE)
    - p/w atrophy, scarring (cicatricial alopecia), **central hypopigmentation w/ hyperpigmented periphery** typically on the scalp, face and **conchal bowls**
    - Labs: ANA positive in 10% of cases

        - Widespread (above and below neck) and childhood DLE regularly has SLE
        - Path: vacuolar interface, epidermal atrophy, BMZ thickening, follicular plugging, superficial and deep PV/PA lymph infiltrate w/ ↑ dermal mucin
        - DIF: LBT+ in 75% of DLE cases: higher sensitivity in **old lesions ("disc-old")**
    - Chilblains lupus erythematosus
        - p/w Circumscribed, dusky-red papules on acral sites precipitated by Cold
        - May be sporadic (adults; a/w anorexia, lymphoma, pregnancy) or familial (child; AD mutation in TREX1 gene which encodes a DNA exonuclease)
        - Chronic relapsing course and persists year-round (vs non-lupus chilblains)
        - Ddx: pernio (chilblains) is less chronic (appears 12–24 hours after cold exposure and is **a/w AI-CTD like SLE,** drugs, CML; Rx: CCBs.), covid-toes (pseudo-chilblains) occurs as a late feature of covid, and ADHD stimulant toes (resolves after discontinuation of amphetamines)
        - Path: features of both chilblains (pap dermal edema + lymphs) and DLE
            - DIF: LBT (+)
        - Rx: topical Corticosteroids, CCBs, Cigarette Cessation, rewarming
    - Tumid lupus erythematosus (TLE)
        - p/w edematous, indurated, erythematous, annular plaques w/ central clearing on the trunk > face; lesions heal in weeks but relapses can occur
        - Jessner's, TLE and reticular erythematous mucinosis are on a spectrum
            - Rx: treat all 3 with antimalarials

        - Path: similar to DLE but w/ massive dermal mucin and no epidermal changes (lacks follicular plugging, vacuolar interface, and BMZ thickening)
    - Lupus profundus (panniculitis)
        - p/w indurated, non-tender SQ nodules/ plaques that heal with atrophy
        - Located on the **upper arms (MC)**, face, upper trunk, breasts, butt, thighs
        - May have overlying discoid changes (scaling, follicular plugging, and scarring)
        - Overlying skin may be "tethered" down creating surface depressions
        - **Path: lymphocytic lobular panniculitis with hyalinized fat necrosis**
    - **Hypertrophic (verrucous) LE**
        - p/w thick, hyperkeratotic **verrucous** scaling plaques on sun-exposed skin (upper half of body vs lower half in hypertrophic LP) **w/ features of DLE**
        - ↑ risk of SCC (like hypertrophic LP)
        - Path: orthohyperkeratosis w/ endophytic buds of hyperplastic follicular epithelium; pseudoepitheliomatous hyperplasia (often mistaken for SCC)
- Labs: ANA and other serologic abnormalities more common w/ widespread CCLE lesions
- Rx (all types of CCLE except chilblains which was discussed above): "SHaQ does Meth"
    - Sun-protection, Steroids (systemic steroids if lesions are widespread), **HCQ**
        - If no response, add Quinacrine; if still no response, add Methotrexate
        - **HCQ takes 3 months to work so wait 4 months until adding quinacrine**

    - Future directions: anifrolumab (inhibits IFN-1 receptor)

Tumid lupus related diseases

- Jessner's lymphocytic infiltrate
  - Photosensitive eruption on a spectrum w/ tumid lupus and REM in adult females
  - p/w **annular red plaques** (may see central clearing) on the face, neck, upper back
  - Path: similar to tumid lupus and REM (superficial and deep PV/PA lymphocytic infiltrate w/ mucin; absent vacuolar interface) but w/ **CD8^{+} T-cells** and less mucin
    - "The word Jessner's has 8 letters in it"
  - Rx: resolution in 1–2 months with sun protection and antimalarials
- Reticular erythematous mucinosis
  - Photosensitive eruption on a spectrum w/ tumid lupus and REM in adult females
  - p/w red papules and plaques in a reticular configuration on the upper back/chest
  - Path: same as tumid lupus but DIF is negative
  - Rx: resolution in 1–2 months with sun protection and antimalarials

Subacute cutaneous lupus erythematosus (SCLE)

- More common in females (4:1) and more common in Caucasians (DLE and SLE are MC in people of color)
- Nearly half of patients will eventually meet criteria for SLE but will have mild disease
- Pathogenesis: **UVB** ("say luBus") > UVA-induced apoptosis → release of nuclear antigens (Ro/La) plus reduced Clearance of these apoptotic cells (due to Complement deficiencies) → loss of immune tolerance and production of proinflammatory Cytokines

- Genetic associations: HLA-B8-DR3; hereditary Compliment deficiencies
  - Whereas Bullous lupus and EBA have DR2 (B is 2nd letter of alphabet), Childhood DM and SCLE have HLA-B8-DR3 (C is 3rd letter of alphabet)
- Complement: SCLE is a/w Complement deficiencies in early intrinsic pathway (C1/C2/C4)
- p/w **Chronic, relapsing** course of psoriasiform or scaly annular (Central Clearing) plaques on lateral face/ Chest (sun-exposed skin) → heals with hypopigmentation but no scarring
  - "Looks like a scaly chronic version of Jessners lymphocytic infiltrate/tumid lupus"
  - Ddx of annular scaly lesions: annular LP (purple plaques w/ white Wickman striae scale), EAC (trailing scale), tinea (peripheral rim of scale), PLC (lesions appear in crops and have central scale), guttate psoriasis (hundreds of small drop-like lesions w/ thicker scale), secondary syphilis (copper-colored lesions involving palms/soles), PR (herald patch, collarette of scale w/ Christmas tree orientation)
- Half of patients have severe **photosensitivity** (a/w the presence of anti-Ro/La Abs)
- MC systemic finding (70%) is **arthritis/arthralgias** ("joints Crack")
- Labs: **anti-Ro** (75–90%), anti-La (30–40%), ANA (70%; usually a speckled IIF pattern)
- Path: hyperkeratosis, epidermal atrophy, vacuolar interface, BMZ thickening, PV/PA lymphoid aggregates (superficial +/- deep dermis) w/ plasma cells and ↑ dermal mucin
- DIF: LBT (+) in 75%
- Rx ("Shaq does meth"): Sun protection, Steroids and (HCQ/chloroquine)

    - Counsel to avoid smoking w/ HCQ as this makes it less effective
- Before treating, consider drug-induced causes as 25% of SCLE cases are drug-induced (anti-Ro/SS-A+); unlike DI-SLE, there is no specific antibody that indicates DI-SCLE
    - "Greasy PATCH" (as the mnemonic progresses, the drugs become more common)
        - Griseofulvin
        - Piroxicam, **PPIs**
        - ACE inhibitors, Anti-histamines, Anti-convulsants, **Aldactone**
        - Terbinafine (**2nd MC**), TNF-α inh. (etanercept is MC), Taxanes (docetaxel)
        - CCBs (Diltiazem is Delayed → has the longest latency until rash onset)
        - **Hydrochlorothiazide** (MCC): careful because the MCC of drug-induced SLE (Hydralazine and procainamide) and DM (Hydroxyurea) all start w/ "Hydr" but HCTZ and SCLE both have 4 letters

SCLE-like syndromes

- Neonatal lupus erythematosus (NLE)
    - Pathogenesis: transplacental passage of maternal anti-Ro (99%) autoantibodies
    - In a healthy Ro (+) mom, baby has 1–2% chance of NLE; in Ro (+) mom w/ CTD, baby has 15% of NLE; mom w/ prior NLE child, **next baby has 25% of NLE**
        - In all cases the MC outcome is healthy baby, **but still order serial fetal US**
    - 50% of mothers w/ NLE baby are asymptomatic at time of baby's birth but half of these mothers later develop SCLE, SLE, or Sjögren's

- Like SCLE, it is MC in Caucasians and p/w a photosensitive papulosquamous annular rash with prominent facial involvement which heals with Color Changes but no scarring (SCLE affects lateral face but NLE affects the central face around the eyes → "**raccoon eyes**"; racoon eyes in neuroblastoma are more bruise-like)
- Systemic findings
  - Cardiac: MC systemic finding; 70% overall; 33% with Congenital 3rd degree (Complete) heart block which p/w irreversible bradycardia
    - "Ro makes the heart go slow"
  - Hepatobiliary disease (50%): elevated LFTs and bilirubin on CMP
  - Hematologic abnormalities: Cytopenias (esp **thrombocytopenia**) on CBC
- 1st test: ECG (electrocardiogram)
- Path: same as SCLE but DIF only shows (+) LBT in 50% (vs 75% in SCLE)
- Labs: anti-Ro/SS-A, ↑ LFTs, Cytopenias (↓ platelets is MC)
- Rx ("Shaq does meth")
  - Skin: Sun protection + topical Steroids
  - Cardiac disease ppx (mom): HCQ + systemic Steroids in pregnancy
    - Consider in Ro (+) moms w/ CTD or if prior baby had NLE
  - Cardiac disease treatment (baby): pacemaker for complete heart blocks
- Prognosis
  - Skin: lesions resolve by 6 months with atrophy, dyspigmentation and telangiectasias which persists for years (but no scarring)
  - Cardiac: complete heart block is irreversible and has a 33% mortality

- Stats to know
  - If mom had prior NLE baby, next baby has a 1 of 4 chance of getting NLE
    - "Sort of like it was an autosomal recessive trait"
  - 1 of 3 NLE babies will get 3rd degree heart block (1 of 3 of these will die)
  - 1 of 2 NLE babies will get hepatobiliary disease
  - 1 of 2 moms with a NLE baby will have no CTD symptoms at time of birth

- Complement deficiencies
  - Pathogenesis (like SCLE): UV-damaged apoptotic keratinocytes express autoantigens (esp. Ro) which cannot be cleared due to complement deficiencies
  - p/w ↑ risk of SLE and ↑ risk of encapsulated bacterial infections (recurrent PNA)
  - **C2 def (MC but least severe)** > C4 > C1s > C1r > **C1q** (least common; most severe)
    - C2 deficiency-associated lupus: p/w **adult-onset** lupus w/ prominent photosensitivity, SCLE-lesions, ↑ bacterial infections but **no renal disease**
    - C1q/r/s and C4 deficiency-associated lupus: p/w **childhood onset** lupus w/ photosensitivity, SCLE/CCLE-lesions, ↑ bacterial infections w/ **severe, recalcitrant renal disease** +/- palmoplantar keratosis (C4 deficiency only; "2 palms + 2 soles are keratotic = 4")
  - Anti-C1q autoantibodies (acquired): arises in nearly ½ of SLE patients (a/w renal disease) and nearly all of "hypoqomplementemic urtiqarial vasqulitis" patients
  - Labs: low or (-) ANA, **(+) anti-Ro** in most, **↓ complement levels** (screen w/ CH50)

Compliment deficiencies: "Compliment Jessica ALBA"

↓C1q: Acquired Angioedema and severe SLE (C1q auto-Ab in SLE and "hypoqomplementemic urtiqarial vasqulitis")

↓C2: MC compliment deficiency in Lupus

↓C3: Barraquer Simons syndrome (acquired partial lipodystrophy) w/ glomerulonephritis

↓C4: seen in all forms of acquired or hereditary Angioedema and in severe SLE w/ PPK

Acute cutaneous lupus erythematosus (ACLE)

- Of the 3 major cutaneous lupus subtypes (DLE, SCLE, and ACLE), ACLE is most strongly a/w SLE
- p/w **transient erythema on the nasal bridge and B/L malar eminence ("butterfly rash")** after sun exposure; **spares NL folds (vs DM)** as sun cannot get into those deep dark folds
    - o Variable morphologies: scaling, papules, poikiloderma, atrophy, dyspigmentation
    - o Rash may involve other sun-exposed sites such as neck, upper back, arms, legs and dorsal hands classically **sparring the knuckles (DM favors knuckles)**
- Path: vacuolar interface, sparse PV lymph infiltrate limited to upper dermis
- DIF: LBT (+)
- Labs: same as in SLE (ANA, dsDNA, CBC, CMP, etc.)
- Rx: ACLE skin lesions correlate w/ systemic disease activity; treat systemic symptoms

Cutaneous lupus variants

- Bullous SLE
    - o MC in females and African Americans (Black people)

- Pathogenesis: Abs vs NC1 and NC2 domains of type VII collagen (same as EBA)
  - "VII" symbol looks like a BED frame: Bullous lupus, EBA, Dystrophic EB
- HLA-DR2 (Bullous lupus and EBA have a B which is the 2nd letter of the alphabet)
- p/w widespread, symmetric eruption of tense, subepidermal Bullae on an urticarial Base +/- mucosal lesions in patients with SLE
- Path: subepidermal bullae with neutrophils at DEJ and in dermal papillae
- DIF: continuous deposition of IgM/G/A and C3 along BMZ; IgG stains floor on SSS
- Labs: same as in SLE (ANA, dsDNA, CBC, CMP, etc.)
- Rx: dapsone (differentiates from EBA: "Extremely Bad Antidotes")

- Rowell's syndrome
  - Anti-Ro (+)
  - EM-like lesions arising in the setting of ACLE, SCLE or DLE
    - ROWELLL: Really Odd Wacky EM-Like Lesions in Lupus
- TEN-like lupus erythematosus
- TEN triggered by excessive UV exposure in pts w/ pre-existing ACLE or SCLE

Systemic lupus erythematosus (SLE)

- MC in females and African Americans
- Pathogenesis: complex but simply put it is a defect of phagocytes to clear apoptotic cells
  - ↑ plasmacytoid dendritic cells (**CD123+**) → ↑ IFN
- Genetics (SLE): multiple genes encoding STAT4, LYN and Early compliment components
- Triggers (SLE): Sunlight (UVB; "say LuBus"), Smoking, Low vitamin D levels, Estrogen
- High yield cutaneous manifestations in SLE include:

  - Sneddon syndrome: APLS + livedo reticularis + ischemic strokes
  - Loops of wandering and dilated glomeruloid-like vessels around the nails
    - vs symmetric dilation and vessel dropout seen in DM and SSc
  - LCV (and other forms of vasculitis like HUV or PNGD) → ulcers, purpura, Dego's
  - **Eruptive dermatofibromas**; malar or palmar Erythema; Erosions in mouth
- Fetal complications (SLE): Slow heart (congenital heart block), Loss of fetus, Early birth
  - Rx: treat mother w/ systemic steroids and HCQ
- Labs: ↑ ESR/CRP, cytopenias, UA, ↓ compliment levels, antibodies to "ABCD KRUSH"
- Path: from ACLE to SCLE to DLE, the vacuolar interface becomes more obvious, lymphoid infiltrate becomes deeper, and epidermis becomes thinner w/ more follicular plugging
- Rx ("ShaQ CRAB"): Sun protection/topical/IL/systemic Steroids, HCQ +/- Quinacrine
  - Recalcitrant disease: Cyclophosphamide, Rituximab, Anifrolumab, Belimumab
- Prognosis: younger onset has worse prognosis; 90% 10-year survival (MCC of death):
  - In First Five years of disease: MCC of death is Inflammatory lesions or Infection
  - Beyond five years: MCC of death is **thromboses** (DVT/PE/MI)
- Workup for SLE: ANA (dsDNA, Sm) UA, CBC, BMP, ESR/CRP, C3/C4, and antiphospholipid Abs
- SOAP BRAIN MD criteria (4 of 11): Serositis, Oral ulcers, Arthritis, Photosensitive rash, Blood/Renal disease, ANA, Immunologic disease, Neurologic disease, and Malar/Discoid rash

Things that erupt: "When coronavirus erupts, Gates HASSS D VAX"
Gryzbowski (eruptive keratoacanthomas)
Generalized eruptive Histiocytosis
Eruptive Aquired nevi (EBA and LS&A)
Eruptive Syringomas (Asians, Downs); Sign of leser trelat (SKs); eruptive SCCs/Kas (BRAF inh)
Eruptive Dermatofibromas (SLE)
Eruptive Vellous hair cysts
Eruptive Acne (conglobata)
Eruptive Xanthomas

Drug-induced SLE (DI-SLE)

- Begins > 1 year after drug initiation and resolves within 1 month of discontinuation
- Usually p/w no skin lesions and only mild lupus symptoms: arthritis/arthralgias, myalgias, fevers and serositis (no severe internal involvement like renal or CNS disease)
  - vs DI-SCLE which only has cutaneous findings and no systemic findings
- Most important implicated drugs: "Dads Tiny Mini Pirate SHIP"
  - D-penicillamine, **TNF-α inh** (Dads Tiny): looks like true SLE (↑ skin involvement)
  - Minocycline, Methimazole, PTU (Mini Pirate): a/w vasculitis and internal disease
  - Sulfonamides, **Hydralazine**, **INH**, **Procainamide** (SHIP): MCC of DI-SLE
- Labs: (+) anti-histone antibodies
  - DI-SLE from D-penicillamine or TNF-α inh: **(+) ds-DNA** and (-) anti-histone
  - DI-SLE from PTU, methimazole, minocycline: **(+) p-ANCA** and (-) anti-histone
  - DI-SLE from sulfonamides, hydralazine, INH, procainamide: **(+) anti-histone**
    - PTU and hydralazine can cause both (+) histone and (+) p-ANCA

Other autoimmune connective tissue diseases and sclerosing dermopathies

Dermatomyositis (DM; Polymyositis)

- F > M; bimodal Peaks (5–14 yo and 45–64 yo)
- Pathogenesis: immune-mediated process triggered by outside factors (malignancy)
  - HLA alleles: DR3, -B8 (juvenile DM), DR52 (anti-Jo Abs), -DR7, -DRw53 (anti-Mi-2)
  - **TNF-**α 308A polymorphism (a/w juvenile DM) → ↑ thrombospondin-1 → clots
  - **Type-1 interferons** are uniquely elevated in skin lesions of dermatomyositis
- p/w symmetric Proximal muscle weakness (lacks muscle pain) mainly affecting the shoulders and the hip girdles (difficulty brushing hair/teeth or walking upstairs)
- Skin findings (compared to lupus, lesions are more **Purpuric, Pruritic and Psoriasiform**)
  - Gottron's sign: macular erythema over joints such as elbows, fingers and knees
  - Gottron's papules: less common but pathognomonic; Purple Paps on knuckles
  - Symmetric confluent macular violaceous erythema (CMVE) of face involving NL folds (vs lupus), eyelids (heliotrope sign), lateral thigh (Holster sign), joints (Gottron's sign; erythema of lupus spares joints) and extensor tendons of hands
  - Photodistributed CMVE ("V-sign"/Shawl sign) and Photodistributed Poikiloderma
  - Mechanics hands: rough hyperkeratosis/fissuring of the lateral and Palmar digits
    - The hyperkeratosis is more prominent on ulnar side of thumb and radial side of index finger (where a mechanic would turn to tighten a knob)

        - Similar lateral hyperkeratosis is seen on the feet ("hiker's feet")
        - a/w anti-synthetase syndrome (anti-Jo-1): "Jo is a mechanic"
    - Nail changes: ragged (hypertrophic) cuticles (Samitz sign), Periungual erythema, dilated capillary loops alternating w/ areas of Proximal nailfold vessel dropout
    - Scalp: Psoriasiform dermatitis and severe Pruritis (vs psoriasis/lupus which have no itch)
    - Calcinosis cutis: seen in juvenile DM; favors elbows, knees and buttocks
        - a/w anti-p140 (NXP-2) autoantibodies
    - Painful Palmar Papules (inverse Gottron's sign): p/w Painful red Palmar Papules
        - a/w anti-MDA5 (CADM-140)
    - Vasculitis: a/w malignancy (in adults) or severe course in kids (Bankers variant)
    - Flagellate erythema (BDSM): Bleomycin, Docetaxel, Dermatomyositis, Diode laser, Stills disease, Mushrooms (shitake), Man-o-war/jellyfish
    - Wong-type DM has overlap features of DM and Pityriasis Rubra Pilaris
        - "Nothing Wong with sliding in her DMs but People Recognize Players"
- Non-muscular systemic findings: diffuse ILD (a/w anti-Jo and anti-CADM-140), heart disease (a/w anti-SRP), arthralgias and non-erosive arthritis
- Subtypes based on autoantibody
    - Anti-CADM-140 (MDA5): vasculopathic DM skin lesions (painful palmar papules, skin ulcers) w/ rapidly progressive ILD but no muscle disease (can affect kids too)
    - Anti-synthetase (anti-Jo): mechanics hands, severe ILD, arthritis and myositis

    - "I imagine an MD named CAD and mechanic named Jo (mechanic hands) in a race making them both SOB (ILD), but whereas CAD is an unathletic MD and falls down early onto his hands (painful palmar papules and skin ulcers) and doesn't finish the race (so his muscles are not weak), Jo the athletic mechanic finishes the entire race (weak muscles)"
- Anti-p155 (TIF-1): MC Ab in juvenile DM (a/w Gottrons papules, photosensitivity, linear extensor erythema), and a/w amyopathic and **cancer-associated DM** w/ severe skin disease (psoriasiform w/ **palmar hyperkeratotic papules**) in adults
    - MC cancers (PLONC): Pancreatic, Prostate, Lymphoma, **Lung**, **Ovarian**, Nasopharyngeal (MC in Asia), Colorectal; also gastric, breast, melanoma
        - **Ovarian (#1) and Lung (#2) are the two MC cancers a/w DM**
            - "The closer to the center of PLONC the more common"
    - **RFs a/w cancer (PLONC): males (Penis), LCV, Old age, skin Necrosis and evidence of Capillary damage on muscle biopsy**
    - **ILD and Raynaud's indicate less than average risk of malignancy**
    - 10–25% of adults w/ DM are diagnosed w/ cancer within 3 years
    - Risk for cancers returns to normal 5 years after diagnosis except the two at the ends of PLONC (Pancreatic and Colorectal stays ↑ beyond 5 years)
- Anti-p140 (anti-NXP2): juvenile DM with calcinosis (peds DM is never a/w cancer)
- Anti-Mi2 (helicase): classic DM skin findings with no visceral disease or cancer

- Anti-SRP: fulminant myopathic DM w/ severe cardiac involvement
    - "Symmetric Rapid Proximal muscle weakness and Severely Rapid Pulse"
- Anti-SAE: classic skin findings, dysphasia, and HCQ-associated skin eruption
- Anti-U1-RNP: DM overlaps with MCTD
- Anti-Ku: DM overlaps with SLE, Sjögren's or scleroderma
- ANA: although not specific, ANA is still the most sensitive antibody in DM

- Juvenile DM: average age is 7 yo; never a/w cancer
    - Brunsting variant: gradual onset of classic skin and muscle disease w/ calcinosis cutis which favors sites of trauma (fingers, elbows, knees); steroid responsive
    - Banker variant: rapid onset of vasculitis (ulcers, livedo reticularis, GI perforation) and severe muscle involvement; poor response to steroids/poor prognosis
- Path: subtle vacuolar interface, ↑BMZ, sparse PV/PA lymph infiltrate, ↑ dermal mucin
    - Looks just like lupus on path but epidermis tends to be more atrophied in DM
- Dx: after confirmatory biopsy evaluate for systemic disease
    - Evaluate for myositis: ↑ muscle enzymes (CK, **aldolase**), EMG, MRI or US of proximal muscles, muscle biopsy (gold standard; triceps muscle is highest yield)
    - Evaluate for cancer (PLONC): CA19-9 (pancreatic), PSA (prostate), CT (lung), **CA125/transvaginal US** (Ovary), FOBT/colonoscopy (colorectal)
    - Evaluate for ILD: **PFTs w/ CO diffusion** (if abnormal → high-resolution chest CT)

    - Evaluate for cardiac (EKG) and esophageal (barium swallow, manometry) disease
- Rx (similar to SLE, we start w/ sun protection and topicals then systemics and rituximab)
    - Non-vasculopathic skin disease: sun protection + topical CS/CNIs
        - IVIG or HCQ (morbilliform drug eruption in 31% of DM pts) if recalcitrant
            - IVIG has great efficacy for esophageal complications (dysphagia)
- Skin and muscle disease: systemic CS (Prednisone) +/- steroid sparing agents
        - IVIG if patient failed therapy w/ steroid and DMARD
    - Vasculopathic skin disease (painful palmar papules; anti-CADM): rituximab + ILK
    - Future directions: JAK3 inhibitor (tofacitinib) is demonstrating great efficacy
- Prognosis: 5-year survival is 63% (MCC of death: cancer, Pulmonary/heart disease, PNA)

Periungual telangiectasias: "These conditions have ↑ ODSS of having periungual vessels"
Osler-Weber-Rendu: ectasia of half of capillary loop DM: **symmetric dilation of vessels w/ vessel dropout** (↓ capillary density) Systemic sclerosis: same as DM but w/ tapered fingers and hyper curvature of the nail SLE: "wandering" dilated **glomeruloid** vessels (normal capillary density just tortuous/dilated)

Drug-induced DM: "Big DISH" (As the mnemonic progresses, the drug is more common)

- BCG vaccine, D-penicillamine, Infliximab (TNF-α inh), Statins, **Hydroxyurea (MC)**
    - Hydroxyurea-induced: Huge (60 month) latency, no myositis, usually ANA (-)

- Non-hydroxyurea-induced (Statins MC): Shorter latency (occurs within 60 days of drug intake), myositis present and has positive Serologies (usually ANA+)

Sjögren's syndrome (RST: "around S in the alphabet)

- Pathogenesis: a/w anti-Ro/SS-A > anti-La/SS-B antibodies which are Ribonucleoproteins
  - Lymphocytic infiltration of Secretory glands (lacrimal and Salivary glands)
  - Mutation in **TNFAIP3** → ↑ risk of MALT-type non-Hodgkin **lymphoma** (like DH)
- p/w triad of xerophthalmia, xerostomia, arthritis ("can't see, can't spit, can't climb up shit")
  - May also see skin xerosis/pruritis (MC skin finding), dyspareunia, neuropathy, **vasculitis**, glomerulonephritis, lymphoma, ↑ risk of baby with neonatal lupus
- Dx (RST): Rose Bengal test and Schirmer Test to detect impaired lacrimal gland function
  - Serologies: **Anti-α-fodrin** (most sensitive and specific), anti-Ro/SS-A, anti-La/SS-B
  - ANA (+) with a Speckled nuclear pattern on IIF
- Rx (RST + SLE Rx): **Suck on candy**, Sialagogue therapy (pilocarpine), artificial Saliva/Tears
  - SLE treatments (ShaQ CRAB): Steroids, HCQ +/- Quinacrine and CRAB for recalcitrant cases (Cyclophosphamide, Rituximab, Anifrolumab, Belimumab)

Relapsing Polychondritis (RP)

- Pathogenesis: Th1 mediated inflammatory disease (IFN, IL-2, and IL-12) that is a/w HLA-DR4
- Autoantibodies against type II Collagen ("car-two-lage") and matrillin-1

- Need 3 of 6 diagnostic criteria: inflammation of joints (non-erosive inflammatory Polyarthritis), Cochlear/ vestibular damage and Chondritis of 4 facial orifices:
  - o Chondritis of both auricles **sparing earlobes** (MC criteria) → "Cauliflower" ears
    - ▪ **Ddx: auricular hematoma in a child (child abuse)**, lobomycosis (keloidal ear lesions), juvenile hyaline fibromatosis (fibrotic nodules on ears)
  - o Chondritis of nasal cartilage: ↓ smell and saddle nose deformity (see below)
  - o Chondritis of ocular structures: conjunctivitis, corneal ulceration, uveitis, iritis
  - o Chondritis of respiratory tract: airway collapse → **Pneumonia (MCC of death)**
- Other features: vasculitis (2nd MCC of death), cardiac valvopathy, aphthous ulcers, EN
- Path: breakdown of normal lacunar cartilage structure with a neutrophilic infiltrate
- Rx: Prednisone is 1st line (MTX is best steroid sparing agent); dapsone for ppx
- MAGIC syndrome (Mouth And Genital Ulcers w/ Inflamed Cartilage) = RP + Behçet's
- Ddx for Nasal destruction (LMNOPqRST): Leishmaniasis (Mucocutaneous), NK T-cell lymphoma, Noma, Olfactory tumors, PLAID, Paracoccidoidomycosis, RP, Rhinoscleroma, Rhinosporidiosis, Syphilis (late congenital or tertiary), Sarcoid, SAVI, and TB (lupus vulgaris)

Conditions with saddle nose deformity: "Saddle GIRL"
Granulomatosis with polyangiitis Idiopathic Relapsing polychondritis, Rothmund-Thompson Late congenital syphilis, Lepromatous Leprosy

Mixed Connective tissue disease (MCTD)

- Mixed features of at least 2 of the following (PqRS): PM/DM, RA, SLE, Scleroderma
- Pathogenesis: a/w HLA-DR4 and autoantibodies against Anti-U1RNP
  - o "The 4th DR has a fast car which goes VVRRUM": Vitiligo, pemphigus Vulgaris, Relapsing polychondritis, RA, Urticaria (chronic idiopathic) and Mixed CTD
- Abs to EBV and CMV cross-react w/ U1RNP, suggesting that Molecular Mimicry related to prior exposure to these viruses may be responsible for anti-U1RNP autoimmunity
- p/w Mixed features of PM/DM (myopathy, DM-rash), RA, SLE (arthritis), and scleroderma (Raynaud's is the MC/earliest sign; pulmonary HTN is the most severe sign of MCTD)
- **DIF: characteristic immune deposits (IgG is MC) within epidermal cell nuclei**
- Dx: ANA (+) w/ a speckled pattern (fluorescent areas Mixed in w/ less fluorescent ones)
- Rx: prednisone (MTX is 1st line for severe arthritis but watch out for pulmonary fibrosis)

Systemic-onset juvenile idiopathic arthritis (Still's disease; "stIL-l disease")

- Still's disease is only 1 of 6 forms of JIA but is the most relevant to dermatologists
- Autoinflammatory syndrome (disorder of innate immune system) w/ **↑IL-1 cytokines**
- p/w **daily high fevers** (evenings) and an associated **transient salmon-pink exanthem** w/ a predilection for the axilla/waist; linear lesions due to köebnerization
  - o Other features include symmetric arthritis, uveitis, LAD/HSM and serositis
- Dx: ↑ESR/CRP, **↑ ferritin** (RF and ANA are negative)

- Rx: NSAIDS, prednisone, MTX, TNF-α inhibitors depending on severity
    - IL-1 (anakinra, **canakinumab**, rilocept) and IL-6 inh (tocilizumab) work well
- Refer to ophthalmology for uveitis screening
- Prognosis: resolves in 50%, exhibits chronic course in 50% and progresses to life-threatening macrophage activation syndrome in 5% (pancytopenia, neurologic issues)

Adult onset Still disease

- Presents in young adults (but not < 16 years old by definition)
- Presents similar to Still's with spiking afternoon fevers w/ an associated transient salmon-pink exanthem +/- persistent papules/plaques, arthralgias and LAD/HSM but is a/w a **flu-like prodrome w/ a sore throat, carpal ankylosis** (limited ROM in the carpal joints) and a more common progression to macrophage activation syndrome (15%)
- Criteria (needs 2 major and 3 minor)
    - Major: fever > 39°C x 1 week, arthralgias x 2 weeks, typical rash, WBC > 10,000
    - Minor: pharyngitis, LAD, ↑ LFTs, negative ANA, and RF, ↑ ferritin
- Dx: labs are like Juvenile Still's
- Path: neutrophil-predominant PV inflammation w/ necrotic keratinocytes in epidermis
- Rx: same treatment as for Juvenile Still's

Rheumatoid arthritis

- a/w HLA-DRB1 (↑ propensity to form anti-CCP antibodies due to molecular mimicry to proteins produced by EBV and E. coli), HLA-DR1, and HLA-DR4
    - BP and DH have epitope spreading; RA and MCTD have molecular mimicry

- Pathophysiology: initiating event is binding of ECM components to TLR → ↑ inflammatory cytokines (TNF-α, IL-1, IL-6) → cartilage break down and B cell activation
    - RANKL binds RANK on osteoclasts (bone erosion)
    - RF and anti-CCP antibodies form immune complexes inside joints → activation of compliment → activation of neutrophils which cause cutaneous findings
- PTPN22 gene confers susceptibility to RA and other autoimmune conditions
- Skin findings (associated with ↑ RF antibody titers)
    - **Rheumatoid nodulosis p/w painless nodules over bony prominences**
    - Accelerated rheumatoid nodulosis p/w sudden appearance of multiple **painful** rheumatoid nodules following initiation of **methotrexate** or TNF-α inhibitors
    - Rheumatoid vasculitis (40% mortality) p/w systemic vasculitis (e.g., neuropathies, carditis) in patients with a long history of severe erosive RA
    - Bywater's lesions p/w nailfold thromboses and **purpuric macules on distal digits**
        - Demonstrates LCV on path but no signs of systemic vasculitis
    - Felty syndrome p/w Low WBCs, Large spleen, Leg ulcers, and Leukemias/Lymphomas
        - Rx: G-CSF or splenectomy
    - Superficial ulcerating necrobiosis (rheumatoid necrobiosis) resembles NLD
    - Rheumatoid neutrophilic dermatosis resembles Sweets syndrome
        - Rx: prednisone or antineutrophilic agents (dapsone, colchicine)
        - Other neutrophilic conditions a/w RA include EED, PG, and IGDA/PNGD

- Path: early lesions resemble IGDA/PNGD (granulomatous or neutrophilic infiltrate) while later lesions show **palisading granulomas surrounding bright Red eosinophilic fibrin**
- Dx: RF (most sensitive) and anti-CCP (most specific)
- Rx (arthritis): NSAIDS, prednisone, DMARDS (MTX, hydroxychloroquine, sulfasalazine leflunomide), or biologics (TNF-α inhibitors, abatacept, tocilizumab)
    - Rheumatoid nodules do not respond to arthritis treatment (consider IL steroids)
- Prognosis: course waxes and wanes; MCC of death is ischemic heart disease

Morphea (localized scleroderma; "Go BLAND and wear hard HATS, SAM")

- Most cases present in childhood w/ F > M (except linear morphea in which M = F)
- Plaque type is MC variant overall and in adults but linear is MC variant in children
- Pathogenesis: genetic predisposition + environmental trigger (**Borrelia afzelii/garinii**) → vascular injury → inflammation → ↑ profibrotic Th2 cytokines (**↑TGF-β**) → ↑ collagen
- Plaque morphea: p/w hairless and indurated hyperpigmented plaques w/ a **lilac** (violet tone on top of pink)**-colored inflammatory border** on the **trunk** or proximal extremities
    - This lilac (pink-purple) color is also the color seen in lupus and dermatomyositis
    - **Ddx: extragenital LS&A favors the breast/chest, back, posterior neck, butt and wrists and has a more porcelain-white and wrinkled center (vs hyperpigmented in plaque morphea) w/ a violaceous border +/- follicular plugging**
- Clinical subtypes of plaque morphea ("Go BLAND")

- Generalized morphea: p/w widespread indurated plaques → muscle atrophy and difficulty breathing (constrictive effect of taut skin on chest); a/w fatigue/malaise
    - Pansclerotic variant: generalized morphea involving deep structures
- Guttate morphea: p/w multiple, small flat or slightly depressed white macules
    - Appears similar to guttate LS&A but lacks follicular plugging
- Bullous morphea: usually only seen in the context of generalized morphea
    - Diffuse sclerosis of skin → lymphatic obstruction → bullae formation
- Linear morphea: p/w linear lesions of sclerosis on the **Legs**
    - a/w serious morbidity (permanent limb undergrowth/joint contractures)
    - Involves deeper (Lower) structures such as muscle, fascia and bone
    - "Lower age, lower extremities, lower structures involved, lower QOL"
    - Melorheostosis (roughened long bones seen underlying linear morphea and in Buschke-Ollendorff): resembles wax dripping off a candle on X-ray
    - Head/neck subtypes of linear morphea
        - En coup de sabre: variant of linear morphea of the scalp
        - Parry-Romberg syndrome: variant of linear morphea of the face
            - a/w epilepsy and eye involvement (**next step is eye exam**)
- Atrophoderma of Pasini and Pierini: superficial variant of plaque morphea

        - p/w large hyperpigmented atrophic plaques w/ sharp "cliff-drop" borders
        - MC location is back and pre-sacral area ("Above the Ass")
    - Nodular or keloidal morphea: keloid-like nodules/ streaks
    - Deep morphea (morphea profunda): p/w pseudo-cellulite look (like eosinophilic fasciitis) due to sclerosis of the deep structures (e.g., fascia, muscle)
        - Difficult to treat: poor response to steroids (vs eosinophilic fasciitis)
- MC associated symptom: **arthralgias** (esp w/ deep, generalized, and linear morphea)
- Path: square punch, eccrine glands "trapped" and compressed by sclerotic collagen
    - Early lesions show a lymphocytic infiltrate w/ plasma cells at the dermal-SQ junction w/ loss of $CD34^+$ dendritic cells (vs ↑ in NSF and scleromyxedema)
- Dx/antibodies ("hard HATS"): all forms lack anti-Scl70/ topoisomerase 1 (vs SSc)
    - Anti-Histone: linear and generalized forms (correlates w/ disease activity)
    - ANA: linear and generalized forms; correlates w/ disease severity/activity
    - Anti-Topoisomerase 2 (Two): all forms
    - Anti-ssDNA: linear form only (correlates w/ disease activity)
- Rx ("SAM"; Steroids, UVA phototherapy, Acitretin, Methotrexate)
    - Superficial localized lesions: topical or IL CS + UVA phototherapy
    - Superficial generalized lesions: UVA phototherapy
    - Deep lesions (linear or deep morphea): **pulsed IV Steroids + MTX**

- Isotretinoin/Acitretin are affective for morphea, LS&A and sclerodermoid GVHD
- Prognosis: superficial plaque morphea is self-limited (resolves in 3 years); spontaneous resolution for deep and generalized morphea is uncommon
- High-yield points: treat deep/severe Morphea w/ MTX (1st line) or Mycophenolate mofetil (2nd line); see Melorheostosis in linear Morphea
  - Rx MCTD w/ MTX also (careful MTX and MCTD both cause pulmonary fibrosis)

↑ TGF-Beta: "BS Moles"
Buschke-Ollendorff syndrome, Scar/keloids (↑ TGF Beta 1 and 2, **↓ TGF Beta 3**) Morphea, Osler-Weber-Rendu (HHT), Loeys-Dietz, Eosinophilic fasciitis, Scleroderma

Scleroderma (systemic sclerosis; SSc)

- Mainly affects F > M in 30–50s but older age, AA race, male sex, truncal distribution, anemia, internal organ involvement (**pulmonary**) and ↑ ESR confers a worse prognosis
  - "Old black males with truncal sclerosis, pulmonary disease and ↑ ESR do worse"
- Pathogenesis: key features include vascular dysfunction (earliest feature), immune activation (↑ Th2 profibrotic cytokines e.g., **TGF-β**, IL-1, -4, -6, -8, IGF) w/ autoantibody production (anti-centromere, anti-Scl70) and deposition of collagen in skin and organs
- SSc subtypes
  - Limited SSc: cutaneous sclerosis limited to face and distal extremities
    - CREST syndrome is a variant: Calcinosis, Raynaud's, Esophageal dysmotility, Sclerodactyly, **flat matted Telangiectasias on face/palms**

        - Ddx: HHT also has matted telangiectasias (but are in the mouth)
      - Lacks severe renal involvement or ILD (**MCC of death is PAH**)
  - Diffuse SSc: cutaneous sclerosis is generalized; a/w poor prognosis
      - a/w severe, rapidly progressive visceral disease (**MCC of death is ILD**)
- Cutaneous features (check the fingers)
  - **Skin thickening of fingers on both hands extending proximal to MCP**
      - **Solely having this feature is sufficient to meet the diagnostic criteria**
      - 3 stages: edema (1st year), induration (1–4 years), atrophy (forever)
  - Sclerodactyly: sclerosis/thickening of fingers distal to MCPs but proximal to PIPs
  - Fingertip lesions: **digital tip ulcers (due to recurrent vasospasm)** → pitting scars
  - Interphalangeal joint ulcers: due to trauma
  - Nail folds capillaries w/ dilated capillary loops alternating w/ areas of vessel loss
      - November 2022 JAAD CME 1 has a great picture of this
  - Pterygium inversum unguis (ventral pterygium) vs dorsal pterygium (seen in LP)
  - Raynaud's phenomenon: MC initial presenting sign of SSc (hand edema 2nd MC)
      - Whereas CCBs and α-blockers help Raynaud's, **β-blockers exacerbate it**
  - Other cutaneous features: mat telangiectasias, calcinosis, **"salt and pepper" pigmentation** (leukoderma w/ perifollicular sparing), microstomia, beaked nose, hyperpigmentation increased at areas of pressure (belt), pruritis and ↓ sweating
- Systemic features

  - Pulmonary disease is MCC of death: (**ILD in diffuse** and **PAH in limited**) and 2nd MC site of visceral involvement (after GI/dysphagia)
  - GI (dysphagia): MC site of visceral involvement (↑ morbidity but no ↑ mortality)
  - Renal: scleroderma renal crisis affects 20% of diffuse SSc (Rx: ACE inhibitors)
  - Other systemic features: restrictive cardiomyopathy, sicca syndrome, tendon friction rubs, arthralgias, proximal muscle weakness and esophageal dysmotility
- Path: same as morphea (differentiate w/ physical exam and autoantibodies)
- Dx: antibodies in systemic sclerosis ("Hard fibrotic CARS")
  - Fibrillarin (U3RNP): a/w diffuse skin disease and pulmonary HTN; poor prognosis
  - Centromere: a/w limited SSc/CREST (a/w pulmonary HTN and digital ulcers) > SSc
  - ANA (nucleolar staining pattern seen on IIF)
  - **RNA polymerase III**: a/w SSc (**Renal**; Rapidly progressive); ↑ risk of cancer
  - Scl-70 (DNA topoisomerase I): a/w SSc (lung disease) > CREST; poor prognosis
- Main ddx ("hard EGGS"): Eosinophilic fasciitis, Eosinophilia-Myalgia syndrome (ingesting L-tryptophan), Generalized morphea, GVHD (chronic), Scleredema, and Scleromyxedema
- Rx (SSc/CREST): **avoid Cold exposure**, Cigarette Cessation and Corticosteroids +/- MTX in SSc (careful because **steroids can exacerbate renal crisis** and **MTX can exacerbate ILD**)
  - Skin sclerosis: **Celcept is 1st line**, Cyclophosphamide, MTX, phototherapy (PUVA/UVA1), CS, rituximab, tocilizumab (IL-6) help; HSCT if severe

- ILD: MMF (**Celcept**) and Cyclophosphamide are first line; rituximab, nintedanib
- Pruritis: Cannabinoid receptor modulator (lenabasum), antihistamines
- Renal disease/HTN: ACE inhibitors (Captopril)
- PAH: PDE5i (sildenafil), ERA (bosentan), and guanylate cyclase stimulator (riociguat)
- Raynaud's: non-cardioselective **CCBs** (nifedipine) are 1st line, PDE5i (sildenafil) and prostanoids (IV iloprost if severe) are 2nd line; botox, SSRIs, ARBS/ACEi help
- Digital ulcers: same as Raynaud's but PDE5i alone or in combo w/ a CCB is 1st line
- GI: PPIs for GERD, prokinetic agents (metoclopramide) for GI dysmotility, nutrient supplementation for malabsorption, antibiotics for bacterial overgrowth
- Calcinosis cutis (poor evidence): Coumadin, CCBs, Cut it out, sodium thiosulfate
- Mat telangiectasias: vascular lasers (**PDL**, KTP IPL), green-tinted camouflage
- Microstomia: IPL, IL hyaluronidase, CO2 laser

• Screening in SSc (**CXCL4** is a new biomarker for PAH and skin/lung fibrosis)
- ILD: **PFTs** at baseline and every 4–6 months for 3 years → high-resolution CT
- PAH (DETECT algorithm): telangiectasias, anti-centromere Ab, BNP, serum urate or EKG w/ right axis deviation → echo-Cardiogram → right heart Catheterization
- Renal: Cr, urea, electrolytes and UA at baseline and annually)

DNA Topoisomerases
Topoisomerase 1 (anti-Scl-70): auto-antibody in diffuse SSc Topoisomerase 2 (DNA gyrase): autoantibody in morphea ("1 more topoisomerase than SSc") Topoisomerase 2 and 4: fluoroquinolones inhibits topo 2 (G- coverage) +/- 4 (G+ coverage)

Eosinophilic fasciitis

- Pathogenesis: unknown but **TGF-β is markedly Elevated**
- a/w **strenuous Exercise** (precedes clinical findings by days to weeks in 30% of cases)
- p/w rapid onset (Eruptive), symmetric (Equal), and Edema in Extremities (**spares hands/feet**)
    - Develops a peau d'orange/pseudo-cellulite look (like deep morphea and NSF) w/ a **"dry riverbed/ groove sign" (linear depressions of veins within indurated skin)**
    - Lacks Raynaud's as it does not involve the hands/ feet (vs SSc)
- a/w joint contractures, arthritis and loss of mobility > lymphoma/leukemia, MGUS, MM
    - "Can't Exercise anymore and they get leuk-E-mias"
- Ddx: SSc (but spares hands), Eosinophilic-myalgia syndrome (but lacks fever/myalgias), and deep morphea (but has excellent response to systemic steroids)
- Path (must obtain deep biopsy to fascia): fibrosis of deep fascia +/- eosinophils
- Dx: **CBC (peripheral Eosinophilia)**, ↑ ESR, ↑ TGF-β and normal ANA
    - **CBC may show pancytopenia due to an associated myelodysplastic syndrome**
        - "If veins are clinically low ("groove sign"), CBC may show low cell counts"
    - MRI or CT may show fascial thickening and eliminate the need for a biopsy

  - **Metalloproteinase inhibitor-1 (TIMP-1)** serves as a marker for disease activity
  - Rx: Excellent response to **systemic steroids** (vs deep morphea) + **physical therapy**

Nephrogenic systemic fibrosis (NSF)

- Nephrogenic disorder (results from gadolinium contrast exposure in setting of AKI/CKD)
  - Pathogenesis: gadolinium leaks into tissues and triggers profibrotic cytokines → circulating fibroblasts ($CD34^+$, Pro-collagen I^+) recruited to skin → ↑ collagen
- p/w pruritis and edema → Stiffening of the skin w/ **Symmetric "ameboid" (Swirvy) plaques** w/ pSeudo-cellulite look MC on the extremities (**always Spares the face**)
  - Puckering/rippling/linear banding is seen due to focal areas of bound-down skin
- Extracutaneous involvement: **Scleral plaques (white-yellow plaques)** > organ fibrosis
- Path: identical to Scleromyxedema (↑ $CD34^+$ Spindled fibrocytes, ↑ collagen, ↑ mucin) except is generally deeper and may see "lollipop bodies" (elastic fibers stick like a lollipop stem out from the center of round osseous metaplasia)
  - vs morphea/scleroderma which has loss of $CD34^+$ cells in dermis (and no mucin)
- Rx: Failure of treatment; Fast death (try to treat kidney disease; physical therapy)

Mucinoses

Scleredema

- p/w erythema and woody induration of skin of face and trunk (distal extremities spared)
- 3 types ("It's probably hard to SKI with scleredema")

  - o Type 1 (55%; a/w **Strep** infection): p/w induration of the cervicofacial region with extension to the trunk and arms; difficulty Swallowing; Self-resolves
  - o Type 2 (25%; a/w **IgGκ** monoclonal gammopathy); a/w a "kronic course"
  - o Type 3 (20%; scleredema diabeticorum; a/w **Insulin dependent diabetes**): p/w erythema/induration of the posterior neck/back; Indolent onset, chronic course
- Path: **wide spaces b/w deep dermal collagen bundles filled w/ mucin** (Ddx: back skin)
- Rx: type 1 is self-limited; treat Type 2 and 3 with phototherapy (UVA1 and PUVA)
- **Workup ("SKI"): next step is SPEP/Immunofixation to look for paraproteinemia**

Scleromyxedema

- p/w widespread **Symmetric Closely aligned papules in a Linear array** on the upper body
  - o Surrounding skin is Shiny and Stiff (Sclerodermoid) w/ **Sclerodactyly of digits**
  - o **Scalp is Spared** (face is spared in NSF; hands are spared in eosinophilic fasciitis)
  - o **Shar-Pei Sign**: deep furrowing of back skin (named after shar-pei breed of dog)
  - o **Donut Sign**: induration of skin w/ **Central Low-lying depression over PIP joint**
- Systemic symptoms: dysphagia, myositis, renal/lung disease, dermato-neuro syndrome (p/w high fever, flu-like symptoms, seizures and coma; this patient will be in the ICU)
- CNS involvement → Coma and Carpel tunnel
- **Leonine faces** (deep furrows of the glabella; "it is like the Shar-Pei sign on the face")
- a/w **IgGλ (Lamda)** paraproteinemia in 90% of patients

- Path: looks Like NSF (↑mucin, ↑collagen, ↑ CD34+ fibroblasts) but not as deep into SQ
- Rx: **IVIG** (1st line; "I looks like a lower-case L"), Systemic Steroids + thalidomide (2nd line)
    - Refractory disease: autologous Stem Cell transplant, bortezomib, melphalan
    - Dermato-neuro syndrome: IVIG + systemic steroids +/- melphalan, bortezomib
- Workup: next step is **SPEP/immunofixation** to look for paraproteinemia
- **Lichen myxedematosus** is a localized variant w/ only the Symmetric Closely aligned Linear papules but w/o the surrounding sclerodermoid changes and systemic symptoms
    - a/w immune Suppression (**HIV**), Hepatitis C or exposure to L-tryptophan/toxic oil

PreTibial myxedema

- p/w waxy indurated Purple-brown Plaques w/ a Peau d'orange look on the Pretibia
- a/w Thyroid excess (**Graves** disease)
- **Path: Tuns of mucin in the dermis w/ attenuation/ fragmentation of collagen fibers**
- Rx: Triamcinolone 10–40 mg/cc or steroids applied under occlusive dressings
- Generalized myxedema is seen in hypothyroid states and typically effects the face

Reticular erythematous mucinosis

- Debatable whether this entity is distinct from tumid lupus
- p/w persistent reticular erythematous plaques in the midline back or chest of women
- Path: small amounts of mucin in the dermis w/ a perivascular and periadnexal infiltrate
- Rx: hydroxychloroquine or chloroquine

Follicular mucinosis

- Primary follicular mucinosis: p/w eruption of several pink plaques composed of grouped Follicular papules w/ **alopecia** on the Face (**eyebrow is MC**) and scalp of children
    - a/w systemic findings such as Fever, arthralgias and carpel tunnel syndrome
- Secondary follicular mucinosis: patients are older; a/w atopic dermatitis or **CTCL**
- Path: **mucin accumulates in the follicular epithelium**
- Rx: no specific treatment; follow patient for CTCL if lesions do not go away

Sclerodermoid syndromes induced by exogenous substances

- These present like SSc but have no antibodies

Chemicals: "Poly's Silly Tryp where she got raped was hard for her"

- Polyvinyl chloride: **slowly progressive** SSc-like syndrome in people who clean autoclaves
    - "Vinyl records are a hard material (sclerosis) and they spin slowly"
- Silica: occupational exposures can induce scleroderma-like skin changes
- L-tryptophan: ingestion caused Eosinophilia-myalgia syndrome in the US in 1989
    - p/w rapidly progressive skin sclerosis, fevers, fatigue, myalgias and eosinophilia
- Rapeseed cooking oil: ingestion caused toxic oil syndrome in Spain in 1981
    - p/w rapidly progressive skin sclerosis, flu-like symptoms, and eosinophilia

Systemic drugs: "Bleo's taxes were hard to file"

- Bleomycin: SSc-like syndrome w/ pulmonary fibrosis and Raynaud's
- Taxanes (e.g., docetaxel): diffuse edema and sclerosis (legs #1 site) → joint contractures

Injectables: "Bleo's Silly opioid-induced anti-vax texts were hard for his ex to understand"

- Bleomycin: sclerosis at injection site
- Silicone: chronic inflammation that leads to skin sclerosis at injection site (face MC)
- Opioids (methadone, pentazocine): sclerosis at injection site
- Vaxines: p/w **sclerosis of upper arm** in a young child
- Texier's disease: form of traumatic panniculitis due to vitamin K (phytonadione) injections which p/w painful sclerotic (often w/ lilac-colored borders) inflamed nodules on the **buttocks and thighs ("cowboy holster pattern"),** which can persist for years
    - Ddx: equestrian panniculitis

Other sclerosing/fibrosing skin disorders

- Radiation-induced morphea: morphea-like plaques in radiation field and beyond it (chest wall is #1 site); MC in breast cancer patients (nipple is often spared)
- Diabetic cheiroarthropathy: symmetric loss of joint mobility in the small joints of the hand with scleroderma-like skin thickening of the dorsal hand; positive "prayer sign"
- PCT: sclerotic plaques in sun-exposed areas w/ hypertrichosis and hyperpigmentation
    - Pseudoporphyria lacks sclerodermoid changes, hyper-trichosis, and -pigmentation
- POEMS syndrome (polyneuropathy, organomegaly, endocrinopathy, M-protein, Skin changes such as sclerotic skin changes on the extremities)

- **Carcinoma en cuirasse: sclerosis of the chest wall due to cutaneous mets (breast CA)**
- Chronic GVHD: may present as lichenoid GVHD or sclerotic GVHD (morphea or EF-like)

Perforating diseases

- Group of papulonodular skin disorders with keratotic plugs characterized by transepidermal elimination of dermal connective tissue
- Diseases can be remembered by "Emergency Room PA": as the mnemonic progresses, the people affected get older and the MC body area affected gets more inferior
  - o EPS, RPC, PCE, Acquired perforating dermatoses
- Path: keratotic plug of collagen/elastin w/ surrounding epithelial hyperplasia (crab-claw)
  - o Verhoeff-van Gieson stain is most helpful (stains collagen red and elastic black)
- Rx: EPS/RPC resolve spontaneously; acquired perforating dermatoses is difficult to treat

Elastosis perforans serpiginosa (EPS)

- Presents in **childhood** (M > F) w/ small keratotic papules arranged in a **serpiginous** or annular pattern most commonly on the **lateral neck** but other flexural sites common
- About 40% of cases occur in association with other genetic disorders: "MAD PORES"
  - o Marfan's, Acrogeria, Down's (#1 cause), PXE, Penicillamine use, Osteogenesis imperfecta, Rothmund-Thomson, Ehlers-Danlos syndrome, Scleroderma
- Path: the keratotic plug is also **serpiginous** (wavy) and contain Eosinophilic Elastic fibers

Reactive perforating Collagenosis (RPC)

- Presents in **Childhood** (usually weeks after **trauma**) with keratotic papules on the **arms**
- Exhibits **Köebner** phenomenon
- Path: keratotic plug is wide and **Cup-like** and contains basophilic Collagen fibers

Perforating calcific elastosis (PCE)

- Presents in middle-aged, obese, hypertensive, **multiparous, black women** with keratotic plaques on the **Periumbilical region**
- Path: keratotic plug w/ calcified elastic fibers (like PXE) evident on von Kossa or VVG

Acquired perforating dermatoses (Kyrle's disease)

- Presents in **Adults** with keratotic papulonodules on the extensor **legs/Ancles**
    - o Patients usually have thyroid disease, diabetes or renal failure requiring dialysis
    - o Drug-induced (BITS of perforations): Bevacizumab, Indinavir, TNF-α inh, Sirolimus
- Path: most resembles RPC
- Rx: UVA/UVB (all other perforating diseases self-resolve)

Abnormalities of connective tissue

Mid-dermal elastolysis

- Acquired disorder w/ loss of elastic tissue in the mid-dermis → **p/w fine wrinkling**
- Pathogenesis: unknown but UV light is thought to play a role
- MC affects middle-aged females on the trunk (mid-body) > lateral neck and arms
- Ddx: anetoderma (upper and mid-dermal elastolysis), cutis laxa (full-dermal elastolysis)

- Path: normal H&E (elastic tissue stains show loss of elastic tissue in the mid dermis only)

Anetoderma (A-F)

- Classifications
  - Primary: inflammatory (Jadassohn-Pellizzari) or non-inflammatory (Schweninger-Buzzi)
  - Secondary: a/w systemic disease (autoimmune disease especially **APLS** > lupus)
- Arms, Back, Chest show Circumscribed areas of slack skin (Depressions or **Elevations**)
  - **Buttonhole sign**: finger sinks in when pressed, bulge reappears when released
- Path: normal H&E (loss of elastin in the papillary + mid-reticular dermis w/ elastic stains)
- EM: Fragmentation of elastic fibers

Striae

- p/w linear atrophic depressions of the skin that form in areas of dermal damage (Marfan's syndrome, topical steroids) or stretching (**puberty**, pregnancy, rapid growth)
- Ddx: linear focal elastosis (p/w rows of yellow striae-like bands on the back of old males)
- Rx (STRIAE): Stretching/massaging skin for prevention; treat w/ Tretinoin and other topical Retinoids, RF, IPL/PDL laser, Ascorbic acid, Alpha-hydroxy acids, and Excimer laser

Atrophoderma of Pasini and Pierini (discussed in section on morphea)

Follicular Atrophoderma (A-F)

- Atrophoderma presents from Birth to early Childhood w/ Dimple-like (ice-pick) Depressions on the Face (cheeks), Feet and Fingers/dorsal hands

- a/w Bazex-Dupré-Christol and Conradi-Hünermann-Happle syndromes
- Atrophoderma vermiculatum is a variant which is a/w loeys-Dietz, Nicolau-Balus and Rombo syndromes and p/w "worm-eaten" atrophoderma on the **cheeks** of a child
    - "There's already worms growing out of his face, just sign the DNR"
- Path: Dilated Follicles with follicular plugging

Piezogenic pedal papules

- Fat herniation through the dermis which p/w pale to skin-colored papules (MC on feet)

Hypertrophic scar/keloid

- Pathogenesis: collagen synthesis by fibroblasts is markedly increased by ↑ expression of TGF-β1 and TGF-β2 whereas **TGF-β3 is a/w a reduction in scarring**
    - Hyper-TROPHIC scar: ↑TGF-β1/ β2, early growth Response protein 1, PDGF, Homeobox B13, IL-6, -8, and COX1 (↓ TGF-β3 and anti-inflammatory cytokine IL-10)
    - **TNF-α is responsible for wound reepithelization whereas TNF-β makes scars**
- Hypertrophic scars are raised and stay confined to wound borders whereas keloids extend beyond the wound borders and are delayed in onset
    - Keloids also have this dog bone/dumbbell appearance where its depressed centrally and more expansile peripherally (lobomycosis and DFSP also do this)
- Path (hypertrophic scars and keloids have ↑ mast cells)
    - Scar: fibroblasts w/ east-west and blood vessels w/ north-south orientation
    - Hypertrophic scar: whorled/nodular proliferation of myofibroblasts

    - Keloid: whorled proliferation of fibroblasts and blood vessels w/ central bundles of amorphous pink "bubble gum" collagen
- Rx (TROPHIC): recombinant TGF-β3 (avotermin), Radiation, Onion extract, Pressure therapy, PDL laser, mannose-6-Phosphate (TGF-β1/2 inhibitor), Human recombinant IL-10, ILK, IL Insulin (inhibits myofibroblasts), Cryotherapy, CO2 laser, Cut it out

Dupuytren's Disease (A-F)

- Triggers (ABCD): Alcoholism, BRAF inhibitor (vemurafenib), Cigarette smoking, Diabetes
- Pathogenesis (E): myofibroblast proliferation → Excess collagen synthesis
- p/w nodule in the Fascia of the palm which causes Flexion of the MCP joint of 4th digit
- Path: nodular lesion consisting of a proliferation of myofibroblasts
- Rx: Fasciectomy/Fasciotomy or IL Collagenase (from Clostridium histolyticum)
    - IL Collagenase (from Clostridium histolyticum) is also used to treat Cellulite

Cutis vertices gyrata (CVG)

- Primary CVG is isolated or a/w neurologic (CNS) or ophthalmologic abnormalities
- Secondary CVG is a/w endocrinopathies (myxedema, **acromegaly**, Graves), genetic disorders (Turner, Klinefelter, Tuberous sclerosis, hyper-IgE syndrome) or vemurafenib
- p/w overgrowth of the scalp that produces **Cerebriform folding of the skin**
    - Terminal hair density is reduced in the folds but not in the furrows
- Ddx (CVG-like conditions) is "Go Bear-Packing"

- Goeminne syndrome: CVG-like scalp + congenital torticollis + keloids + cryptochordism + renal dysplasia
- Beare-Stevenson (FGFR2 mutation): furrowed skin on head/neck, trunk, palms/soles + AN + prominent **umbilical stump** ("um-beare-ical stump")
- Pachydermoperiostosis (SLCO2A1): hypertrophic osteoarthropathy of head (CVG) and hands (clubbing of the fingers), periostosis (subperiosteal new bone formation seen on X-ray) of the long bones, and painful arthropathy (Rx NSAIDS)

Elastoma/collagenoma (discussed in section 4.1)

3.6 Granulomatous/Histiocytic Disorders

Non-infectious granulomas

- All of these disorders (except NLD and cutaneous Crohn's) p/w non-scaly purple plaques

Sarcoidosis

- More common and severe in African Americans (highest incidence in Sweden)
- Bimodal incidence peaks (around age 30 and in 50s)
- Multisystem granulomatous disease caused by ↑ cell-mediated immunity ($CD4^+$ Th1 cells) → ↑IL-12, IFN-γ, TNF-α and monocyte chemotactic factor → granuloma formation
- Most patients do not have skin lesions but when seen they p/w red-brown to violaceous papules and **annular** plaques near antigenic entry sites (nose, mouth, sites of trauma such as **tattoos**, piercings, scars); lesions produce an "apply jelly" color on diascopy

- Specific variants include lupus pernio, papular/plaque sarcoidosis, hypopigmented macules, ulcerative lesions, psoriasiform sarcoidosis and scalp sarcoidosis
- **a/w erythema nodosum (like in coccidioidomycosis it predicts a benign course)**
- Leading cause of death is **lung** (MC; pulmonary HTN/ fibrosis) and **heart** (2nd MC; arrythmias, CHF) and so related signs such as digital clubbing predicts a poor prognosis
    - Heart disease also predicts poor prognosis in dermatomyositis and scleroderma
    - Screen sarcoid, dermatomyositis and SSc w/ **PFTs** and high-resolution CT if (+)
- May see **nail changes** (clubbing, onycholysis, subungual hyperkeratosis) and oral lesions
- Other areas of involvement: lungs and hilar LAD (90%), eyes (anterior uveitis), heart, CNS, liver/spleen, kidneys, endocrine, BM and joints
- Path: naked (epithelioid) granulomas +/- Asteroid bodies (star-shaped eosinophilic collagen inclusions) and Schaumann bodies (basophilic calcium inclusions)
- Workup: Kveim-Siltzbach test, CXR, CT, **PFTs**, ↑ calcium, ↑ ACE levels, **Hep C antibody**
- Follow-up: monitor eyes (**eye exams**), lungs (CXR/ **PFTs**), heart (EKG, holster, cardiac PET)
    - **Notice that you should get PFTs both at baseline and at regular follow-ups**
- Rx (like-SLE; "SHaq does meth"): **Steroids** +/- steroid sparring agent (methotrexate best)
    - Use chloroquine or HQC for chronic skin-predominant disease
        - Refractory: TNF-α, JAK (tofacitinib), MMF (Celcept), thalidomide, PDE inhibitors (apremilast, pentoxyphylline), allopurinol
- "SARCLE" may help you remember the high-yield aspects of sarcoidosis

 - Schaumann bodies, Kveim-Siltzbach test, "SHaQ does meth" to treat
 - Asteroid bodies, AA, Annular lesion, Anterior uveitis, Apple-Jelly diascopy, ↑ ACE
 - Restrictive pattern on **PFTs** due to lung fibrosis (honey-comb pattern on CT)
 - Calcium ↑, hep C association, CD4+ Th1 cells upregulated, CXR/CT, nail Clubbing, systemic Corticosteroids for systemic disease or Chloroquine for skin disease
 - **Lung (90%) and hilar or paratracheal LAD (90%)** are the MC organs affected
 - Lung is MCC of death (heart is #2) and involvement predicts a poor prognosis
 - **Erythema nodosum signifies a benign course**

Sarcoid variants ("DUMBELL")

- Darier-Roussy: Deep SQ (vs dermal) sarcoid which p/w multiple firm, painless, Deep-seated mobile nodules with hilar LAD; a/w a good prognosis
- Uveoparotid fever (Heerfordt's syndrome; "PUFF"): Parotid gland enlargement + Uveitis + Fever + **Facial nerve palsy**
- Mikulicz's syndrome: bilateral sarcoid of parotid, submandibular and lacrimal glands
  - "Licz sounds like licks which reminds me of parotid and salivary glands"
- Blau syndrome: sarcoid in a child; NOD2/CARD15 mutation
- Exogenous causes (drug-induced sarcoid): hepatitis C drugs (**IFN**, ribavirin) > melanoma drugs (ipilimumab, nivolumab, vemurafenib), HIV drugs, TNF-α inhibitors
- Löfgren's syndrome (LOFGRENS): LAD (hilar), **Ocular disease (uveitis)**, Fever, Good prognosis, Roaming polyarthritis, **Erythema Nodosum**, Scandinavian whites are affected

- Lupus pernio: p/w violaceous (rather than red-brown) lesions on the Lower nose (**nodules and/or notching of alar rim**) and ear-Lobes → resolves with scarring
    - Strongly a/w chronic **Lung disease** → poor prognosis

Granuloma Annulare (GA)

- Pathogenesis similar to sarcoid: Th1 delayed reaction to an unknown antigenic trigger
    - In GA, monocytes release lysosomal enzymes which degrade elastic fibers
    - Diffuse/generalized and familial GA is a/w **HLA-Bw35**
- Adolescents are most commonly affected (2/3rds arise Before 35)
    - This fact also helps me remember that generalized GA is HLA-Bw35
- Drug-induced GA: Gold, Allopurinol, Amlodipine, **TNF-Alpha inhibitors (MC)**
- p/w Asymptomatic non-scaly Annular plaques in an Acral distribution that self-resolves
    - Sites: isolated hands/arms (60%), legs/feet (20%), trunk (5%)
- Variants ("GA lesions have central DIPS")
    - Diffuse/generalized GA: later onset (50s); p/w numerous small violaceous papules coalescing into small annular plaques on the trunk/proximal extremities
        - a/w **Dyslipidemia (MC)**, DM, Drugs > thyroid, HIV, hematologic cancers
    - Patch GA: p/w patches of erythema on the trunk/ extremities (dorsal foot is MC)
        - Need path to diagnose which will show an interstitial GA pattern
    - Perforating GA: small keratotic papules w/ **central umbilication** on dorsal hands

- Paraneoplastic GA-like eruption: p/w **Painful** lesions on unusual locations (**Palms and soles**); a/w solid organ tumors and lymphomas (CTCL, Hodgkin's and NHL)
    - Acanthosis nigricans on the palms/soles is also paraneoplastic (gastric)
- Subcutaneous (deep) GA: p/w large nodules ("pseudo rheumatoid nodules") on the **dorsal foot** > palms, buttocks, scalp in **children**; 50% also have classic GA
- Other scenarios include GA in herpes zoster scars, HIV (generalized or photodistributed GA), Hepatitis B or C and drug-induced (TNF-α inhibitors)

- Path: all forms show a granulomatous dermal infiltrate with ↑ mucin and eosinophils
    - Interstitial (MC; 70%): histiocytes and ↑ mucin between collagen bundles
    - Palisaded (25%): palisaded granulomas around dermal mucin
    - Sarcoidal pattern (5%): well-formed epithelioid histiocytic nodules
    - Deep GA: palisaded granulomas around mucin in SQ (vs pink fibrin in RA nodule)
- Rx
    - Localized disease: steroids (IL/topical), lasers, cryotherapy, niacinamide
    - Severe: PUVA, Antimalarials, triple Antibiotic (minocycline, ofloxacin, rifampin)
- Prognosis: spontaneous resolution in 2 years in 50% of pts but recurs in 40% of pts

Annular elastolytic giant cell granuloma (AEGCG; actinic granuloma)

- GA variant affecting **chronically sun exposed skin** (head/neck) of middle-aged adults
    - GA is never on the face

- p/w large annular plaques w/ raised erythematous borders and a slightly atrophic center
- Path (optimal site: edge): interstitial > palisaded granulomatous infiltrate w/ histiocytes and multinucleated foreign body giant cells which demonstrate **elastophagocytosis** (phagocytosed elastic fibers); lacks mucin; VVG stain shows absence of elastic fibers
- Rx: persistent condition that responds poorly to GA therapies

Necrobiosis lipoidica (NLD)

- Most NLD patients do not have diabetes and only 1% of diabetics will have NLD
- Unknown pathogenesis but diabetes-related dermal ischemia is thought to play a role
    - o **TNF-α** is found in high concentration in skin and sera
- p/w shiny red-brown patches on B/L shins → yellow atrophic plaques w/ telangiectasias
    - o Minor trauma results in **ulceration** (MC complication)
- Path: square punch w/ a "layered cake" of palisaded granulomas and plasma cells
- Rx: potent topical steroids (early lesions); ILK into the active border (established lesions)

Cutaneous Crohn's disease

- About 1/3rd of Crohn's patients have mucocutaneous findings
- Pathogenesis: exaggerated Th1 and Th17 response to altered gut flora → granulomas
- High-yield clinical features: "Crohn's CAPE"
    - o Mucosal Cobblestoning; Colossal Crotch **(vaginal/ scrotal edema)**
    - o Cheilitis granulomatosa: idiopathic lip swelling (granulomas) seen alone (Crohn's, sarcoid) or in the

Melkersson-Rosenthal triad (facial palsy, plicated tongue)
  - Acrodermatitis enteropathica due to zinc deficiency; Aphthae-like oral ulcers
  - Anogenital erythema/**linear "knife-like" ulcers** (specific); **perianal Acrochordons**
  - **Pyostomatitis vegetans** (UC > Crohn's): multiple painless (HSV and aphthae are painful) pustules on a red base w/ **shallow snail-track (serpentine/ linear) ulcers**
  - Pyoderma gangrenosum (**UC** > Crohn's)
  - Epidermolysis bullosa acquisita (**IBD is strongly a/w EBA**); Erythema nodosum
  - Extragenital ("metastatic") Crohn's: p/w dusky plaques → ulcerates → draining sinuses → scars; MC site is the lower Extremities/soles
- Path: non-caseating sarcoidal granulomas w/ lymphocytes and Langhan's giant cells
- Workup: **Colonoscopy** w/ biopsy if high suspicion for IBD
- Rx
  - Localized disease: topical or IL Corticosteroids + PO metronidazole
  - Severe disease: PO Corticosteroids, sulfasalazine, 6-MP, TNF-α inhibitors, IL-23s

Reactive granulomatous dermatitis (RGD)

- New designation unifying the older terms of interstitial granulomatous dermatitis and arthritis (IGDA), palisaded neutrophilic and granulomatous dermatitis (PNGD)
- Pathogenesis: palisaded granulomatous inflammatory reaction in response to collagen degeneration from low-intensity autoimmune disease-induced vasculitis; ANA+ in 50%

- Classically p/w linear Red to violaceous palpable cords on the lateral trunk ("Rope sign")
  - MC systemic symptom is "R-thritis"
- a/w **autoimmune disease (esp RA and SLE)**, **vasculitis**, drugs and hematologic cancers
- Path: histiocytes surrounding necrobiotic collagen; intense neutrophilic infiltrate +/- LCV
- Rx: treat underlying disease; remission is expected in 2/3rds of patients
- Workup: look for autoimmune (ANA, RF), vasculitis, hematologic cancer (SPEP) triggers

Interstitial granulomatous drug eruption (also under the new umbrella term of RGD)

- p/w asymptomatic erythematous-violaceous plaques distributed in an annular pattern on the inner surface of the limbs and thighs and in intertriginous zones
  - Clinically and histologically resembles RGD (IDGA/PNGD)
- MC implicated drugs ("grandmas CATS"): CCBs, ACE inhibitors, **TNF-α inhibitors**, Statins

Foreign body reactions

- Tattoo inks
  - Red ink (mercuric sulfide/cinnabar) causes lichenoid reactions (MC), pseudolymphomatous reactions, delayed reactions and eczematous reactions
  - Yellow ink (cadmium sulfide; "yellow cab") is MCC of photoallergic reactions
    - "The sun is yellow"
  - **Gray ink**: increasingly recognized cause of atypical **mycobacterial** infection (not a foreign body) as gray ink is obtained by diluting black ink in contaminated water

        - p/w lichenoid paps/pustules in gray area of tattoo weeks after procedure
    - Aluminum (tainted ink) causes granulomatous reactions
    - Path: black material in the dermis (melanin and hemosiderin are brown)
    - Dx: rule out sarcoid (CXR) and TB (tissue culture) in sarcoidal granulomas
    - Rx: laser tattoo removal not recommended in active disease; IL 5-FU
- Silica (Silicon dioxide): p/w nodules or indurated plaques within a Scar 25 years after (Slow incubation) penetrating injuries involving Sand, Soil, rocks, glass (motor accidents)
    - Path: Sarcoidal granulomas containing colorless birefringent crystalline particles
    - Rx: Surgical excision
- Talc (hydrous magnesium silicate): p/w sarcoid-like papules after using white dusting powders (intertriginous areas of obese patients) or injection sites of IV drug users
    - Path: sarcoidal granulomas w/ white birefringent crystals on polarized light
        - "Don't talc to white cops"
- Zirconium: p/w soft, brown papules in the axilla after using antiperspirants (ZeroSweat)
    - Path: sarcoidal granulomas; no (Zero) polarizable particles seen
- Beryllium: p/w nodules at site of puncture of a **fluorescent light Bulb**
    - Systemic beryllosis is due to inhalation (Dx: Bronchioalveolar lavage)
    - Path: caseating granulomas w/ no polarizable particles seen
- Aluminum: p/w SQ nodules at vaccine injection site or in tattoos (tainted ink)

- Path: granulomas w/ no polarizable particles seen
  - **Topical aluminum chloride (Drysol) can cause a granulomatous reaction w/ histiocytes containing prominent basophilic granules**
- Zinc: p/w furuncles at injection site of zinc-containing insulin shots
  - Path: dense neutrophilic infiltrate w/ birefringent **rhomboidal** crystals
- Starch: p/w nodules from contamination of wounds w/ starch lube on Surgical gloves
  - Path: foreign body granulomas w/ ovoid basophilic **PAS+** starch granules
- Cactus (Opuntia): p/w papules w/ central black dot in those who peel prickly pear fruit
  - Path: sarcoidal or foreign body granulomas w/ PAS+ spines
- Jellyfish, coral or sea urchin spines: p/w linear or flaggelate pruritic plaques
  - Path: lichenoid dermatitis w/ birefringent calcite crystals (sea urchin spines)
- Keratin: p/w inflammatory nodule
  - Path: foreign body granulomas w/ birefringent keratin flakes
- IL steroids: p/w skin-colored to yellow-white papules at site of prior IL-steroid injection
  - Path: foreign body granulomas w/ pale bubbly bluish material **(resembles mucin)**
- Suture: p/w inflammatory papule in wound that opens to form a fistula
  - Path: foreign body granulomas w/ birefringent suture material within a scar
- Wood splinter/cactus spine: p/w papule w/ central black dot
  - Path: PAS+ birefringent material made of regularly sized cells in cross section

- Arthropod parts: p/w papule w/ central black dot
  - Path: PAS+ birefringent material

Refer to pathology section for foreign body granulomas due to filler material

Diagnostic tools to diagnose foreign body granulomas
Birefringence: all are birefringent except aluminum, beryllium, zirconium (all end in …ium → "I, umm, am not Bi")
PAS: Arthropod parts, Aluminum, Starch, cactus Spines and wood Splinters are PAS+

Histiocytoses

- Group of proliferative disorders that share a common $CD34^+$ progenitor cell in the BM
- This common ancestor cell turns into the histiocytoses ("Dermal Macrophage Lineage")
  - Dermal dendrocyte (two "Dos" types)
    - Type 1: found in papillary dermis and stains for factor 13a
    - Type 2: found in the reticular dermis and stains for CD34
  - Macrophage: found in dermis and stains for CD68 and HAM56
  - Langerhans cell: found in epidermis and stains for CD1a, S100 (1 looks like L) and Langerin (CD207; most specific and stains the Birbeck granules seen on EM)

Langerhans Cell Histiocytosis (LCH)

- Oncogenic **BRAF V600E** (50%; like in melanoma) and MAP2K1 (25%) mutations are found → clonal proliferation of LCs in various organs (skin and bones are MC)
- LCs stain for **S100** (also like melanoma)**, CD1a, langerin (CD207)**

- Poor prognostic factors: high risk organs (liver, spleen, BM) and BRAF-V600E mutation
- MC organs affected: bone (75%), skin (40%), LNs (20%), liver/spleen/lungs (15%) > CNS
    - o Half of patients have single system and half have multisystem disease
    - o In children MC bone affected is skull (40%) and MC in adults is the jaw (30%)
- MC complications of LCH Disease: Lytic bone lesions, Chronic otitis media, Hematologic cancers, Diabetes insipidus, **Deafness**
- Four overlapping clinical variants which may be becoming outdated: "Langer-Hand CEll"
    - o Letterer-Siwe: presents before 2 y/o w/ disseminated seborrheic papules, crust, pustules or vesicles on the scalp, flexures and diaper area → **petechia, purpura**
        - ▪ Poor prognosis: Low platelets/RBCs and Lytic bone Lesions
    - o Hand-Schuller-Christian: presents from 2–6 y/o with the triad of Osteo-Lytic bone lesions (cranium is MC), Diabetes insipidus, Exophthalmos ("hand hOLDEr"); skin disease is like Letterer-Siwe but with oral mucosa disease
        - ▪ Rx: vasopressin ("hands holding are pressin against each other")
    - o Congenital self-healing reticulohistiocytosis (Hashimoto-Pritzker): presents at birth w/ rapidly resolving skin-limited disease (e.g., widespread purple papules)
    - o Eosinophilic granuloma: presents in 6–12 y/o w/ bone-limited disease (cranium)
- Path: dense proliferation of langerhans cells (reniform nuclei) in dermis which cross into the epidermis (vs mastocytosis) as LH cells normally reside in the epidermis

- EM shows racquet-shaped intracytoplasmic Birbeck granules
- Workup (LCH Disease): skeletal survey (Lytic bone lesions), audiology exam (Chronic otitis), CBC (Hematologic cancers), CMP (Diabetes insipidus), audiology exam (**Deafness**)
- Rx
  - Skin-limited disease: topicals (steroids, nitrogen mustard, UVB phototherapy)
  - Multisystem LCH: **vinblastine** + prednisone (BRAF inhibitors if mutation present)
    - "Rx of LCH is LCV": Light (UVB), Corticosteroids, **Vinblastine**, Vemurafenib

Non-Langerhans Cell Histiocytosis

- All are **CD68 positive** with variable positivity of **HAM56**, CD163, CD11, CD14, and factor 13a
  - All negative for CD207, S100 (except Rosai-Dorfmin & ICH), and CD1a (except ICH)
- Variants: "BIG JEN listens to XM Radio" ("BIG" lesions are clinically and histologically identical, no internal organ/mucous membrane involvement and **no touton giant cells**)
  - Benign Cephalic histiocytosis (BCH): presents in **Babies** w/ numerous red-brown macules and papules which are Cephalad (**face**/neck) and which **self-resolve**
    - **Path: dermal proliferation of histiocytes with no touton giant cells**
    - **EM: Comma-shaped/worm-like bodies**
  - Indeterminate cell histiocytosis (ICH): presents like BCH but in any age
    - **S100 and CD1a positive** (like LCH) **but CD207 negative** and CD68 positive
  - Generalized eruptive histiocytosis (GEH): presents in **adults** w/ recurrent lesions identical to BCH and

ICH clinically and on path, but has **axial** distribution (trunk)

- Juvenile xanthogranuloma (JXG): like BIG, it self-resolves (**no Rx**) but unlike BIG, lesions are **one** to few (vs numerous), yellow (vs red), located on head, there are **touton giant cells on path** and there is internal involvement (but just the eye)
  - "JIANT": **JXG/JMML/NF1** triple association, **Iris** is MC eye structure affected, occurs in Infancy, Anterior chamber of eye pools with blood (hyphema → glaucoma blindness), a/w NF-1, Touton giant cells
- Erdheim-Chester: presents in adults w/ the same triad as seen in Hand-Schuller (hand hOLDEr) → Osteo-Lytic bone lesions, Diabetes insipidus, Exophthalmos
  - Also like Hand-Schuller (LCH), most cases a/w **BRAF V600E mutation**
  - Skin involvement in 25% of pts (brown-red to yellow papules/plaques)
    - Xanthelasma-like lesions are typical
  - Path: monotonous, foamy histiocytes in the dermis
  - Rx: BRAF inhibitors
- Necrobiotic xanthogranuloma (NXG): presents in adults with **yellow**-brown xanthomatous nodules that can become necrotic; MC in a periorbital distribution
  - Like JXG, it is a/w ophthalmic complications (50% vs only 0.5% in JXG)
  - IgG kappa paraproteinemia (> 80%): "neKrobiotic xanthoGranolma"
  - Ddx: plane xanthomas are commonly periorbital but are flat (vs nodular), yellow (vs yellow-brown) and are never necrotic

        - The MC paraproteinemia for both is IgG kappa
    - Path: "X" shaped (NXG) areas of palisaded necrobiosis, cholesterol clefts and huge bizarre multinucleated giant cells
- Xanthoma Disseminatum: usually presents before age 25 with eruption of numerous red-brown or yellow papules coalescing into oddly patterned xanthoma-like plaques on the flexures and intertriginous sites (eruptive xanthomas occur in older patients and usually affect extensor surfaces)
    - Triad: cutaneous Xanthomas, mucosal Xanthomas, Diabetes insipidus
    - a/w monoclonal gammopathy (get SPEP/ immunofixation)
- Multicentric reticulo-Histiocytosis: presents in adults with red-brown or yellow nodules on acral sites (Head and dorsal Hands), lesions in the Mouth/Mucosal lesions (50%), **arthritis Mutilans** (45%) and **solid organ Malignancy** (30%)
    - Bronchial, breast, stomach and cervical carcinomas are MC solid tumors
    - a/w autoimmune disease (**Hashimoto's thyroiditis**, Sjögrens, vitiligo, IBD)
    - a/w abnormalities of the Heart (CHF, pericarditis, cardiomegaly)
    - **"Coral bead" appearance of small papules aligned MC along the nailfold** (Hands) but also ears/nasal ala (Head), when in this latter location can be confused w/ the papules of scleromyxedema or Birt-Hogg-Dubé
    - Path: histiocytes w/ two-toned cytoplasm ("reticulohistiocy-two-sis")
    - Workup: age-appropriate cancer screening +/- CT abdomen/chest/pelvis

- Rosai-Dorfman: presents between 10–30 yo w/ massive but asymptomatic B/L cervical LAD, B symptoms, polyclonal hypergammaglobulinemia; self-Resolves
  - Skin involvement is rare but when seen is MC on the eyelids/malar cheek
  - Rare familial form due to mutation in SLC29A3
  - **a/w HHV6** (cause of Roseola infantum)
  - Path: infiltrate of large foamy **S100**$^{+}$/CD68^{+} histiocytes w/ emperiopolesis (lymphs passing through histiocytes) and **numerous plasma cells**

3.7 Monoclonal Gammopathies in Dermatology

- Often arise in the setting of plasma cell dyscrasia or multiple myeloma
- Workup: the most sensitive test for detecting a monoclonal gammopathy is a **serum immunofixation** but serum free light chains and serum protein electrophoresis work too

Monoclonal Gammopathies in Dermatology: "SPACE X"
Scleromyxedema (IgG lamda), Scleredema (IgG-k: kappa), Schnitzler (IgM-k), Sneddon-Wilkinson/Subcorneal pustular dermatosis (IgA; neut diseases are IgA), Sweets (IgA) PEOMS (IgG, -A but always **lamda**), PG (IgA), Paraneoplastic Pemphigus, IgA Pemphigus (IgA) Acquired Angioedema, Amyloidosis, AESOP Cryoglobulinemia (IgM): monoclonal IgM (type 1), monoclonal IgM to polyclonal IgG (type 2) EED (IgA), EBA Xanthoma disseminatum, diffuse plane Xanthoma (IgG-k), NXG (IgG-k)

3.8 Xanthomas and Hyperlipoproteinemias

Xanthomas

- Develop as a result of lipid deposition in the dermis (macrophages > extracellularly)
- Signals the presence of an underlying **hyperlipidemia** or **monoclonal gammopathy**
- May be 2° to primary biliary cirrhosis (p/w severe pruritis, hyperpigmentation, jaundice)
    - o Dx: various penias, hyperbilirubinemia, transaminitis, antimitochondrial antibody
    - o Rx: ursodeoxycholic acid
- Xanthoma variants ("Plane VET")
    - o Plane xanthomas ("DIXX"): p/w yellow-orange macules/papules/patches/plaques
        - ▪ Diffuse plane xanthoma: a/w **IgG paraproteinemia**; no lipid abnormalities
        - ▪ Intertriginous plane xanthomas: when located on **antecubital fossae** or **web spaces of fingers** it is pathognomonic for type 2 lipoproteinemia
            - "We have 2 antecubital fossae and make peace signs w/ 2 fingers"
        - ▪ Xanthoma striatum palmaris: plane xanthomas on palmar crease (type 3)
            - "We have 3 main palmar creases"
        - ▪ Xanthelasma: plane xanthomas on the eyelids (**most are normolipemic**)
    - o Verruciform xanthoma: Verrucous plaques in the **mouth** (MC) or **genitals** (Vulva)
        - ▪ Not a/w lipid abnormalities (normolipemic) but is a/w CHILD syndrome
        - ▪ **Path: looks like a "wart on fire" w/ foam cells in dermal papillae**

- Eruptive xanthomas: p/w numerous small red-yellow papules on Extensor surfaces of Extremities, buttocks and hands
  - Occurs when triglycerides Exceeds 3000 mg/dl usually because they are fat (obesity, **DM**, ↓ thyroid), POOR (Protease inhibitors, Olanzapine, OCPs, Retinoids) and have hyperlipoproteinemias (type 1, 4, 5)
- Tuberous xanthomas: p/w large yellow-pink indurated nodules on **elbows/knees**
  - a/w hyperlipoproteinemias type 2 and 3 (Two and Three)
- Tendinous xanthomas: p/w firm nodules on achilles tendon and hand tendons
  - a/w hyperlipoproteinemias type 2 > 3 (**Two** and Three)

- Path: foam cells (plane/tendinous/tuberous) +/- extracellular lipid (eruptive xanthoma)
- Rx: lipid lowering agents and destruction (lasers, cryotherapy, chemical agents like TCA)
- Workup: lipid panel, glucose level, TSH, UPEP/SPEP

Lipoproteinemias

- Type 1 (familial lipoprotein lipase deficiency; familial hyperchylomicronemia; Apo C-II deficiency): AR lipoprotein lipase (LPL) gene defect
  - "The 1 looks like the l and i"
- Type 2 (familial hypercholesterolemia): AD **LDL receptor defect** or apo B-100 defect
  - "LDL recep-two-r defect" and "B in B-100 is the 2nd letter in the alphabet"
- Type 3 (familial dysbetalipoproteinemia; apo E deficiency): AR apo E gene mutation
  - "The letter E (Apo E deficiency) has 3 horizontal lines"

- Type 4 (familial hypertriglyceridemia): AD mutation in multiple genes; a/w DM, obesity
- Type 5: multiple causes including diabetes mellitus
- Just remember that type Two and Three cause hypercholesterolemia/atherosclerosis and produce Tuberous, Tendinous (2 > 3), intertriginous planar (2 > 3) and palmar (3 > 2) xanthomas, while the others (1, 4, 5) cause hypertriglyceridemia which result in eruptive xanthomas but no coronary disease (however, type 4 and 5 do have metabolic disease)

3.9 Urticaria and Angioedema

Urticaria

- The range delineating acute from chronic urticaria is **6 weeks** ("wheals has 6 letters")
    - o Acute intermittent urticaria lasts longer than 6 weeks but w/ disease-free gaps
- F > M (except for delayed pressure urticaria in which males are more affected)
- ABCD triggers (Autoimmune, Bug, Cancer, Drug): in children MCC is viral and idiopathic
- Pathogenesis: mast cells are the primary cell responsible (basophils and eos contribute)
    - o Contain preformed (histamine, proteases, heparin) and newly formed (prostaglandin D2, leukotrienes C4/D4/E4, platelet-activating factor, TNF-α, IL-1, -4, -5, -6, -8 and other cytokines) proinflammatory mediators
        - "Preformed mediators are short words, newly formed have numbers"
- Stimuli that release these mediators have immunologic and non-immunologic causes ("When you go to CAMP Pack your DARN SOCKS")

- Immunologic: **autoantibodies against FcεRI or Fc portion of IgE** caused by Cephalosporins, AutoAbs, Asparaginase, Minocycline/Medical devices, PNCs
- Non-immunologic: Polymyxin B, Dietary pseudo-allergens, ASA, ACEI (↑ bradykinin), Radiocontrast media, Nettle stings/NSAIDS, Substance P (and other neuropeptides), Opiates, C5a anaphylatoxin, KIT ligand (Stem cell factor)

- p/w transitory pruritic wheals (swelling and erythema from plasma leakage in dermis)
  - Acute vs chronic urticaria ("submit your IRB in APA format")
    - Acute: MCC is Idiopathic > Respiratory infections > β-lactams
      - **Urticaria starts 1 day after drug and 1 week after a viral infection**
    - Chronic: **MCC is Autoantibodies against FcεRI or Fc portion of IgE (50%)** > Physical (35%); **a/w Autoimmune disease (thyroid is MC)**
- Physical urticarias: "I physically want to see D CASH"
  - Dermatographism (MC): urticaria develops seconds after scratching
  - Delayed pressure urticaria: as name implies it is delayed (12 hours after stimuli) from pressure (commonly on waistline); more painful and a/w flu-like symptoms
  - Cold urticaria: urticaria after cold contact (Dx: ice-cube test)
    - **Primary cold contact urticaria**: urticaria on exposed areas (face/hands)
      - **Positive ice Cube test: wheal develops upon rewarming**
      - **Do not let them swim alone** (fatal shock may occur in cold water)

        - Rx: doxepin or **Cyproheptadine**
      - Secondary cold contact urticaria: Cryoglobulinemia, hep C, blood Cancers
        - Do not do ice cube test as it can precipitate vascular occlusion
      - Reflex cold urticaria: widespread urticaria after cooling of body
      - Familial cold autoinflammatory syndrome: p/w urticaria w/ cyanotic centers and blanched white halos that burn (rather than itch)
        - Negative ice cube test
    - Cholinergic urticaria: papular wheals after heat/sweating (exercise, emotions)
    - Aquagenic urticaria: lesions similar to cholinergic but in response to water
    - Adrenergic urticaria: blanched halos around pink wheals (test w/ NE injections)
    - Heat-induced: urticaria after a few minutes of contact w/ heat (very rare)
- Urticarial vasculitis (UV): unlike urticaria, lesions last > 24 hours, hurt (vs itch) and bruise
    - Systemic symptoms: **arthralgias (#1)**, GI disease, obstructive pulmonary disease
    - a/w **AI-CTD**
    - Path: LCV
    - Rx: **NSAIDS** (1st line) but may need other meds (colchicine, dapsone, steroids)
- Schnitzler's syndrome (SCHNI): Sore bones/joints, Chronic urticaria, High temp/ESR, Non-pruritic wheals, Neutrophils on path, **IgM gammopathy**; Rx IL-1 blockers (anakinra)
    - "Spell it like SchMitzler's to remind you it's an IgM gammopathy"
- Diseases that p/w urticarial lesions and systemic symptoms (fever/arthralgias) → "puss"

   - Periodic fever syndromes, UV, Serum sickness-like reaction, Stills, Schnitzler's
- Path: scant perivascular and interstitial neutrophilic infiltrate (invisible dermatosis)
- Dx
   - Acute: RAST and intradermal skin prick testing to identify environmental allergen
   - Chronic: CBC, ESR/CRP, C4, thyroid antibodies, anti-FcεRI, anti-IgE antibodies
- Rx: avoid triggers; **H1 antihistamines** (2nd generation non-sedating antihistamines can be **↑ to 4x normal daily dose**; if still no improvement can add H2 antagonist ranitidine)
   - If recalcitrant consider doxepin, systemic steroids, montelukast, omalizumab
- **Workup for chronic urticaria: if no improvement w/ trial of antihistamines then you can do bloodwork described above (CBC, ESR, C4, anti-FcεRI) but if wheals last greater than 24 hours you can go straight to biopsy to rule out urticarial vasculitis**

Angioedema

- Like acute urticaria, the MCC is idiopathic but physical stimuli and ABCD triggers (Autoimmune disease, Bug/Bites, Cancers of blood and Drugs) are common causes
   - Pathogenesis: similar to urticaria, but for **angioedema lacking urticaria (HAE, AAE, ACE inhibitor-induced), ↑ bradykinin is the cause**
- Hereditary angioedema (HAE): starts in 1st to 2nd decade of life (all forms are AD)
   - Type 1 HAE (MCC): mutation in C1 inhibitor → ↓ C1 inhibitor levels
   - Type 2 HAE: mutation in C1 inhibitor → ↓ C1 inhibitor function
   - Type 3 HAE: mutation in Hageman factor ("happen later when you are a man")

- Acquired angioedema (AAE): occurs in adulthood
  - Type 1 AAE: consumption of C1 inhibitor (**B-cell lymphoproliferative disorders**)
    - Type 1 cryoglobulinemia also is a/w lymphoproliferative disorders
  - Type 2 AAE: autoantibodies against C1 inhibitor (AI-CTD; au-two-immune")
    - Type 2 cryoglobulinemia also is a/w AI-CTD (also Hep C and cancers)
- Labs
  - All forms of HAE and AAE: ↑ bradykinin and ↓C4 levels ("screen 4 angioedema")
  - All forms of AAE (acquired angioedema): ↓C1q and ↓ C1 inhibitor levels
  - Type 1 HAE: ↓ C1 inhibitor levels; type 2 HAE: normal/↑ C1 inhibitor levels
- Drug-induced Angioedema: MCC is ACE-inhibitors (5x ↑ risk in AA patients); occurs within 3 weeks of drug onset due to ↑ **bradykinin**
  - Other drugs are in "When you go to CAMP Pack your DARN SOCKS" mnemonic
- Angioedema p/w painful deep swelling of skin/mucosa (deep dermis/SQ/submucosa)
  - MC affects lips, eyelids, throat ears, nose
  - **Lasts 2–5 days** and is **a/w urticaria (except in HAE/AAE/ACEI)**, GI pain, N/V/D
- Rx: similar to urticaria treatment; should carry an epipen for throat swelling
  - Type 1 HAE (C1 inh def): danazol (ppx) and FFP/C1 inh concentrate (acute attack)
    - Icatibant is a new bradykinin B2 receptor antagonist
- Anaphylaxis is a life-threatening reaction to drugs ("CAMP/DARN SOCKS") that p/w skin (urticaria/angioedema) and systemic (hypotension) findings minutes after exposure

- Rx: hospitalization + systemic steroids + SQ 1:1000 epinephrine

- Angioedema mnemonic (A-F)
  - ACEI (MC drug; 5x ↑ risk in AA patients); AI-CTD (type 2 acquired angioedema)
  - B-cell lymphoproliferative disorders/Blood cancers (type 1 acquired angioedema)
  - ↑ Bradykinin (ACE inhibitor-induced and HAE/AAE); β-lactams (2nd MC drug)
  - ↓C1 inhibitor level (type 1 HAE/AAE), ↓C1q (AAE), ↓C4 (all HAE/AAE)
  - Danazol (prophylaxis for type 1 HAE; **works by ↑ plasma levels of C1 inhibitor**)
  - Exogenous C1 inhibitor concentrate (acute attacks of type 1 HAE)
  - Fresh frozen plasma (acute attacks of type 1 HAE)
- Workup: manage angioedema w/ wheals as you would for urticaria (see above), but for angioedema w/o wheals immediately order C4 (screen 4 angioedema) +/- C1q or C1 inh

Compliment deficiencies: "Compliment Jessica ALBA"

↓C1q: Acquired Angioedema (C1q autoAbs in SLE and hypocomplimentemic urticarial vasc)
↓C2: MC compliment def. in Lupus
↓C3: Barraquer Simons syndrome (acquired partial lipodystrophy) w glomerulonephritis
↓C4: seen in all forms of acquired or hereditary Angioedema (C4 is screening test of choice)

3.10 Neutrophilic Dermatoses

- These disorders display pathergy: wounding (e.g.,needle-stick) → disease-specific lesions

Sweet's syndrome (acute febrile neutrophilic dermatosis)

- Subtypes: Classic (65%) > Malignancy-associated > Infectious/Inflammatory-associated > Drug-induced > Pregnancy-associated ("Classic MID-Pregnancy Sweet's syndrome")
- Classic Sweets affects F > M (4:1) but M = F for cancer-associated ("Women are sweet")
- p/w rapid onset tender ("sweet and tender") red edematous/"juicy" ("sweet and juicy") "mountain range morphology" plaques that favor the head, neck and upper extremities
    - Lesions display pathergy, last for 1–3 months and recur in 30% of patients
    - Bullous, oral (Buccal mucosa), ulcerative (Bloody) lesions are **a/w Blood cancers**
        - In PG, the mucosal and bullous lesions are also most a/w blood cancers
- MC extracutaneous features: **fever** ("sweet and hot") > ↑WBCs, arthralgias, eye disease
- Labs show a "left shift" ("sweet women tend to lean left politically")
- ABCD (Autoimmune, Bug, Cancer, Drug) triggers
    - MC autoimmune disease is **IBD** > RA
    - MC bug is streptococcus ("she's sweet and she strips")
    - MC cancer is acute myelogenous leukemia ("sweet and cute")
    - MC drugs are **G-CSF/GM-CSF** ("colonies are sweet") > OCPs ("contraceptives are sweet"), trimethoprim-sulfamethoxazole ("meth is sweet"), **minocycline** ("minos are sweet"), NSAIDS ("NSAIDS are sweet after a hangover")
    - Other common triggers are pregnancy, HIV and other autoimmune CTDs
- Path: dense neutrophilic infiltrate w/ papillary dermal edema

  - The papillary dermal edema gives it a pseudo-bullous appearance clinically
- Rx: prednisone ("it is sweet how great prednisone works")
- Workup: **colonoscopy**; **fecal calprotectin** is an extremely sensitive/specific test for IBD; anti-saccharomyces cerevisae Abs is less sensitive as it is only a/w Crohn's
- Marshall syndrome: children with Sweet's-like lesions that resolve with acquired cutis laxa lesions at affected sites ("marSHALL: Sweet's Has Acquired cutis Laxa Lesions")

Pyoderma gangrenosum (PG)

- Like Sweet's, it usually affects middle age females and has similar triggers such as **IBD, RA** and blood cancer such as AML and IgA monoclonal gammopathy (CML also common)
- Mutation in PSTPIP1/CD2BP1 (same as PAPA syndrome: Pyogenic arthritis, PG, Acne)
- Can exhibit Pathergy
- When it involves the breast it often spares the nipple
- Drug induced PG: rituximab, imatinib, sunitinib
- Subtypes ("PG PUBS"): Pustular, Ulcerative (classic), Bullous, Superficial granulomatous
  - Pustular: a/w IBD; p/w multiple Pustules that do not ulcerate (looks like Sweet's)
  - Ulcerative (classic): a/w IBD; p/w Painful Papulopustule/bulla → **Painful ulcer with undermined (overhanging) Purple border w/ a Purulent base and Peripheral satellite lesions** which eventually fuse with main central ulcer; variants include Pyostomatitis vegetans (a/w IBD; chronic vegetative lesions of oral mucosa) and Peristomal PG (a/w IBD; PG lesions around ostomy)

and Pediatric PG (a/w IBD or leukemia; MC on head and anogenital region)
    - Bullous: **a/w Blood cancer** (AML); p/w widespread Bullae
    - Superficial granulomatous (vegetative): not a/w systemic disease; p/w superficial painless cribriform ulcers on trunk that usually arises after trauma (Surgery)
- Path: dense dermal neutrophilic infiltrate w/ papillary dermal edema
- Dx: biopsy (Path) of active border, sterile tissue culture/ PCR, (r/o infectious cause), stool for occult blood, CBC, serologic studies (SPEP, ANA, ANCA), CXR, UA
- Rx: Prednisone, **Infliximab** and Cyclosporine are 1st line therapies: "take a PIC of PG"
    - Dapsone, topical steroids and topical CNIs work well for more mild disease
- Workup: SPEP/immunofixation and refer to GI for colonoscopy if not already done

Neutrophilic dermatosis of the dorsal hands
- p/w PG or Sweet's-like ulcer on the dorsal hand (makes for a good Kodachrome)
- Rx: **prednisone**

VEXAS syndrome
- 1st described in 2020
- Stands for Vacuolization of cells on bone marrow biopsy, E1 enzyme, X-linked, Adult-onset Autoinflammatory disease caused by Somatic mutation in UBA1
- p/w relapsing polychondritis (> 50%), PAN-like vasculitis and tender Sweets-like plaques
    - Whereas MAGIC is Behçet's + RP, VEXAS is Sweets + PAN + RP
- Rx: systemic steroids

Behçet's disease ("Ms. Behçet")

- M > F; highest prevalence in Middle Eastern and Mediterranean populations
- Strongly a/w **HLA-B51** ("5+1=6 and there are 6 letters in Behçet")
- Need one major and two minor criteria to diagnose
  - Major: recurrent aphthous stomatitis of **Mouth (first and MC symptom)**
    - Aphthous ulcers: painful, round white ulcer w/ red halo on the anterior non-keratinized oral mucosa (labial and buccal mucosa, ventral tongue)
      - HSV: anterior keratinized ("Hard") mucosa (Hard palate, gingiva)
      - Herpangina: posterior non-keratinized mucosa (uvula, soft palate)
  - Minor: 1.) ocular Mucosal issues; 2.) genital Mucosa/skin ulcers; 3.) acrofacial (**body Margins**) papulopustules; 4.) lesions have positive pathergy to needle Stick
- Multiorgan disease: #1 cause of morbidity is ocular Mucosal lesions (90%; posterior uveitis is MC) but also can affect joints, CNS, vascular (SVT thrombosis), kidneys and GI
- Dx: positive pathergy test (papule or pustule develops within 2 days of needle prick)
- Rx: dapsone, colchicine, TNFi; topical steroids (Mild Mouthwashes) for aphthous ulcers
- MAGIC syndrome (Mouth And Genital Ulcer w/ Inflamed Cartilage): Behçet's + RP

Bowel-Associated Dermatosis Arthritis syndrome (Bowel Bypass syndrome): "1st letters in ABCs"

- **Occurs After Bypass surgery** → Blind loops of Bowl → Bacteria overgrowth immune complexes with bacterial antigens are deposited into skin, subcutis and joints

- Constitutional symptoms (e.g., Arthritis, Chills) precede Classic rash which consist of red to purpuric **papulo-pustules on the proximal extremities/trunk (body Center near bowl)**
  - Lesions of Behçet's have a similar morphology but are located on body margins
- Other features include Diarrhea and tender EN-like lesions on the trunk and extremities
- Rx: Excision of blind bowel loop, steroids or antibiotics such as Doxy, Clinda or Flagyl

Neutrophilic eccrine hidradenitis

- Toxic injury to eccrine glands MC from chemo (**cytarabine**, daunorubicin, bleomycin, cyclophosphamide) but also from acetaminophen, carbamazepine, G-CSF and cancers
- Classic presentation is in AML patients receiving cytarabine
- p/w **fever, neutropenia and pruritic, painful red-purple papules and plaques** MC on face, back, trunk and extremities (esp hands/feet) 10 days after drug exposure
- Dx: biopsy (neutrophils in eccrine coils) and CBC (neutropenia)
- Rx: self-limited; topical steroids is usually sufficient

3.11 Eosinophilic Disorders

Eosinophilic folliculitis ("Eosinophils foll into a NAP")

- Neonatal eosinophilic pustular folliculitis: self-limited crops of pruritic vesiculopustules on **scalp** (head/Neck) > trunk/extremities of infants

    - Rx: do Nothing (topical steroids/tacrolimus or PO antihistamines to control itch)
- **AIDS-associated** eosinophilic folliculitis: **persistent** (Always exist) pruritic paps in AIDS pt
    - Rx: **ART**; antihistamines +/- topical steroids
- Pustular eosinophilic folliculitis (Ofuji's disease): young Japanese adults (M > F) with **recurrent** (every month) crops of intensely Pruritic Papulopustules in a figurate/serpiginous distribution typically on the face; Rx: indomethacin
    - OFUJI: crops Of Figurate pustules on Upper body in Japanese men; Indomethacin
- Path: all forms show spongiosis w/ eos and lymphs in the follicular epithelium

Papuloerythroderma of Ofuji

- Elderly Japanese men with generalized pruritic red papules (no pustules) → erythroderma with **islands of sparing in the skin folds ("deck chair sign")**
    - "I imagine an old Japanese man sitting outside in a chair all day, so he gets sunburnt everywhere except in his skin folds"
- **a/w malignancy (T-cell lymphoma, gastric cancer)**, infection (Hep C, HIV) or drugs (ASA)
- Dx: CBC (lymphopenia, eosinophilia), hep panel, HIV studies
- Rx: **systemic steroids** ("we usually treat erythrodermas with steroids")

Wells' syndrome (eosinophilic cellulitis)

- Inflammatory dermatitis that is often misdiagnosed as infectious cellulitis
- p/w **recurrent** painful/pruritic edematous (early) to indurated (late) red plaques on the extremities that resolve in 4–8 weeks; various triggers (e.g., arthropod bite) involved

- Path: papillary dermal edema w/ many eosinophils (acute), "flame-figures" consisting of collagen fibers and eosinophilic granules (subacute); vasculitis is absent
- Labs: peripheral eosinophilia seen in half of patients in the acute phase
- Rx: systemic steroids work very "Well" (dramatic response within a few days); dapsone

Hypereosinophilic syndrome (HES)

- 3 criteria of Hyper-EOSinophilic Syndrome
  - o Hypereosinophilia > 1500/mm^3 for > 6 months
  - o Exclusion of Other Stuff (e.g., infectious, allergic or other underlying causes)
  - o Signs/Symptoms of end organ involvement
- Most have mucocutaneous lesions (itchy red papules/ nodules and mucosal ulcers)
- **CHF is #1 cause of death** in HES followed by sepsis
- Two major subtypes
  - o Myeloproliferative (neoplastic, primary) HES
    - **FIP1L1-PDGFRA fusion gene → clonal proliferation of eosinophils**
      - Same fusion gene as in Mastocytosis that caused clonal mast cells
    - Striking Male predominance (> 90%)
    - Myocardial fibrosis/cardiomyopathy and hepatosplenomegaly on echo
    - **CD25+ atypical Mast cells on bone Marrow biopsy**
    - Rx: **imatinib** if fusion gene present, Mepolizumab/reslizumab (anti-IL-5 antibodies), prednisone or dapsone if fusion gene absent
      - Endomyocardial disease may worsen during the 1st weeks of imatinib therapy

so troponin and BNP levels should be monitored

- Lymphocytic (reactive, secondary) HES
  - Hypereosinophilia is cytokine driven (not a clonal proliferation of eos)
  - **Clonal T-cell proliferation** (↑ Th2 cyotokines → ↑ IL-5 → ↑ eosinophils)
  - Benign course (Low mortality) with eczema and ↑ IgE
  - ↑ risk of T-cell Lymphoma
  - Workup: if negative for FIP1L1-PDGFRA fusion gene then evaluate for peripheral blood T-cell population w/ flow cytometry, T-cell receptor gene rearrangement analysis or IL-5 level (if positive treat w/ prednisone)
  - Rx: **prednisone** (first line) or imatinib, mepolizumab/reslizumab
- Granuloma faciale: discussed in section 3.22

3.12 Figurate Erythemas

Erythema annulare centrifigum

- Immune reaction to ABCD trigger: Autoimmune, Bug (**tinea pedis**), Cancer, Drugs
- p/w erythematous papule that **advances peripherally** (millimeters per day) to form **arcuate or annular plaques** w/ central clearing and **trailing scale** on the thighs/hips (#1)
  - Ddx: when on the chest it can look like SCLE so look for that trailing scale
  - There is a deep variant which p/w infiltrative annular plaques without scale
- Path: mild spongiosis, focal parakeratosis, dense PV lymphocytic infiltrate ("coat sleeve")

- Rx: spontaneous resolution is common but can treat w/ steroids, TCIs, PUVA, antifungals

Erythema marginatum

- Primarily seen in children in developing countries who are not treated for strept throat
- Seen in the setting of rheumatic fever (JONES criteria): painful Joints, imagine an O shaped like a heart for carditis, SQ Nodules, Erythema marginatum, Sydenham's chorea
- p/w expanding erythematous annular/polycyclic patches/plaques (centimeter per day)
- Dx: plasma Abs to strept (ASO) > throat culture or rapid antigen test; EKG/echo
- Rx: Penicillin is given but has not been proven to alter long-term outcomes

Erythema migrans

- MC in US and Europe (hosts of Borrelia are white-footed mice and white-tailed deer)
- Pathogenesis: ixodes tick transmits Borrelia species → Lyme disease
- p/w large annular red expanding "Bulls-eye" patch at site of tick bite (not always seen)
- Lyme disease symptoms: flu symptoms (early localized disease), Bell's palsy/AV-block (early disseminated disease), arthritis/acrodermatitis chronica atrophicans (chronic dz)
- Labs: tissue/fluid culture, tissue/fluid PCR, anti-Borrelia Abs via ELISA or Western blot
  - Agar for Borrelia is Barbour-Stoenner-Kelly medium
  - Peak IgM response occurs 3–6 weeks into infection (low sensitivity early on)
- Rx: doxycycline (amoxicillin if pregnant or less than 8 yo; ceftriaxone in Lyme meningitis)

- It is now acceptable to use doxycycline regardless of age (but not in pregnancy)

Dermatologic diseases with Bell's palsy: "Bell LUV's Melkerson-Rosenthal"
Lyme, Uveoparotid fever, Varicella (esp Ramsey-Hunt syndrome), Melkerson-Rosenthal

Erythema gyratum repens

- Paraneoplastic disorders due to tumor-associated antigenic trigger
- "Here's my LGBTQ PITCH"
  - MC cancers in order of frequency (LGBtq): **Lung** (#1) > GI, Breast
  - a/w (PITCH): Psoriasis, PRP, Ichthyosis, Tb, CREST, **Hypereosinophilic syndrome**
- p/w multiple polycyclic ("wood grain") concentric rings w/ rapid expansion (1cm/day)
  - Kodachrome can look very similar to tinea imbricata but is less scaly (get KOH)
- Rx: look for (if still unknown) and treat underlying neoplasm

Necrolytic migratory erythema

- Para-neoplastic eruption highly suggestive of a **glucagonoma** of the pancreas
  - 50% of patients have hepatic metastasis by the time of diagnosis
- p/w eczematous and **erosive** lesions w/ a distinct scalloped border that crust over
  - Peripheral expansion and central clearing → serpiginous or arcuate morphology
  - Affects flexural areas as well as lateral neck and genitals
- Ddx: necrolytic acral erythema (a/w Hep C; lesions are more hyperkeratotic and MC affect the dorsal feet, hands and genitalia) and acrodermatitis chronica

enteropathica (a/w zinc def; lesions are more eczematous and MC affect face, hands/feet, genitals)

- Dx: ↑ glucose and **glucagon** levels (1000X normal limit) → **CT abdomen**
- Path: pale vacuolated keratinocytes and epidermal necrosis/separation
- Rx: resection of tumor if localized; somatostatin and zinc supplements may be helpful
- Prognosis: 50% of patients die in 5 years

3.13 Follicular and Eccrine/ Apocrine Disorders

Acne vulgaris

- Pathogenesis: abnormal follicular keratinization and formation of the microcomedo → comedo rupture with release of keratin and sebum (sebum is overproduced due to ↑ androgens such as DHT and DHEA) → inflammatory papule/pustule/nodule/cyst
  - The G+ rod Cutibacterium acnes contributes to the pathogenesis by "12345"
    - Produces lipases which breaks down triglycerides into free fatty acids (1 fatty acid) which are comedogenic and proinflammatory
    - Activates **TLR-2** which induces inflammatory cytokines (IL-1α, -8, -12)
    - Produces **coproporphyrin 3** which fluoresces coral-red under woods lamp
      - Coproporphyrin 3 also causes fluorescence in erythrasma and hereditary coproporphyria (vs protoporphyrin 9 in PDT and EPP)

    - Activates NOD-like receptor protein 3 (NLRP3) of the inflammasomes
    - C. acnes ribotypes 4 and 5 are more frequently found in skin with acne
  - Diet also plays a role: dairy and foods with a high glycemic load are contributory
- p/w open and closed comedones, inflamed papules/pustules/cysts and scars in sebaceous skin (face, neck, upper trunk); females may flare 1 week before menstruation
- Path: follicle filled with laminated keratin +/- suppurative inflammation
- Rx: use topicals (ABCDE'S) for comedonal and mild to moderate inflammatory acne
  - Amzeeq (4% minocycline foam): no risk of minocycline pigmentation
  - Adapalene and other topical retinoids (trifarotene, tazarotene, tretinoin): ↓TLR2
  - Azelaic acid: dicarboxylic acid that ↓ tyrosinase (↓ pigment) and kills C. acnes
  - Benzoyl peroxide: kills C. acnes by oxidation (no bacterial resistance reported)
  - Blue light: at home treatment using light-emitting diodes which have anti-inflammatory effects and reduces pore size through ROS-induced apoptosis
  - Clascoterone: topical androgen inhibitor (unlike spironolactone, can use in men)
  - Dapsone: inhibits myeloperoxidase (↓ neuts) and dihydropteroate synthetase
  - Erythromycin/clindamycin: binds to 50s subunit of ribosome → kills C. acnes
  - Sodium Sulfacetamide: ↓ bacterial dihydropteroate synthetase → kills C. acnes
  - Sulfur and Salicylic acid

- Rx: use systemic agents for severe nodulocystic acne
  - Antibiotics: minocycline, doxycycline, saracycline, sulfonamides, erythromycin
  - Androgen antagonists: → ↓ sebum
    - Spironolactone (HAH): Hyperkalemia, Ataxia, Huge breast (gynecomastia)
      - No need to check baseline potassium levels in healthy patients
    - OCPs: **norgestimate**-ethinyl estradiol (Ortho Tri-Cyclen), **norethindrone** acetate-ethinyl estradiol (Estrostep), **drospirenone**-ethinyl estradiol (Yaz)
      - CI: **smoker > 35 y/o**, HTN of >160/100, active liver disease, severe headaches w/ neural symptoms, current breast cancer, pregnancy
  - Isotretinoin +/- prednisone (discussed in detail in section 2.1)

Acne variants

Acne Fulminans

- Polymorphisms in TLR-4 (Four) are protective against acne fulminans
- Males around Fourteen to Fifteen years old
- p/w severe acne (acute suppurative nodules with hemorrhagic crusts) and **systemic symptoms (Fever, sterile osteolytic bone lesions on the sternum and clavicle)**
- Dx: ↑ WBC and ↑ ESR
- Rx: 4 weeks of high-dose prednisone followed by low dose isotretinoin (0.1mg/kg)
  - Gradually taper prednisone and increase isotretinoin

Acne Conglobata

- p/w severe acute nodulocystic acne but without any systemic manifestations (**no fever**)
    - o Large Cysts and Comedones on acne prone sites (Chest, back, face, arms)
- Rx: 2 weeks of PO Corticosteroids followed by 6 months of oral isotretinoin (0.5–1mg/kg)
- PAPA syndrome: Pyogenic Arthritis, PG, Acne conglobata (can see HS too → PAPASH)

Solid facial edema in acne

- p/w woody non-pitting swelling (peau d'orange) in midline face and cheeks presenting years after severe acne due to disruption of lymphatics
- Rx: isotretinoin

Acne mechanica

- Mechanical pressure and obstruction of the pilosebaceous units (e.g., helmets, collars)
- p/w acne in unusual patterns based on the external cause

Acne excoriée (de jeunes filles)

- Young women with underlying psychiatric disorders
- p/w self-mutilation of perceived or mild acne → crusted excoriated lesions
- Rx: antidepressants and psychotherapy

Neonatal acne ("Mother's androgens")

- Appears within 1 Month and resolves in 3 Months
- Occurs in 20% of healthy babies (M > F)
- Pathogenesis: Maternal androgens transiently stimulate sebaceous glands
    - o Variant termed Neonatal cephalic pustulosis (NCP) is due to Malassezia (a/w AD)

- p/w follicular-based inflammatory papules/pustules on Nasal bridge and around Mouth
    - NCP is more pustular, inflammatory and monomorphic and is not follicular based
- Rx: **do Nothing/observe** (topical ketoconazole in NCP variant)

Infantile acne ("Child's androgens")

- Appears around 3 months and resolves around 3 years (early Childhood); M > F
- Relatively rare (affects < 2% of babies) and is caused by hyperandrogenism of the baby
- p/w inflammatory lesions and **Comedones** on the face which can result in scarring
- Dx: endocrine eval (DHEAS, 17-OH-progesterone, LH, FSH, testosterone, bone age)
- Rx: topical acne treatments (Clindamycin/benzoyl peroxide); oral erythromycin if severe

Transverse nasal crease

- A horizontal anatomic demarcation line on the nose w/ milia, cysts, comedones in kids

Acne in setting of endocrinologic abnormality

- ↑ androgens may be due to PCOS (teenage girls), CAH (children), tumors or Cushing's
- p/w acne, hirsutism and menstrual irregularities
- Dx: ↑ testosterone (ovarian source), ↑ DHEA/17-hydroxyprogesterone (adrenal source)
    - Consider 21- or 11-hydroxylase levels (↓ in CAH), prolactin, cortisol, FSH/LH
- Rx: treat underlying cause; OCPs or spironolactone

Pomade acne

- Monomorphic closed comedones on forehead of AA pts that use greasy hair products

Chloracne (A-E)

- Occupational exposure to Aromatic Chlorinated hydrocarbons
    - Agent orange was contaminated w/ 2,3,7,8-tetrachlorodibenzo-p-dioxin (**Dioxin**)
- p/w Acne on the Axilla, Balls (scrotum), Dick, **retroauricular Ears** weeks after exposure
- Rx: Accutane

Radiation acne

- p/w acne-like papules in radiated skin (appears as radiation dermatitis resolves)

Drug-induced acne ("JAK has Big PIMPLES")

- JAK inhibitors (especially upadacitinib)
- vitamin B2, **B6**, B7, B12; BRAF inhibitors
- Prednisone and other Post-**transplant** drugs (cyclosporine, sirolimus)
    - **p/w abrupt-onset monomorphous papules w/ no comedones**
- Proteosome inhibitors (Bortezomib, carfilzomib)
- Iodides (and other halogens including bromides), Isoniazid, Imiquimod (cysts/milia)
- Marijuana (cannabinoids), MEK inhibitors (trametinib)
- Progesterone only contraceptives, **Phenytoin**
- **Lithium**
- **EGFR inhibitors (cetuximab)**: ppx w/ doxy or minocycline
- Steroids (anabolic); Sirolimus (mTOR inhibitors)

SAPHO syndrome

- Synovitis, Acne, Pustulosis, Hyperostosis, Osteitis
- p/w acne (any entity in follicular occlusion tetrad), pustulosis (pustular psoriasis) and bone disease (sternoclavicular area is MC; "bulls head" may be seen on X-ray)

- Rx: bisphosphonates, TNF-α inhibitors, IL-1 inhibitors, MTX, NSAIDS, prednisone

PAPA syndrome

- Pyogenic Arthritis, PG, Acne conglobata (also known as PAPASH if you add HS)
- AD mutation in CD2BP1 (PSTPIP1; proline-serine-threonine phosphatase) → ↑ IL-β1
- Rx: **Anakinra** or Adalimumab (Arthritis/PG); Antibiotics or Accutane (Acne)

HAIR-AN syndrome

- Hyper-Androgenism, Insulin Resistance, Acanthosis Nigricans
- Rx (same as for PCOS): metformin, OCPs, spironolactone

Rosacea

- Most common in middle-aged Caucasian women
- Pathogenesis: genetic predisposition plus environmental triggers (heat, alcohol) causes neurovascular dysregulation and aberrant innate immunity → "STUCK with rosacea"
  - Skin barrier dysfunction
  - TRVP (transient receptor potential vanilloid) and TLR2 (toll-like receptor 2) are ↑
  - UV radiation
  - Cathelicidin is ↑ and is converted to its active form (LL-37) by Kallikrein 5
  - Kallikrein 5 is ↑
- Variable presentation depending on subtype
  - Erythematotelangiectatic: p/w permanent flushing, telangiectasias +/- stinging
  - Papulopustular (inflammatory): p/w persistent central facial erythema and transient papules/

pustules (presents similar to acne vulgaris but no comedones)
  - Phymatous: p/w thickening of the skin due to overgrowth of sebaceous glands
  - Ocular: half of rosacea patients are affected; p/w dryness, foreign body sensation, blepharitis, recurrent chalazion; Rx: doxycycline/minocycline
    - MC eye findings: lid margin telangiectasia, meibomian gland dysfunction
- Path: PV/PF lymphohistiocytic infiltrate with vascular dilation and sebaceous hyperplasia
- Rx: "Must Always STICK to this rosacea regimen"
  - Microencapsulated Benzoyl peroxide and Minocycline 1.5% are new topicals
  - Metronidazole (topical or systemic)
  - Alpha agonists: Brimonidine ($\alpha 2$ agonist; B is 2nd letter in ABCs), Oxymetazoline (mostly an α-One agonist but also a partial $\alpha 2$ agonist); Azelaic acid
  - Sunscreens; Sodium Sulfacetamide; Sulfur
  - Trigger avoidance (UVR, heat, stress, alcohol, spicy foods); **TCNs (all forms)**
  - Ivermectin (topically); IPL (for telangiectasias); Isotretinoin (for phymatous form)
  - Clindamycin (topically); Cyclosporin (ocular form); CO_2 laser (phymatous form)
  - KTP laser (for phymatous form)
- Workup: if patient is not improving on traditional therapy, perform a scraping of pustules to look for demodex mites → should respond better to ivermectin
- Boards pearl: Haber's ("Haver") syndrome is a genoderm w/ Verrucous lesions + rosacea

Rosacea variants

Solid facial edema in rosacea (Morbihan disease and rosacea lymphedema)

- Pathogenesis: chronic inflammation → obstruction of lymphatic vessels
- **p/w hard non-pitting edema in forehead, glabella, nose and cheeks**
- Worse in the Mornings
- ↑ Morbidity: spontaneous resolution does not occur; ↓ vision (if eyelids involved)
- Rx: **isotretinoin +/- ketotifen**

Pyoderma Faciale (rosacea Fulminans)

- Females in their 20s to 30s
- p/w Fast onset erythematous nodules, plaques and draining cysts on Face → scarring
  - **Characteristically spares the nose (vs lupus) and trunk (vs acne fulminans)**
  - Unlike acne fulminans there are no comedones present
- Systemic symptoms: Fever, myalgias, ↑ ESR, ↑ WBCs
- Rx: same treatment as acne Fulminans (**prednisone taper and isotretinoin**)

GranulomatouS rosacea

- p/w discrete (Separated) Small Skin-colored to brown papules on the face → Scarring
- Spontaneously resolves in a few years
- Path: Sarcoidal (non-caseating epithelioid) granulomas
- Rx: Systemic rosacea treatments (**TCNs and isotretinoin**)

Lupus miliaris disseminates faciei (LMDF)

- Many authors consider it a severe form of granulomatous rosacea that affects **Asians**

- p/w discrete red-yellow-brown firm papules on the face with a predilection for the **eyelids** ("LMD faci-eye") → heals with scarring
- Rx: same treatment as granulomatous rosacea

Perioral/periorificial dermatitis

- Inflammatory condition of adult females and children related to rosacea
- Mostly attributed to use of **topical (MCC)**, nasal and inhaled corticosteroids but facial cosmetic products, fluorinated toothpastes and chewing gum have also been implicated
- p/w burning sensation and clusters of erythematous papules which surround the eyes, mouth and nose but leave an unaffected "Grenz zone" of skin around the vermillion lip
- Ddx: in contrast to steroid-induced rosacea, perioral derm spares the cheeks/forehead
- Rx: taper off steroids otherwise similar to rosacea → avoid triggers (e.g., topical steroids, cosmetics), **TCNs (erythromycin for peds),** topical metronidazole, topical clindamycin

Folliculitis

Superficial folliculitis

- Culture of pustule is usually negative (when positive it is most likely S. aureus)
- p/w perifollicular pustule on a red base in hair bearing sites (scalp, beard, trunk, thighs)
- Rx: based on culture or treat empirically with benzoyl peroxide, topical/oral antibiotics

Gram Negative folliculitis

- p/w worsening centrofacial "acne" in those on long-term TCNs

- Nares become colonized with gram negative organisms → p/w pruritic pustules on an erythematous base that fans out from the Nose
- Rx: TOC is isotretinoin (topical gentamycin or PO ciprofloxacin may help)

Pityrosporum folliculitis

- Intensely pruritic eruption caused by Malassezia furfur
- p/w follicular papules and pustules on the **upper trunk** > head/neck of young adults
- a/w immunocompromise including **diabetes**, HIV, Down's and systemic candidiasis
- Rx: combination of oral and topical antifungals

Hot tub folliculitis

- Gram negative folliculitis due to pseudomonas aeruginosa
- p/w perifollicular papules and pustules on a red base on the trunk days after hot tub use
- Rx: self resolves (if immunocompromised treat with ciprofloxacin)

Eosinophilic folliculitis ("Eos foll into a long NAP")

- Neonatal eosinophilic pustular folliculitis presents in early infancy with multiple pruritic pustules on a red base which crust over; course is cyclic and may recur in crops for years
  - MC location is the **scalp** (Head/Neck > trunk, extremities)
  - Rx: do Nothing/self-limited (symptom control w/ topical steroids, antihistamines)
- AIDS-associated eosinophilic folliculitis: p/w extremely pruritic follicular papules on the scalp, face or upper trunk of AIDS pts; lesions are **persistent** (Always present), not cyclic

    - Rx: ART +/- symptom control (topical steroids, antihistamines)
- Pustular eosinophilic folliculitis (Ofuji's disease): p/w recurrent **crops** of pruritic follicular papules and pustules that extend centrifugally and display central clearing, giving rise to annular, arcuate or figurate configurations on the face or trunk in young Japanese males
    - Labs: CBC shows peripheral eosinophilia; get HIV to rule out AIDS-associated EF
    - Rx: ToC = indomethacin (symptomatic treatment with antihistamines)
    - OFUJI: crops Of Figurate pustules on Upper body in Japanese man; Indomethacin

Disseminate and recurrent infundibulofolliculitis

- Idiopathic disorders which results in numerous monomorphic skin-colored, follicular-based papules resembling goose-bumps on the trunk > proximal extremities in AA males
- Ddx: papular eczema
- Rx: topical corticosteroids, lactic acid, urea

Pseudofolliculitis barbae

- MC in African Americans who shave their beards
- Pathogenesis: hairs curve back into skin after being shaved → foreign body reaction
- p/w hyperpigmentation, inflammatory papules, scars and even keloids on the neck
- Path: suppurative folliculitis + naked hair shafts in the dermis
- Rx: stop shaving (if they must then shave in direction of hair growth, use short strokes), laser hair removal (Nd:YAG safe in POC), antibiotics, retinoids and corticosteroids

Acne keloidalis

- MC in African American males
- p/w follicular papules → keloidal papules → plaques on the posterior neck or occiput
- Dx: bacterial culture from any site of drainage (antibiotics based on sensitivities)
- Path: suppurative folliculitis + naked hair shafts + scar tissue
- Rx: ↓ any mechanical occlusion (e.g., hats, high sweaters); topical retinoids
    - o Inflamed papules/pustules: topical or PO antibiotics
    - o Keloidal papules: potent topical steroids/ILK or punch excision
    - o Keloidal plaques 1 to 1.5 cm in vertical diameter: excision w/ primary closure
    - o Keloidal plaques > 1.5 cm in vertical diameter: excision to level of fascia or deep SQ and left to heal by second intention; CO_2 laser w/ post-op ILK is an option

Follicular occlusion tetrad

- "To remember the follicular occlusion tetrad, you need to get your PhD in Acne"
    - o Pilonidal cyst, HS, Dissecting cellulitis of the scalp, Acne conglobota
- Pathologic event causing each is follicular hyperkeratinization

Pilonidal cyst

- Most common in young adult males with curly hair, obesity and poor hygiene
- p/w painful draining sinus in sacrococcygeal region
- Rx: oral antibiotics, I&D and surgical excision

Hidradenitis suppurativa (HS; acne inversa)

- Onset at puberty; F > M (but males have more severe course); predilection for AAs
- Pathogenesis: occlusion of follicular infundibula + immune dysregulation → follicle rupture → chemotaxis of WBCs → abscess and sinus tract formation → scarring
- Overproduction of TNF-α, IL-1β, -2, 12, -17, -23 in lesional skin (**IL-2** c/w disease severity)
- Associations: obesity (metabolic syndrome) and smoking
- p/w recurrent painful inflammatory nodules/sterile abscesses in the apocrine-rich folds (axilla, groin, inframammary) → sinus tracts (**double-ended pseudocomedones**) → scars
- Complications ("ALFAS"): Amyloidosis, Lymphedema, Fistulas (e.g., bladder), **Anemia**, **SCC**
- Path: heavy mixed inflammatory infiltrate in the lower dermis +/- abscesses (may connect to epidermis via sinus tracts); fibrosis with follicular destruction (later)
- Staging of HS
  - Hurley staging: stage 1 (abscesses w/o sinus tracts or scars); stage 2 (abscesses, sinus tracts and scars widely spaced); stage 3 (interconnected sinus tracts; scars)
  - Sartorius staging: examines anatomic site, # of lesions, space between lesions
- Rx: weight reduction if overweight, smoking cessation, antiseptics, ↓ friction/moisture
  - Hurley stage 1: ILK, topical/oral antibiotics, oral antiandrogens (e.g., finasteride)
    - "Treat the abscesses in stage 1 like acne"
  - Hurley stage 2: stage 1 therapy + acitretin, TNF-α, IL-1s, IL-17s, apremilast, surgery (marsupialization/ CO_2/Nd:YAG) w/ second intention healing

        - "Treat stage 2 like acne (stage 1) and severe psoriasis (stage 2)"
    - Hurley stage 3: stage 1 and 2 therapy + wide surgical excision
        - "Treat stage 3 like acne (stage 1), psoriasis (stage 2) and cancer (stage 3)"

Dissecting cellulitis of the scalp explained in section 3.25

Acne conglobota explained earlier in this section

Other diseases of eccrine and apocrine sweat glands

Hyperhidrosis ("CHAMPS sweat a lot")

- Nerves which control sweating are anatomically sympathetic but functionally cholinergic
- Primary hyperhidrosis: MC form; MC on the palms, soles > axilla > face
    - B/L and symmetric sweating present for > 6 months w/ no secondary causes
- Secondary hyperhidrosis ("CHAMPS")
    - Cortical hyperhidrosis: disorders of Cornification and other genodermatoses
    - Compensatory hyperhidosis: anhidrosis in one area cause hyperhidrosis in others
        - Seen in miliaria, diabetic neuropathy and with sypathectomies
    - Hypothalamic (thermoregulatory) hyperhidrosis: due to ↑ body temperatures (e.g., chronic infections, cancers, thyroid, drugs); may be nocturnal (night sweats)
    - Autonomic dysreflexia: direct stimulation of a sympathetic Axon (e.g., electrical, physical, drugs) or inflammatory skin disease (e.g., AD); cause localized sweating

- Medullary (gustatory) hyperhidrosis
    - Physiologic: any food or drink that stimulates taste buds may cause sweating (face) due to crossed afferent impulses from taste bud receptors which travel via the **glossopharyngeal nerve** to nuclei within the medulla oblongata (hence the term "medullary" hyperhidrosis)
    - Pathologic: disrupted nerves for sweat and salivation aberrantly connect
        - Frey syndrome: **auriculotemporal nerve** injured after Parotid surgery → parasympathetic fibers innervate sweat glands of the overlying skin → sweating on cheek or neck after eating/drinking
            - Rx: botox injections and topical antiperspirants
        - Chorda tympani syndrome: salivary stimuli to the submandibular gland induce sweating on the chin/jawline ("chorda chin-pani")
- Spinal (cord transection) sweating: massive sweating may occur around the injured level with a lack of thermal sweating below the injury
- Systemic drugs: cholinesterase inhibitors, α/β agonists, insulin, stimulants

• Dx ("CHAMPS"): CBC, Catecholamines, HbA1c, ANA, Med rec, PPD, Sed rate
    - Starch iodine test (starch powder + iodine solution): sites w/ sweating turn black

• Rx
    - Topical: aluminum chloride (salt), glycopyrronium/sofpironium (anticholinergic)
        - CI to anticholinergics ("Forrest GUMP"): Glaucoma, Urinary retention, toxic Megacolon, Myasthenia gravis, Paralytic ileus

- Oral: oxybutynin glycopyrrolate (anticholinergic), clonidine (α_2-agonist)
- Tap water iontophoresis (may be done at home if patient buys device)
- OnabotulinumtoxinA: prevents release of acetylcholine from neurons
  - This helps me remember that sweat glands are functionally cholinergic
- Surgical treatment: thermolysis of the sweat glands by Nd:YAG, dissection, curettage, liposuction or excision of axilla; sympathectomy is the last resort

Hypohidrosis and anhidrosis

- Major categories
  - Central and neuropathic diseases (e.g., brain tumors, spinal injuries) or meds that disrupt neural impulses (anticholinergics, α-blockers, clonidine, CCB, topiramate)
  - Peripheral (non-neural) alterations in the gland itself via congenital alterations (ectodermal dysplasias), obstruction (ichthyosis) or acquired destruction (burns)
- p/w ↓ sweating → hyperthermia
- Dx: review meds, starch-iodide test, biopsy may identity sweat gland abnormalities
- Rx: instruct to keep cool, D/C offending med, gentle exfoliation (duct obstruction)

Miliaria

- MC in neonates with immature eccrine ducts > adults in hot-humid climates
- Pathogenesis: excessive sweating causes maceration of the stratum corneum sufficient to block eccrine duct → sweat retention in duct
- 3 types distinguished by level of obstruction noted in parentheses

  - Miliaria Crystallina (stratum Corneum): p/w non-pruritic small Clear vesicles
  - Miliaria Rubra (mid-epidermis; "Right in the middle"): p/w pruritic small non-follicular Red papules with punctate vesicles/pustules in the center
  - Miliaria profunda (profunda means Deep in Spanish; DEJ/upper Dermis): p/w non-pruritic deep-seated white to skin-colored papules
- Dx: biopsy will show keratinous obstruction of sweat ducts
- Rx: place patient in cool environment

Bromhidrosis

- Eccrine bromhidrosis (3 types)
  - Keratogenic: bacterial degradation of macerated keratin in stratum corneum
  - Metabolic: abnormal secretion of amino acids as seen in metabolic disorders (musty odor in phenylketonuria, sweet odor in maple syrup urine disease)
  - Exogenous: foods (garlic, asparagus, curry), drugs (bromides), chemicals (DMSO)
- Apocrine bromhidrosis: bacteria degrade odorless Axillary apocrine sweat into Ammonia

Chromhidrosis

- Eccrine Chromhidrosis: results from Contamination of colorless eccrine sweat by a Chromogen on the skin surface such as dyes or pigments from microorganisms (3 colors)
  - Blue sweat: Copper or Corynebacterium (may be black pigment also)
  - Brown sweat: o-chronosis or dihydroxyacetone in sunless-tanning products
  - Red sweat: bacterial infection or patients taking rifampin or Clofazamine

- Aprocrine chromhidrosis: much more common and usually intrinsic in origin
    - Yellow sweat from axilla: lipofuscin ("wear-and-tear" pigment) in apocrine sweat

Fox-Fordyce disease (apocrine miliaria)

- Females 15–35 years old
- Pathogenesis: obstruction of apocrine glands from ↑ keratin in follicular **infundibulum**
    - The miliaria equivalent for the apocrine glands
- p/w **pruritic** dome-shaped, skin-colored Follicular papules in apocrine regions (Folds)
- Rx (Rx similar to acne but commonly Fail): topical/IL steroids (1st line), topical and oral retinoids, topical and oral antibiotics, pregnancy and oral contraceptives (**estrogen**)

Granulosa Rubra nasi

- Rare AD inherited disorder which starts in childhood and usually resolves in puberty
- p/w hyperhidrosis of tip of nose for years followed by Redness of the nose > cheeks
- May also see primary hyperhidrosis of the palms and soles with pernio and acrocyanosis
- Rx: drying lotions (aluminum chloride), Reassurance that it Resolves in puberty

Idiopathic palmoplantar hidradenitis

- Disease of healthy children
- Pathogenesis: vigorous physical activity → eccrine gland rupture due to trauma
- p/w multiple tender erythematous nodules on palms or soles
- Path: neutrophilic infiltration of secretory and ductal components

- **Spontaneous resolution** in days to weeks; can have recurrences

3.14 Drug Reactions

- The most common medications to cause cutaneous drug eruptions (CDEs) are the **aminopenicillins** ampicillin and amoxicillin (8% of those on drug develop rash) > anticonvulsants (5%) > TMP/SMX (4%) > NSAIDS (0.5%)
    - In the HIV population (↑ incidence of CDEs), **TMP/SMX** is the MCC (40%), but dapsone, β-lactams, nevirapine, abacavir and anticonvulsants are also common
- The most common morphologies are morbilliform (92%) > urticarial (6%) > vasculitis
- Immunologically mediated drug reactions
    - IgE dependent drug reactions (type 1): urticaria, angioedema, anaphylaxis
        - Occurs within 24 hours of drug intake
    - Cytotoxic drug reactions (type 2; antibody against a fixed antigen): petechia
    - Immune complex mediated (type 3): vasculitis, serum sickness, SLE
    - Delayed type/cell mediated (type 4): morbilliform, FDE, SJS/TEN, lichenoid drug

Morbilliform (exanthematous/maculopapular) drug eruption

- By far the most common CDE ("Morbilliform is much more common")
- Similar to SJS/TEN, onset is 1–2 weeks and culprit drugs include Antibiotics (sulfonamides and β-lactams), Anticonvulsants, Antiretrovirals, Allopurinol

- p/w **pruritic maculopapular** rash starting in groin and axilla ("morbilli-folds") of an adult then spreads (ddx: viral rash is a non-pruritic macular rash in a child)
- Should not see painful/dusky skin w/ mucosal lesions (SJS/TEN) or facial edema (DRESS)
- Path: vacuolar interface, spongiosis, necrotic keratinocytes, PV infiltrate w/ lymphs/eos
- Rx: supportive (D/C drug but may attempt to treat through if drug is essential)

Urticaria, angioedema and anaphylaxis (see section 3.9)

Drug-induced hypersensitivity syndrome/drug reaction with eosinophilia and systemic symptoms (DIHS/DRESS)

- 10% mortality ("1 out of every 10 women in a DRESS will end up killing you")
  - Fulminant **hepatitis** is the MCC of death
- Develops **2–6 weeks** after drug initiation ("takes 2–6 weeks to kiss the girl in the DRESS")
  - Drugs similar to morbilliform/SJS/TEN (sulfonamide **A**ntibiotics, **A**cetaminophen, **A**nticonvulsants, **A**ntiretrovirals, **A**llopurinol) but also Dapsone and Minocycline
    - "Don't forget to DM the girl in the DRESS"
    - MCC in order of frequency: **phenytoin**, carbamazepine, acetaminophen
      - "In regard to the girl in the DRESS, fun (phen) cars get you ass"
      - MC in HIV-patients: **abacavir** (MC; "baby got back") > nevirapine
- p/w morbilliform rash that starts on face and top half of body then becomes edematous (facial edema in 30%) w/ follicular accentuation; mucosal lesions (oral) in 25% of cases
  - "The girl in the DRESS first puts red blush on her face but later she becomes fat (edema), hairy (fol-

licular accentuation) and only gives oral sex 25% of the time"

- The most common symptoms include **fever** (85%, "The girl in the DRESS is almost always hot") > morbilliform rash (75%) > LAD, arthralgias and multi-organ involvement
    - **Liver is most common and most severe**, followed by kidneys
        - "In regard to the girl in the DRESS, you most likely will live with her (liver; MC organ affected) and then you'll have kids (kidneys; 2nd MC organ)"
        - But may affect any organ: colitis, myocarditis, pneumonitis, encephalitis
- Late sequela includes **thyroiditis/Graves**, cardiomyopathy and DM (requires monitoring)
    - "The girl in the DRESS might get diabetes and thyroid disease later in life"
- Risk factors
    - HLA-A*3101 (Northern Europeans on carbamazepine)
        - "Europeans eat 3101 carbs/day"
    - HLA-B*5801 (Han Chinese exposed to allopurinol)
        - "The Han Chinese eat all things, about 5801 things"
    - HLA-B*5701 (**abacavir**): causes DRESS >> SJS
        - Abacavir is 100 back from the Han Chinese HLA (5801-100=5701)
    - HLA-A*3201 (vancomycin-induced DRESS)
    - Inability to detoxify arene oxide metabolites in aromatic anticonvulsants
        - "Don't give the girl in the DRESS an oxidized ring or she may convulse"
    - Slow acetylators (Sulfonamide-induced DRESS)
    - Likely role of HHV-6 > HHV-7, CMV, EBV

    - "Be careful, the girl in the DRESS likely has herpes 4, 5, 6 and 7"

- DRESS variants
  - Anticonvulsant hypersensitivity syndrome: cannot detox arene oxide metabolites in anticonvulsants due to **epoxide hydrolase deficiency**; liver involvement is MC
    - Switch to valproic acid or levetiracetam
  - Allopurinol hypersensitivity syndrome: seen in renal failure pts or Han Chinese with HLA-B*5801; common liver and kidney involvement, pancreatitis and DM
    - "Han Chinese eat all (5801) things and this syndrome effects all organs"
  - Sulfonamide hypersensitivity syndrome: ↑ risk in Slow acetylators
  - Dapsone hypersensitivity syndrome: p/w hemolysis/icterus; lacks eosinophilia
  - Minocycline hypersensitivity syndrome seen in young females w/ **glutathione** S-transferase deficiency: interstitial eosinophilic pneumonia and liver involvement
    - "The girl in the DRESS has miniature glutes"
- J-SCAR diagnostic criteria ("FRAIL"): Fever, HHV-6 Reactivation, maculopapular Rash developing > 3 weeks after starting drug, prolonged symptoms After discontinuation, Internal organ abnormalities, Leukocyte abnormalities (↑ eos, atypical lymphs) and LAD
- Rx: prolonged steroid taper (esp. if lung and heart involvement) and D/C offending med
- Workup: CBC w/ diff, peripheral smear for atypical lymphs, BUN/Cr, UA, LFTs, CK, lipase, CRP, TSH, fasting glucose (in anticipation for steroids) +/- EKG, PCR for HHV6

- o Follow TSH for 2 years and CBC, BUN/Cr, UA, LFTs for at least 1 year

Acute generalized exanthematous pustulosis (AGEP; A-G)

- Acute febrile, pustular eruption usually caused by Azithromycin and β-lactams > CCBs > Chloroquine/hydroxyChloroquine Drugs
- Edematous skin, Fever and **sterile pustules** develop Fast (within Four days of starting drug); starts on the Face and Folds (intertriginous sites) and Generalizes within hours
- Non-drug causes: mercury and viruses (enterovirus) cause it in kids
- Path: Intraepidermal pustule (clinically and histologically mimics generalized pustular psoriasis but eos, necrotic keratinocytes and mixed PV inflammation points to AGEP)
- Rx: D/C med and supportive treatment w/ topical steroids and antipyretics
- Workup: may show neutrophilia, hypocalcemia and a positive patch test

Photosensitive drug reactions

- Photosensitivity caused by an exogenous photosensitizing agent
- Phototoxic: more common; occurs in anyone who receives drug (**usually PO**) and UVR
    - o Caused by UVR (**UVA**) interacting with drug free radicals → damages skin
    - o Presents as a **painful and exaggerated sunburn reaction** limited to sun-exposed skin which happens hours after sun-exposure and heals with hyperpigmentation
    - o Path: necrotic keratinocytes ("sun-burn cells") and a superficial dermal infiltrate
    - o My FAV TAN is a PhotoToxic Sunburn

    - **Methotrexate**
    - **Fluoroquinolones**, Furocoumarins (celery, parsnips, figs, citrus), **5-FU**
    - Amiodarone: p/w gray hyperpigmentation
    - Voriconazole (XP-like presentation w/ aggressive SCCs), Vemorafenib
    - TCNs (demoxycycline > doxycycline > tetracycline >> minocycline)
    - Azines (**chlorpromazine** and prochlorperazine)
    - NSAIDS
    - **Psoralens (MCC in US from a topical)**
    - Thiazides (esp HCTZ), Tar, TCAs (**imipramine**)
    - **St John's wort**, Sulfonamides
  - Less common manifestations of phototoxicity
    - Pseudoporphyria: skin similar to PCT but lacks sclerodermoid features, hypertrichosis and hyperpigmentation ("not hard, hairy or hazel")
      - Causes are similar to "FAV TAN" but NSAIDS (**naproxen**) is #1
    - Photo-onycholysis: TCNs and Psoralens ("TP touches nails when wiping")
      - Taxanes result in painful hemorrhagic onycholysis
    - Photo-lichenoid eruption: HCTZ and "ENSAIDS" are MC
    - Slate gray hyperpigmentation: TCAs, Amiodarone, Diltiazem
      - "The drug that gave you a sunburn also turned you a TAD gray"
    - UV recall: reaction in area of previous burn after starting drug (MTX)
    - Phytophotodermatitis: furocoumarin containing plants
- Photoallergic: less common but more chronic; only occurs in sensitized patients (delayed type hypersen-

sitivity) who receive drug (usually **topical**) and UVR (UVA)

- Caused by UVR (**UVA**) interacting with drug turns it into a photoallergen
- Requires sensitization with a 7–10-day incubation period
- Presents as an **eczematous** eruption on sun-exposed areas → later spreads
- Path: non-specific spongiotic dermatitis w/ eosinophils present
- Most common drugs to cause a photoallergic reaction: M-T
    - Musk ambrette, Methyl-coumarin (fragrances)
    - NSAIDS (piroxicam and ketoprofen)
    - **Oxybenzone (benzophenone-3) is #1 cause**
    - Piroxicam (patch test positive to thimerosal), PABA
    - Quinidine (antiarrhythmic), Quinine (malarial), Quinolone (antibacterial)
    - **gRiseofulvin**
    - Sandalwood oil (fragrance), Sulfonamides, Salicylates
    - Thiazide diuretics, Tricyclic antidepressants
- Dx: photopatch test (each allergen has 2 chambers, one w/ UV and one without)
    - Photoallergy: only the UVA exposed chamber cause a reaction
    - Contact allergy: both non-exposed and UVA-exposed chambers react

Drug-induced pigmentary changes

- Hyperpigmentation: often photodistributed; a/w melanonychia and oral pigmentation
    - Drugs that cause hyperpigmentation due to More than just Melanin (Ms): Malarials (stains w/ both

perls and Fontana Masson), Minocycline (type 1 and 2 stain with Perls and Fontana Masson), Metals (stains w/ neither Perls nor Fontana Masson except for arsenic which stains with Fontana Masson)

- Most drugs cause ↑ melanin in basal keratinocytes (A-F): Arsenic, Amiodarone, AZT, Anti-psychotics (chlorpromazine), Anti-depressants (TCAs), Bimatoprost, BCNU (carmustine), Bleomycin, Busulfan, Cyclophosphamide, Diltiazem, Dactinomycin, Doxorubicin, Estrogen (OCPs), 5-FU, (also psoralens, hydroxyurea)
  - These will stain w/ Fontana Masson (↑ melanin in basal keratinocytes)
- Clofazimine causes orange-brown hyperpigmentation due to Ceroid lipofuscin
- Rx: stop drug; Q-switched lasers

• Hypopigmentation: frequently due to tyrosine kinase inhibitors (imatinib) and various topical meds → phenols/catechols (hydroquinone and MBEH), sulfhydryls, steroids, azelaic acid, benzyl alcohol (MBEH is only one that is irreversible and affects distant skin)

<u>Drugs that cause hyperpigmentation due to something More than just an ↑ in Melanin (M's)</u>

Minocycline-induced pigmentary changes

- In addition to skin, can affect oral **mucosa, sclerae (1st site affected)**, nails, bones, teeth
  - Fetal exposure to Minocycline affects Mid-portion of teeth while Tetracycline affects the gingival 1/3rd (Top of the teeth on the Top row)
- Types
  - Type 1: blue-gray hyperpigmentation in areas of inflammation or scars (**acne**)
    - Path: perivascular pigment deposits in the **dermis** and in macrophages

        - Stains w/ **Perls** (iron) > Fontana Masson (melanin)
  - Type 2: blue-gray hyperpigmentation on the **B/L shins** ("you have 2 shins")
    - Path: brown-black granules free in the dermis and within macrophages distributed around the vasculature and sweat gland coils
      - Stains w/ Pers (iron) and Fontana Masson (melanin); "2 stains"
  - Type 3: diffuse muddy brown pigment in sun-exposed areas ("sun has 3 letters")
    - Path: increased epidermal basal cell pigmentation
      - Stains w/ **Fontana Masson** (sun-exposed makes me think melanin)
  - Type 4 (rare): circumscribed blue-gray pigmentation on acne scars on the back
    - Path: **calcium**-containing melanin-like substance without iron

Anti-malarial-induced pigmentary changes

- Occurs in 25% of patients w/ long-term use; does not fully resolve after discontinuation
- CQ/HCQ: p/w blue-black to gray pigmentation on **lower leg** (mimics type 2 minocycline)
- Quinacrine: p/w diffuse yellow brown discoloration of skin and eyes (mimics jaundice)

Heavy metal-induced pigmentary changes

- Arsenic: "rain-drops" of hypopigmentation on a hyperpigmented background mimicking the "salt and pepper" pigmentation of scleroderma (**PPK/SCCs arise decades later**)
  - Path: only metal that shows ↑ melanin in basal keratinocytes

- Bismuth: generalized Blue-gray pigmentating on the head/neck, dorsal hands, mouth
  - Path: dermal bismuth deposits
- Gold (chryiasis): permanent blue-gray hyperpigmentation on face (periocular is MC; "eyes on gold") and other sun-exposed sites (rare as we no longer use gold for RA)
  - Path: gold deposits found in Giant cells/macrophages which have a Gold-red-orange birefringence on polarized light
    - Deposits do not bind to BMZ or eccrine membrane propria (vs argyria)
- Silver (argyria): diffuse slate-gray pigmentation which is ↑ in sun-exposed areas
  - Silver is found in silver sulfadiazine (burn wounds) and in elixirs
  - Path: silver deposits bound to BMZ and membrane propria of **eccrine glands**
    - "Since silver is cheaper than gold, you will be able to accumulate it in your basement membrane and eccrine gland membrane propria"
- Iron: pigmentation occurs after Monsel's use, sclerotherapy and in stasis dermatitis
  - Path: hemosiderin (Perl's +) deposits in dermis and in macrophages
- Lead: lead lines on gingival margins
  - Path: subepithelial lead deposits
- Mercury: slate gray discoloration from ointments containing mercury (no longer used); also causes acrodynia (painful dusky-red swelling of hands and feet) and baboon syndrome (morbilliform eruption w/ accentuation in groin and thighs)
  - Path: huge (Massive) deposits of brown-black mercury granules in Macrophages

Drugs that cause hyperpigmentation due to an ↑ in melanin (A-F)

Amiodarone

- p/w phototoxic eruption (50% in 6 months; face is MC) → **slate-gray discoloration**
- Path: PAS+ **yellow-brown granules of lipofuscin (Fontana Masson+) in macrophages**
- EM: **lipid-like lysosomal inclusions**

AZT (zidovudine)

- Widespread pigment w/ accentuation in sun-exposed skin; **longitudinal melanonychia**
  - o Path: dermal melanophages w/ ↑ melanin in keratinocytes

Anti-psychotics (phenazothiazines: chlorpromazine) and anti-depressants (TCAs: imiprimine)

- **p/w blue-gray hyperpigmentation in photo-exposed skin**
- Path: refractile golden-brown granules (Fontana Masson+) in macrophages
- SEs of TCAs (4 Cs): Cardiac, Convulsions, anti-Cholinergic and Color changes

Bimatoprost/latanoprost (prostaglandin analogs)

- p/w **periocular and iris hyperpigmentation**

BCNU (carmustine) and nitrogen mustard (mechlorethamine)

- p/w pigment at sites of topical application ("mustard only stains the skin it touches")
- Path: ↑ melanocytes and melanin in keratinocytes

Bleomycin

- **Linear or flagellate hyperpigmented patches on trunk**, transverse melanonychia, sclerodermoid

changes, **hyperpigmentation of palmar ("pelmar") crease** and digital ulcers
  - o Flagellate hyperpigmentation/erythema looks like BDSM whip marks
    - **Bleomycin**, Docetaxel, Dermatomyositis, Diode laser, Stills disease, Mushrooms (shi-take), Man-of-war/jellyfish
- Path: ↑ melanin in keratinocytes

Busulfan
- p/w generalized hyperpigmentation ("the entire bus gets darker/dirtier w/ time")
- Pulmonary fibrosis
- Path: ↑ melanin in keratinocytes

Cyclophosphamide
- p/w diffuse mucocutaneous hyperpigmentation or localized to nails, teeth, palms/soles
- Ifosfamide is related to cyclophosphamide and p/w hyperpigmentation in the Flexures, Feet, under Occlusive dressings (just like thiotepa) and Scrotum

Diltiazem
- Occurs in **Dark-skinned patients (AAs)**
- p/w slate-gray discoloration in sun-exposed skin w/ reticular or perifollicular pattern
- Notice how ditiazem, antipsychotics (…azines), AZT and amiodarone all cause hyperpigmentation in sun ("Zun")-exposed skin → p/w gray-blue discoloration of the face w/ sparring of the lower eyelids, philtrum and sub-mental area
- Path: lichenoid dermatitis w/ melanophages

Dactinomycin and doxorubicin (anthracyclines)
- p/w hyperpigmentation on the face (dactinomycin) or hands (doxorubicin)

    - "You shake your head "no" with your face and you rub your hands"
    - **The pigmentation in doxorubicin is over the hand joints so it looks like Gottron's sign of DM**, but the lesions are blue-gray, not the lilac color of AI-CTD
- May also see hyperpigmentation in the mouth (tongue), transverse melanonychia and extravasation reactions (ulceration and induration at chemo infusion site)
- Path: ↑ melanocytes and melanin in keratinocytes

Estrogen (OCPs/pregnancy)

- p/w melasma, nipple hyperpigmentation and darkening of nevi
- Path: ↑ melanocytes and melanin in keratinocytes

5-fluorouracil

- PO: phototoxic dermatitis and later replaced by hyperpigmentation
- IV: **Serpentine hyperpigmentation overlying veins** ("5 is a Serpentine number") and extravasation reactions w/ ulceration or indurated red plaques at chemo infusion site
    - Infusion of docetaxel can also cause serpentine hyperpigmentation
        - "F U (5FU) taxes (taxanes)! The IRS are snakes (serpentine pigmentation)"
- Path: necrotic keratinocytes and ↑ melanin in keratinocytes

Hydroxyurea

- p/w DM-like eruption over joints on dorsal hands ("like-mechanics Hands"), diffuse mucocutaneous Hyperpigmentation (longitudinal melanonychia,

Hyperpigmentation of lunulae;) and lower leg ulcers (classically on the lateral malleolus just lateral to Heel)

Methotrexate

- p/w phototoxic dermatitis → post-inflammatory hyperpigmentation (like 5-FU)
- UV recall: weeks after chemo, a phototoxic rash will occur in previously sunburnt sites
    - o Initially described w/ MTX but also seen w/ gemcitabine, etoposide and taxanes
- Necrosis of psoriatic plaques is another high-yield SE

Triethylenethiophosphoramide (thiotepa)

- p/w hyperpigmentation at sites occluded by adhesive-containing material

Psoralens

- p/w diffuse (PUVA) or focal (topical PUVA/phytophotodermatitis) hyperpigmentation
- Path: ↑ melanin in keratinocytes

Pigmentary changes besides hyperpigmentation

Clofazimine

- p/w diffuse orange-pink and later blue-brown Color of skin and Conjunctivae
- Birefringent red Crystals (seen with fresh frozen tissue) and PAS+ brown granular pigment within foamy macrophages (H&E; "drug-induced lipofuscinosis")

Imatinib (Gleevac)

- Gingiva/teeth/nails hyperpigmentation
- Loss of pigment in skin (due to c-KIT blockade)
- Eye edema (periorbital edema)

Sunitinib/Sorafenib (multi-targeted kinase inhibitors which target VEGF, PDGFR, CEGFR)

- **Hand-foot-Skin reaction**: painful hyperkeratotic plaques on pressure areas of Sole
- Stomatitis, Seb derm-like facial rash, KP-like eruption, Subungual splinter hemorrhages, SCCs, benign dyskeratomas, **yellow (sun is yellow) skin pigmentation, lightening of hair**
    - o Quinacrine also causes yellowing of the skin and lightening of hair
- Scrotal reactions: Scrotal ulcers w/ pain (Sunitinib); Scrotal eczema w/o pain (Sorafenib)
    - o All-trans-retinoic acid also causes scrotal ulcers (foscarnet causes penile ulcers)
- Bevacizumab is a VEGF multikinase inhibitor which cause **Bleeding/ulceration of striae**

Drug-induced nail pigmentation

- Every med we have discussed in this section can cause melanonychia ("Ms and ABCs")
    - o Drug-induced melanonychia can be diffuse, longitudinal or horizontal
- Favipiravir (medication for COVID-19) has caused greenish florescence of nails

Chemotherapy-specific cutaneous reactions

Hand-foot-syndrome (HFS; palmoplantar erythrodysesthesia)

- MC drugs: **cytarabine**, anthracyclines (doxorubicin), 5-FU/capecitabine, MTX, taxanes
- **p/w prodrome of pain and dysesthesia followed by symmetric, sharply demarcated patches of diffuse erythema on the palms and soles**
    - o Taxanes cause unique type of hand-foot-syndrome w/ erythema and dysesthesia on the **dor-**

sal hands w/ hemorrhagic onycholysis termed "PATEO syndrome"

- Rx: **topical steroids**, NSAIDS, icepacks (only severe cases need drug holiday)
- Preventative measures: localized cryotherapy (frozen gloves/socks) during infusion
    - o Similar to "cold caps" pts can wear to prevent chemotherapy-induced alopecia
- When it involves the ears (redness/swelling) it is known as Ara-C ears (cytarabine is MC)

Hand-foot-Skin reaction (HFSR)

- Less severe acral dysesthesia and swelling compared to HFS but w/ **painful hyperkeratotic plaques on pressure areas of hands/Soles**
- MC drugs: mutikinase inhibitors (Sunitinib, Sorafenib)
- Rx: high potency topical Steroids, topical retinoids, urea

Neutrophilic eccrine hidradenitis

- p/w erythematous papules and plaques on the extremities and trunk
- MC drug: cytarabine

Actinic keratosis inflammation in patients on systemic chemotherapy

- Originally described w/ 5-FU but also seen in doxorubicin, dactinomycin, dacarbazine, cisplatin, fludarabine and vincristine

Alopecia

- Most chemotherapy agents will cause anagen effluvium but it can be irreversible w/ **Busulfan**, Cisplatin, **Docetaxel**, Etopiside ("You may Always have Alopecia w/ B-E drugs")

- May be prevented w/ cool caps worn at time of infusion which limits absorption in hair

Mucositis

- Most chemotherapy agents will cause mucositis (stomatitis is MC) but is particularly common w/ 5-FU, etoposide and methotrexate → p/w mouth ulcers
    - o Fascarnet is a high-yield cause of penile erosions
- Begins 5–10 days after initiation of chemotherapy and lasts 7–14 days

Extravasation reactions

- Vesicant (blister-causing) chemotherapy agents such as **anthracyclines** (esp doxorubicin) cause ulceration and necrosis of skin when inadvertently administered into tissue
- MC locations are chest (port) or arms (lines)
- Rx: stop infusion immediately; DMSO (free radical scavenger)

Chemotherapy recall

- p/w tender nodules overlying superficial veins at a location previously used for infusion
- Has been reported w/ 5-FU, mitomycin C, paclitaxel, doxorubicin and epirubicin

Cutaneous side effects of monoclonal antibodies

EGFR inh (cetuximab, erlotinib, pertuzumumab, necitumumab, panitumumab; PRIDE syndrome)

- **Papulopustular rash**, Pyogenic granulomas/ Paronychia, Regulatory change in hair (**trichomegaly**), Itchiness and Dryness (painful fissures of fingers/toes) caused by EGFRs
- Acneiform rash occurs early (3 weeks) post therapy in 90% of pts (**portends a good prognosis for the**

cancer; **use TCNs**, topical clinda/steroids, not topical retinoids)
- Oral: mucositis, aphthae, xerostomia

Bruton tyrosine kinase (ibrutinib)
- **SEs: purpura (Bruising), petechia**, folliculitis, nail changes

Proteosome inhibitors (bortezomib, carfilzomib)
- SEs: morbilliform exanthem, pruritis, acneiform eruption (folliculitis), EM/SJS/TEN, Sweets, small vessel vasculitis and increased risk of herpes zoster and cutaneous lupus

mTOR inhibitors (sirolimus, ererolimus, temsirolimus)
- SEs: stomatitis, facial hair growth/trichomegaly, paronychia, periorbital edema, morbilliform exanthem, pruritis, acneiform eruption, small vessel vasculitis, xerosis, eczematous eruptions, yellow fragile nails, angioedema, bruising

Other high-yield medication side effects

Ichthyosis
- MC drugs: **nicotinic acid** (vitamin B3), Cholesterol-lowering meds (e.g., statins), Cimetidine, Clofazimine, Hydroxyurea and Triparanol

Exogenous ochronosis
- MC drugs: topical phenol, resorcinol or hydroquinone; mercury or antimalarials

Coumadin-induced skin necrosis
- Hemorrhagic bullae and ulcers on fatty areas 2–5 days after starting coumadin
- Main risk factor is protein C deficiency

- Path: Coagulation of blood vessels
- Rx: wound care, stop coumadin, start vitamin K, heparin, and IV protein C
- Not the same as warfarin blue toe syndrome (anticoagulant-induced cholesterol emboli)

Heparin-induced skin necrosis (heparin-induced thrombocytopenia with thrombosis syndrome)

- Autoantibodies to heparin/platelet factor 4 complexes lead to ↓ platelets, thrombosis and cutaneous necrosis days after starting unfractionated heparin
- Rx: **stop heparin and start a direct thrombin inhibitor or factor Xa inhibitor**

Radiation recall/radiation enhancement

- Acute inflammatory reaction confined to previously irradiated areas that can be triggered when chemo agents are administered after radiotherapy
- Seen MC w/ doxorubicin, taxanes, gemcitabine, capecitabine, MTX

Baboon syndrome

- Systemic contact dermatitis to mercury, antibiotics, nickel, heparin or food additives
- p/w symmetric diffuse exanthem on the butt, anogenital area, flexures of extremities
- Baboon syndrome has historically been equated w/ mercury-induced exanthem
- Symmetric drug-related intertriginous exanthema (SDRIFE) specifically refers to drug-induced baboon syndrome in which **Beta-lactam antibiotics (amoxicillin) are the MCC**

Red-man syndrome

- p/w flushing, pruritis and hypotension 10 minutes after infusion of vancomycin

- Rx: slow infusion and pretreat w/ antihistamines

Bromoderma and iododerma

- p/w acneiform or vegetating lesions after chronic exposure to bromide, radiocontrast, amiodarone, SSKI or povidone-iodine
- Path: pseudoepitheliomatous hyperplasia w/ puss (neutrophilic microabscesses)

Cutaneous side effects of CCBs ("calcium channel blockers block the GATE")

- Granulomatous drug reactions, Gingival hyperplasia, **AGEP, Telangiectasias**, **Eczema**

Eczematous drug reaction ("U ITCH")

- Ustekinumab, IVIG, TNF-alpha, CCBs, HMG-CoA-reductase inhibitors (statins)

Sticky skin syndrome

- p/w sticky feeling of skin (most pronounced on acral surfaces)
- MC drugs ("Sticky DIK"): **Doxorubicin, Isotretinoin, Ketoconazole**

Gingival hypertrophy

- MC meds: **Phenytoin (MCC)** > CCB (esp. nifedipine) > Cyclosporine
  - "PC Culture" will make you bite your tongue, and gums b/c of how big they are"

Serum sickness

- Drug-induced CSVV (circulating immune complexes) which p/w fever, arthralgias, LAD, renal disease and hypocomplementemia
- MC meds: anti-thymocyte globulin, infliximab, minocycline

Serum sickness-like reaction

- p/w fever, polyarthralgias and an urticarial rash (often w/ a bruise-like quality) in a kid
- MC med: **cefaclor** ("fac I have serum sickness-like reaction")
- Rx: self-limited; antihistamines, NSAIDS

Side effects from injections

- Texiers disease: sclerotic plaques due to vitamin K injections (can see on leg of newborn)
- Nicolau syndrome (embolia cutis medicamentosa): vessel occlusion due to IM injection
    - p/w severe pain, ischemia and pallor within minutes of injection → ulceration

3.15 Photodermatoses

Sunburns/pigment darkening

- SunBurns (reddening): p/w erythema: peaks at 12–24 hours post **UVB** > UVA exposure
    - UVA penetrates deeper into the dermis and is responsible for photo-Aging
- Pigment darkening (tanning): p/w darkening of the skin
    - UVA causes immediate pigment darkening in **mins** d/t **melanin redistribution**
    - UVA causes **persistent pigment darkening** within **hours** d/t **melanin oxidation**
    - **UVB** light causes **Delayed pigmentation** (tanning) **Days** after exposure to light which is due to ↑ **Synthesis of Melanin** ("Keep it straight w/ BDSM mnemonic")

Photo-Aging (dermatoheliosis; solar elastosis): A-F

- Actinic elastosis (solar elastosis): p/w dyspigmentation, wrinkles, telangiectasias and AKs
- Acrokeratoelastoidosis: **p/w waxy papules on lateral fingers**
- Beaded striated lines: hyperplastic sebaceous glands (chronic sun damage causes them to be visualized) that form **parallel beaded lines on the lateral neck**
- Citrine skin of Milian: wrinkled, inelastic, red and yellow skin w/ telangiectasias
    - Non-atrophic variant: p/w yellow leathery facial skin w/ deep furrows and scales
    - Atrophic variant: p/w **telangiectasias** and hyperplastic sebaceous glands w/ erythema and yellowing of skin (deep furrows/wrinkling is uncommon)
- Cutis rhomboidalis nuchae: thick leathery and coarsely wrinkled skin on nape of neck
- Colloid milium: p/w 1–2 mm white-yellow SQ papules on sun exposed skin
- Poikiloderma of Civatte: p/w reticular red patches on the neck (submentum spared)
- Elastoma of Dubreuih: yellow-brown papules/plaques on forehead, cheeks and neck
- Elastotic bands: cord-like bands extending around the flexure aspect of forearms
- Elastotic nodules of the ear: p/w asymptomatic papules on the bilateral helix/antihelix
- Erosive pustular dermatosis: pustules, crusts and erosions on the scalp of old bald men
    - Rx: potent topical steroids
- Favre Racouchot: severe solar elastosis w/ cysts on the temples/upper lateral cheeks
    - Actinic comedonal plaques is a variant (identical path) that p/w confluent nodules pierced w/ numerous tiny holes on the face > chest, forearms
    - Rx: I&D, topical retinoids, CO2 laser

Clues to the diagnosis of specific photodermatoses in adults
Presents with urticarial lesions within **minutes** of sun exposure • Solar urticaria: lesions lasts < 24 hours and are painful/smarting Presents with pink to red edematous papules and plaques within **hours** of sun exposure • PMLE: lesions last days to weeks and are pruritic • Cutaneous lupus: lesions lasts weeks to months and are non-pruritic Presents with eczematous lesions in sun-exposed areas • Photoallergic contact dermatitis • Photoallergic drug eruption • Photoaggrevated dermatosis (e.g., AD) • Chronic actinic dermatitis: sharp cutoff at clothing lines with profound lichenification Presents with a sunburn • Phototoxic drug reaction due to systemic medications • Phototoxic contact dermatitis due to topical medication or chemical

Polymorphous light eruption (PMLE)

- Common UV induced eruption hours to days after sun-exposure in the spring or summer
- **Delayed (type 4) hypersensitivity reaction** to an unidentified photo-induced allergen
- p/w non-scarring Pruritic Pink Papules, Papulovesicles or Plaques which last weeks
- Path: Perivascular lymphocytes (CD4 in hours; CD8 in days) w/ Papillary dermal edema
- Rx: PhotoProtection with broad-spectrum sunscreens and prevention via Plaquenil or "hardening" (Phototherapy in the spring w/ Prednisone to ↓ exacerbation)

Juvenile spring eruption ("Juvenile spring Ear-uption")

- Presents like PMLE but occurs in **young boys** (Juvenile) not young adult females
- Like PMLE it occurs in the Spring
- **Ears are the MC site**

Actinic prurigo ("ACTS")

- MC in Native American children caused by UVA > UVB light
- HLA-DR4 DRB1*0407 polymorphism present in majority of cases
- p/w intensely pruritic Crusted papulonodular eruption usually on sun-exposed skin
  - o Dyspigmentation and scarring are common (vs PMLE)
- **Actinic Cheilitis** (path: lymphoid follicles) and **actinic Conjunctivitis** are characteristic
  - o Path of non-mucosal lesions are less specific (superficial PV lymphoid infiltrate)
- Chronic Course that Continues until adulthood
- Rx: TOC is **Thalidomide** (↓TNF-α and IFN-γ); otherwise same treatments as PMLE
  - o If considering thalidomide, refer to neurology for peripheral neuropathy testing
- Flares in Spring and Summer (but unlike PMLE, it does not completely remit in Winter)

Hydroa vacciniforme (HYDROA V)

- Hours after sun exposure children p/w stinging skin → **Hemorrhagic crusts**
- Lymphoproliferative disorders w/ EBV association (may progress to NK T-cell lymphoma)
  - o Pathogenesis: activation of EBV-infected T cells by UV light
- **Dorsal hands and face** show pink macules → papules → vesicles → crusting
- **Resolves** at puberty but leaves punched out varioliform scars; Refractory to treatment
- Reticular keratinocyte degeneration w/ spongiosis and EBV RNA on path
- Ocular involvement (photophobia, keratoconjunctivitis, uveitis) → **refer to Ophtho**

- **UVA** photoprovacation testing helps confirm diagnosis
- **Varioliform scars** remain after resolution of active lesions; EBV association
- Rx: similar to PMLE but w/ acyclovir and treatment of lymphoma if present

Chronic actinic dermatitis (CAD)

- Like PMLE it likely represents a DTH reaction to endogenous photoinduced antigens
- Like PMLE the action spectrum is mostly UVA (UVB and visible light to a lesser degree)
- Breaking up the words tells you everything you need to know
    - Chronic: chronic lesions in old men (50% resolve over 15 years)
    - Actinic: effects sun-exposed skin (**spares sun-protected sites like upper eyelids, nasolabial folds and retroauricular/submental regions**); worse in the summer
    - Dermatitis: p/w eczematous or lichenified plaques; patients have pre-existing **Allergic/photoallergic Contact Dermatitis** (+ Patch tests: e.g., Compositae, PPD)
- May be a presenting sign of **AIDS** (consider HIV testing)
- Dx: phototesting shows ↓MED to UVA and UVB; 75% have positive patch test
- Path (non-specific): spongiosis, superficial PV lymph infiltrate w/ CD8 predominance
- Ddx: CTCL (but presents on sun-exposed sites not sun-covered sites), pellagra
- Rx: photoprotection, avoidance of allergens and immunosuppressants (Corticosteroids for acute exacerbations or **Azathioprine** if long-term treatment is needed)

Photosensitivity in HIV patients

- Photosensitivity resembling PMLE, actinic prurigo or CAD occurs in 5% of HIV patients
- Commonly a/w photosensitizing medications (NSAIDS, efavirenz, TMP-SMX) but eruption often does not improve w/ discontinuation of the medication
- Rx: thalidomide may be effective

Solar urticaria

- Pathogenesis: immediate (type 1) hypersensitivity reaction (crosslinking of circulating IgE antibodies to a UV-induced photo-allergen → mast cell degranulation)
- p/w pruritic urticarial lesions minutes after sun-exposure that last for < 24 hours
- Action spectrum is mostly **visible light** (like porphyrias; in fact, solar urticaria is a/w EPP)
- Drug-induced solar urticaria: chlorpromazine, tar, benoxaprofen and reprinalast
- Rx: physical blockers to protect against visible light; antihistamines or omalizumab

Porphyrias w/ cutaneous* manifestations: "Curing Hepatic Porphyrias Help Vampires Evolve"

	Curing ***	Hepatic	Porphyrias	Help	Vampires	Evolve
	Congenital erythropoetic porphyria (Gunthers)	Hepato-erythropoietic porphyria	Porphyria cutanea tarda	Hereditary coproporphyria	Variagate porphyria*****	Erythropoietic porphyria (EPP) and XLDPP
Inheritance	**AR**		Acquired >> AD mutation in C282Y	AD	AD	AD
Deficient enzyme	Uroporphyrinogen III Cosynthase	Uroporphyrinogen III decarboxylase (Homozygous in HEP)		Coproporphyrinogen III oxidase	Proto-porphyrinogen oxidase	ferrochelatase
Built up porphyrin	hydroxymethylbilane	Uroporphyrinogen III		Coproporphyrinogen III	Proto-porphrinogen IX	Proto-porphyrin IX
Onset	Infancy		3rd–4th decade	1st–2nd decade	2nd–3rd decade	childhood
Clinical	Most severe; photosensitivity to point of mutilation; sclerodermatous changes; severe scarring; red urine/ teeth (teeth fluoresce w/ woods lamp); splenomegaly; cholelithiasis		Milia, scarring, blisters hypertrichosis, Pigmentation, erosions	Neurovisceral attacks + skin findings similar to PCT		Sting/burn/itch **minutes** post sun exposure; crusts/scars; **cholelithiasis****
CBC	Severe hemolytic anemia; ↓ platelets	No hemolytic anemia	↑ iron and RBCs			Hemolytic anemia
Urine	20:1 (uro:copro) ↑ uro and copro in urine, stool, plasma	5:1 (uro:copro) ↑ urogen (fluoresce w/ Woods lamp) ↑ urine isocoproporphrin in HEP		1:1 (uro:copro) ↑ALA, ↑PBG in acute attacks	1:2 (uro:**copro**) ↑ALA, ↑PBG in acute attacks	Normal urine "EPP stands for Empty PP"
Stool******	↑ uro and copro	↑**isocoproporphrin** ("iso-crap-o")		Copro > Proto	**Proto > Copro**	
Plasma peak fluorescence	Floret band and 620 nm**** (plasma)	Floret band and 620 nm (plasma)		Floret band and 620 nm (plasma)	626 nm (plasma)	**Fluorescent RBCs (636 nm)**
Rx: all must avoid sun	Blood transfusions Vit C (ascorbic acid) Vit E (α-tocopherol)	No treatment besides sun protection	Phlebotomy to Hgb <10 low dose Plaquenil (if Hgb already < 9)	Supportive care in the ICU (acute attacks) Prophylaxis with hemin (hematin) Avoid antimalarials in acute attacks		**afamelanotide (α-MSH analog)** → ↑ melanin (FDA approved)
Interesting facts		Clinically like Gunthers but labs like PCT	↑ risk of hepatocellular carcinoma	Coproporphyrinogen III synthesized by C. minutissimum and P. acnes	MC in **South Africa** (A is an upside down V)	MC porphyria in children; **protoporphyrin 9 used in PDT**

*Acute intermittent porphyria (AD defect in porphobilinogen deaminase) and ALA dehydratase deficiency p/w neuropathy, seizures, and abdominal pain during acute attacks but no skin findings (Absent skin findings)
**Hydroxymethylbilane, uro-, copro- and proto- porphyrinogen are hydrophilic/water soluble (results in blisters)
**Protoporphyrin is lipophilic (results in burning/erythema) and since protoporphyrin is not water soluble, EPP has "Empty Pee Pee"
***The first 3 ("Curing Hepatic Porphyrias") happen in the Cytosol, the last 3 ("Help Vampires Evolve") happen in the mitochondria
****All porphyrins are activated by **visible light** (red and blue spectrum) and absorb light in the Floret band (400–410 nm) and from 500–650 nm
*****Variagate porphyria variaties from the others as it is the only one w/ copro > uro in urine and only one with peak fluorescence at 626 nm
******They all have Uro > Copro in the urine ("U > C him pee") except variegate porphyria
*******All porphyrias toxic effects on the skin are due to oxidative damage from ROS generated by protoporphyrins in the skin

Porphyria precipitants: "He BEGS for Alcoholic Drinks"
Hemochromatosis (**iron** overload), Hepatitis C, HIV, Hemodialysis Barbiturates, Estrogen (OCPs), Griseofulvin, Sulfonamides, Alcohol abuse, Diabetes mellitus

*In addition to sun protection w/ physical blockers, all these factors should be avoided in the porphyrias

3.16 Amyloidosis

- Amyloid is composed of a fibril protein (major component; Aker, AL or AA) in a **cross-β-pleated sheet** and stains w/ PCT (PAS, Crystal violet, Congo red, Thioflavin T)
- Amyloid demonstrates **apple green birefringence on Congo red stain w/ polarized light**
- AA amyloid loses Congo red affinity after exposure to "PP" (Potassium Permanganate)
- Types of amyloidosis include Localized cutaneous (LMNo), Primary systemic (P), (skip Q and R), Secondary

systemic (S) and genetic/autoinflammatory Syndromes (S)

Localized cutaneous amyloidosis (LMNo)

- MC in those of LMnO (Latinos, Middle Easterners, Oriental) descent
- Lichen amyloidosis p/w rippled, hyperpigmented pruritic papules/plaques (MC on shins)
  - a/w EBV infection and MEN2A (Sipple syndrome; "ripple rhymes w/ Sipple")
  - Deposition of **Aker protein** derived from **keratinocyte** tonofilaments (keratin 5)
  - Path: amyloid deposits in papillary dermis w/ overlying orthohyperkeratosis
  - Rx: treat the itch w/ potent **topical steroids** or UVB
- Macular amyloidosis p/w pruritic hyperpigmented patches (MC on interscapular back)
  - Exists on a spectrum w/ lichen amyloidosis
  - Deposition of **Aker protein** derived from **keratinocyte** tonofilaments (keratin 5)
  - Path: amyloid in superficial papillary dermis
  - Rx: same as for lichen amyloidosis
  - A rare variant is amyloidosis cutis dyschromica (OSMR gene) which p/w generalized Mottled hyper- and hypopigmented macules in children
- Nödular amyloidosis p/w pink to yellow waxy Nodules MC on acral areas (esp face)
  - a/w AI-CTD esp **Sjögren's** (get ANA, alpha-fodrin, SS-A/Ro)
  - May progress to systemic amyloid or MM (**get CBC, UA, SPEP/immunofixation**)
  - Deposition of **AL protein** derived from **Ig light chains**
  - Path: large amyloid deposits in reticular dermis and vessel walls

- Rx: hard to treat (PDL, excision, steroids, treat associated condition e.g., Sjögren's)

Primary systemic amyloidosis (AL amyloidosis)

- Deposition of **AL protein** derived from **Ig light chains** (usually λ subtype)
- Poor Prognosis (especially if cardiac involvement)
- Due to underlying Plasma cell dyscrasia (MC is **multiple myeloma**)
- p/w Purpuric Papules, **Pinch Purpura (Periorbital), Protruding tongue (macroglossia),** alopecia, waxy thickening of scalp, shoulder Pad sign (enlargement of anterior shoulder)
  - **Purpura can also be elicited by trauma (e.g., under EKG leads)**
  - Peripheral neuropathy due to carpal tunnel, renal and cardiac involvement
- Path: amyloid throughout entire dermis, subcutis, in sweat glands and in vessel walls
  - In the absence of skin lesions, a blind biopsy from the abdominal SQ fat (best; 80% sensitive), rectum or salivary glands can show amyloid deposits
- Labs: UPEP/**SPEP** or immunofixation electrophoresis, echo, UA (Proteinuria)
- Rx: chemo prior to autologous stem cell transplant (melphalan is the standard conditioning agent used prior to autologous stem cell transplant)
  - Multidisciplinary approach including oncology, cardiology, nephrology
- Scleromyxedema also has a IgGλ plasma cell dyscrasia, carpal tunnel and melphalan Rx
  - However we only use melphalan in severe cases as it has severe cardiac toxicities

Secondary systemic amyloidosis (AA amyloidosis)

- Deposition of **AA protein** derived from **SAA (Serum Amyloid A)**
- Sequela of Severe chronic Systemic diseases (e.g., ankylosing Spondylitis, Scleroderma)
- Skin is Spared (but involves organs such as kidneys, liver, spleen, adrenals and heart)
    - Amyloidosis of hemodialysis is a subtype w/ deposition of β_2**-microglobulin**

3.17 Pruritis, Psychodermatology, and Trauma

Pruritis

Mediators of itch

- Nerve fibers: C and Aδ nerve fibers in skin produce itch sensation ("δ looks like an h")
- Primary mediators of itch ("ITCH"): **IL-31, Tryptase, Cathepsin S, Histamine**
- 2° mediators (O-PINS): (Opioids, Prostaglandin E, IL-2, Nerve-growth factor, Substance P)
- Histaminergic pathway: histamine is secreted by mast cells, basophils and keratinocytes
    - Histamine binds to H1/H4 receptors on histaminergic nerves, activating TRPV1
- Neuropeptides involved in itch: Substance P and Calcitonin gene-related protein (CGRP)
- Cytokines: Th2 (IL-4, 13), gastrin releasing peptide pathway (IL-17, 22), uremic (IL-2, 31)
- Opioids: **itch is induced by mu-opioid activity and suppressed by k-opioid activity**

- Proteases: kallikrein, tryptase, trypsin and cathepsin bind to protease activating receptors (PARs) which are G protein-coupled receptors to induce itch

Epidemiology of itch

- Chronic itch affects up to 25% of the elderly population due to ↑ incidence of xerosis, neuropathy, drugs (CCBs, HCTZ), psychiatric diseases, poor skin barrier and Th2 shift
- POC are more likely to seek care for itch (PIH is more distressing)
- 10–25% of people w/ generalized pruritis have an associated systemic condition

Internal causes of pruritis ("ITCH")

- Thyroid/endocrine: p/w localized genital (DM) or generalized pruritis (hyperthyroidism)
    - Rx: correct thyroid hormone and glucose level
- Chronic kidney disease: intractable pruritis worse at night and 2 days post-hemodialysis
    - Rx: UVB, gabapentin (inhibits calcium channels), renal transplant, difelikefalin (k-opioid agonist) and naltrexone (mu-opioid blocker) all work for uremic pruritis
- Cancers: **intractable and abrupt pruritis** without primary skin lesions in the elderly
    - MC in polycythemia vera (67%) but also common in Hodgkin's and NH lymphoma
    - Polycythemia vera: p/w aquagenic pruritis (within minutes of water contact)
    - Rx: determined by heme-onc (phlebotomy, ASA, Chemo, stem cell transplant)
        - Carbamazepine (inhibits Na channels) works for hematologic cancer itch
        - Neurokinin-1 inhibitors: aprepitant/serlopitant (itch in Sézary syndrome)

- Hepatobiliary pruritis: pruritis starts on Hands and generalizes due to biliary obstruction
  - Dx: LFTS, bilirubin level; abdominal imaging to look for obstruction/cancer
  - Rx ("Cirrhotics Scratch Real Nebulously"): Cholestyramine (1st line), Sertraline (2nd line), Rifampin, (3rd line), and Naloxone (4th line)

Drug-induced pruritis ("ITCH")

- Many causes: Iron deficiency, Tylenol, Checkpoint inhibitors (EGFR, PD-1, and CTLA-4), Clonidine, Chloroquine, HCQ, Hydroxyethyl starch, HIV medications, and Heavy metals
- MCC of xerotic pruritis are **β-blockers** (perhaps due to ↓ blood flow to the skin)
- MCC of drug-induced eczematous dermatitis are CCBs
- Rx: D/C inciting med, Burrow's solution (aluminum acetate)

Neurocutaneous dysesthesias

Scalp dysesthesia (burning scalp syndrome)

- p/w burning, itching, stinging on the scalp in the absence of primary cutaneous disease
- Thought to be caused by either psychiatric conditions or nerve trauma
- Rx: gabapentin, topical steroids, antidepressants (doxepin, amitriptyline, venlafaxine)

Trigeminal trophic syndrome

- p/w self-inflicted face ulcer (**nasal ala** MC) from damage to **trigeminal nerve (V2 is MC)**
- **Tip of the nose is spared** which is innervated by the anterior ethmoidal nerve, not CN V
- Rx: keep nails short, wear gloves at night, apply a barrier to affected area and medical therapy w/ gabapen-

tin, carbamazepine, pregabalin or pimozide; **surgery** works well

Meralgia paresthetica

- p/w paresthesia on the lateral thigh from lateral femoral cutaneous nerve damage
- Rx: avoid compressive clothing, weight loss, capsaicin cream, lidocaine patch, injection of steroid, lidocaine or botox, PT/chiropractor, acupuncture, pulsed RF ablation

Notalgia paresthetica

- p/w dysesthesia on the upper back between the vertebra and scapula (T2-T6) due to alteration of the cutaneous sensory nerves in this region
- a/w MEN2A (consider checking calcitonin levels in the pediatric population)
- Rx: capsaicin cream, lidocaine patch, gabapentin, amitriptyline, transcutaneous electrical muscle/nerve stimulation, PT, osteopathic manipulative medicine

Brachioradial pruritis

- p/w pruritis on the dorsolateral arm (MC) due to solar damage or cervical spine disease
- Rx: topical amitriptyline/ketamine combination > capsaicin; PO gabapentin, lamotrigine, amitriptyline, carbamazepine, NSAIDS; PT/chiropractic, acupuncture, surgery can help

Pruritis ani

- Pruritis of anus affecting M >> F
- May be primary or secondary to hemorrhoids, irritation from stool, ACD, infections, degenerative changes of the lower spine (L4-S2)

- Dx: KOH prep, bacterial culture, clear adhesive tape (pinworms), Wood's lamp (erythrasma), biopsy (Paget's) and patch testing (ACD)
- Rx: ("I had an itchy butthole in SCHool"): Sitz baths, topical Steroids, Sarna (menthol), Sarna Sensitive (pramoxine), Strontium (Dermeleve); topical CNIs, CeraVe anti-itch (pramoxine), Capsaicin, good Hygiene and treat any underlying disorders
    - Also instruct patient to avoid prolonged sitting, nylon underwear and spicy food

Pruritis scroti/vulvae

- Pruritis of scrotum or vulva which p/w lichenification due to repeating rubbing
- May be acute (infections, ACD/ICD) or chronic (cancer, radiculopathy, psychogenic)
- Rx: specific to underlying etiology but similar to pruritis ani

Aquagenic Pruritis and aquadynia

- p/w severe pruritis after water contact (irrespective of temperature) which begins within 30 minutes of contact and lasts up to 2 hours with no visible skin changes
- May be primary but usually secondary to systemic disease (Polycythemia vera, CF)
- Rx: Alkalization of bath water to pH 8, Antihistamines, PUVA, Propranolol

Prurigo nodularis (PN)

- Results from chronic scratching/picking of the skin due to a primary cutaneous disease (AD is MC) or secondary to a systemic disorder (lymphoma, liver/renal disease, HIV)
- a/w AA race, middle aged pts (5th-6th decade), females, HIV, ESRD, depression/anxiety

- p/w multiple hyperpigmented dome-shaped papulonodules symmetrically distributed on extensor extremities with sparring of hard-to-reach mid-back ("butterfly sign")
- Path: regular epidermal acanthosis (w/ no spongiosis), hyperkeratosis, hypergranulosis, vertical dermal collagen streaking, mixed inflammatory infiltrate (eos, mast cell, lymphs)
    - ↓ density of intraepidermal nerve fibers in lesional and nonlesional skin
- Rx: super potent topical or IL steroids, topical capsaicin/calcipotriene, phototherapy, SSRI/TCAs, doxepin, MTX, cyclosporine, pregabalin, **thalidomide**
- Workup: biopsy (H&E/DIF), CBC, TSH, Cr, LFTs +/- HIV, Hep panel, stool for ova/parasites

Lichen simplex chronicus (LSC)

- p/w lichenified plaques (MC on the posterior neck, shins/ankles, anogenital skin, hands)
- Path: same as for PN
- Rx: avoidance of scratching/rubbing, topical/intralesional steroids, menthol, pramoxine

Treatment of chronic neuropathic itch

- Capsaicin: locally desensitizes peripheral nerve fibers by depleting substance P
    - Limiting factor is transient nature and need for application 5 times a day
- Lidocaine and pramoxine: topical anesthetics
- Menthol: activates TRPM8 channels which stimulates Aδ fibers that transmits cold stimulus (cold can reduce itch)
- Topical strontium (Dermeleve): calcimimetic that blocks calcium channels
- Carbamazepine and lamotrigine: block voltage-dependent Na channels

- TCAs: inhibits 5-HT and NE reuptake; blocks Na and Ca channels and NMDA receptors
- Gabapentin: blocks the $\alpha 2\delta$ subunit of the voltage gated calcium channel

Cutaneous manifestation of psychiatric illness and physical trauma

Delusions of Parasitosis

- The delusion that one is infested w/ bugs
- p/w excoriations and "matchbox sign" (pt brings in samples of their skin to show you)
- Commonly seen w/ use of **amphetamines** and cocaine
- Dx: examine patient samples under the microscope
- Rx: relay desire to help pt; 2nd generation antipsychotics like **risperidone** and olanzapine are considered 1st line due to less extra-Pyramidal SEs, Q-T Prolongation, drug-drug interactions, anticholinergic effects and Prolactin secretion than Pimozide
- Workup: referral to Psychiatry is warranted but only after establishing rapport

Body dysmorphic disorder

- The fixation on the mild flaw in appearance (very common in derm offices)
- Do not perform unnecessary cosmetic treatments
- Assess for suicidality (strong link) and consider psych eval after rapport is established

Cutaneous findings in anorexia and bulimia

- MCC cutaneous finding is **xerosis** (nearly 100%) followed by diffuse hypertrichosis (70%)
- **Russell sign** (30%): dorsal hand calluses from teeth contact during self-induced vomiting

Erythro-Melalgia

- SCN9A gene mutation in familial form (encodes voltage-gated Na channel alpha subunit)
- p/w erythema, tenderness and burning of the extremities (exacerbated by heat)
- May occur secondary to **Myeloproliferative disease** (thrombocytosis and PV)
- Ddx: hand-foot reaction (toxic erythema of chemotherapy)
- Rx: Misoprostol, SSRIs

Cutaneous disease caused by external/ environmental factors

Lichtenberg's figures

- Branching pattern of cutaneous marks pathognomonic for Lightening injury

Coining

- Not a psychiatric illness but it is an external insult from cultural practices
- p/w linear ecchymosis in a "pine-tree" pattern from rubbing the skin w/ a coin
- Ddx: child abuse, Gardner diamond syndrome, psychogenic purpura
- Similar cultural practices include cupping (local suction → round purpuric patches) and moxibustion (dried plant material is burned into skin → vesicles, bulla and burns)

Skin picking disorder

- Individuals repeatedly pick their skin, leading to noticeable tissue damage
- Rx: N-acetylcysteine (glutamate modulator)

Onychotillomania

- Repetitive rubbing or picking of the proximal nail fold
- p/w multiple transverse grooves in the nail plate in a "fur-tree pattern"
- Rx: reassurance, behavioral modification, cover nail w/ bandage, SSRIs

3.18 Acquired Palmoplantar Keratodermas

- a/w malignancy except aquagenic PPK, keratoderma climactericum and punctate PPK
- Dx: clinical diagnoses and no further testing is necessary except aquagenic (CF workup) or if worried for malignancy (cancer-screenings)
- Rx: we treat PPKs w/ keratolytics, emollients and acitretin if severe

Aquagenic keratoderma ("Aquagenic keratoderman")

- p/w thickened **white pebbly papules** or plaques on the palms after water immersion
  - "I think of Aquaman → Disney superheroes are almost always white"
- Burning and pain which resolves after drying of the skin is characteristic
- Found in about 25% of **carriers of cystic fibrosis** and very common in CF patients
- Ddx: aquagenic urticaria (seen in CF); aquagenic pruritis (no skin findings; seen in PV)
- Workup: cystic fibrosis transmembrane conductance regulator **(CFTR) mutation screen**

Keratoderma climactericum

- p/w **hyperkeratosis over the pressure points** (esp heels) in post-menopausal women

  - o "I imagine a woman climaxing to remind me the PPK is at points of pressure"
- Ddx: sorafenib-induced hand-foot-skin syndrome

Punctate keratosis of the palmar creases

- **p/w small keratotic plugs in the creases of the palms/fingers seen in AA patients**
- Ddx: punctate porokeratosis, arsenic keratosis (these are not in palmar creases)
- a/w Dermatitis herpetiformis, Dupuytren's contracture, Knuckle pads, Psoriasis, Pterygium inversum unguis ("Dotted Keratoses of the Palmar crease")

Circumscribed palmoplantar hypokeratosis

- p/w well-defined circular depressions on palms (esp thenar) or soles (esp medial)
- Path: focally ↓ stratum corneum and stratum granulosum w/ underlying angioplasia

Malignancy associated PPK

- PPK may be seen w/ various carcinomas (e.g., lung), as a precursor to carcinoma in various genetic syndromes (Rothmund-Thompson), a/w malignancy in some genetic syndromes (Howell-Evans → esophageal carcinoma; dyskeratosis congenita → oral SCCs or AML) or precursor to SCC w/ arsenic exposure (selenium is used to bind arsenic in exposed pts)
- Tripe palms: hyperkeratotic corrugated palms most a/w **gastric** (+AN) or lung cancer
- Rx: keratolytic agents, Co2 laser
- Workup: age-appropriate cancer screenings; malignancy workup based on presentation

3.19 Nutritional Disorders

- Consider vitamin deficiency in fad diets, GI surgery, IBD, alcohol use or eating disorders
- Kwashiorkor: protein deficiency; due to **rice milk** diet or babies weaned from breast milk
  - p/w distended pot belly, peripheral (leg) edema w/ red-brown desquamation ("flakey paint") which heal w/ hypopigmented patches and dyschromia
    - "Wash that ugly red-brown flakey paint to reveal the white underneath"
  - Diffuse alopecia w/ alternating bands of light and dark hair ("**flag sign**")
    - We see flag sign w/ PIBIDS, Pilli annulate, ↓ Protein (Kwashiorker), MTX
  - Dx: low albumin and glubulins
  - Rx: protein and vitamin supplementation; zinc paste to flakey eroded skin
- Marasmus: ↓ energy/caloric intake; infants in developing countries (very rare in US)
  - p/w dry, loose, wrinkled skin w/ emaciated appearance (loss of SQ fat/Muscle)
    - "Monkey appearance" due to loss of buccal fat pads
  - Rx: nutrition replacement
- Essential fatty acid deficiency: ↓ arachidonic, linoleic and linolenic acid (major constituent of the stratum corneum and help maintain skin barrier)
  - Deficiency is rare but may be seen in Anorexia, Alcoholics, Low fat diets, nephrotic syndrome, CF or GI disorders/surgeries resulting in fat malabsorption
  - p/w dry, **Leathery skin**, intertriginous erosions, Alopecia, Light hair and petechia
  - Dx: ↓ plasma arachidonic, linoleic, linolenic acid; ↑ palmitoleic and oleic acid and the presence

of 5, 8, 11-icosatrienoic acid which is normally undetectable
    - Rx: topical, oral or IV essential fatty acids; topical moisturizers
- Anorexia: MC finding is **xerosis** (97%), diffuse hypertrichosis w/ lanugo-like hairs (70%), white dermographism (70%), acrocyanosis, telogen effluvium, scars, decayed teeth
- Bulemia: knuckle callus ("Russell's sign"), large salivary glands, erosion of tooth enamel
- "Know your Russell's"
    - Russel sign: calluses/scars on dorsal hands seen in bulimics
        - Russel Silver: genodermatosis w/ CALMs
        - Russel bodies: intracytoplasmic immunoglobins in plasma cells seen in rhinoscleroma
        - Russel viper venom: specific test for anti-phospholipid syndrome

Vitamin deficiencies

Vitamin A

- Dietary vit A obtained as retinoids in animal products or B-carotene from plant products
- The role of vitamin A in the skin is **keratinization**
- Excess: p/w desquamation, xerosis, cheilitis, epistaxis, alopecia (think SEs of Accutane)
- Deficiency (phrynoderma): p/w keratotic follicular papules ("toad skin") and eye issues
    - Bitot's spots are keratin buildups on the conjunctiva (ddx: scleral plaque in NSF)
    - Rx: 50,000 IU daily w/ food (as it is a fat-soluble vitamin)

Beta-carotene (pro-vitamin A)

- Excess (Carotenemia): yellow discoloration on skin of **Central face** and palms/soles
  - Seen in vegetarians, **hypothyroidism**, diabetes, hepatic or renal disease
  - Ddx: lycopenemia (orange-yellow discoloration from eating lots of tomatoes) and yellow discoloration from quinacrine (sclera and dorsal hands involved)

Selenium ("Selena Gomez is pretty hypopigmented for a Latina")

- Deficiency: p/w generalized **hypopigmentation** of skin, hair, **nails** +/- cardiomyopathy
  - a/w HIV and hemodialysis; predisposes to intrahepatic cholestasis of pregnancy
  - Dx: serum selenium < 8 ug/dL

Vitamin B1 (thiamine; "B1 deficiency is 1 B, aka Beriberi")

- Deficiency (Beriberi): Wernicke's **encephalopathy** (psychosis, ataxia, ophthalmoplegia) and peripheral neuropathy (dry Beriberi) or dilated cardiomyopathy (wet Beriberi)
  - All B vitamin deficiencies p/w cheilitis (cracked-lip) and glossitis (smooth tongue)
  - Alcohol use disorder is the MCC in the US
  - Dx: thiamine blood levels not reliable (thiamine diphosphate is more accurate)
  - Rx: best to treat empirically if suspected (10mg x 1 week then 2–5 mg x 6 weeks)

Vitamin B2 (riboflavin; "B2 deficiency is 2 C's)

- Deficiency (oculo-orogenital syndrome): **Corneal neovascularization and Cheilitis**
  - Seb derm-like rash that is classically on the **scrotum**/genitals (but spares midline)

- In the US seen mostly w/ restrictive **vegan diet**, IBD, alcoholics, anti-epileptic use
- Dx: erythrocyte glutathione reductase activation Coefficient > riboflavin levels
- Rx: 10 mg PO until symptoms resolve

Vitamin B3 (niacin, aka nicotinic acid; B3 def is 3 D's): "Just saw a prostitute w/ nice Double D's"

- May be synthesized endogenously from tryptophan (**utilizing B6 and B2 as cofactors**; "6 divided by 2 endogenously makes 3") or absorbed from dietary intake
- Excess: **flushing** due to ↑ prostaglandins (pretreat w/ aspirin)
  - Ddx: red man syndrome (vancomycin) caused by ↑ histamine (Rx: antihistamine)
- Deficiency (Pellagra): p/w 3 D's (**photosensitive Dermatitis**, **Diarrhea**, **Dementia**)
  - p/w symmetric, well-demarcated erythematous rash on sun exposed skin **("glove" distribution on hands is 1st sign**, "Casal's necklace", "malar rash") w/ hyperpigmented hyperkeratotic eruption over boney prominences
  - Due to ("Casal's necklace has 5-CHAINs"): **5-FU, Carcinoid syndrome, Carbamazepine**, Chloramphenicol, Crohn's, Hypothyroidism, **Hartnup disease**, AIDS, **Azathioprine**, Anorexia, Alcoholism, Isoniazid, Nutritional deficiency)
  - Rx: sun avoidance and **nicotinamide** (does not cause flushing like giving niacin)

Vitamin B6 (Pyridoxine)

- Excess: acneiform lesions
- Deficiency: glossitis w/ smooth Painful red tongue, oral ulcers, cheilitis, seb derm-like rash, **Peripheral neu-**

ropathy and all things seen in B3 deficiency (B6 is a cofactor for B3)
  - o Classically due to isoniazid but theophylline, penicillamine and OCPs are others
  - o Dx: plasma level of Pyridoxal Phosphate (active form)
  - o Rx: 50–100 mg PO QD

Biotin (B7): "Botox the DAOs"

- Excess: Dermatitis, Acne, Allergic reactions, Odd lab values (looks like hyperthyroidism)
- Deficiency: **Dermatitis (periorificial),** Alopecia, Optic atrophy/neuro effects/hypotonia
  - o Inherited in biotinidase (childhood) or carboxylases (neonates) deficiency but can also be acquired by diets rich in raw egg whites ("avidin avidly binds biotin")
  - o Dx: urine testing for metabolites is more sensitive than serum testing
  - o Rx: skin lesions respond in days to oral or IV supplementation

Vitamin B9 (folic acid)

- Deficiency: B9 and B12 deficiency p/w **hyperpigmentation** (esp. on knuckle pads), **melanonychia** (longitudinal and total), hair/nail changes, angular cheilitis/stomatitis w/ a beefy red tongue and GI symptoms (N/V/D and abdominal pain)
- Dx: B9 and B12 deficiency cause megaloblastic anemia (other B vitamins are microcytic)
  - o Normal homocysteine and MMA levels (vs ↑ in B12 deficiency)

Vitamin B12 (Cobalamin)

- Very similar to B9 deficiency (Color/pigmentation of skin/nails) but w/ **CNS symptoms**

- **Metformin** use in diabetics is a/w B12 deficiency
- Downs syndrome get angular cheilitis due to deficiency in **B12** (also vit C and A)
- Dx: megaloblastic/macrocytic anemia; ↑ homocysteine and MMA levels

Vitamin C (L-ascorbic acid)

- Deficiency (scurvy): **epistaxis, gingival bleeding** (rarely gingival hyperplasia), **Corkscrew hairs w/ perifollicular petechiae**, splinter hemorrhages and vascular fragility (purpura)
    - Gingival hypertrophy mnemonic ("PC Culture will make you bite your tongue and gums"): Phenytoin (MCC), CCBs, Cyclosporine, vit C deficiency
- RFs: elderly, alcoholics, Cigarette smoking, restrictive diets ("tea and toast" diet)

Vitamin D

- Deficiency (Ricket's): bone deformities/osteomalacia and **alopecia**
    - "Not getting enough D will make women lose their hair"
- Rx: D_2 (ergocalciferol) or D_3 (cholecalciferol) are both effective
    - D_2 comes from plants and would be the preferred supplement in vegan patients

Vitamin E

- Excess: Excess/Elevated vitamin E causes Ecchymosis/petechiae

Vitamin K: "K, you're Pretty (P-T)"

- Deficiency: p/w purpura/hemorrhage ("K Kancels Koagulation" so ↓ K → bleeding)
    - RFs: infants (life-threatening bleeding due to low placental transmission of vit K), antibiotics (kills

gut bacteria which produce vitamin k), CF, Crohn's, short gut
  - Dx: ↑ **PT** and normal PTT
  - Rx: FFP (life-threatening bleeding) or oral/IV **Phytonadione** (vitamin K)

Zinc

- Excess: impairs copper absorption → iatrogenic copper deficiency
- Deficiency (acrodermatitis enteropathica; ADE): AR mutation in **SLC39A4**
  - Or secondary to **cystic fibrosis**, alcoholics, anorexia, preterm infants, infant who breastfeeds from zinc deficient mothers, **infant when weaned off breast milk**
  - p/w triad of ADE: **Alopecia + Diarrhea + Erosive vesiculopustular Eczematous lesions** involving Acral sites, Diaper area, peri-oral region (where they Eat)
    - Perioral rash spares upper lip → **horseshoe ("U-shaped") configuration**
  - Dx: ↓ Alkaline phosphatase which is a zinc-Dependent Enzyme (and ↓ zinc < 70)
    - **Early morning plasma zinc level** is the recommended diagnostic modality
  - Rx: 3 mg/kg elemental zinc for ADE; 0.5–1 mg/kg for acquired zinc deficiency

Copper

- Important role in skin for wound healing and melanin synthesis
- Deficiency: skin hypopigmentation ("cops are white") and kinky hair ("cops are kinky")
  - Microscopy of hair shows pili torti ("cops are twisted")

  - Inherited in Menkes (ATP7A gene) and acquired in IBD, **excess zinc intake**, cirrhosis, parenteral nutrition, low birthweight infants exclusively fed cow's milk

Iron deficiency

- p/w angular stomatitis, glossitis and **koilonychias**

3.20 Depositional and Calcification Disorders

Gout

- Giant cells surround negatively birefringent amorphous material with needle-like clefts
- Obesity and Over-drinking are the main risk factors
- Urate crystals deposit in tissues years after acute gout attacks (in which MTP joint is MC) to produce gouty tophi indicative of chronic gout (helix of ear is MC)
- Tophi p/w smooth firm white-yellow dermal or SQ papules over the helix or small joints
  - Filled w/ a chalky white substance very similar to calcinosis cutis
- "DR. FAUCI knows how to diagnose and treat gout"
  - De Galantha stain and 20% silver nitrate will stain crystals black
  - Refractile negatively birefringent needle-like crystals seen under polarized light
  - Febuxistat (xanthine oxidase inhibitor): 1st line for chronic gout
  - Allopurinol (xanthine oxidase inhibitor): 1st line for chronic gout
  - Uricosuric agents (probenecid): 2nd line for chronic gout
  - Colchicine and Corticosteroids (oral/IL): acute gout

  - Indomethacin/Ibuprofen: acute gout
- Labs: ↑ **uric acid** (↑ ESR and ↑ WBC during acute attacks)
- Path: if placed in formalin, the urate crystals wash out and instead of polarizable needle shaped crystals, you get whispy amorphous deposits; so placing in **alcohol** is better
  - "You must get Dr. Fauci drunk (alcohol) for him to give you correct information"

Pseudogout

- Presentation and treatment same as gout but there is deposition of **calcium Pyrophosphate crystals** which exhibit **Positive birefringence** under polarized light and are short and rhomboidal (Pudgy) as opposed to the negatively birefringent long needle-like crystals in gout; the calcium pyrophosphate stains a dark blue on path

Colloid Milium

- Adult type (MC) presents in Middle-aged Males w/ severe photodamage and p/w Multiple tiny dome-shaped translucent yellow papules in areas of chronic sun exposure
- Whereas in lichen amyloid the amorphous material is due to degenerated keratin intermediate filaments, in colloid milium it is due to degenerated elastic fibers
- Path: amorphous pink nodular material in superficial dermis and solar elastosis
- Stains like amyloid (PAS, Crystal violet, Congo red, Thioflavin T) but is cytokeratin (-)
- Other types of colloid milium include juvenile, pigmented and nodular

Calcinosis cutis

- Deposition of cutaneous calcium salts in the skin and SQ (5 broad categories)
  - o **Dystrophic calcinosis: Damage to skin results in calcium deposits (e.g., AI-CTD)**
  - o Metastatic calcification: result of a systemic Metabolic disorder (sarcoid, ESRD)
  - o Iatrogenic, idiopathic and mixed are other broad categories
- p/w small firm white papules/nodules that may ulcerate and extrude chalk-like material
  - o Mostly seen w/ AI-CTD e.g., DM (MC on knees/elbows) or CREST (MC on hands)
- Scrotal calcinosis: benign entity of unknown pathogenesis in which painless white nodular lesions aggregate on the scrotum; Rx: surgical excision
- Subepidermal calcified nodule (Winer's nodule) is a solitary nodular congenital calcification on the head/neck (esp ears) in an otherwise healthy infant
- Workup: after biopsy confirms diagnosis search for underlying cause (calcium, phosphate, parathyroid hormone, vitamin D3, BUN, CBC, CK, aldolase, ANA)

Calciphylaxis

- Pathogenesis: Chronic renal failure leads to chronic ↓ Ca → ↑ PTH → recruitment of calcium and phosphate from bone; hyper-Coagulable states also thought to play a role
- a/w CKD on **hemodialysis**, hyperparathyroidism, DM, Cancer, female gender, age > 60, obesity, liver disease, Coumadin and Calcium/vitamin D supplements
  - o Non-uremic calciphylaxis has been reported in Cancers and drugs such as **Corticosteroids and Coumadin** due to ↑ NFkB
- p/w exquisitely painful, indurated stellate ulcers w/ necrotic eschar on fat-bearing areas

- Criteria (requires these 3 clinical features or 2 clinical features and classic histopath)
    - Patient on hemodialysis or glomerular filtration < 15 mL/min
    - ≥ 2 painful skin ulcers w/ painful purpura
    - Painful ulcers on the trunk, extremities or penis along w/ purpura
- Path (**wedge excision** or telescope punch): Calcification of SQ vessels w/ necrosis of skin
    - Calcification occurs in more Central layers of BVs such as the intima (vs media/middle layer calcification in atherosclerosis)
- Labs: protein C, CBC, Calcium, Cr, Cryoglobins, Coagulation factors, hep C antibodies
- Imaging: x-ray ("net-like pattern"), bone scintigraphy and CT can also detect calcification
- Rx (according to 2022 CME): TOC is IV **sodium thiosulfate** w/ dialysis
    - Stop triggers: calcium, vit D, **warfarin** (switch to heparin), iron, systemic steroids
    - Vitamin K supplements may be of benefit as it works antagonistically to warfarin
    - Maintain serum calcium/phosphate (phosphate binders) and PTH (cinacalcet)
    - Consult: nephrology, palliative care/pain management, wound care

Osteoma cutis: "They say he's Pretty FAT, but I think he's big boned (bone in skin)"

- Plate-like osteoma cutis: p/w shiny firm plaque in infancy MC on scalp; Rx: excision
- Progressive osseous heteroplasia: p/w tender papules coalescing into plaques in infancy
- Fibrodysplasia ossificans progressiva: p/w lesions in deep connective tissue/skeletal muscle, dystrophic great toes, deafness and MR

- Albright hereditary osteodystrophy: p/w multiple firm plaques in infancy
- **TCN-induced miliary osteomas of the face**: lesions develop in **acne** scars and are blueish

Terra firma-forme dermatosis

- Results from extensive retention hyperkeratosis in those w/ poor hygiene
- p/w dark dirt-like discoloration of the skin; hard to reach mid-back location is common
- Dx: **alcohol swab** will remove the discoloration

Arsenic dermatoses

- Sources: occupational exposure (smelting industry) and contaminant of drinking water
- Skin: hyperpigmentation on areas not exposed to sunlight (back and upper chest are MC), raindrop hypopigmentation, acral arsenical keratoses, Bowens/SCCs
- Nails: Mees lines (transverse white bands in fingernails)
- CNS: peripheral sensory neuropathy in a stocking-glove distribution
- Rx: selenium (chelates arsenic)

3.21 Ulcers

Common ("venous ulcer LAND"): venous ulcer, Lymphedema, Arterial, Neuropathic, Decubitus

- Venous ulcers: shallow ulcer with irregular/Variable borders classically on the medial malleolus on a background of Venous stasis changes and Varicosities
    - Dx: duplex US ("VS") or Venography help to obtain CEAP score
    - Rx (ABCD): Antibiotics (only if infection suspected), **Aspirin**/pentoxyfylline, Biologic dressings, **Compression** (r/o arterial insufficiency first),

Debridement, and moisture-retentive **Dressings** (hydrocolloids, hydrogels, and foams)

- Lymphedema: ascending pitting edema → induration/ ulceration → elephantiasis nostras verrucosa (chronic lymphedema w/ skin fibrosis and verrucous changes)
  - Ddx: lipidemia looks similar but spares the feet ("cuff-sign")
  - Rx: compression to ↓ lymph accumulation; urea for any hyperkeratosis
- Arterial: painful deep punched out ulcer classically on the lateral malleolus ("arterial and lateral have same letters except for i") on a background of Atrophic skin and Absent hair
  - Dx: Absent/↓ pedal pulses; ABI
  - Rx: Angioplasty (**refer to vascular surgery**); do not do sharp debridement
- Neuropathic (diabetic): Non-painful, punched out, smelly ulcer w/ wet base and **callused borders** (from trauma) on pressure points of feet in a setting of peripheral Neuropathy
  - Dx: MRI may show osteomyelitis (bone biopsy or culture to confirm)
  - Rx: **off-loading** or Negative pressure therapy; becaplermin gel
- Decubitus: ulcer from prolonged pressure from immobility MC on the sacrum and heels
  - Four stages: I) non-blanchable erythema ("none-blanchable"); II) loss of epidermis +/- dermis (erosion/shallow ulcer); III) skin + SQ damage ("3 letters in fat"); IV) tissue necrosis to muscle or bone ("4 letters in bone")
  - Rx: Debridement and moisture-retentive Dressings

The rare, but highly testable, **leg ulcers**: "Dermal Damage PARKS BetWeeN Her Legs"

- Diffuse Dermal angiomatosis: violaceous patches/ ulcers on the legs, forearms and **pendulous breasts** (DD = breasts) strongly a/w atherosclerosis and smoking
- PAN: Palpable Purpura, Painful SQ nodules, livedo reticularis and ulcers on legs
- PG: Painful undermined ulcer w/ irregular "gun metal gray" border
- Panniculitides: variable presentations
- Prolidase deficiency: AR mutation in PEPD; Progressive leg ulcers w/ recurrent infections, Photosensitivity, diffuse telangiectasias and hypertelorism
- PXE: AR mutation in ABCC6 that affects connective tissue → ↑ risk of leg ulcers
- Arteriosclerotic ulcer of Martorell: painful blisters → purpura → ulcers on lower legs of women w/ **HTN**; calcinosis/hyalinization/thickening of media on path
- Rheumatoid arthritis: Felty syndrome and Rheumatoid necrobiosis, aka superficial ulcerating necrobiosis both p/w ulcers that resemble NLD (see below)
- Rothmund-Thomson: AR mutation in RECQL4 ↑ risk of leg ulcers
- Klinefelter's syndrome: XXY genotype that commonly p/w leg ulcers
- Sickle cell anemia and clotting abnormalities: prevents proper tissue oxygenation
- Scleroderma: lower extremity ulcers occur in 4% of scleroderma patients
- Bart's syndrome: AD mutation in COL7A1 → dystrophic EB + ACC of legs of baby
- Werner syndrome: AR mutation in REQQL2 w/ accelerated aging and leg ulcers
- NLD: erythematous rim w/ atrophic yellow center; minor trauma cause ulcers

- Homocystinuria: AR mutation in CBS w/ skin/hair Hypopigmentation, brittle hair, malar erythema, livedo reticularis and leg ulcers
- Hydroxyurea side effect: painful ulcers over malleoli and tibial crest
- Livedoid vasculopathy (atrophie blanche): burning pain along the ankle → painful and irregular leg ulcers → porcelain-white scar; a/w hypercoagulation

Treatment for ulcers

- Dressings
    - Dressings based on absorbency
        - **Provides moisture: hydrogel**
        - Maintains moisture: film and hydrocolloid
        - **Absorbs moisture/dries out the ulcer**: Foam, **Alginate** and Gelling fibers
            - "A FAG (old term for cigarette) dries your mouth if you smoke"
    - Hemostatic dressings (for bloody ulcers): alginates
    - Dressing may be impregnated w/ silver, iodine or honey in infected ulcers
- Debridement
    - Surgical debridement: fastest method but is painful
    - Mechanical debridement: the use of wet-to-dry dressings but is painful and it does not distinguish between viable and non-viable tissue
    - Autolytic debridement: the use of an occlusive dressing which promotes the lytic enzymes that accumulate in wound fluid
    - Enzymatic (chemical) debridement: topical agent which can supplement autolytic debridement (collagenase, aka Santyl is FDA approved)

3.22 VASCULAR DISORDERS

Important vascular morphologies

- Livedo reticularis: partial or intermittent reduction of cutaneous blood flow leading to transient or persistent dusky **ring-like** patches (livedo racemosa has broken ring pattern)
  - Seen in AI-CTD, sepsis, rheumatoid vasculitis, PAN, ANCA vasculitis, thrombosis
  - Get a deep biopsy from Lateral purpuric rim if possible
  - Amantadine is a well-recognized cause of drug-induced livedo reticularis
- Retiform Purpura: specific morphology which develops when cutaneous blood vessels are compromised, resulting in downstream ischemia, purpura, and **necrosis** of the skin which p/w Persistent hemorrhagic Purple Patches/Plaques in a branched configuration
  - Seen w/ wall damage (vasculitis/angio-invasive organism) or vessel occlusion

Vasculitis

Categories of vasculitides by vessel size

- Cutaneous small vessel vasculitis (CSVV): p/w palpable purpura
  - "Small vessel vasculitis is A HUGE Sickness": Acute hemorrhagic edema of infancy, Henoch-Schönlein purpura, Urticarial vasculitis, Granuloma faciale, EED, Serum Sickness, Secondary CSVV (ABCD trigger; Autoimmune, Bug, Cancer, Drug)
- Mixed small and medium vessel vasculitis: p/w a mix of small and medium vasculitis
  - Examples: mixed cryoglobulinemia and ANCA-associated vasculitis

- Medium vessel vasculitis: p/w SLURD → **SQ nodules** (best to biopsy), Livedo reticularis, Ulcers (red rim is 3rd best), Retiform purpura (2nd best to biopsy), Digital necrosis
- Large vessel vasculitis: p/w ulceration on frontotemporal scalp (temporal arteritis) or SQ nodules and PG-like lesions on extremities (Takayasu arteritis)

Cutaneous small vessel vasculitis ("I PAC'D Prednisone")

- Pathophysiology ("I"): Immune complex deposition in post-capillary venules activate complement which attract neutrophils → vessel damage and tissue ischemia
- Presentation ("P"): Pruritic or Painful **Palpable Purpura** +/- erythematous Papules or Pustules occurring days after exposure to trigger and lasting for weeks
    - o Systemic symptoms such as fever and arthralgias occur only in 5–25% of patients so if seen consider a systemic vasculitis
- Triggers ("A"; secondary CSVV; ABCD): Autoimmune (RA is MC), Bug (GAS is MC bacteria whereas Hepatitis C > B > A is MC viral), Cancer, Drug (Antibiotics like β-lactams and sulfonamides, Anti-inflammatories like NSAIDS, TNF-Alpha inhibitors and many others)
- Path (lesional skin > 72 hours old): leukocytoclasia and fibrinoid necrosis of vessels
- DIF ("C"; need fresh lesion < 24 hours old or you risk false negative; need proximal lesion as dependent areas can result in false positive): perivascular **C3** > IgM > IgA/IgG
    - o Perivascular IgA: HSP
    - o Prominent IgM: cryoglobin or rheumatoid vasculitis
    - o Positive around blood vessels and BMZ: HUV
    - o Negative: ANCA-vasculitis

- Rx (C'D prednisone): D/C trigger; 90% self-resolve (treat symptoms w/ NSAIDS); consider Colchicine, Dapsone or Prednisone in chronic (> 4 weeks) or more severe disease
  - Go straight to treatment for urticarial vasculitis (indomethacin, dapsone, and steroids), EED (dapsone, IL steroids), ANCA vasculitis (steroids + rituximab)
- Workup: **CBC, BMP, UA**, **cryoglobulins**, stool guiac, ESR, and hepatic panel

Subtypes of CSVV ("A HUGE Sickness")

- Acute hemorrhagic edema of infancy: like other CSVV it is due to immune complex deposition in small blood vessels due to various triggers (A, B >> C, D) p/w self-resolving annular or **targetoid/cockade hemorrhagic plaques on the head (cheeks/ears)** and extremities of **healthy appearing** male children < 3 years of age
  - Dx: Path may show LCV; DIF can have IgA deposits (but it is usually negative)
  - Rx: supportive therapy with antihistamines
- Henoch-Schönlein purpura (ABC): IgA deposition in blood vessels occurs 1–2 weeks after URI trigger (GAS is MC) causing **Arthralgias (80%)**, palpable purpura on Buttocks (100%), Colicky abdominal pain (60%; GI bleeding in 30%) and renal disease (40%; hematuria > proteinuria) progressing to Chronic renal failure (2%) in male Children < 10 years old
  - Adult HSP (rare) has more frequent vesiculobullous lesions and cutaneous necrosis, associated cancer (**lung is MC**; "Schön-lung") and a higher chance of IgA glomerulonephritis (especially if palpable purpura is located above waist) → CRF
  - Path (shows LCV): PV neutrophilic infiltrate w/ karyorrhexis and fibrin in vessels

        - A lack of eosinophils triples the risk of renal involvement
    - DIF: IgA > C3 in BV walls
    - Rx (similar to CSVV): supportive; colchicine, dapsone or prednisone if severe
    - Workup: CBC, CMP, **UA (if + send to nephro),** stool guaiac (if + send to GI to r/o intussusception) and **serial urinalysis and BP monitoring for 6 months**
- Urticarial vasculitis (UV): immune complex deposition in small BVs due to various triggers (**Autoimmune** >> B, C, D) → p/w **painful/burning** urticarial plaques **lasting > 24 hours** which resolves w/ **hyperpigmentation** or **purpura** MC in females > 50 years old
    - Normocomplemententemic UV (75%; NUV) is skin-limited and idiopathic
    - Hypocomplemententemic UV (25%; HUV) is systemic and a/w systemic disease
        - IgG antibodies bind C1q → ↓ **serum levels of C1q ("C One q")**
        - MC triggers are autoimmune (**SLE and Sjögren's**)
            - "UV makes me think of UV light which makes me think of SLE"
        - Systemic symptoms are similar to lupus (fever, arthralgias, GI, renal, ocular) but in HUV, pulmonary involvement (e.g., **COPD**), angioedema and ocular manifestations are much more common
        - MSK (e.g., arthralgias) and ocular are MC extracutaneous manifestations
    - Diagnostic criteria for HUV syndrome (HUVS): requires 2 major and 2 minor
        - Major: urticaria x 6 months and hypocomplementemia

    - Minor: vasculitis on path, arthralgias/arthritis, uveitis/episcleritis, glomerulonephritis, recurrent abdominal pain, low C1q level
  - Path (like LCV, best taken from new lesion < 24 hours old): subtle LCV
  - DIF: perivascular immunoglobins, C3 or fibrinogen +/- lupus band
  - Labs: (HUV): ANA+ (strongly a/w SLE), ↓CH50/C3/C4, anti-C1q antibodies, ↑ESR
  - Rx: **indomethacin**, colchicine, dapsone, prednisone, IVIG, rituximab
    - "Get away from UV light by going indoors (indomethacin)"
    - Indomethacin was also the treatment for Eosinophilic folliculitis of Ofuji
  - Workup: **evaluate for monoclonal gammopathy** (see Schnitzler's below)
  - Schnitzler's syndrome ("SCHMItzler's"): Sore bones/joints, Systemic symptoms, **Chronic urticaria (typically HUV) + IgM gammopathy**, Rx: IL-1 blockers
- Granuloma faciale ("FACIALE")
  - Face has red-brown papules and plaques with **Follicular openings**
    - Collagenomas (cephalic plaque of TS) also have this pebbly appearance
  - Asymptomatic lesions w/ no systemic symptoms or associated systemic disease
  - Path: Chronic LCV (grenz zone separates infiltrate from epidermis and follicles)
  - DIF: granular IgG, IgA, IgM and/or C3 in blood vessel walls
  - Rx (often recalcitrant to treatment): Cryotherapy, **Intralesional triamcinolone,** UVA, Antibiotics (TCNs), Lasers (CO2, PDL), Excision

    - One of the IgG4 related diseases: "Rosey, Kimmy, Angy and my Granny are 4 Gs"
        - Rosai-Dorfman, Kimura disease, Angiolymphoid hyperplasia w/ eosinophilia and Granuloma faciale
- Erythema elevatum diutinum (ABCD): same CSVV pathogenesis
    - a/w **AIDS/HIV**, **IgA gammopathy**, chronic GAS infection, Hep B, TB and syphilis
    - p/w Brown to Blue papulonodules on extensor surfaces near joints
    - Path: Concentric onion skin fibrosis w/ LCV more prominent in early lesions
        - Ddx: sclerotic fibroma has a similar concentric fibrosis but is said to have "plywood-like collagen" and there is no inflammation
    - Rx: **Dapsone** is TOC
    - Workup: **SPEP/immunofixation**, hep panel, HIV, quant gold, RPR/VDRL, CBC
- Serum Sickness: similar pathogenesis to all other CSVV (immune complexes)
    - p/w Systemic Symptoms (arthritis, fever) and **purpuric urticarial rash in adults**
    - Caused by vaccines (rabies), immune modulating meds (infliximab), anti-venoms
    - Rx: Self-resolves but can treat Symptomatically (NSAIDS and antihistamines)
- Secondary CSVV is due to the "ABCD" triggers discussed above

Mixed small to medium vessel vasculitis

- Wegener's (granulomatosis with polyangiitis; "wecgener's"): triad of necrotizing Granulomas in the upper and lower respiratory track and Glomerulonephritis
    - If you draw a "C" on a stick figure the top of the "C" will go over his face (nasal and sinus inflamma-

tion, rhinorrhea), the middle will go over his lungs (cough, hemoptysis) and the bottom will go over his kidneys (glomerulonephritis)
        - **The presenting sign is the top of the "C" (sinusitis) but the most likely to kill them is the bottom of the "C" (glomerulonephritis)**
    - In addition to this triad, CNS involvement is common
    - Skin: palpable purpura (MC), oral ulcers, and **PG-like nodules and strawberry Gums**
    - Labs: c-ANCA, CXR, CT sinus, UA, and RF
    - Path (LCV w/ stellate abscesses): palisaded Granuloma w/ central neutrophils ("blue granulomas") and Giant cells; ANCA-associated vasculitides are DIF (-)
    - Rx: Cyclophosphamide + Corticosteroids
- Microscopic polyangiitis: pulmonary, renal and CNS involvement (no nasal involvement)
    - Males > females; a/w Meds and Malignancy
    - **MCC of pulmonary-renal syndrome (focal segmental necrotizing GN)**
    - p/w Mixture of small (palpable purpura) and medium ("SLURD") vessel disease
    - Labs: p-ANCA (**anti-MPO by ELISA** or p-ANCA by IIF) in 60%
    - Path: LCV w/ no granuloma formation (unlike Wegener's and Churg-Strauss)
        - "Out of the three main ANCA+ vasculitides, this is Missing the granuloma"
    - Rx: same treatment as Wegener's but should use MTX in remission
- Churg-Strauss syndrome (A-G)
    - Adult-onset **Asthma/Allergic rhinitis (1st stage of disease)**
    - B-anca (just kidding, its p-ANCA, aka anti-MPO)
    - **Cardiomyopathy (MCC of death)**

  - Drops (foot drop/wrist drop)
  - Eosinophilia (get CBC) and ↑IgE
  - Feet/hands p/w numbness and tingling
  - GI symptoms/Glomerulonephritis (limited renal involvement)/ "red Granulomas"
  - Leukotriene inhibitor (montelukast) and anti-IgE Ab (omalizumab) are triggers
  - Path: LCV w/ stellate abscesses (palisaded granuloma w/ central eosinophils)
  - Rx: corticosteroids (add cyclophosphamide if internal organ involvement)
- General workup for ANCA-associated vasculitides
  - Labs: IIF followed by confirmation w/ antigen-specific ELISA (PR3 or MPO)
  - Rule out drug-induced causes of ANCA+ vasculitis: IVIG, PTU, hydralazine, TNF inh, sulfasalazine, d-penicillamine, minocycline and levamisole tainted cocaine
    - Only high dose IVIG is a/w c-ANCA (all other are more likely p-ANCA)
  - Rule out other causes of ANCA vasculitis: mixed Cryoglobulinemia, RA, sepsis
  - Workup: CBC (eos), sinus CT, chest CT/CXR, UA, EKG, skin biopsy (granuloma)
  - Rx: **rituximab** is becoming the new best modality for the ANCA vasculitides
- Type 2 and 3 cryoglobulinemia: discussed below

Medium vessel vasculitis

- Polyarteritis nodosa
  - Childhood PAN: mutation in CECR1 that encodes ADA2 (expressed in monocytes)
  - Classic PAN triggers (BCDE): **Hep B** > Hep C, IBD and hairy cell leukemia ("hair-E")
  - Cutaneous PAN triggers (PAM'S): Parvo B19, AIDS, **Minocycline**, Strept throat

  - p/w (SLURD): SQ nodules, Livedo reticularis, Ulcers, Retiform purpura, Digital necrosis
  - Classic PAN has multi-organ involvement: orchitis (esp w/ Hep B infection), GI disease, renovascular HTN but no glomerulonephritis; pulmonary disease is rare
  - Dx: renal angiography, ANCA (only + in cutaneous PAN), **Hep B**/C, ASO, UA, CBC
  - Path: LCV with necrotizing arteritis of medium sized arteries in the superficial SQ
  - Rx: consider penicillin in children; corticosteroids + cyclophosphamide in adults
- Kawasaki disease: discussed in section 5.1

Large vessel vasculitis

- Temporal arteritis (giant cell arteritis)
  - Granulomatous vasculitis of the temporal artery
  - p/w Tenderness and erythema along Temple/Temporal scalp, unilateral HA, loss of Temple pulse, **vision loss**, jaw claudication, **ulcer of anterior Tongue** and polymyalgia rheumatica (**limb and girdle pain and weakness**)
    - Behçet's will also p/w tongue ulcers/vision loss but not muscle weakness
  - Labs: ↑ ESR; temporal artery biopsy shows a granulomatous large vessel arteritis
  - Rx: ASA + steroids; IL-6 blocker Tocilizumab is approved for large vessel vasculitis
  - Workup: MRI of head or cranial duplex US may be more sensitive than biopsy
- Takayasu's arteritis
  - Granulomatous vasculitis involving the aorta and its main branches
  - **p/w loss of pulse in the extremities**, EN, PG-like lesions and digital gangrene
  - Labs: ↑ ESR; MRA of aortic arch

- o Rx: 1-year taper of prednisone +/- steroid sparring agent

Vasculopathies

Cryoglobulinemia

- Cryoglobulins are immunoglobins that precipitate at Colder temperatures
- **Type I: ↑ monoclonal IgM** → vessel occlusion with hyaline material → p/w Raynaud's, gangrene, livedo Reticularis, ulceration, **acrocyanosis (commonly helices)**
  - o a/w **hematologic Cancer** like MM (makes sense as this will ↑ monoclonal IgM)
  - o Dx: CBC, CMP, UA, SPEP, immunofixation, serum and urine free light chains
- **Type II and III (mixed type): monoclonal IgM (type 2) or polyclonal IgM (type 3) complexes against polyclonal IgG** to form complexes that occlude vessels → trigger Complement → LCV → p/w palpable purpura and a systemic vasculitis
  - o a/w AI-CTD (RA), Bugs (**Hepatitis C in 9/10 cases,** HIV), Cancer (**NHL** in MC)
  - o MC systemic findings are arthralgias (70%), peripheral neuropathy (40%), GI disease/hepatitis (30%) and membranoproliferative glomerulonephritis (25%)
  - o Labs: ↑ Cryoglobins, **hypo-Complementemia/ ↓C4, Hep C and RF (+)**
- Path: vessels occluded by pink jelly (Type 1) or LCV (Type 2/3); perivascular IgM on DIF
  - o LCV in types 2 and 3 affects both small and large vessels but mostly small vessels
- Rx: treat underlying disease (IFN-α +/- ribavirin for HCV related disease); Rituximab

Thrombosis and thrombotic syndromes

- Anti-phospholipid syndrome (APLS): p/w Arthritis, Premature birth/PE, Labile BP, Stroke
  - Cutaneous features of APLS: Atrophie blanchie, retiform Purpura, **Livedo reticularis (MC finding)**, Leg ulcers and Splinter hemorrhages
  - MC association of APLS is SLE
  - Lab findings of APLS is ABC'S: lupus Anticoagulant, anti-β2-glycoprotein I (most specific), anti-Cardiolipin (most sensitive), False (+) Syphilis serologies
  - Dx of APLS can only be made if 1 or more Abs are positive on two separate occasions at least 12 weeks apart (transient positivity in thrombotic states)
  - Rx: anticoagulation
- Thromboangiitis obliterans (Buerger's disease): arteries and veins in the hands and feet get inflamed and blocked w/ blood clots (thrombi) → digital gangrene
  - Rx: **TOC is smoking cessation**; prostacyclin analogs and sympathectomy also help
- Livedoid vasculopathy ("ABCs of Atrophie Blanchie"): chronic thrombo-occlusive disease
  - p/w B/L Ankles w/ Burning pain prior to a painful/irregular Cutaneous ulcer
    - Atrophie Blanchie in later lesions: p/w porcelain-white scar
  - a/w AI-CTD (**APLS**), Blood vessel sclerosis, **Coagulation disorders (MCC)**
  - Path (Biopsy ulcer Border): **"Crayon-pink" hyalinization of vessel walls/lumen**
    - The fibrinoid material is PAS+ and diastase resistant
  - Rx: ASA, Betamethasone (steroids), **anti-Coagulants** (e.g., rivaroxaban), Danazol
  - Workup: AI-CTD workup (ANA), hep B/C, CBC, **Coagulation workup** (protein C/S)

- Cholesterol Emboli: p/w **livedo reticularis** > retiform purpura, digital gangrene, ulcer
    - Clinical setting: post-Catheterization, CAD (MC association), anti-Coagulation
    - Path: Cholesterol Clefts in small vessels
    - Rx: no therapy alters prognosis, but aim is to Enhance Circulation; **wound Care**
    - Workup: ↑ Creatinine, ↑ ESR, **Eosinophilia**, Eye exam may show cholesterol emboli in the retinal circulation and Echo may show atheromatous lesions
- Pigmented purpura (capillaritis; "I bet you can't even SPELLL capillaritis")
    - Schamberg's: cayenne-pepper purpura on LEs in older adults
    - Purpura annularis telangiectodes of Majocchi: annular patches of petechiae
    - Eczematoid-like purpura of Doucas and Kapetanakis: scaly eczematous petechiae
    - Lichenoid dermatitis of Guogerot and Blum: rust-colored lichenoid papules
    - Lichen aureus: solitary golden or rust-colored patch on LEs
    - Linear pigmented purpura: U/L linear eruption of yellow-brown macules in kids
    - Path: PV lymphocytic infiltrate w/ extravasated RBCs in the papillary dermis
    - Rx: topical steroids, PUVA/NB-UVB, pentoxifylline, rutoside + ascorbic acid
- Hypergammaglobulinemic purpura of Waldenstrom: p/w crops (Waxes and Wanes) of stinging ("Waah this hurts") petechiae/purpura (**Wide petechia**) on the LEs of Women
    - a/w a polyclonal gammopathy (in the name) and/or AI-CTD (**Sjögren's** > RA, SLE)

- Rx: compression socks, treat any underlying diseases, avoid prolonged standing
- Workup: CBC (anemia), ↑ESR, SPEP, AI-CTD workup (anti-Ro, RF)

- Levamisole-induced vasculitis (A-E)
  - **ANCA (+) vasculitis** (p-ANCA > c-ANCA); Arthralgias (MC systemic manifestation)
  - Blood vessel thrombosis w/ LCV on path; Bullous necrotic plaques seen on trunk
  - Cocaine may by contaminated by levamisole (get a urine toxicology)
  - **Decreased blood cells (neutropenia)**
  - **Ears** and legs are MC locations which show retiform purpura (ddx for retiform purpura in acral locations includes APLS, cholesterol emboli, cryoglobulinemia)
  - Dx: Anti-HNE-ANCA (human neutrophil elastase) can help aid in the diagnosis
  - Rx: stop cocaine; supportive treatment
- Dego's disease (malignant atrophic papulosis; ABC)
  - Adolescent men; ASA +/- pentoxifylline (steroids worsen disease) is treatment
  - **Bowel perforation (MCC of death is from sepsis 2° to peritonitis; consider EGD)**
    - CNS and eye disease are also common so consider eye exam/brain MRI
  - p/w Crops of rose-colored papules that develop **a Central porcelain white depression with surrounding telangiectasias** on the trunk or extremities
  - Path: wedge-shaped area of dermal changes (edema, mucin, sclerosis) w/ sparse perivascular infiltrate and overlying atrophic epidermis
- Sneddon syndrome (Sneddon the SNAIL won the race): Stroke, Neuro issues (dementia), **APLS**, Increased BP,

Intimal smooth muscle proliferation on path, **Livedoid racemosa**

- Hyperoxalosis: AR metabolic disorders w/ ↑ serum oxalate → deposition in tissue
    - p/w recurrent urolithiasis, renal failure, **livedo reticularis**, calciphylaxis-like presentation, Raynaud's and acral cyanosis/necrosis
    - Path: characteristic yellow-brown, birefringent crystal deposits around vessels

Endocarditis

- Inflammation of the endocardium (usually due to infection)
- Cutaneous manifestations
    - Janeway lesions: **painless** red macules on the palms/soles ("Ms Janeway is nice")
    - Osler nodes: **painful** red papules on the finger pads ("Mr Osler is mean")
    - May also see conjunctival or splinter hemorrhages (nails) and retiform purpura
- Systemic symptoms: cough, dyspnea, fever, chest pain
- Workup: CBC (leukocytosis), blood cultures and echocardiogram
- Rx: IV antibiotics

3.23 Panniculitidies and Lipodystrophies

Panniculitis

- Ideal biopsy technique for panniculitis is deep incisional biopsy (can use 6mm punch)

Erythema nodosum (EN)

- MC panniculitis (esp women in 2nd to 4th decade of life)

- Pathogenesis: DTH response (Th1 cytokine pattern) to various antigens (I remember them by saying, "it Sarcs when Crony COPS Strep search you and Touch yer cock"
  - o Autoimmune: Sarcoidosis > Crohn's
    - ▪ Löfgrens syndrome (sarcoidosis): LAD, öcular symptoms, Fevers, Good prognosis, Roaming polyarthritis, EN, Scandinavian whites affected
  - o Drugs (COPS): Contraceptives/estrogen, OCPs, Penicillins, Sulfonamides
  - o Bugs: **Strep infections** (MC overall antigen) > TB, Yersinia, coccidioidomycoses
- EN is a/w a **good prognosis** in patients with **sarcoidosis** and coccidioidomycoses
  - o "These are the first and last words in the mnemonic above"
- p/w bilateral tender erythematous SQ nodules on the shins (> thighs and forearms) that never ulcerate and resolve in days to weeks with bruise-like patches but no scarring
- A chronic variant exists called subacute nodular migratory panniculitis (erythema nodosum migrans) with migratory nodules that expand in a centrifugal manner (central clearing) and may assume a yellow or morpheaform appearance; Rx: potassium iodide
- Path: septal panniculitis with Miescher's granulomas
- Rx: treat underlying cause/stop implicated drug, bed rest/leg elevation/compression, NSAIDS, salicylates, SSKI, colchicine (if a/w Behçet's) or TNF-α inhibitors (if a/w IBD)
- Workup: look for cause (ASO for strept, GI consult for IBD, CXR for coccidioidomycosis)

Alpha-1 Antitrypsin deficiency (AAD)

- Inborn error of metabolism causing release of proteolytic enzymes and fat necrosis

- Severe disease is due to homozygous mutation in the Z allele of SERPINA1 gene (PiZZ)
- Clinical features ("over-ZEALOUS"): Z allele has severe phenotype, **Emphysema**, SQ **Atrophy** upon resolution, Liver disease (cirrhosis), **Oily discharge from skin**, nodular **Ulcers**, Underwear distribution (flanks, buttocks, upper thighs), Scarring upon resolution
- Path: liquefactive necrosis of SQ fat + neutrophilic lobular panniculitis
  - "I'M A neutrophilic panniculitis": **Infectious, Myelodysplastic syndrome, AAD**
- Rx: IV alpha$_1$-antitrypsin enzyme replacement; liver transplant

Pancreatic panniculitis (OPqRST)

- Pathogenesis: hydrolysis of the fat by ↑ levels of lipase, amylase and trypsin
- p/w SQ nodules of the legs (MC) that **may ulcerate and produce an Oily discharge**
- a/w Pancreatitis, Pancreatic carcinoma, Pancreatic Psuedocysts and Pancreus divisum
- Lesions Resolve over weeks with hyperpigmented Scars
- **Systemic Symptoms** common (fever, abdominal pain, arthritis, ascites, pleural effusions)
- **Schmid's triad ("Pencreatic Penicullitis"): Polyarthritis + Eosinophilia + Nodular lesions**
  - **a/w a worse prognosis**
- Path: Septal panniculitis (early); Saponification of fat by calcium Salts (later)
- Rx: treat underlying pancreatic disease; Somatostatin analog (Octreotide)
- Workup: **abdominal CT** to look for pancreatitis or pancreatic neoplasm

Erythema induratum of Bazin/nodular vasculitis (A-F)

- p/w Annular erythematous nodules in cases involving TB (Erythema induratum of Bazin) or tender non-annular nodules on the **Calves** in the idiopathic (nodular vasculitis) form
    - o Like α_1-antitrypsin def and pancreatic panniculitis, lesions ulcerate, drain, scar
- Path: Cutaneous SVV of the medium sized vessels with Coagulative/Caseous necrosis
- Dx: **CXR**; DNA of mycobacterium may be detected in skin lesions by PCR
- Rx: treat Erythema induratum like TB (RIPE therapy), otherwise treat like EN
- Represents a type IV (Four) cell mediated response to an antigen; occurs MC in Females

Post-steroid panniculitis

- p/w SQ nodules on the cheek, arms and trunk after rapid withdrawal of steroids in kids
- Path: needle-shaped clefts (SQ fat necrosis and Sclerema neonatorum look identical)
- Rx: spontaneous resolution (treatment unnecessary)

Subcutaneous fat necrosis of the newborn and Sclerema neonatorum discussed in 4.1

Lupus panniculitis

- p/w tender SQ nodules and plaques arising on the **face, proximal arms and upper trunk** that heals with atrophy in an adult (Perry-Romberg disease is a child with facial atrophy)
- a/w discoid lupus in 1/3rd of cases and SLE in 15% of cases
- Path: lobular panniculitis w/ **lymphoid aggregates and hyaline necrosis of fat lobules**
- Rx: **antimalarials**

Traumatic panniculitis

- Cold panniculitis: painful **red nodules on the Cheeks** (MC) seen after Cold exposure
    - o Variants include popsicle panniculitis (seen on the cheeks and chins of infants) and equestrian panniculitis (seen on the thighs of young women equestrians) Path: lobular panniculitis + pernio (sup and deep lymphs + pap dermal edema)
- Sclerosing lipogranuloma: due to injection of oil-based material on the Shaft of the penis
    - o Path: vacuolated Spaces with a "Swiss-cheese" appearance
- Texier's disease: form of traumatic panniculitis due to vitamin K (phytonadione) injections which p/w painful sclerotic (often w/ lilac-colored borders) inflamed nodules on the buttocks and thighs ("cowboy holster pattern") which can persist for years
    - o Ddx: equestrian panniculitis

Lipodermatosclerosis (LIPODermatosclerosis)

- Lower Legs show Induration, hyperpigmentation and "Inverted wine bottle" sclerosis
- Venous Insufficiency is MCC
- Path: Ischemic necrosis of fat lobules lipomembranous changes ("frost on a window")
- Rx: Pentoxifylline + anabolic steroids (Oxandrolone or Danazol); elevation/compression

Lipodystrophies

- All present with metabolic syndrome → **diabetes (MC), HSM (2nd MC), ↓ leptin**, ↑ triglycerides, PCOS or menstrual issues in women) and **severe acanthosis nigricans (AN)**
    - o Rx: leptin replacement helps metabolic issues but not the cosmetic issues like AN

- The congenital/familial forms are a/w big organs (e.g., enlarged female genitalia, HSM, **hypertrophic cardiomyopathy** and fat loss gives appearance of muscular hypertrophy)
- Acquired forms are preceded by panniculitis/infection (kids) or AI-CTD (adolescence)

Congenital generalized lipodystrophy (Berardinelli-Seip syndrome; ABC)

- AR mutation in AGPAT2, BSCL2 or CAV1
- Only lipodystrophy to present at Birth; highest frequency in Brazil
- ↓ fat in skin, viscera and Bone marrow (acquired generalized form preserves BM fat)
    - Results in osteosclerotic and lytic Bone lesions
- As stated above, metabolic syndrome (severe AN) and big organs (HSM, **HCM**) present

Familial Partial lipodystrophy (Köbberling-Dunnigan syndrome; LMNoP)

- AD mutation in LMNA (same gene that is mutated in Progeria) > PPARG > PLIN1
- Subtype with Mandibuloacral dysplasia (LMNA or ZMPSTE24 genes): Mandibular, digital and clavicular hypoplasia, scleroderma-like lesions with Mottled hyperpigmentation
- Muscular hypertrophy appearance due to loss of fat on trunk and extremities
- Moon faces and ↑ Neck fat (double chin) due to ↑ fat on head/neck
- Starts at Puberty

For the acquired forms the letter in the name helps you remember the salient points of the other acquired form (e.g., acquired Generalized form has Preceding Panniculitis and acquired Partial form is a/w membranoproliferative Glomerulonephritis, DON'T get this confused!)

Acquired Generalized lipodystrophy (Lawrence syndrome)

- Unknown gene (occurs after Preceding **Panniculitis**, infection or AI-CTD)
- Loss of fat on skin (everywhere including Palms/soles) and viscera but BM fat Preserved

Acquired Partial lipodystrophy (Barraquer-Simons syndrome)

- AD mutation in LMNB vs sporadic due to infections or AICTD (Girls >> boys)
- Pathogenesis: complement hyperactivation → compliment-mediated fat destruction
- Whereas familial partial form has ↑ fat on head/neck and ↓ on trunk/extremities, acquired partial form has ↓ fat on head/neck (cadaveric faces) initially and spreads down stopping at the trunk **(↑ fat in Gluteal region and hips**)
- **a/w membranoproliferative Glomerulonephritis and dermatomyositis**
- IgG autoantibodies against the alternative pathway (↑ C3 nephritic factor) → activation of alternative compliment pathway → **↓C3** → **Neisseria infections (e.g., N. Gonorrhoeae)**

Localized lipoatrophy/lipohypertrophy

- The MCC of localized lipoatrophy are from AI-CTD (Parry-Romberg syndrome and lipoatrophy following lupus panniculitis), pressure and iatrogenic medications
    - o Lipohypertrophy (SHIP): Steroids, HIV/ART (PI), Insulin (IM), Pegvisomant (IM)
    - o Lipoatrophy (SHIP): **Steroids**, HIV/ART (esp NRTIs), Insulin (IM), Penicillin (IM)

- Rx: treat associated metabolic syndrome; poly-L-lactic acid/calcium hydroxyapatite filler

3.24 Dermatoses of Pregnancy

Pemphigoid gestationis (herpes gestationis; "CHERPES G")

- Due to IgG1 antibodies against Collagen 17 (BP180); a/w **Choriocarcinoma**
- linear **C3** along BM zone on DIF (otherwise it's the same as BP on path and SSS)
- a/w HLA-DR3 and HLA-DR4; p/w Herpetiform blisters that **begins in umbilical Hole**
- Exacerbation around the time of birth; **ELISA** is a sensitive test
- **Recurs** in ½ of future pregnancies (high-risk OB care in next pregnancy) or with OCP use
- **Preterm** labor; Premature infants
- Exanthem in 10% of infants (only pregnancy dermatoses that affects newborn skin)
- Small for gestational age infants; eruption in the Second half of pregnancy
- Rx: **Steroids** (topicals for mild disease and systemic for widespread/severe disease)
- a/w **Graves disease/hyperthyroidism** in mother; IgG1 antibodies to BP180

Polymorphic eruption of pregnancy

- Pathogenesis: due to stretching of the skin so it makes sense it is seen in **primiparous women**, **↑ risk in multiple-gestation pregnancy**, and seen in the **third trimester**
- p/w urticarial, pruritic papules that start in the peri-umbilical striae (**spares umbilicus**)
    - May generalize but resolves in 1 month and **does not recur** in future pregnancies

- Dx: path is non-specific, DIF is negative, labs are normal
- Rx: resolves in 4 weeks but treat symptomatically (topical steroids and antihistamines)

Intrahepatic Cholestasis of pregnancy ("ABCD")

- ABCB4 mutation (**encodes Bile transporter proteins**) → failure to excrete Bile Acids
- Country with the highest incidence is Chile > Bolivia; Hepatitis C is a risk factor
- p/w extreme pruritis (beginning on palms/soles) in **third trimester** but no primary rash
- Cholestasis steatorrhea → vitamin k deficiency → postpartum hemorrhage/**Bleeding**
- Dx: ↑ AST/ALT, ↑ Bilirubin, ↑ serum Bile acid levels (>11 mmol) due to ↓ excretion
- Fetus: **prematurity, still-Birth, meconium stains, fetal Distress** (↑ risk w/ ↑ bile acids)
- Rx: **Early Delivery (if possible), ursodeoxy-Cholic acid (1st line)**, Cholestyramine (2nd line)
- Recurs in future pregnancies or with oral Contraceptive use

Atopic Eruption of pregnancy (prurigo of pregnancy)

- **MC pruritic disorder in pregnancy**
- Pathogenesis: shift from Th1 to Th2 during pregnancy
- Occurs **Early in pregnancy** (usually first trimester)
- p/w Eczematous papules and plaques in typical atopic places (flexures of Extremities)
- Dx: ↑ IgE levels
- Rx: symptomatic control w/ Emollients and topical steroids; recurs in future pregnancies

Pustular Psoriasis of Pregnancy (impetigo herpetiformis was the old name)

- Presents in the third trimester with generalized **Pustular** Psoriasis starting in the groin and extending symmetrically to the trunk; systemic symptoms (fever, N/V/D, seizures)

- Commonly occurs after rapid taper of Prednisone
- Placental insufficiency (monitor w/ **uterine doppler US**) → stillbirth/neonatal death
- Dx: ↓ **calcium**, ↓ vitamin D levels, hypoalbuminemia, leukocytosis, ↑ ESR
- Rx: Prednisone, Infliximab and Cyclosporine are 1st line (same Rx as PG)
    - o "Take a PIC of PG and Pustular Psoriasis of Pregnancy"
- Workup: hospitalize to closely monitor electrolytes, CBC, CMP and calcium
- Resolves with delivery but typically recurs in future Pregnancies or with OCPs

3.25 Hair Disorders

Non-scarring alopecia

Androgenetic alopecia (pattern alopecia; AGA)

- MC form of alopecia in men and women (80% of men and 50% of women by age 70)
- Pathogenesis: 5α-reductase converts testosterone to dihydrotestosterone (DHT)
    - o Type 1 5α-reductase: predominant in **sebaceous glands** and the liver
    - o Type 2 5α-reductase: predominant in **prostate**, seminal vesicles and **hair follicles**
- p/w frontotemporal recession w/ vertex thinning (men) vs preserved frontal hairline w/ vertex thinning and ↑ central part width in a "Christmas tree" pattern (women)
- Path: ↑ vellus and miniaturized (previously large hairs) leads to **Anisotrichosis** (↑ variability of hair shaft

diameter); **shortened anagen phase → ↓anagen/telogen ratio ("A Girly Anagen phase")** due to "catagen/telogen shift" → ↑ fibrous streamers

- o The small vellus or miniaturized hairs are surrounded by relatively larger sebaceous glands and so this scalp biopsy will look like a biopsy from the face

- Rx: topical and oral minoxidil, 5α-reductase inhibitors (finasteride inhibits type 2 and dutasteride has dual action of type 1 and 2), red light therapy, PRP and hair transplant

Catagen/telogen shift (↑ % of catagen/telogen hairs): "All Tricky tracks tell the same pattern"
"All Tricky Tracks" (huge "catagen/telogen shift"; > 50% of hairs in catagen/telogen phase)
Alopecia areata, Trichotillomania and Traction alopecia
"Tell the same Pattern" (mild "catagen/telogen shift"; 20–50% of hairs are catagen/telogen)
Telogen effluvium and Pattern alopecia (AGA)

*All of these forms of alopecia also show ↑ fibrous streamers (except telogen effluvium)

Telogen effluvium

- Pathogenesis: ↑ hair shedding (telogen shift) due to thyroid abnormalities and …
  - o Stressors (SIP): Surgery, Illness, Post-Partem
  - o Malnutrition (ZIP): ↓ Zinc ↓ Iron, ↓ Protein
  - o Drug (CIP): antiCoagulants, antiConvulsants, IFN, Isotretinoin, PTU (thyroid med)
- p/w diffuse shedding of hairs that occurs 4 months after inciting event (subsides in 1 yr)
  - o Positive hair pull test (will see club shaped telogen hairs on trichoscopy)
- Path: mild ↑ in catagen/telogen hairs (20–50%); normal # of total hairs

- Rx: self-limited; D/C potential drugs and correct iron, zinc or thyroid abnormality

Trichotillomania

- p/w large, **irregular, geometric** areas of alopecia on scalp, eyebrows or genital hair w/ adjacent areas of normal hair (affected areas contain hairs of varying length)
- Affects young girls (MC) and is a/w trichophagy and GI obstruction from trichobezoars
- Path: huge catagen/telogen shift (> 50%), many irregularly shaped catagen hairs w/ apoptotic keratinocytes, **tracheomalacia** (distorted hair shafts), **pigmented melanin casts** in follicular canals and empty anagen follicles due to hair shafts being pulled out
- Dx: hair growth window (will grow back normal after shaving/occluding an area)
- Rx: **behavioral treatment/habit reversal training** is TOC; SSRIs, clomipramine, NAC

Traction alopecia

- MC in AA females who use Tight braids, elastic bands, tight rollers, cornrows, hot combs
- p/w **fringe sign** (Tuft or cluster of unaffected Terminal hairs at the frontotemporal edge)
    - o vs lonely hair sign in frontal fibrosing alopecia: one or few isolated terminal hairs
- Path: same as trichotillomania except chronic traction alopecia you see **"naked sebaceous lobules"** as hair is wiped out but sebaceous glands are not
- Rx: discontinue any manual traction, IL/topical steroids, topical minoxidil, Tetracyclines

Alopecia areata: "VISTA → you will have a good VISTA (means view in Spanish) of the scalp"

- Pathogenesis (VISTA)
  - Viruses (HCV, CMV) have historically been thought to play a role (poor evidence)
  - **IL-15** (working through JAK-STAT) is significantly elevated
  - Susceptibility genes (HLA DRB1, **NKG2D**, PTPN22, filaggrin gene mutation)
  - T-cell mediated (CD8 > CD4) disease with ↑ **Th1 cytokines** (IL-2, IFN-γ, TNF-α)
  - Autoimmune disease where the hair follicles experience loss of immune privilege
- p/w sudden onset round patches of alopecia (**regrown hair comes in gray/white**)
  - Alopecia totalis (entire scalp) vs alopecia universalis (scalp and body)
  - Ophiasis (band-like loss across occipital/temporal scalp) vs Sisapho (opposite)
  - **Exclamation point hair**: hairs are broader distally and tapered towards the scalp
  - Nails: trachyonychia or geometric pitting of the nails
- Drug-induced AA: immune checkpoint inhibitors (CTLA-4, PD-1), TNF-α inhibitors
- a/w VISTA: **Vitiligo (MC)** > IBD, SLE, autoimmune Thyroid disease, **Atopy** (bad prognosis)
- Path: lymphoid inflammation at level of hair bulb ("swarm of bees"), miniaturization, huge catagen/telogen shift, empty dilated follicular infundibula ("swiss-cheese sign") and lymphocytes, eosinophils and melanin in fibrous tract remnants
- Rx (VISTA): UV light, Immunotherapy w/ squaric acid or diphencyprone (best for face) to induce a contact dermatitis, topical/IL/systemic Steroids, Tofacitinib (and

other oral JAKs such as ritlecitinib, ruxolitinib, baricitinib), Anthralin, Antihistamines
- Poor prognosis (VISTA): Vaginas (females), Infantile/young onset w/ long duration, ↑ Surface area (most important), Temporal (ophiasis), Trachyonychia/nails, Atopy

Temporal triangular alopecia
- p/w triangular patch of **non-scarring hair loss at or just behind frontotemporal hairline**
- Presents at birth and **persists throughout life**
- Rx: hair transplant

Atrichia with papular lesions ("hairless cystic D")
- AR defect in zinc finger domain of **Hairless gene**
- Failure to grow hair after initial shedding of hair after birth
- Papular cystic lesions erupt within the first year of life
- Hereditary vitamin D-dependent rickets type 2A has an AR mutation in the vitamin D receptor and presents identical except they also have rickets (osteomalacia, etc.)

Cicatricial alopecia

Central Centrifugal Cicatricial Alopecia (A-F but skip B)
- Mutation in **PADI3** (peptidyl arginine deiminase type 3)
- Pathogenesis: **Early Desquamation of inner root sheath**
- MC in AA patients (F > M) and is **a/w uterine leiomyomas and uterine Fibroids**
- a/w Chemical relaxers, hot Combs or other traumatic Cosmetic hairstyling practices
- p/w Cicatricial alopecia in Center of scalp (Crown) and spreads Centrifugally

    - Polytrichia ("Doll hairs"): multiple hair shafts from same infundibulum
- Path: perifollicular Concentric lamellar Fibrosis, Eccentric thinning of ORS
    - Perifollicular inflammation is not as dense as seen in lichen planopilaris
- Rx: anti-Androgens, Corticosteroids, Cyclosporine, Chloroquine/HCQ, Doxycycline, Eliminate traumatic hair grooming practices, Finasteride, minoxidil, and hair transplant

Lichen planopilaris

- MC in white females (a/w autoimmune conditions such as vitiligo and hypothyroidism)
- p/w scalp pruritis/tenderness w/ **perifollicular erythema and keratotic plugs** at the margins of the expanding scarring alopecia +/- mucocutaneus LP (15%)
    - **Frontal fibrosing alopecia**: variant w/ hairline recession; **> 50% w/ eyebrow loss**
        - Lonely hair sign: isolated hairs spared at anterior hairline (vs fringe sign in traction alopecia that has a band of unaffected hairs on anterior hairline)
        - Gram-Little syndrome: LPP (scarring hair loss on scalp) + non-scarring hair loss on axilla and pubic area + KP-like follicular papules on trunk
- End stage LPP is known as pseudopelade of Brocq: described as "footprints in the snow"
- Path: **dense perifollicular lichenoid interface dermatitis at the level of the infundibulum**, civatte bodies in the follicular epithelium, perifollicular melanophages, perifollicular concentric fibrosis and loss of sebaceous glands and arrector pili muscles
    - Ddx: DLE has dense infiltrate at all levels of follicle and b/w follicles along the DEJ

- DIF: cytoid bodies w/ shaggy fibrin deposition at the DEJ
- Rx: **antimalarials** (generally considered 1st line for severe disease), topical/IL/oral steroids, mycophenolate mofetil, cyclosporine, pioglitazone, doxycycline, acitretin
    - Finasteride is another good option for Frontal Fibrosing alopecia

Folliculitis decalvans

- Scarring alopecia w/ highly inflammatory papules and pustules +/- tufted hairs
- Dx: culture often reveals S. aureus
- Rx: oral antibiotics (tetracyclines, rifampin, clindamycin)

Hypertrichosis and hirsutism

Hypertrichosis

- Defined as excessive hair growth anywhere on the body (vellus > terminal)
- Most testable forms
    - Acquired hypertrichosis lanuginosa ("LGBtq")
        - **Lanugo** (long, fine) hair appears quickly (esp. face → simian appearance)
        - Paraneoplastic disease a/w Lung, GI and Breast cancer
    - Acquired generalized hypertrichosis
        - **Terminal** hairs slowly grow on forehead, temples, trunk and extremities
        - "Going to CAMP will put terminal hairs on your chest (and head/arms)"
            - Cyclosporine, Anorexia, Minoxidil, Phenytoin, POEMS, Porphyria
    - Acquired trichomegaly (primarily of eyelashes): "Huge Pretty Eye-Lashes"

        - HIV, Prostaglandin F-2α, EGFR inh. (**cetuximab**), Latanoprost/bimatoprost
    - Anterior Cervical hypertrichosis: rare form of congenital localized hypertrichosis
        - a/w neuropathy/optic atrophy (get CNS eval/Eye exam) and hallux valgus
    - Other forms of localized hypertrichosis: Becker's nevus, hair collar sign, repeated trauma/friction, plaster casts for fractured limb, prostaglandin analogs
- Rx: electrolysis, laser, eflornithine cream

Hirsutism

- Defined as male pattern hair growth in a female (e.g., chin, chest, back, abdomen)
- Related to ↑ androgens from adrenals (↑ DHEA-S) or ovaries (↑ **androstenedione**)
- General rules
    - Rapid onset hirsutism is due to tumors (e.g., adrenal, ovarian, pituitary)
    - Non-tumoral Adrenal source: Central hirsutism (Central abdomen, Chest, Chin); a/w low weight and Amenorrhea ("low letters → low # of pounds and periods")
    - Non-tumoral Ovarian source: Lateral hirsutism (lateral face/neck, areola); a/w Obesity and Polymenorrhea ("high letters → high # of pounds and periods")
- Major forms
    - PCOS: cysts in ovaries, secondary amenorrhea or menstrual irregularities
        - a/w HAIR-AN: Hirsutism (90%), AGA, Acne (70%), Insulin Resistance, AN
        - Rotterdam criteria (need 2 of 3 so pelvic US is not required for diagnosis)

        - Oligomenorrhea (< 9 cycles/yr) or anovulation (≥3 missed menses)
        - Biochemical (see below) or clinical signs of hyperandrogenism
        - Polycystic ovaries (> 12 follicles) or ovarian volume > 10 cc on US
    - Biochemical signs: ↑ **total T**, androstenedione and DHEA-S
        - Also order 17-OH-progesterone (normal) to rule out CAH
  - CAH: 21-hydroxylase deficiency (95% of CAH) → both sexes p/w salt wasting (hyponatremia, hyperkalemia) in first 2 weeks and pre-pubertal virilization
    - Male infants: large hyperpigmented penis
    - Female infants: ambiguous genitalia (but normal internal structures)
    - Labs: ↑ **17-OH-progesterone**, ↑ DHEA-S, ↑ ACTH, **normal testosterone**
  - Neoplastic: p/w abrupt virilization + very high testosterone levels (> 200 ng/dL)
    - Testosterone > 200 (usually > 600) but normal DHEA-S → ovarian tumor
    - Testosterone > 200 And high DHEA-S (> 600 mcg/dL) → Adrenal tumor
- Rx: **antiandrogens (spironolactone, OCPs)**, 5-α-reductase inhibitors, laser, eflornithine
  - CAH in infants is treated w/ systemic hydrocortisone (but not by derms)

Hair shaft abnormalities

Discussed in section 4.7

3.26 Nail and Mucosal Disorders

Nail matrix injury ("The Matrix was a True TOP Boxoffice Knock-Out" → "True" is a defect in distal matrix, "TOP Boxoffice" is a defect in proximal matrix, "Knock-Out" is defect in both)

- True leukonychia: white color that does not fade w/ pressure; grows out w/ nail
    - Can be diffuse which is congenital (Bart-Pumphrey), punctate from trauma, striate from manicures or thallium/arsenic exposure (Mees lines)
        - "It's true that Bart, a man, can't look at tha arse w/o getting Mee too'd"
- Trachyonychia (sandpaper nails): rough longitudinally ridged nails: "Sandy APLE"
    - **Alopecia areata (MCC)** > Psoriasis, Lichen planus, and Eczema
- Onychorrhexis (**longitudinal ridging**/brittle nails): longitudinally ridged nails ("BRITTLE")
    - Bullemia; -Rhexis/Ridging or fissuring of nail plate; due to Impaired vascular supply; a/w Trauma or Tumor compressing nail matrix, LP and Elderly patients
- Pitting: Proximal matrix defect w/ Parakeratosis in superficial nail plate
    - Psoriasis (irregular pits), alopecia areata (geometric, grid-like pits)
- Beau's lines: horizontal indentions from temporary arrest of growth of proximal matrix
    - Stress on Body (systemic illness, chemotherapy, child-Birth, major injury)

- Koilonychia (spoon nails): nail is "KonKave" instead of convex
    - a/w Plummer-Vinson syndrome (iron def anemia, esophageal web) and amyloid
- Onychomadesis (nail shedding; "onycho-made-a-new-nail"): proximal separation of nail plate from nail matrix due to temporary arrest of growth of proximal and distal matrix
    - Same causes as Beau's lines w/ the addition of Coxsackievirus infection

Injury to the nail bed ("An ASS lys in my bed")

- Apparent leukonychia: white color that fades w/ pressure: "ABCD"
    - Hypo-Albuminemia: Muehrcke's nails (horizontal white bands)
        - Mee's lines are the true leukonychia counterpart
    - Nail Bed edema causes apparent leukonychia
    - Chemotherapy
    - Cirrhosis: Terry's nails (leukonychia of most of the nail plate; "I imagine a fat white guy w/ cirrhosis named Terry that takes up most of the bed")
        - CKD patients on Dialysis: half-and-half nails/ Lindsay's nails (leukonychia on half of nail plate; "kidneys are located in the body's half-way point")
- Subungual hyperkeratosis (onychauxis): thickened TOP of nail
    - Tinea, Onychomycosis, Psoriasis
- Splinter hemorrhages: damage to nail bed capillaries: "STOVE TOP"
    - Proximal: Systemic disease, Trichinosis, Oral meds, Vasculitis, **Endocarditis**
    - Distal: Trauma, Onychomycosis, Psoriasis

- Onycholysis: distal nail plate detachment: "TOP"
    - Trauma, Thyroid disease, Onychomycosis, Psoriasis
    - Photo-onycholysis: Taxanes (painful hemorrhagic onycholysis), Tetracyclines, flouroquinolones, chloramphenicol, Psoralens + UV

Other high-yield nail disorders

- Nail changes in COVID19: transverse erythronychia (red half-moon sign)
    - Seen early (Beau's lines and onychomadesis are seen > 6 weeks post COVID)
- Onychocryptosis (ingrown nail): excess lateral nail-growth into nailfold; Rx matricectomy
- Longitudinal erythronychia: long red band → think Dariers disease if on multiple nails or onychopapilloma (MC), glomus tumor, Bowen's or amelanotic melanoma if on one nail
    - SCC is MC malignancy that p/w erythronychia but would also p/w hyperkeratosis
- Longitudinal melanonychia: longitudinal brown band: "MAGA HATS"
    - Melanoma/nevus, Minocycline, Antimalarials, Gold (metals), AZT, HIV, Laugier-Hunziker syndrome, Addison's disease, Tinea rubrum, Scytalidium spp.
- Horizontal or diffuse melanonychia: "A-H but skip vowels and G"
    - Bleomycin, Cyclophosphamide, Doxorubicin, **5-Flourouracil**, Hydroxyurea
- Hutchinson's sign (melanoma): proximal nail fold pigment w/ longitudinal melanonychia
- Black nails: proteus mirabilis or T. rubrum infection (Rx: pigmented fungal nail infections must be treated w/ **itraconazole** because the melanin makes terbinafine not work)

- Green nail syndrome: green staining of nails from pseudomonal pyocyanin
    - Rx: topical gentamicin, vinegar soaks, consider oral ciprofloxacin if severe
- Yellow nail syndrome: thickened yellow nails w/ absent cuticle
    - **Lung/heart issues** (bronchiectasis, pleural effusions, **chylothorax**), Lymphedema
- Blue lunulae: "democrats (blue) say Make America Great Again HOW?"
    - Minocycline, Antimalarials, Gold, Argyria, Hydroxyurea, Ochronosis, Wilson's
- Red lunulae: "red hot COAL"
    - CO poisoning, Organ failure (heart, COPD, cirrhosis), Autoimmune (SLE, RA, DM, vitiligo), Alopecia areata, Lymphogranuloma venereum, LS&A, Lichen planus
- Brachyonychia (racquet thumb): shortening of distal phalanx (e.g., Rubinstein-Taybi)
- Clubbing: soft tissue growth in distal phalanx → large Curved Club-like distal digit
    - a/w Cutis vertices gyrate, heart/lung issues and **Graves (thyroid achropachy)**
- Nail-Patella syndrome ("NAIL"): Nephropathy (**get UA; glomerulonephritis in 40%**), Nail changes, Absent patella, Iliac horns (seen on X-ray), **Lunula is triangular, Lester iris** (hyperpigmentation of inner margin/pupillary side of the iris), LMX1B gene mutation
- Darier's disease (keratosis follicularis): multiple red and white longitudinal streaks ("candy cane nails"), "V-nicking" and fissuring at the distal margin of the nail plate
- Acute paronychia (< 6 weeks): p/w pain, redness, swelling of nail fold; MC is S. Aureus
- Chronic paronychia (> 6 weeks): classically due to Contact dermatitis or Candida

- Habit-tic deformity: Horizontal ridges/depressions due to manipulation of cuticle
- Pincer nails: over-curvature of nail plate which may be painful: Rx matricectomy
  - Seen in Pachyonychia congenita
- Onychomatricoma: tumor which produces thick yellow nail plate w/ multiple longitudinal hollow spaces (holes) seen on frontal view of the nail free margin
  - "Onyc-hole-matric-hole-ma"
- Onychopapilloma: p/w **longitudinal erythronychia** and v-shaped distal nail splitting
- Subungual exostosis: boney growth at tip of the distal phalanx (under distal nail plate)
  - Next step is get an **X-ray** (not a biopsy)
- Myxoid cyst (digital mucous cyst): translucent nodule just proximal to proximal nail fold
- Periungual fibroma: skin colored papule on proximal nail fold +/- longitudinal groove
  - Multiple seen with Tuberous sclerosis (Koenen's tumor)
- **Glomus tumor**: **painful** bluish subungual papule +/- nail dystrophy
  - Love test: pain while applying pressure to the tumor
  - Hildreth sign: reduction in pain with the love test when using a tourniquet
- Pterygium unguis (dorsal pterygium): proximal nail fold fuses w/ the underlying matrix
  - **Lichen planus** > pemphigus/pemphigoid, GVHD, TEN, radiodermatitis
- Pterygium inversum unguis (ventral pterygium): hyponychium expands and anchors to the undersurface of the nail plate; seen in AI-CTD (esp. **scleroderma**)
- **SCC: p/w subungual verrucous mass; MC malignant tumor of the nail; HPV 16 is MC**

- Drugs that cause paronychia and periungual pyogenic granulomas: "SCREAM"
  - Sirolimus, Capecitabine, Retinoids, EGFR inhibitors, ART, MTX; mTOR inhibitors

High-yield mucosal disorders

- Recurrent aphthous Stomatitis: Small Sharply defined Shallow painful ulcers with a white/gray base and red border on the **anterior non-keratinized** ("Soft" → Soft palate, ventral tongue, buccal/labial mucosa, floor of mouth) **oral mucosa**
  - a/w Systemic disorders (iron/vit B deficiencies, stress, HIV, Behçet's disease)
  - Rx: topical Steroids
- **Herpangina** (MCC is coxsackie): looks like aphthous ulcers but are on the **posterior non-keratinized oral mucosa** (tonsils, uvula, soft palate) and p/w febrile illness
  - Hand-foot-mouth disease is also caused by coxsackie → skin and mouth lesions
- HSV: grouped painful erosions on **keratinized (Hard) mucosa (lips, Hard palate, gingiva)**
- Fordyce granules: ectopic ("free") sebaceous glands which p/w multiple yellowish papules on the buccal mucosa and upper vermillion lip
  - Ectopic sebaceous glands: "Five Mucosal Triglyceride Making Zones"
    - Fordyce granules (mouth), Meibomian (eyelid tarsal plate), Tysons (labia minora, prepuce), Montgomery (areolae), Zeis (eyelid margin)
- Geographic tongue (migratory glossitis): well-demarcated migratory patches of atrophy (loss of papilla) surrounded by a layer of red and a layer of white; a/w psoriasis

- Fissured (scrotal) tongue: deep grooves on dorsum of tongue
    - o a/w "MAD BV": Melkersson-Rosenthal, Acromegaly, Downs, Bazex, P. Vegetans
- Hairy tongue: yellow to brown-black (from bacterial porphyrins) Hypertrophic papillae on mid dorsal tongue from keratin build-up; a/w bad oral Hygiene/ smoking, Hot drinks
- Smooth tongue (atrophic glossitis): atrophy of papillae → p/w red painful tongue
    - o a/w vitamin deficiencies (iron, folate and other B vitamins)
- Central papillary atrophy (median rhomboid glossitis): p/w Circumscribed smooth area on Central dorsum of tongue (anterior to Circumvallate papillae); a/w oral **Candidiasis**
- Necrotizing ulcerative gingivitis (trench mouth): Necrotic painful ulcerative "punched out" lesions on gingiva due to Normal oral flora (mixed bacteria); a/w poor Nutrition
- Desquamative gingivitis: Diffusely eroded gingiva seen in immune-mediated Disease (LP)
- Fibroma: "I call it a bite fibroma because it occurs on the buccal mucosa at the bite line"
    - o #1 tumor of the oral cavity ("Fibroma is First"); MC in middle-aged Females
- Morsicatio buccarum: white surface changes on buccal mucosa from habitual chewing
    - o "Morder" in Spanish means to bite or to chew
- White sponge nevus: appears similar to morsicatio buccarum but with less-defined margins and can also involve the tongue, gingiva, palate; **a/w Keratin 4 and 13 mutation**
- Gingival hyperplasia: **Phenytoin (MCC)**, CCB (nifedipine), Cyclosporine, vit C deficiency

- "PC Culture" will make you bite your tongue, and gums b/c of how big they are"
- Contact stomatitis (mouth ACD): erosions due to Cinnamon flavoring or Dental Amalgam
- Eosinophilic ulcer of the oral mucosa (traumatic eosinophilic granuloma): enlarging ulcer of Tongue (MC) covered by a white layer of fibrin ("pseudomembrane"); a/w Trauma
  - Say "Teosin-ophilic" b/c Teosin, Tongue and Trauma have 6 letters and start w/ T
- Cheilitis granulomatosa (CG): p/w episodic **non-tender** swelling of lips (**upper** > lower)
  - a/w **Melkersson-Rosenthal syndrome: CG + fissured tongue + facial nerve palsy**
  - Chronic lesions: lip is **dry,** fissured, painful, scaly w/ a consistency of firm rubber
- Cheilitis glandularis: inflammatory hyperplasia of the lower labial salivary glands seen in a/w actinic cheilitis (occurs exclusively on lower lip) which p/w **tender** swelling of **lower lip** w/ **pinpoint erythema** and a sticky **wet** film (viscous fluid expressible through ducts)
- Granulomatosis with polyangiitis ("wecgener's"): c-ANCA+ vasculitis effecting nasal/oral cavity, lungs, kidneys (Glomerulonephritis) w/ PG-like nodules + **"strawberry Gums"**
- Oral leukoplakia/erythroplakia: white/red premalignant plaques in mouth, respectively (leukoplakia is more common, erythroplakia is more likely to become malignant)
- Leukoedema: gray-white buccal mucosa that becomes less apparent when stretched
- Mucocele (ranula when on floor of mouth): disruption of minor salivary gland → mucus spills into submucosal tissue → blue pseudocyst located **MC on the lower labial mucosa**

- Angular Cheilitis/perleche (A-F): a/w AIDS, B_{12} deficiency, Candida, Downs, **Dentures**
  - p/w Erythema and Fissuring of the oral commissures
- Pyostomatitis vegetans (oral variant of PG): **Pinpoint yellow Pustules in a serpentine pattern** on a red background on the labial/gingival/buccal mucosa → "snail-track" ulcers
  - a/w IBD (UC > Chron's)
  - Dx: peripheral eosinophilia; get **colonoscopy**
  - Rx: treat IBD w/ immunosuppressants
- Oral manifestations of Crohn's: linear ulcerations in the buccal vestibule
- Cutaneous Sinus of dental origin: untreated dental infection which spreads to the skin
  - Mandibular region such as chin and **Submental region** are most common
  - Rx: perform oral exam/referral to dentist for Surgery/extraction and antibiotics

High-yield genital/penile disorders

- Zoon's balanitis: p/w single chronic red patch on glands/foreskin in uncircumcised men
  - Ddx: erythroplasia of Queyrat, psoriasis, LP, eczema
  - Path: band-like infiltrate of plasma cells, hemosiderin laden macrophages and numerous capillaries in the upper dermis w/ epidermal atrophy
  - Rx: topical steroids can help; circumcision is curative
- Sclerosing lymphangitis: p/w linear (parallel to corona) cord-like distal penile Shaft mass
  - Pathogenesis: thrombosed/Sclerosed lymphatic vessels due to trauma during Sex
  - Rx: resolves in weeks if patient is able to Stop rough and vigorous Sex

- Median raphe cyst: p/w smooth small cyst (solitary > multiple) b/w the urethra and anus
  - Path: pseudostratified columnar epithelium
  - Rx: surgical excision
- **Genital ulcers**
  - EBV: non-sexually active immunocompetent adolescents; MC on labia minora
    - Dx: EBV PCR or serology
    - Another common cause of non-sexually related genital ulcers is Behçet's or idiopathic aphthous genital ulcers (p/w recurrent **round or oval** ulcer w/ peripheral rim of erythema and adherent yellow exudate centrally)
  - CMV: recalcitrant genital ulcers in immunocompromised patients
    - Dx: CMV PCR
  - HSV: MCC of sexually related genital ulcers
    - Dx: HSV PCR is better than viral culture
- Penile carcinoma: 95% are SCCs but others include erythroplasia of Queyrat, verrucous carcinoma, melanoma, metastatic tumors, Kaposi's, extramammary Paget's and BCC
  - RFs: **chronic dermatitis (9x)**, HPV 16 (6x), no circumcision (3x), smoking (2.8x)

3.27 Pigmentary Disorders

Disorders of hypopigmentation and depigmentation

Vitiligo

- Pathogenesis: melanocytes are destroyed by immune cells by this proposed mechanism
  - IFN-γ → JAK1/2 → STAT1 → CXCL10 → CXCR3 on Th1, Th17 and cytotoxic T cells

    - **IL-15** is involved in memory T-cells (vitiligo returns in same spots after treatment due to these lurking memory T-cells) and represents a future target of therapy
        - Alopecia areata has a pathogenesis involving Th1 cells and IL-15 also which may explain why the MC association of alopecia areata is vitiligo
- p/w well-circumscribed amelanotic (depigmented) macules/patches which have a predilection for the face, dorsal hands, nipples, axillae and sacral/inguinal/genital areas
    - Generalized vitiligo (MC): Universal (> 80% of skin affected), **Vulgaris** (affects those common sites described above) or Acrofacial (affects face, hands and feet)
        - "Treat generalized vitiligo with UVA (just a mnemonic, UVB is better)"
    - Localized vitiligo: Focal (affects one area but not clearly in a segmental distribution), Segmental/unilateral (unilateral and stops at midline; corresponds to path melanocytes take during embryogenesis; MC in children; this form is stable and rarely develops new lesions in new areas, but original spot can grow)
        - "Treat localized vitiligo with Formulations of Steroids"
- Exhibits Köebner phenomenon (develops in areas of trauma such as surgical sites/burns)
- Other clinical variants: vitiligo punctué (confetti-like), inflammatory vitiligo (erythema at margins), trichrome vitiligo (hypopigmented zone b/w normal and depigmented skin)
- Associated disorders
    - Autoimmune disease: **thyroid** is MC but also APECED, alopecia areata and LS&A

- Vogt-Koyanagi-Harada ("Vitiligo Kan't Hear"): **vitiligo and B/L deafness > uveitis**
- Alezzandrini ("Alezzandruni"): unilateral variant of Vogt-Koyanagi-Harada
- **Deafness**: vitiligo is a/w hearing loss (may want to send to an audiologist)

- Path: ↓ **or absent melanocytes** highlighted through MART-1, MITF or HMB45 stains
- Dx: depigmented lesions seen w/ woods lamp (365 nm; "no one gets wood 365 day/yr")
- Rx: difficult to treat so combination therapy is always best
    - Generalized vitiligo: 1st line is nbUVB 2–3x a week (endpoint is mild erythema)
    - Localized vitiligo: alternate high-potency topical steroids with TCIs +/- nbUVB
    - PO pulsed steroids x 3 months in active disease (trichrome/inflammatory vitiligo)
    - Monobenzyl ether of hydroquinone is an FDA approved treatment which causes irreversible full body depigmentation (Michael Jackson did this); major SE is ICD
    - Topical and Oral JAK inhibitors are FDA approved
    - Consider surgical modalities such as melanocyte keratinocyte transplant
- Prognosis: "SMOKE is a/w a worse prognosis"
    - **Symmetric** (non-segmental)/Mucosal lesions, Old age, Köebnerization, Extremity
        - vs poor prognosis in AA (VISTA): Vaginas (female), Infantile/young onset w/ long duration, ↑ Surface area, Temporal scalp, Trachyonychia, Atopy

Halo nevus

- MC in children and young adults on the trunk (back is MC); a/w vitiligo and melanoma

- Path: dense band-like infiltrate of lymphocytes surrounding nest of melanocytes

Chemical and pharmacologic hypomelanosis

- Three major groups of depigmenting compounds
  - Phenols/catechols: monobenzyl ether of hydroquinone and rhododenol
  - Sulfhydryls: mercaptoethylamine hydrochloride, methimazole, sulfanilic acid
  - Miscellaneous: mercurials, arsenic, cinnamic aldehyde, PPD, azelaic acid, imiquimod, corticosteroids, benzyl alcohol, tyrosine kinase inhibitors (imatinib)

Idiopathic guttate hypomelanosis

- ↑ incidence with age (thought to be related to sun exposure, aging and genetics)
- p/w small well demarcated hypopigmented macules (MC on extremities)
- Path: ↓ **melanocytes**

Progressive macular hypomelanosis (PMH)

- ↑ incidence in darkly Pigmented women from tropical regions; **a/w P.acnes**
- p/w Poorly defined, nummular, non-scaly hypopigmented macules/patches on the trunk
- Woods lamp: lights up (Pink/orange Punctate macules) due to copro-Porphyrin 3
- Path: **normal number of melanocytes** but they have ↓ melanosomes/melanin
- Ddx: hypopigmentation of tinea versicolor (yellow-orange patches on woods lamp)
- Rx: P. acnes treatments (topical clindamycin, benzoyl peroxide) +/- Phototherapy

Wood's lamp fluorescence pattern
Vitiligo/ (depigmentation): blue-white
Nevus depigmentosus (hypopigmentation): dull off-white
Erythrasma (Corynebacterium): Coral-red plaque from Coproporphyrin 3
PMH/acne (Pimples): Punctate orange-red-Pink follicular fluorescence from Copro-Porphyrin
Pseudomonas: green from pyoverdine
Tinea versicolor (Yeast): Yellow-orange patches from the porphyrin pityrialactone
Tinea capitus: blue-green vs yellow-green vs no fluorescence
Head lice: pale-blue

*Wood's lamp can also be used to delineate cancer margins before surgery (e.g., dark brown/black fluorescence in lentigo maligna melanoma and coral-red fluorescence when using methyl aminolevulinate (MAL) cream in BCCs)

Nevus depigmentosus

- p/w well-defined congenital **hypomelanotic** mosaic areas (rather than depigmented as the name would suggest), often breaking apart into smaller macules at the periphery
- Woods lamp: dull-off white due to a ↓ in melanin
- Path: **normal number of melanocytes** but they have ↓ melanosomes/melanin
- Ddx: may look like a spot of vitiligo on a Kodachrome but **vitiligo is depigmented**

Leukodermas without hypomelanosis (related to vasoconstriction; **path is 100% normal**)

- Woronoff's ring: White/blanched halo which surrounds psoriatic lesions after treatment
- Nevus anemicus: p/w pale area w/ peripheral erythema on the trunk at birth; lesion becomes indistinguishable from surrounding skin on diascopy (vs nevus depigmentosus)
    - Pathogenesis: localized hypersensitivity of blood vessels to catecholamines

  - o Dx: application of heat or an ice-cube will often accentuate the lesion
- Angiospastic macules (**Bier spots**): pale macules on distal extremities of young women
  - o May be a/w systemic disease but unless history/PE warrants further workup, **no laboratory investigations are indicated**
  - o BASCULE (Bier Anaemic Spots, Cyanosis w/ Urticarial-Like Eruption) syndrome: irregular white macules on a background of cyanosis that appear after minutes of immobile standing followed by the appearance of pruritic, orange-red papules superimposed on the white macules; resolves w/ sitting or walking
    - a/w orthostatic hypotension (consider performing tilt test)

Pigmentary mosaicism

- Hypomelanosis of Itö: unilateral or bilateral hypopigmented streaks along Blaschko's lines evident at birth +/- CNS, MSK, **eye abnormalities and hypodontia**
  - o "I put an umlat over the 'ö' in Ito because it looks like eyes and a mouth"
- Nevus depigmentosus: discussed above
- **Rx: observe only (workup only if symptomatic)**

Nutritional hypomelanosis

- Kwashiorkor (severe protein deficiency): thick brown-red desquamation ("flakey paint") which leave behind hypopigmented patches, mostly at sites of friction/pressure
  - o "Wash that ugly red-brown flakey paint off to reveal the white underneath"
- Diffuse pigmentary dilution can also be seen in deficiencies of copper and selenium

Hypomelanosis secondary to cutaneous inflammation (post-inflammatory hypopigmentation)

- Cutaneous inflammation alters melanosome and melanin biogenesis and transport
- Path: normal # of melanocytes

Infectious and parasitic hypomelanosis

- "These bugs result in LOST Pigment"
    - Leprosy: multiple hypopigmented, slightly scaly anesthetic macules and patches
    - post-kala-azar Leishmaniasis: hypomelanotic macules and papules that usually start around the mouth and later spreads out in a symmetric distribution
        - Pts have recovered from visceral leishmaniasis and are otherwise well
    - Onchocerciasis: punctate hypomelanotic macules on shin ("leopard skin")
    - Syphilis and other treponematoses: secondary syphilis ("necklace of Venus"), pinta (vitiligo-like areas over bony prominences), yaws (hypomelanosis on wrists)
    - Tinea versicolor: slightly scaly hypopigmented macules on the chest, back, face
    - Progressive macular hypomelanosis: non-scaly hypopigmented patches on trunk

Disorders of hyperpigmentation

Post-inflammatory hyperpigmentation (PIH)

- Acquired excess of pigment after cutaneous inflammation MC in those with dark skin
- Pathogenesis
    - Epidermal PIH: ↑ in melanin production and/or transfer to keratinocytes
        - MC from acne, AD, psoriasis and PR

  - Dermal PIH: melanin falls into dermis via damaged BM and stay in melanophages
    - MC from dermatoses w/ BM damage (LP, lichenoid drug rash, DLE, FDE)
- p/w tan to dark brown (epidermal PIH) or gray-blue (dermal PIH) macules/patches
- Path: ↑ pigment in keratinocytes (epiderma PIH) or dermal melanophages (dermal PIH)
- Rx: hydroquinone, cysteamine, kojic acid, L-ascorbic acid, licorice, mequinol, niacinamide, retinoids, steroids, soy, arbutin, azelaic acid, glycolic acid, salicylic acid

Melasma (chloasma, Mask of pregnancy)

- More common in women of childbearing age with darker skin
- p/w symmetric hyperpigmented macules/patches w/ "Moth-eaten" edges (MC on face)
- Pathogenesis: UVR/**visible light** or hormones activate hyperfunctional melanocytes
- Exacerbating factors: UVR, estrogen, thyroid dysfunction and meds (phenytoin)
- Path: ↑ Melanin in all layers of epidermis (esp. basal layer), ↑ dermal Melanophages
- Dx: epidermal areas are accentuated with woods lamp, areas of dermal pigment are not
- Rx: same treatment as PIH + diligent sun protection and discontinue OCPs
  - Systemic tranexamic acid works well (SE is thrombosis such as PE/MI/DVT)
  - Tinted sunscreens w/ iron oxide and titanium dioxide offer better protection against visible light than micronized nanoparticles of zinc and titanium

Arsenical melanosis

- p/w hyperpigmentation on areas not exposed to sunlight (back and upper chest are MC)
- May see other signs of arsenic poisoning (raindrop hypopigmentation, acral arsenical keratosis), Mee's lines (transverse white bands in fingernails), Bowens/SCCs

Lichen planus pigmentosus

- Variant of LP in adults with darker skin
- p/w oval brown to gray-brown macules/patches in sun-exposed or intertriginous areas
- Path: mild lichenoid infiltrate w/ dermal melanophages

Linear and whorled nevoid hypermelanosis

- Sporadic skin condition with clones of skin cells which have ↑ pigment production
- p/w hyperpigmented linear (Blaschkoid) streaks presenting in infancy
- May be a/w systemic findings (CNS, MSK, **deafness or cardiac**)
    - "Linear and whorled hypear-melanosis affects the heart and ears"

Prurigo pigmentosa

- Classic patient is a young adult Japanese female
- p/w **pruritic erythematous reticulate papules/plaques** which rapidly involute leaving behind residual **reticulate macular hyperpigmentation** MC on upper back (scapula)
- a/w keto diet and other low carb states (fasting, DM, **post-bariatric surgery**, anorexia)
- Ddx: REM (erythematous phase) or CARP (pigmented phase)

- Path: neutrophilic infiltrate w/ necrotic keratinocytes (red papules) or lymphocytic infiltrate with numerous melanophages (hyperpigmented patches)
- Rx: doxycycline or dapsone
    - Prurigo pigmentosa rap: pt is a jap, p/w red pap on scap, treat with doxy or dap

Familial progressive hyperpigmentation

- AD gain of function mutation in KIT ligand gene (KITLG)
- p/w diffuse hyperpigmented patches on palms, soles, lips and conjunctiva in infancy

Pigmentary demarcation lines

- Demarcation lines b/w dorsal and ventral skin surfaces where dorsal side has ↑ pigment
- These lines are B/L, symmetric, present during infancy and are located at various sites:
    - Group A is Arms (MC demarcation line site) so B must be legs
    - Group C is midline Chest so D must be midline back
    - Group E is lateral chest (from medial clavicle to ipsilateral nipple on both sides)
    - Group F, G, H are on the Face

3.28 Cutaneous Manifestation of Systemic Disease

Endocrine disorders

Hypothyroidism and hyperthryroidism

- p/w lethargy, thin hair, edematous face, large tongue and cold, dry, pale skin that may have a yellowish hue (esp around palms, soles, and NL folds) from carotenemia ("pseudojaundice"; can distinguish from true jaundice by sparing of sclera)

- Alopecia involves lateral eyebrow in 50% of patients (Hertoghe or Queen Anne sign)
- May see generalized myxedema due to deposition of glycosaminoglycans ("puffy eyes")
    - In hyperthyroidism there is ↑ glycosaminoglycans synthesis → thyroid acropachy (digital clubbing), pretibial myxedema and exophthalmos
- Dx: TSH

Diabetes mellitus

- Skin manifestations strongly a/w diabetes mellitus
    - **Acanthosis nigricans**: velvety hyperpigmented thick skin folds; 75%; MC finding
        - **Rx**: improve insulin resistance (diet), topical retinoids, keratolytics
    - **Xerosis**: 2nd MC skin manifestation; 50%
    - **Diabetic dermopathy**: small, well-demarcated red to brown atrophic macules on the shins ("I think of it as a macular version of necrobiosis lipoidica")
    - Sceroderma-like skin changes: thick skin, sclerodactyly w/ periungual telangiectasias), "prayer sign" (inability to press palmar surfaces together)
    - **Bullosis diabeticorum:** rapid onset tense non-inflammatory blisters on legs (MC)
    - Scleredema diabeticorum: induration of upper back skin; a/w IgG-k gammopathy
    - Necrobiosis lipoidica: well-demarcated atrophic yellow plaques on shins; F > M
- Non-specific dermatologic signs and symptoms: ichthyosiform changes on the shins, acquired perforating dermatosis, eruptive xanthomas, acrochordons, pruritis, finger pebbles ("pebble sign" or "Huntley sign"), KP, PPD, palmar erythema, Rubeosis facei (facial flushing;

a/w retinopathy), yellow skin/nails, onychocryptosis (ingrown nails)
- Dermatologic diseases a/w diabetes: GA, psoriasis, LP, vitiligo, HS, glucagonoma
- Neuropathic ulcers: painless ulcers surrounded by callused rim at pressure sites
- Infections: mucocutaneous candidiasis, diabetic foot ulcers are often infected w/ pseudomonas, staph (MC bacterial infection), mucormycosis, necrotizing fasciitis

Addison's disease
- Adrenal glands unable to produce sufficient minerocorticoids and glucocorticoids
- p/w fatigue, ↓ axillary/pubic hair and **hyperpigmentation** of sun-exposed areas, palmar creases, frictional surfaces (axilla), scars, vermillion border, areola, nails and oral mucosa

Organ failure

Renal disease
- Non-specific signs: xerosis, half-and-half nails, pruritis, yellow skin, hyperpigmentation, ecchymosis, PCT/ pseudoporphyria, calcinosis cutis
- Specific signs: acquired perforating dermatoses, calciphylaxis, NSF, uremic frost
- Genoderms: nail-patella syndrome, Reed syndrome, tuberous sclerosis, Lesch-Nyhan syndrome, LUMBAR syndrome, NF1 and recessive dystrophic EB

Liver disease
- MC cutaneous symptom is pruritis which is often protracted and disabling
    - Rx ("Cirrhotics Scratch Real Nebulously"): Cholestyramine (1st line), Sertraline (2nd line), Rifampin, (3rd line), Naloxone (4th line)

- Others include jaundice, spider angiomas/telangiectasias classically over upper trunk and face, palmar erythema, dilated abdominal wall veins, gynecomastia, xanthelasma
- Nails: clubbing, thickening, ridging, white bands (Muehrke's), Terrys nails, blue lunulae
- Steatorrhea cause malabsorption and vitamin deficiencies: vitamin A (xerosis, phrynoderma), vitamin D (alopecia), vitamin K (purpura), vitamin B (glossitis, seb derm)

Malignancy (not covered elsewhere)

- **Dx: if there are signs of malignancy (e.g., ulcerative skin lesion, weight loss) then do a malignancy workup (e.g., LN exam, pelvic US, CXR, abdominal CT)**
- **Rx: always treat underlying malignancy**

Cutaneous signs associated with malignancy ("LGBTQ")

- Hypertrichosis lanuginosa acquisita ("LGB"): Lung > colon cancer (GI) > Breast
  - p/w sudden onset of long lanugo-like hairs which start on face and spread down
- Tripe palms ("LG"): Lung cancer or Gastric/GI (tripe palms + acanthosis nigricans)
- Acanthosis nigricans (without tripe palms): a/w gastric cancer (MC)
  - p/w AN in unusual locations such as the mouth (p/w cobblestone lips/tongue)
- PPK ("LLG"): Lung cancer, Lymphomas, GI (esp esophagus) and many others
- Eruptive SKs (Sign of Leser-Trélat; LGBTQ): **Gastiric** cancer is MC
- Paraneoplastic sign of multiple myeloma: p/w small hyperkeratotic spicules on the nose

Cutaneous signs of metastases ("LGBTQ")

- Lung, GI and Breast ("LGB") are the 3 MC primary sites of skin metastases: Lung is MC in men (except men < 40 years old where melanoma is MC) while Breast is MC in women
    - p/w red violaceous papules and nodules
- Sister Mary Joseph nodule: metastasis from the pelvis or abdomen (GI > GU)
    - p/w palpable nodule bulging into the umbilicus
- Alopecia neoplastica (localized scarring alopecia): a/w Breast mets ("Breast = Bald")
- Carcinoma en cuirasse (hard peau d'orange texture) and carcinoma erysipeloides (raised red plaque) occur on the chest from metastatic Breast cancer infiltrating lymphatics
- Highly vascularized papules/nodules on the head/neck: renal metastasis
    - But the MC scalp mets are more likely to be from Lung (men) or Breast (women)

Paraneoplastic syndromes

- Acquired angioedema ("L"): a/w Lymphoproliferative disease
- Acquired ichthyosis ("L"): **Lymphoma** (Hodgkin/non-Hodgkin) > lung and breast
    - If it is scaly (PPK/ichthyosis) the "L" stands for Lymphoma in addition to Lung
- Anti-epiligrin cicatricial pemphigoid ("LG"): Lung and GI adenocarcinoma > uterine
- Erythema gyratum repens ("LGB"): Lung > GI and Breast
- Dermatomyositis ("PLONC"): Pancreas, Lung, **Ovarian** (MC), NHL, Colorectal
- Juvenile xanthogranuloma: juvenile myelomonocytic leukemia (and NF1)
- MEN2A (sipple): medullary thyroid, pheochromocytoma, hyperparathyroidism

- Necrolytic migratory erythema: pancreatic glucagon-secreting tumor

High-yield genoderms that are a/w malignancy (refer to chapter 4 for mnemonics)

- Birt-Hogg-Dubé: renal cancer, medullary thyroid cancer, colon cancer
- Pachydermoperiostosis: bronchogenic carcinoma
- Peutz-Jeghers: GI, ovarian, breast, pancreatic and endometrial carcinoma
- Carney complex: atrial and skin myxoma, psammomatous melanotic schwannomas, testicular tumors, pigmented nodular adrenocortical disease, pituitary adenoma
- Gardners: pilomatricomas, skull osteomas, desmoid tumors
- Dystrophic EB: SCCs
- Tuberous sclerosis: astrocytomas, cardiac rhabdomyomas, renal angiomyolipomas
- Muir-Torre syndrome: **GI > GU**
- Cowden: breast and thyroid cancer

Florid cutaneous papillomatosis (Schwartz-Burgess syndrome)

- Paraneoplastic disease characterized by rapid and widespread eruption of verrucous skin-colored papules over the entire body (MC on dorsal hands and wrists)
- a/w **GI adenocarcinoma (MC)** > lung, breast, bladder, liver, prostate, ovary, uterus
- May occur w/ other paraneoplastic signs (AN, tripe palms, PPK, sign of Leser-Trélat, etc.)
- Path: wart-like (hyperkeratosis, papillomatosis, acanthosis) but there are no koilocytes
    - o HPV can be ruled out by immunofluorescence or DNA hybridization studies

Carcinoid syndrome

- p/w head, neck and upper trunk **flushing**, pellagra-like rash (niacin is ↓ as tryptophan is diverted to serotonin production), diarrhea, **wheezing/Coughing,** CV disease
- Typically occurs when a **midgut (small intestine)** tumor metastasizes to liver (95%), but foregut (bronchial and gastric) tumors cause carcinoid syndrome w/o liver metastases
- Dx: ↑ 5-HIAA in urine, abdominal imaging (CT is best)

Acrokeratosis paraneoplastica (Bazex syndrome)

- p/w Acral, psoriasiform plaques on hands, feet, nose and ears ("acro-keratosis")
- Longitudinal and horizontal ridging of the nails is seen in 75% of patient
- a/w malignancies of the upper Aerodigestive tract (e.g., **laryngeal** cancer)

Extramammary Paget's disease (EMPD)

- p/w slowly expanding red plaque w/ scattered white scale and erosions ("**strawberry and cream**") located MC on the **vulva of women** or **perianal area of men** but can occur in axillae, ear canal (ceruminous glands), eyelid (Moll gland) or scalp; F > M
    - o 5x risk of internal malignancy w/ **perianal** location
- Primary EMPD (75%): whereas neoplastic cells in Paget's migrate to the epidermis from **lactiferous ducts, in EMPD they begin in the epidermis ("adenocarcinoma in situ")** from toker cells (apocrine sweat glands); **GCFDP-15+, CK20-**
- Secondary EMPD (20%): direct extension or mets from visceral malignancy: **GI/GU** > prostate, endometrial, ovarian adenocarcinoma; **GCFDP-15-, CK20+ (also CK7+ if GU)**

- Mnemonic in order from MC to least common ("R U COPEing w/ EMPD?"): Rectal (colonoscopy), Urothelial (cystoscopy) > Cervical or Ovarian (pelvic exam), Prostate (PSA/prostate exam), Endometrial (pelvic exam)

- **Path: large cells with ample cytoplasm (glandular differentiation apparent)** spitting into the epidermis and crushing the basal layer; normal maturation of keratinocytes
  - IHC: EMA, PAS (diastase resistant), CEA, CK7, gross cystic protein (GCDFP-15)
    - "EMA passed by and resisted a sea of 7 cocks, gross!
    - Disease extending from internal cancer is **CK20**$^{+}$, CK7^{-} and **GCDFP-15**$^{-}$
      - "But internally EMA wanted 20 cocks and did not find them gross"
- Rx: **MOHs w/ CK7 immunostaining** and **WLE w/ 5 cm margins** offer 97% cure rate
  - MOHs w/o IHC and WLE w/o large margins have a 23–33% recurrence rate
  - Non-surgical options ("PRICE"): PDT, Radiation, Imiquimod, CO2, Efudex
- Workup: **colonoscopy and urethral cystoscopy**, PSA/ prostate exams, pelvic exam/US)
- NCCN screening guidelines: follow-up q 6 months for 3 years, then annually for 10 years

Paget's disease

- Neoplastic cells in Paget's migrate to the epidermis from **lactiferous ducts**
- p/w chronic, scaly, eczematous plaque on the nipple and later involves the areola
- Path: **CEA and CK7-positive** large, ovoid, pleomorphic cells w/ pale-staining cytoplasm and hyperchromatic nuclei throughout all layers of the epidermis

- Workup: **refer to breast oncologist** to rule out invasive ductal carcinoma

POEMS syndrome

- Rare Paraneoplastic syndrome caused by a lamda-restricted Plasma cell dyscrasia
- MC initial symptom is **Peripheral sensory/motor neuropathy**
- The acronym POEMS helps to remember some findings but it does not tell you enough
    - Polyneuropathy, Organomegaly, Endocrinopathy, M-protein, Skin changes
- Criteria: must hit both mandatory major criteria, 1 non-mandatory major and 1 minor
    - Mandatory major: **Polyneuropathy, Plasma cell dyscrasia** (always lamda)
    - Major (not in mnemonic): **Castleman** (MC cancer), sclerotic bone lesions, ↑VEGF
    - Minor: organomegaly, volume overload (Pleural effusions, edema), endocrinopathy (hypogonadism > thyroid), skin changes (**hyper-Pigmentation** is MC, glomeruloid hemangiomas are classic but cherry angiomas are MC, leukonychia, sclerodermoid, hypertrichosis), Papilledema, Polycythemia
        - There is a strong association w/ skin lesions and abnormal PFTs
- Workup: **↑VEGF**, TSH, glucose, SPEP/UPEP shows lamda phenotype, LN aspirate shows HHV8-negative multicentric Castleman's disease, CT shows sclerotolytic bone lesions

Chapter 4: Pediatric dermatology

4.1 Neonatal Dermatology

Physiologic phenomena of the newborn

Transient vascular phenomena: related to immature autonomic control of the vasculature

- Cutis marmorata: reticulate bluish mottling of the skin which **resolves with warming**
  - Persistent/Durable Cutis Marmorata: a/w Downs, Cornelia de Lange, Menke's
- Harlequin color change: reddening of one Half of the body (sharp midline demarcation) w/ simultaneous blanching of the other Half when infant lies on their side (ddx: CHILD)
- Acrocyanosis: bluish discoloration of the extremities brought on by cold and crying and which disappears on warming or when baby stops crying

Neonatal desquamation

- Occurs within the 1st 24–48 hours and can take up to 3 weeks to complete
  - "Desquamation normally occurs on Day Dos (2 in Spanish) of life"
  - Persistence can be a sign of ichthyosis
- Desquamation at birth can be a sign of postmaturity, intrauterine anoxia or ichthyosis
  - When diffuse must be distinguished from CIE (CIE is more erythematous)
- Premature infants would not show desquamation until several weeks after delivery

Bronze baby syndrome

- Grayish-brown discoloration of skin, serum and urine after phototherapy

Newborn injuries: "Injured long before they ever went to SCHool"

- Subcutaneous fat necrosis: **healthy** full-term neonates p/w indurated red SQ nodules localized to only fat-rich sites (back, cheek, buttocks, thighs) in the first week of life
    - Pathogenesis: ↑ Saturated to unsaturated fatty acid ratio in infants
    - Path: needle shaped clefts in fat w/ Surrounding granulomatous inflammation Dx: Screen for **hypercalcemia** for Six months (granulomas cause hypercalcemia)
    - Rx: Supportive care; treat associated hypercalcemia if present; avoid vitamin D
- Sclerema neonatorum: Sick/**debilitated preterm** neonates p/w Sudden appearance of Symmetric widespread Stone-hard Skin in 1st weeks of life (spares genitals/hands/feet)
    - Ddx: diffuse hard skin in newborn ("Really Hard Skin") Restrictive dermopathy, Hutchinson-Gilford progeria, Stiff skin syndrome and Sclerema neonatorum
    - Path: needle shaped clefts in fat **w/o surrounding granulomatous inflammation**
        - Baby is too sick to mount an immune response
    - Dx: metabolic acidosis, hyperkalemia
    - Rx: Supportive care in NICU (Steroids controversial)
    - Prognosis: most die of **Sepsis and Shock**
- Subgaleal hematoma: massive bleeding into the subgaleal space after traumatic delivery

  - o Dependent edema over a Sizeable area; crosses suture lines; **anemia, DIC, Shock**
  - o Rx: Supportive care in NICU (fluids and blood products as indicated)
- Cephalohematoma: blood between the Cranium and the periosteum (**sub-periosteal**)
  - o p/w U/L > B/L swelling over the scalp (**parietal MC**) that **do not cross suture lines** (**sharp Cliff drop visible**, usually from a swollen parietal to a normal frontal scalp)
  - o Dx: CBC may show mild anemia
  - o Rx: resolves in weeks w/o treatment
  - o Baby at risk for Calcification, hyperbilirubinemia and infection
- Caput succedaneum: edematous fluid in scalp (below skin) due to pressure from cervix
  - o p/w diffuse swelling of the scalp which crosses suture lines
    - "Caput Can Cross whereas Ceph (S sound) Stays inside Suture line"
  - o Rx: resolves in days w/o treatment
- Halo scalp ring: annular alopecia that p/w a circumferential ring around the scalp
  - o Occurs after caput succedaneum due to a pressure necrosis phenomenon

Transient neonatal eruptions: "Mild Transient Neonatal Eruptions" (none require Rx)

- Milia (congenital): up to half of newborns p/w tiny white smooth milia on their **face**
  - o Bohn's nodules and Epstein's pearls are the oral counterpart of congenital milia
    - Bohn's nodules: alveolar ridge ("right next to teeth; teeth are like bones")

        - Epstein's pearls: palatal raphe ("Can also remember they are on roof of mouth because Epstein hung himself from the roof of his cell")
- Miliaria Crystallina: due to intra-Corneal obstruction of eccrine ducts
    - p/w fragile, Clear-colored "dew-drop" vesicles on the upper half of the body
- Miliaria Rubra: deeper intraepidermal obstruction of eccrine ducts
    - p/w Red papules MC in **intertriginous sites** of babies
- Transient Neonatal Pustular melanosis (TNPM): seen at Time of birth in **AA** Term infants
    - Three stages: Pustules → **collarettes of scale** → Pigmented macules
    - Dx: Wright's stain of pustule reveals **neutrophils**
    - Ddx: ETN has pustules w/ red halo 1–3 days after birth and never on palms/soles whereas TNPM has pustules w/ no red halo present at birth that becomes hyperpigmented and can be anywhere, including on palms/soles
- Transient myeloproliferative disorder of Downs syndrome: vesiculopustular eruption on the face > trunk or extremities that occurs in 10% of neonates with Downs syndrome
    - The skin lesions resolve in months but babies are at ↑ risk of myeloid leukemia
- Neonatal acne (due to hormonal influences of not yet involuted sebaceous glands) and Neonatal cephalic pustulosis (NCP; due to Malassezia; affects up to 50% of term infants)
    - p/w small follicular-based inflammatory papules (neonatal acne) or non-follicular-based papules/pustules (NCP) on the cheeks > chin and forehead
        - Unlike infantile acne, neither has comedones

- o Rx: resolves in months but topical antifungals can lead to a more rapid resolution
- Erythema toxicum neonatorum (ETN): affects 50% of full-term infants
  - o p/w **Erythematous** macules, papules, pustules and wheals (described as **"flea-bitten"**) anywhere **Except palms/soles** which **starts 24–48 hours after birth**
  - o Dx: Wright's stain of pustules reveals Eosinophils +/- peripheral Eosinophilia
  - o Ddx
    - ▪ ETN: widespread (spares palms/soles) vesiculopustules on red base
    - ▪ Neonatal cephalic pustulosis: papules/pustules on cheeks and forehead
    - ▪ TNPM: widespread pustules/collarette of scale/pigmented macules
    - ▪ Acropustulosis of infancy: crops of vesicopustules on the hands/feet
    - ▪ Eosinophilic folliculitis: crops of itchy vesicopustules on the face/scalp

Congenital infections

- Neonatal Candidiasis ("k sound"): common infection acquired during delivery/postnatally
  - o p/w monomorphic paps/pustules in diaper area (Crotch) and thrush at 1–2 weeks
  - o Dx (for all candida infections): KOH shows budding yeast and pseudohyphae
  - o Rx: topical anti-yeast medication (imidazole; Ketoconazole)
- Congenital candidiasis: uncommon in-utero infection (so it presents at birth)
  - o p/w widespread monomorphic papules **at birth** → pustules → desquamation

        - Characteristic yellow-brown papules may be found on the umbilical cord
    - RFs: foreign body in uterus/cervix (IUD) and history of vaginal candidiasis
    - Rx: IV antifungals if baby is ill, preterm or low-birth weight (otherwise topical)
- Invasive fungal dermatitis: occurs in very-low-birth-weight newborns 1 week after birth
    - p/w widespread "burn-like" erythema w/ erosions and a sepsis-like illness
    - MC pathogen is Candida albicans > Aspergillus
    - RFs: very low birth weight infants; antibiotic and central catheter use in the NICU
    - Dx: blood culture is gold standard; labs show neutropenia and thrombocytopenia
- Neonatal varicella: maternal primary VZV infection 7 days before to 2 days after delivery
    - Presents at 0–14 days w/ widespread vesicles on a red base ("looks like chicken pox"); may be severe w/ pneumonia, hepatitis, coagulopathy and death
    - Dx (for all herpes infections): Tzank prep, DFA, viral culture, or serologies
    - Rx: VZIG + IV acyclovir
- Congenital varicella ("looks like a chicken"): infection in first 20 weeks of gestation
    - Most women who contract varicella during pregnancy have asymptomatic babies
    - Presents at birth with **limb hypoplasia** ("arms look like a chicken"), mental retardation ("IQ of a chicken"), Chorioretinitis/Cataracts/nystagmus ("chickens have poor eye site"), deep stellate scars, microphthalmia and hydro-Cephalus
    - Rx: VZIG + IV acyclovir
- Neonatal herpes Simplex: infection during birth which presents 1–2 weeks later w/ CNS disease and vesicles/

erosions that favors the Scalp and torso (skin in contact w/ vagina)

  - Dx: biopsy, Tzanck, DFA, PCR or viral culture
  - Rx: IV acyclovir (does not help with the CNS/neurologic sequelae)

- Congenital (intrauterine) herpes simplex: primary or secondary maternal infection causes baby to be born w/ **widespread lesions** (vesicles/pustules/erosions/scars); scalp is often affected by **aplasia Cutis**-like areas; Chorioretinitis; microCephaly; 66% mortality
  - Dx: Tzanck, DFA, PCR or viral culture
  - Rx: IV acyclovir + oral acyclovir therapy for 6 months
- Congenital rubella (ABCDE): maternal infection (most severe if acquired in 1st trimester)
  - **patent ductus Arteriosus** (and other forms of congenital heart disease)
  - Blueberry muffin baby: purple papules d/t extramedullary hematopoiesis (EMH)
  - **Cataracts**, intra-Cranial Calcifications
  - **Deafness** (MC symptom)
  - Dx: Erythroid precursors (nucleated RBCs) and megakaryocytes
  - Rx: prevention w/ vaccine (manifestations of congenital rubella are lifelong)
- Congenital toxoplasmosis ("Cox"): Consumption of un-Cooked meats + exposure to Cats
  - p/w Chorioretinitis, hydro-Cephalus, intra-Cranial Calcifications, blueberry rash
  - Rx: pyrimethamine, sulfadiazine and folinic acid x 1 year
- Congenital CMV: primary maternal (most severe) or postnatal infection
  - Most common infectious cause of congenital... "MR DICS"

        - Mental Retardation, Deafness, Intracranial calcifications, Cutaneous blueberry muffin rash (extramedullary hematopoiesis), Seizures
    - Dx ("FIST"): human Fibroblast culture (gold standard), Intranuclear "owl's eye" inclusion in endothelial cells on path, Shell vial assay, Tests such as serology/PCR
    - Rx: IV ganciclovir
- Congenital syphilis: presents at birth when mother has primary or secondary syphilis
    - Early congenital Syph (< 2 y/o): Skin (vesiculobullous eruption, macular copper-colored papulosquamous lesions, mucous patch), Snuffles, pseudo-paralysis
    - Late congenital syph (> 2 y/o; "not skin"): Hutchinson's triad (interstitial keratitis, Hutchinson's teeth, 8th nerve deafness), Hyperplastic first molar (Mulberry's molar), Higoumenakis sign (**U/L thickening of the dominant sides clavicle**), linear rhagades at oral commissures, High-arched palate, saber shins, Clutton's joints
    - Dx: path or dark field exam of skin lesions, DFA or serologies (IgM FTA-ABS)
    - Rx: parenteral penicillin (prognosis for promptly treated syphilis is very good)

Bedside tests for the diagnosis of vesicles or pustules in a newborn

Wright or Giemsa
- Eosinophils: widespread lesions (ETN), linear streaks (incontinentia pigmenti), lesions on scalp with pruritis (eosinophilic pustular folliculitis)
- Neutrophils: widespread pustules (TNPM), hands/feet (infantile acropustulosis)
- Large histiocytes with reniform nuclei: Langerhans cell histiocytosis
- Immature myeloid cells: transient myeloproliferative disorder

Gram stain shows bacteria: bacterial infection (e.g., staph impetigo)
KOH prep or PAS stain shows yeast forms: candidiasis or neonatal cephalic pustulosis
Tzanck smear shows multinucleated giant cells: herpes
Mineral oil/KOH/water prep shows mites, feces or eggs: scabies

Birthmarks (not discussed in neoplastic dermatology chapter)

- Connective tissue nevus (CTN): hamartoma of elastin or collagen
  - p/w skin-colored to yellowish plaques/nodules w/ p'eau d'orange texture
  - a/w genoderms ("Tubby Men are Pro Busch light which makes them connect")
    - Tuberous sclerosis: Shagreen patch (pebbly plaque MC on lower back)
    - MEN-1: pedunculated collagenomas + facial angiofibromas
    - Proteus syndrome: cerebriform plantar CTN
    - Buschke-Ollendorf: either collagenomas or elastomas + osteopoikilosis
  - Path
    - Collagenoma: haphazard, thickened collagen bundles
    - Elastoma: ↑ elastic fibers (changes are subtle, need VVG stain)
- Congenital smooth muscle hamartoma: hamartoma of erector pili muscle

- p/w hyperpigmented plaques w/ hypertrichosis on **lower back/lumbosacral area**
- Overlap w/ Becker's nevus but arises at birth not in puberty, located on lower back not upper trunk and is not a/w hypoplasia of underlying structures

- Nevus simplex (salmon patch): benign transient vascular ectasia of capillary bed
  - p/w pink macules and patches on glabella ("angel kiss"), eyelids and occiput ("stork's bite"); they all resolve over months to years except stork's bite
- Supernummary/accessory nipple (polythelia)
  - p/w asymptomatic brown macule w/ central papule located anywhere along the "milk line" (from axilla to groin) but are MC directly below their normal location
  - Path: epidermal hyperplasia and central duct w/ surrounding smooth muscle

Developmental anomalies (list is from superior to inferior for MC location affected)

Risk of cutaneous sign's being indicative of occult spinal dysraphism
• High risk ("'i' is 2nd or 2nd-last letter"): **midline… lipoma (MC),** dermoid cyst, sinus tract, acrochordons, **vestigial tail**, large hemangioma (>2 cm), aplasia cutis congenita or having ≥ 2 lower risk stigmata • Intermediate risk ("H"): faun tail Hypertrichosis, small Hemangioma, large dimples/Holes (> 5 mm) which are > 2.5 cm superior from anal verge • Low risk: PWS, dimples, CALM, mongolian spot or nevus depigmentosus

- Aplasia cutis congenita (ACC; superior scalp near hair whorl is MC): localized absence of skin which resolves w/ alopecic scar; often w/ hair collar sign → ring of course hair around a congenital scalp nodule (marker for spinal dysraphism/ectopic neural tissue)

- If ACC is midline, atypical, a/w hair collar sign or skull defect → get an **MRI**
- If ACC is typical (no PWS/hair collar/normal PE) and not midline → wound care
- High yield facts of ACC: "MBA"
  - **MRI**/US can diagnose intracranial extension (only use US if < 6 months)
  - Methimazole/carbimazole: mother took during pregnancy → ACC in baby
  - Bart syndrome: aplasia cutis of lower leg + DDEB (blisters at birth)
  - Adams-Oliver syndrome: Aplasia cutis + CMTC + heart and limb defects
    - O represents a heart (like in mnemonic for JONES criteria)
  - Congenital (intrauterine) HSV infection is another common cause
- Dx: **MRI**; **US if < 6 months old** (vertebrae do not ossify until > 4 months of age)

- Meningocele/encephalocele (<u>occiput</u> MC): herniation of Cranial Contents through skull
  - **Compressible** SQ midline mass that **transilluminates** (light Comes through)
  - Compression of jugular vein (and Crying) causes it to expand (+ Furstenberg test)
    - Dermoid cyst and nasal glioma also p/w midline mass but are firm, non-compressible and do not expand w/ crying or compression of jugular vein
  - Midline mass (lipoma) > hair collar sign is highly suspicious for cranial dysraphism
  - Workup: radiologic imaging w/ MRI needed before surgical planning
- Dermoid cyst (upper lateral forehead/<u>eyebrow</u> is MC): p/w firm SQ nodule

- **On the nose they can p/w protruding hair (sinus ostium) →** pathognomonic
- Unlike encephaloceles, there is a negative Furstenberg test (non-compressible)
- They continue to grow and affect nearby structures, so excision is recommended
- Workup: **get MRI if** Midline; if on Eyebrow and can palpate posterior aspect you can proceed w/ Excision, but deep orbital lesions also require imaging

- Nasal glioma (root of nose): p/w firm, non-compressible, non-pulsatile SQ nodule
  - Workup: imaging to rule out intracranial extension before surgical excision
- Transverse nasal crease/transverse nasal milia: **represents embryonic fusion planes**
- Accessory tragus (pre-auricular region to angle of mouth): 1st brachial arch defect
  - a/w Goldenhar (oculoauriculovertebral syndrome): U/L facial asymmetry, ocular, **renal**, cardiac and otorhinolaryngological defects (cleft lip/palate, **deafness**)
    - Rx: continues to grow so excision is recommended
      - MC complication of surgery is **chondritis**
    - Workup: next step after finding an accessory tragus is acoustic testing
- Thyroglossal duct cyst (midline neck): moves w/ swallowing; MC congenital neck mass
  - Path: variable lining w/ bright pink thyroid follicles in the wall
  - Workup: for all these congenital neck cysts, get US/MRI and ENT for excision
- Branchial cleft cyst (anterior border of SCM in neck): 2nd cleft (MC) fails to obliterate

    - Workup: for all these congenital neck cysts, get US/MRI and ENT for excision
- Congenital rests of neck/wattle (anterior border of SCM): remnants of branchial arches
    - **Composed of Cartilage**; considered the cervical variant of accessory tragus
    - Workup: excision after imaging to rule out sinus or fistula
- Midline cervical cleft (midline neck): midline cervical papule ("nipple-like") superior to a linear sinus tract that forms due to impaired fusion of 1st and 2nd branchial arch
    - Workup: imaging prior to excision (to prevent cervical contracture)
- Bronchogenic cysts (midline over clavicle): midline inferior neck at suprasternal notch
    - Path: ciliated columnar epithelium w/ cartilage, smooth muscle and goblet cells
    - Workup: excision after imaging
- Umbilical granuloma (umbilicus): red friable papule (granulation tissue after losing cord)
    - Rx: use Silver Nitrate to cauterize Umbilical Granulomas (SNUG)
- Umbilical Polyp (umbilicus): p/w pink red nodule w/ **Persistent drainage** in umbilicus
    - Patent urachus: US shows incomplete obliteration of the urachus
        - Path: bladder epithelia (flat cuboidal cells)
    - Patent omphalomesenteric duct: incomplete obliteration of vitelline duct on US
        - Path: GI epithelia (goblet cells)
- Amniotic band syndrome: constricting band around distal extremity → Amputation
- Congenital Hemi-Hypertrophy: one side of the body is longer than the other

  - a/w cutaneous findings: Hyperpigmentation, Hypertrichosis, telangiectasias
  - a/w anomalies in 50% (Half): ear (Hearing) and eye deformities, GU anomalies
  - a/w tumors: Hepatic (Wilm's tumor) > kidney and adrenal tumors

4.2 Viral Exanthems of Childhood

Rubeola (Measles, "first disease")

- RNA virus; paramyxovirus family
- Transmission: respiratory droplets
- p/w fever, prodrome of 3 Cs (cough/coryza/conjunctivitis) and **Koplik spots (gray/white papules on buccal Mucosa)** which resolve before rash but 3 Cs stay
  - Morbilliform rash starts around the hairline and spreads cephalocaudal
    - Patients are infectious 3–5 (Multiple) days before rash
- Labs: MC lab abnormality is **lymphopenia**
- Rx: **vitamin A**; MMR vaccine (within 3 days of infection); immunoglobin (within 6 days)
  - WHO recommends **200,000 IU** vitamin A daily x 2 days for acute measles
- Prevention: MMR vaccine (first dose at 12–15 months; second dose at 4–6 years)
- Complications: URI, otitis Media, Myocarditis, and subacute sclerosing panencephalitis (late)

Rubella (German measles, "Three-day measles", "Third disease")

- RNA virus; Togaviridae family
- Important to avoid infection during pregnancy (TORCH syndrome)
- Like measles but milder → transmitted the same; same morbilliform cephalocaudal rash

  - o Infectious 1 day before rash
  - o Forchheimer's spots (petechiae on the palate)
  - o Generalized painful LAD (suboccipital/postauricular/anterior/posterior cervical)
- Labs: MC lab aberration is **Thrombocytopenia** (makes sense they get palatal petechiae)
- Complications: arthritis (females), thrombocytopenia, myocarditis, encephalitis
- Congenital rubella (ABCD): PDA, Blueberry muffin rash, Cataracts, Deafness
- Rx: supportive (immunoglobin for exposed pregnant women)

Erythema infectiosum ("slapped cheek disease, Parvovirus, "fifth disease")

- Caused by parvovirus B19; single stranded DNA virus ("part of a DNA")
- Transmission: respiratory droplets, blood and vertical transmission
- Initial viremia resolves w/ the development of IgM; IgG coincides with rash and arthritis
- Virus is tropic to BM (**giant Pronormoblasts on BM biopsy**) and replicates in **erythroid Precursors** (binds globoside blood group P antigen) → transient **anemia** during viremia
  - o BM may be chronically infected in the immunocompromised → Pancytopenia
- Rash/arthritis develops 1 to 1.5 weeks after viremia (fever, myalgias, HA during viremia)
  - o **No longer contagious once rash/arthritis develops** (IgG has already developed)
- The different presentation of Parvovirus B19: "Parv has the HERP"
  - o Hydrops fetalis (neonate)
  - o Erythema infectiosum (children): slapped cheeks or lacy Erythema of Extremities

- o RA-like (adult females): small joint-predominant arthritis
- o Papular purpuric gloves and socks syndrome (young adult): **Petechiae and Purpura with sharp demarcation at the wrists and ankles**
    - **Unlike other presentations, pts are infectious when this rash is present**

Exanthem Subitum (HHV-6/HSV-6, roseola infantum, "Sixth disease")

- Six to twenty-Six months of age; occurs mostly in Spring
- Caused by **HHV-6** (Six) > HHV-7 (Seven); DNA virus
- Transmitted by oral Secretions
- High fever up to 5 days (common cause of **febrile Seizures**); **fever resolves as rash starts**
    - o Subtle maculopapular rash with truncal predominance which lasts 2–3 days
    - o **Nagayama's Spots**: red macules on Soft palate/uvula (ddx: Forchheimer's spots)
- Virus remains latent in CD4+ T cells → reactivation a/w **DRESS, PR** and **Rosai-Dorfman**
    - o EBV, CMV, HHV-6, HHV-7 a/w DRESS ("Herpes 4, 5, 6 & 7 are under the DRESS")

Hand-foot-and-mouth disease

- Caused by **Coxsackie A16 virus** > Coxsackie A6 virus and Enterovirus 71
- Transmitted by fecal-oral and respiratory routes
- Febrile prodrome → erosive oral lesions w/ vesicular eruption on palms, soles, buttocks
    - o Discrete vesicles (not grouped like HSV) w/ erythematous border and gray center
    - o Erosive lesions are in the posterior mouth (vs anterior mouth in herpes)

- **Onychomadesis,** aka nail shedding ("made" new nails) is a common sequala
- **Coxsackie A6** has these 6 presentations: "COXSACKIE
  1. Cutaneous purpuric eruption
  2. **Onychomadesis**
  3. X-treme and Severe/widespread vesiculobullous eruption
  4. Atypical hand-foot-and-mouth disease: fever, vesicles, rash on butt, face, and trunk
  5. **Gianotti-Crosti-like eruptions**
  6. **Eczema coxsackium:** does not p/w punched out erosions like eczema herpeticum but instead p/w papules and vesicles in eczematous skin (commonly perioral)
- **Rx: reassurance** (coxsackie infections are self-limited)

Gianotti-Crosti syndrome (papular acrodermatitis of childhood)

- Occurs before age 5
- Exanthem arises after viral trigger: **EBV** #1 cause in US; **Hepatitis B** #1 cause worldwide
- p/w nonpruritic symmetric monomorphic pink papules on the face (esp. cheeks), buttocks ("four-cheeks") as well as extremities (**makes for a good Kodachrome**)

Unilateral laterothoracic exanthem (asymmetric periflexural exanthem of childhood)

- Occurs before age 5; female > males; probable viral origin
- p/w unilateral erythematous macules and papules which start in the axillae and lateral trunk ("Statue of Liberty sign": arm raised to show the rash; good Kodachrome)

4.3 Inherited Pigmentary Disorders

- For all inherited conditions, get in the habit of noticing what systemic involvement they have and send them for appropriate screening/workup (e.g., eye exam in OCA)

Hypo-/depigmentation

- Defects in **melanin synthesis** enzymes: oculocutaneous albinism ("white like TP")
  - o OCA1A/1B (Tyrosinase), OCA2 (P gene), OCA3 (TYRP), and OCA4 (MATP/SLC45A2)
- Defects in **melanosome synthesis** > transfer: Hermansky-Pudlak syndrome
- Defects in **melanosome trafficking/transfer** → Griscelli and Chediak-Higashi syndrome
  - o "Greasy Hashish drug traffickers"
- Defect in **melanocyte migration** (C-Kit): piebaldism ("here kitty kitty makes cat move")

Oculocutaneous albinism (OCA)

- AR disorders w/ abnormal melanin or melanosome biosynthesis and transport
- p/w pigmentary dilution (skin, hair, eyes), **photophobia, nystagmus, ↓ visual acuity**
- ↑ risk of skin cancers (**SCC** > BCC > melanoma)
- Path: ↓ melanin content w/ normal number of melanocytes
- 4 high yield forms: genes can be remembered by mnemonic, "white like TP"
  - o OCA types: 1 (Tyrosinase gene), 2 (P gene), 3 (TYRP gene), and 4 (MATP/SLC45A2)
  - o OCA 1 and 3 (genes start w/ T) has Tyrosinase Trapped in the rough ("Tough") ER

- OCA1a: complete loss of tyrosinase activity results in white phenotype (white hair/skin)
  - Highest risk of SCCs and eye abnormalities
- OCA1b: decreased tyrosinase activity but enough to produce some pheomelanin
  - Yellow phenotype: no pigment at birth, but w/ time, skin becomes yellow
  - Temperature-sensitive phenotype: tyrosinase functions at lower temperatures causing arm/leg hair to be brown, scalp hair to be red and axilla hair to be white
    - "Like a Siamese cat w/ the dark hair peripherally and light hair centrally"
- OCA2 (P gene): normal tyrosinase levels; most Prevalent form and particularly common in POC (People of color)**;** p/w Pink to cream-colored skin
  - a/w Prader-Willi and Angelman ("happy Puppet") disease
- OCA3 (TYRP gene): red phenotype ("picture a red-headed TwYRP")
- OCA4 (SLC45A2/MATP gene): exceedingly rare except in **Japan**

Hermanansky-Pudlack syndrome (HPS; "ABC")

- AR mutation in many genes: **HPS1 (MC)**, AP3B1, BLOC1S3; **MC in Puerto Ricans**
  - Makes proteins needed for synthesis > trafficking of melanosomes
- p/w **OCA, Bleeding diathesis and lysosomal Ceroid accumulation**
  - OCA: pigmentary dilution in skin (SCC), hair, and eyes (Photophobia, nystagmus)
  - Bleeding diathesis: p/w ecchymoses, nosebleeds, and menorrhagia (avoid aspirin)

    - Ceroid accumulation: p/w granulomatous Colitis (like Crohn's), Cardiomyopathy and **Pulmonary fibrosis (MCC of death)**
- Labs: platelet count is normal but they are dysfunctional (**absent Platelet granules**)
- EM: absence of dense bodies in platelets

Silvery hair syndromes

- Includes Griscelli syndromes (GS) and Chediak-Higashi syndrome (CHS): both are AR
- Genes encode proteins important in **transport/trafficking** of lysosomes/melanosomes
    - Griscelli and Chediak-Higashi affects trafficking: "Greasy Hash drug traffickers"
- All have pigmentary dilution of skin and hair w/ immunologic and neurologic features
- GS1 (Elejalde syndrome; MYO5A gene): severe **neurologic** impairment in early childhood
- GS2 (**RAB27A gene**): combined T and B cell **immunodeficiency** (p/w pyodermas) → hemophagocytic syndrome (pancytopenia, bleeding and death)
- GS3 (MLPH gene): least severe subtype with primarily cutaneous findings
- CHS (**LYST gene**): in addition to pigmentary dilution (silvery skin and hair), pyodermas, neurologic deterioration and severe immunodeficiency w/ hemophagocytic syndrome (which is seen in the various forms of GS), CHS also gets **photophobia** (w/ normal visual acuity), acral hyperpigmentation (**dark ears**), prolonged bleeding time (**ecchymoses**), severe gingivitis/ **periodontitis** and early dementia if they survive into adulthood
- Peripheral smear: PMNs appear huge in CHS and are normal in GS (Chediak "Huge" gashi)
- Melanocytes: melanosomes are huge in CHS and are normal in GS (Chediak "Huge" gashi)

- Trichoscopy: melanin clumps are small and spaced regular in CHS vs large/irregular in GS

Piebaldism

- AD defect in c-KIT ↓ migration of melanoblasts from neural crest to ventral midline
    - "Saying here KITy KITy makes cat migrate to your ventral midline"
- p/w white forelock (poliosis) and congenital ventral midline patches of leukoderma
    - Leukoderma has islands of sparring (makes for good kodachrome)

Waardenburg syndrome (WS)

- AD > AR mutation in PAX3 (WS1), MITF (WS2), PAX3 (WS3), and SOX10/endothelin (WS4)
    - "Pack your mittens, pack your socks"
- WS1 (classic): white forelock, synophorys (unibrow), heterochromia irides, dystopia canthorum (eyes appear widely spaced) and low risk of deafness (20%)
- WS2: similar to WS1 but **deafness** is more common and there is **no dystopia canthorum**
    - "MITF defect is strongly a/w deafness so I imagine mittens covering the ears"
- WS3: similar to WS1 but has **upper limb defects** (hypoplasia, syndactyly, and contractures)
- WS4: similar to WS1 but has **Hirschsprung's disease**
    - WS type 2 to 4 (type 1 is classic): "Can't hear, can't grip, can't take a shit"

Hyperpigmentation

McCune-Albright syndrome

- **Non-inherited postzygotic somatic activating mutation in GNAS1**

- o Gene makes G-protein which stimulates adenylate cyclase (**signal transduction**)
- Females >> males ("Happens in girls with vaGNAS with no family history of the disease")
- "I call it McCalm Al-bone endocrinopathy"
  - o Café au lait macule which is segmental and has a jagged "coast of Maine" border
  - o Bone lesions: polyostotic fibrous dysplasia (bone pain, bone deformity, and fractures)
  - o Endocrinopathy: precocious puberty, hypophosphatemic rickets, and Cushing disease

Genodermatoses with Rickets: "PAM'S rickets"
Phakomatosis pigmentokeratotica, Atrichia with papules, McCune-Albright, Shimmelpenning

Acropigmentation of Dohi (Dyschromatosis symmetrica hereditaria)

- AD mutation in ADAR (SRAD) gene which encodes an RNA-specific adenosine deaminase
- Most cases in Chinese and Japanese patients ("Dohi is a Chinese/Japanese name")
- p/w Dyschromia (hypo- and hyperpigmentation) on Dorsal extremities and face in kids

Dyschromatosis universalis hereditaria

- AD/AR mutation in ABCB6 (Harlequin ichthyosis was ABCA12 and PXE was ABCC6)
  - o **These genes encode ATP-dependent transporters**
- p/w generalized or torso-predominant mottled dyschromia and nail dystrophy

Genoderms w/ reticulate hyperpigmentation: "X-DR ENDs career" aka he retires → reticulate
X-linked reticulated pigmentary disorder (POL1A)
Dowling-Degos/ Galli-Galli disease (KRT5)
Reticulate acropigmentation of Kitamura (KRT5 or ADAM10)
EBS with mottled pigmentation (KRT5)
Naegeli-Franceschetti-Jadassohn syndrome (KRT 14)
Dermatopathia pigmentosa (KRT 14)
Dyskeratosis congenita (DKC1 > TERT, TERC)

*All are AD except the first and last in the mnemonic which are X-linked

X-linked reticulated pigmentary disorder

- XLD mutation in POL1A → aberrant immune response (type 1 interferon production)
- Males: **generalized reticulate hyperpigmentation**; early death due to failure to thrive
- Female carriers: streaky hyperpigmentation (similar to stage 3 of IP)
- Other features: recurrent respiratory infections, blonde unruly hair and photophobia
- Path (males): **dermal deposits of amyloid**
- Rx: largely supportive but recent reports show success w/ JAK inhibitors

Dowling-Degos and Galli-Galli disease

- AD mutation in Keratin 5
- **Adult-onset reticulate hyperpigmentation of the axilla**, groin > other skin folds
- Comedone-like lesions on back of neck, **pitted peri-oral scars**, epidermoid cysts, HS
- Path: SK-like pigmented epithelial strands (w/ horn cysts) hanging off hair follicles
- Galli-Galli disease is clinically identical but shows **acantholysis** on path
- Rx (variable success): hydroquinone, topical retinoids, topical steroids, and lasers

Reticulate acropigmentation of Kitamura

- AD mutation in Keratin 5 or ADAM10 ("Kit-adam-ura")
  - EDS, dermatosparaxis was ADAMTS-2 mutation
- Childhood onset reticulate hyperpigmentation on dorsal hands/feet (good kodachrome)
- Other features: **linear palmar pits** ("Pit-amura")
- Ddx: acropigmentation of Dohi has dyschromia (hyper- and hypopigmentation)

EBS with mottled pigmentation (discussed in section 4.4)

Naegeli-Franceschetti-Jadassohn syndrome

- AD mutation in keratin 14
- Childhood onset reticulate hyperpigmentation (abdomen MC); improves at puberty
- Other findings: acral bullae in newborn, heat intolerance (↓ sweat gland function), **absent dermatoglyphics**, PPK, **severe dental anomalies** (loss of death)
  - "I think of Nigel Thornberry from the Nickelodeon show who is always hot, has really bad teeth and has no reticulate hyperpigmentation (improved at puberty)"

Dermatopathia pigmentosa reticularis (DPR)

- AD mutation in keratin 14
- Triad: **persistent** reticulate hyperpigmentation, **non-scarring alopecia**, onychodystrophy
  - "Nigel Thornberry has hair so DPR is the one with alopecia"

Dyskeratosis Congenita (ABCD; Zinsser-Engman-Cole syndrome)

- **XLR mutation in DKC1** > AD mutation in TERT, TERC; involved in **telomere maintenance**
- Males > females
- Main features: Anonychia + BM failure + oral SCCs + skin Dyspigmentation

    - Anonychia or onychodystrophy (longitudinal ridging/splitting, pterygium)
    - BM failure: Fanconi's-type pancytopenia → infection, hemorrhage, leukemia
    - Oral SCCs which arise from **premalignant leukoplakia**
    - Reticulated Dyspigmentation and poikiloderma on neck, chest, upper arms
- Other features (ABCD): Absent teeth, non-scarring Alopecia, frictional Bulla, Blepharitis, Conjunctivitis, Continuous lacrimation (epiphora), Cirrhosis, PPK, and hyperhidrosis
- Prognosis: death (avg 16 y/o) from cancer (SCC > AML), BM failure or pulmonary fibrosis

Tongue Trivia
Dyskeratosis congenita: premalignant leukoplakia
Pachyonychia congenita and Howel-Evans: non-premalignant leukoplakia (+ focal painful PPK)
Riley-Day (Familial Dysautonomia): absent fungiform papillae on tongue (smooth tongue)
Cowden and Dariers (Keratosis follicularis): Cobblestoned/bumpy tongue ("k sounds")
MEN2b: mucosal neuromas which p/w localized bumpy tongue and thickened lips
Melkerson-Rosenthal, Acromegaly, Downs, Bazex, p. Vegetans: scrotal tongue ("MAD BV")

Macroglossia (large tongue): "He got BLAMED for not biting his big tongue"
Beckwith-Wiedemann, Lipoid proteinosis ("wooden tongue"), Amyloidosis, Acromegaly, Angioedema, Mucopolysaccharidosis, Edentulism, Downs

Lentiginoses syndromes: "Big Lentiginosis Problems require TLC" (All are AD inheritance)

Bannayan-Riley Revulcaba syndrome

- Mutation in **PTEN** which encodes a **phosphatase** involved in tumor suppression

- **p/w penile lentigines**, lipomas, MR, macrocephaly, ↑ risk for cancer
    - "Penises look like bananas"

Laugier-Hunziker syndrome

- p/w lentigines on lips, mucosa, genitals; melanonychia in 50%; no ↑ risk for malignancy
- Laug-Hun: Lentigos on Lips And Under Genitals; Half Under Nails (melanonychia in 50%)

Peutz-Jeghers syndrome

- Mutation in STK11/LBK1 which is a tumor suppressor gene
- p/w lentigines on the **lips** (100%; first sign), **mucosal surfaces, palms/soles** and nails
- Hamartomatous polyps and adenocarcinoma → **intussusception**, GI bleeding, anemia
- **Colorectal and breast cancer** are the MC cancers but ovarian and pancreatic also occur
    - "When you eat steak of lamb (STK11/LBK1) you get brown sauce on your lips, mouth and hands and the food goes right to your colon and breasts (cancers)"

Touraine's syndrome (centrofacial lentiginosis)

- p/w lentigines on nose and cheeks (T-zone of face) in the first year of life, sacral hyper-Trichosis, MR, Teeth abnormalities and congenital Tricuspid/mitral valve stenosis
    - Don't confuse w/ Christ-Siemens-Touraine syndrome (XLR ectodermal dysplasia) which has hypo-Trichosis + Teeth abnormalities + ↓ sweating → hyper-Thermia

LEOPARD, aka Noonan w/ multiple lentigines syndrome

- Mutation in PTPN11/SHP2; SHP-2 is a protein that regulates the **RAS/MAPK pathway**
  - o Same gene as noonan syndrome → "PuT leopard in the PeN or SHoP at noon"
- p/w lentigines on the face/neck/trunk, large dark café noir spots and multiple CALMs
  - o **"Leopards have spots on their bodies but not on mucosa"** (vs Carney complex)
- Other features: hypertrophic cardiomyopathy ("leopards have a lot of heart"), facial dysmorphism ("leopards have strange faces"), genital abnormalities like hypospadia ("get your leopard spayed"), joint hyperextensibility ("leopards are flexible"); granular cell myoblastoma ("even leopard's tumors have spots"), deafness
  - o LEOPARD: Lentigos, **EKG abnormalities**, Ocular hypertelorism, **Pulmonary stenosis**, Abnormal genitalia, Retarted growth, **Deafness**

Carney complex ("Car")

- Mutation in PRKARIA ("PaRK cAR") → makes protein kinase A involved in cell division
- p/w **periorificial and conjunctival lentigos** and large epithelioid blue nevi
  - o "When you go fast in a car/bike, your eyes and mouth open wide and you'll get hit by brown bugs in the face/mouth/eyes; large blue bugs may hit your body"
- Cardiac (and mucocutaneous) myxomas ("driving fast gets your heart pumping")
- Endocrine tumors: primary pigmented adrenocortical disease (p/w **Cushing's**), pituitary (acromegaly), thyroid and testes/ovaries (Sertoli cell tumor)
  - o "Driving fast gets your endocrine glands, such as adrenals and testes, pumping"

- Nerve tumors: psammomatous melanotic schwannoma ("gets your nerves pumping")

Cronkite-Canada syndrome ("CAANADA")

- Circumscribed **Acral lentigines (hands/feet/mouth), Alopecia, Nail dystrophy**
- Adenomatous GI polyps (no risk of cancer) → Diarrhea and Abdominal pain

4.4 Epidermolysis Bullosa (EB)

- Group of inherited mechanobullous disorders with defects in different levels of the BMZ
- Hemidesmosome-anchoring filament complex from top down ("Peanut Butter BIL"): Plectin, BPAG1, BPAG2, Integrin α6β4 and Laminin 332
  - EBS: defects in K5, K14 in basal keratinocytes or plectin in the hemidesmosome
    - Plectin (and BPAG1) in the hemidesmosomal plaque connect keratin intermediate filaments of the basal keratinocytes to the hemidesmosome
  - JEB: defects in BPAG2, Int α6β4, Lam 332 in **anchoring filaments** (lamina lucida)
    - "BIL rhymes with fil" (laminin 332 is really in the lamina densa not lucida)
      - Diseases with Collagen 17 (BPAG2) defects is "called 17 times and no answer, what a Judgmental BICH": Junctional EB, BP, linear IgA, Cicatricial pemphigoid, Herpes gestationis
  - DEB: defects in Collagen 7 of the anchoring fibrils in the sublamina densa
  - Kindler syndrome: Defect in FERMT1 (kindlin) involved in keratinocyte adhesion

- H&E biopsy: perform on a freshly induced blister
- Workup: immunofluorescence antigenic mapping (place sample in Michel's/Zeus medium) or transmission electron microscopy (place sample in glutaraldehyde) from an **induced**, rather than a preexisting blister; can do next generation sequencing panel also

EB Simplex (EBS): MC form of EB; intraepidermal split; all are **AD inheritance w/ a Keratin 5,14** defect except EBS w/ muscular dystrophy and EBS w/ pyloric atresia (AR; plectin), all present at birth (except EBS localized and EBS w/ mottled pigmentation) and all have **PPK/nail dystrophy**

- EBS localized (previously Weber-Cockayne)
  - Presents in childhood after prolonged walking in heat w/ bullae on pressure area of soles → compensatory painful hyperkeratosis/**callus on heels/ balls of feet**
    - "Web should make you think web spaces of hands and feet"
    - Ddx: Howel-Evans, pachyonychia congenita and Clouston also p/w PPK in childhood which is worse on pressure areas of soles
  - Worsened by heat, tight shoes and walking but patients have a normal life span
- EBS generalized intermediate (previously Koebner)
  - Presents at birth or infancy with tense bullae at any site of friction ("Kontact")
  - May have oral blisters, PPK and nail dystrophy but patients have normal life span
- EBS generalized severe (previously Dowling Meara or EBS herpetiformis)
  - Presents at birth w/ **generalized blisters** which become **clustered**/herpetiform
  - Oral blisters, PPK and nail dystrophy common
  - Clumped tonofilaments on EM

  - Patients generally have a normal life span but may die early due to sepsis
    - "Dowling reminds me of Bowling: you bowl in groups (clustered blisters, grouped tonofilaments) and bowling gives you PPK and nail dystrophy"
- EBS with mottled pigmentation
  - Presents in childhood with acral blisters, mottled hyperpigmentation on the trunk and limbs, punctate PPK and nail dystrophy
- EBS with muscular dystrophy
  - **AR**; plectin mutation (not AD mutation in K5,14 like the others)
  - p/w **generalized bulla at birth** and **muscular dystrophy later** in life
  - a/w nail hyperkeratosis, dental abnormalities, and cerebral/cerebellar atrophy
- EBS with pyloric atresia
  - **AR**; plectin mutation
  - Presents at birth w/ generalized blisters, pyloric atresia (mother may p/w polyhydramnios) and aplasia cutis congenita → death within the 1st year of life

Junctional EB (JEB): rarest form of EB; level of split is in the lamina lucida; **all AR**; all present at birth w/ "Jeneralized" blisters; all have **enamel hypoplasia/pitting** and Jaw issues (tooth loss)

- JEB generalized intermediate (previously JEB Non-Herlitz)
  - Defect in BPAG2/collagen 17 (like classic cicatricial pemphigoid) or Laminin 332
  - Generalized blisters at birth but improves with time
  - Nail dystrophy, corneal erosions and scarring alopecia ("No hair") common

    - Most likely form of EB to get **eruptive benign Nevi** which occur at sites of previous blisters and are clinically large and atypical
- JEB with pyloric atresia
    - Defect in Integrin α6β4 (like ocular cicatricial pemphigoid)
    - p/w **rudimentary ears**, pyloric atresia (inability to pass an NG tube) and ureteral stenosis (polyhydramnios in utero and hydronephrosis later)
        - The "I" in Integrin reminds me of "eye" (ocular CP) and "I" is a skinny letter to remind me of skinny malformed ears, atresias and stenoses"
- JEB generalized severe (previously JEB Herlitz)
    - Defect in Laminin 332 (like anti-epiligrin CP a/w malignancy) or BPAG2
        - Premature termination codon (Halted gene transcription)
    - Generalized blisters at birth w/ large areas affected → electrolyte imbalances
    - **Hoarse cry** as a result of laryngeal involvement respiratory failure
    - **Granulation tissue** ("G next to H in alphabet") around the mouth/butt ("Holes")
    - Rx: Gentamicin induces Laminin 332 and improves JEB w/ nonsense mutations
    - Prognosis: death by 1 year due to respiratory failure, sepsis or FTT

Dystrophic EB (DEB): split is in the sublamina densa; coll 7 mutation; AD (mild) and **AR (severe)** forms; all present w/ generalized blisters at birth that heal w/ **atrophic scarring and milia**

- Dominant DEB (DDEB)
    - Missense mutation in COL7A1 gene
    - Cockayne-Touraine type: generalized bullae most prominent on Distal arms/legs

  - Pasini type: similar to Cockayne-Touraine but w/ "albopapuloid papules" on trunk
  - **Nail Dystrophy** common in both and disease activity improves over time
- Recessive DEB (RDEB), generalized severe (previously known as Hallopeau-Siemens)
  - Premature Stop codon in COL7A1 → complete lack of anchoring fibrils
  - **PseudoSyndactyly** (mitten deformities) common and pathognomonic
  - Contracture (Shortening) of digits/limbs, Scarring alopecia, esophageal Strictures
  - Aggressive **SCCs (#1 cause of death)** and Renal failure (#2 cause of death)
    - Rx: Ruxolitinib shows promise for treating SCCs
  - Dx: CBC shows anemia
  - Rx: gentamicin induces type 7 collagen in RDEB cells w/ nonsense mutations
- RDEB, generalized intermediate (previously known as non-Hallopeau-Siemens)
  - AR; COL7A1 gene; non-specific; may be difficult to distinguish from DDEB
- Bart syndrome is DDEB with aplasia cutis congenita (absent skin) of **legs**
  - ACC is MC w/ dystrophic EB but can be seen in EB simplex or junctional EB also
- DEB pruruginosa: p/w extremely pruritic linearly arranged papules on the legs

Kindler syndrome (acrokeratotic poikiloderma)

- AR; loss of function mutation in FERMT1 (previously kindlin-1)
- Presents with **poikiloderma**, photosensitivity, SCCs, skin fragility w/ acral blisters (which can lead to "cig-

arette paper" skin atrophy and webbing of digits) and PPK

  - "As a parent you need to be FERM but kind so your children don't pick up bad habits like not wearing sunscreen (poikiloderma, photosensitivity), not washing their hands (acral blisters, PPK) and not brushing their teeth (oral SCCs)"

- Dx: **EM shows duplication of the lamina densa**; path shows absence of elastic fibers

4.5 Tumor Syndromes

- These are all a result of loss of function mutation in a tumor suppressor gene except…
  - Gorlin's: loss of function of PTCH-1, -2, SUFU, or a **gain of function of SMO**
  - MEN2A and 2B: gain of function of the RET tyrosine kinase receptor
- All these syndromes are AD except Bazex-Dupré-Christol syndrome (XLD)
- For all of these entities, the workup will include at a minimum taking a detailed personal and family history and sending for age-appropriate cancer screenings

Basal cell nevus syndrome (Gorlin's syndrome)

- Hedgehog pathway (Hp): in the normally functioning Hp, patched (PTCH) normally binds and inhibits smoothened (SMO); when this pathway is activated, Hp proteins bind to the transmembrane PTCH receptor which ↓ the inhibition of PTCH on SMO, allowing SMO to activate a downstream cascade (e.g., GLI) that results in cell proliferation
  - Even without smoothened, GLI is normally inhibited in the cytoplasm by SUFU

- AD mutation in PTCH (encodes the Patched **Transmembrane** Tumor suppressor)
    - o Patched normally inhibits smoothened (**G-protein coupled receptor**) but if mutated it activates GL1/2 transcription factors → cancer growth
        - "The 2 Vegetarian PA's attach to the smooth doctor (who is such a G) and inhibits him from doing his cancer research"
            - **Erivedge** (vismodegib), **Patched,** CycloPAmine bind/inhibit SMO
            - Itraconazole also inhibits the sonic hedgehog pathway
- SUFU is another common mutation (lacks jaw cysts but has ↑ risk of medulloblastoma and exclusively develops infundibulocystic BCCs)
- Major criteria are multiple BCCs (or 1 BCC ≤ 20 years old), family history and "PORC"
    - o Palmoplantar pits (> 3)
    - o Odontogenic keratocysts of the jaw (**earliest sign**; requires annual dental x-rays)
    - o Ribs are splayed (bifid ribs)
    - o Calcification of the falx cerebri
- Minor criteria (BCC): Big head (macrocephaly, meningioma, medulloblastoma → requires annual brain MRI until 8), frontal Bossing, Broad nasal root, congenital Blindness (strabismus/colobomas), Bent vertebra (scoliosis), ovarian/cardiac fibromas
    - o Ovarian fibromas are the MC tumor a/w Gorlin's syndrome (25% of patients)
- Dx: panorex (dental x-rays will show jaw keratocysts); brain MRI for medulloblastoma
- Rx: surgery and vismodegib
    - o MC vismodegib SEs (MAD): **Muscle spasms (MC)** > Alopecia > Dysgeusia
    - o Gain of function mutations in SMO oncogene can confer vismodegib resistance

Birt-Hogg-Dubé syndrome "Hog makes you think of a FAT PORC"

- AD mutation in BHD gene which encodes Folliculin
- Skin (FAT): **Fibrofolliculomas**, Acrochordons, Trichodiscomas
    - o These are **small smooth white** papules on face (trichilemmomas in Cowdens are verrucous; cylindromas in Brooke-spielger are large pink and smooth)
- Internal (PORC): **Pneumothorax/Pulm cysts**, Oncocytic renal tumor, **RCC** > Colon cancer
- Workup/screening: **yearly abdomen/pelvic MRI** (RCC) and monitor for pulmonary cysts

Brooke-Spiegler syndrome ("C is after B, and T is after S in alphabet")

- AD mutation in CYLD tumor suppressor gene
    - o CYLD normally interacts with NEMO to downregulate **NFkB** expression
    - o CYLD loss of function leads to constitutively active NFkB
- Skin: presents in adolescents w/ BCCs, Cylindromas, Spiradenomas, Trichoepitheliomas
    - o Density of trichoepitheliomas is always greatest in the Central face
- Extracutaneous findings: **Salivary**/parotid gland tumors (may be malignant)
- Workup: close follow-up to monitor for adenocarcinomas of the parotid/salivary gland

Muir-Torre syndrome (variant of Lynch syndrome)

- AD mutation in **MSH2** > MSH6, MLH1, PMS-2 (**genes involved in DNA mismatch repair**)
    - o Tumors show loss of MSH2/MSH6/MLH1/PMS2 uptake on IHC

- "Muire-Torre is more SICK"
    - Sebaceous neoplasms: p/w yellow facial papules (extra-facial lesions are strongly associated)
    - Internal malignancies: **Colon** (MC) and genitourinary cancers (2nd MC)
    - **KA w/ sebaceous differentiation (seboacanthoma) are pathognomonic**
- Workup: biennial colonoscopy, serial US, UA, CBC, and age-appropriate cancer screenings

Multiple endocrine neoplasia (MEN) syndromes

- MEN I (Wermer)
    - AD mutation in MEN1 gene (encodes the tumor suppressor menin)
    - Skin (TS-like): facial angiofibroma (MC), collagenoma, gingival papules, CALMs
    - Tumors (PPP): Pituitary (Prolactinoma is MC; **acromegaly** may be seen due to pituitary adenomas), Parathyroid (p/w hypercalcemia), Pancreas (may p/w necrolytic migratory erythema due to glucagonoma)
- MEN IIA (Sipple)
    - AD mutation in the RET oncogene on chromosome 10
    - Skin: **Lichen amyloidosis** > Macular amyloidosis and Notalgia Paresthetica
        - Lichen amyloid has a rippled appearance ("ripple rhymes w/ Sipple")
    - Tumors: medullary thyroid cancer, parathyroid hyperplasia, and pheochromocytoma
- MEN IIB (Multiple Mucosa neuroma syndrome)
    - AD mutation in the RET proto-oncogene on chromosome 10
    - Skin: **Multiple Mucosal neuromas on tongue/lips**/eyelids → Massive lips/eyelids

- Other findings: Marfanoid habitus, Medullary thyroid carcinoma (MTC; occurs in 100% of patients and fatal if not caught early), **pheochromocytoma,** ganglioneuromatosis (Megacolon, diarrhea, constipation), internal Malignancies
- Labs: **hypocalcemia** (MTC is from perifollicular C cells of thyroid → ↑ calcitonin)
- Rx: **early thyroidectomy** (< 1 year)

Cowden syndrome

- AD defect in tumor suppressor PTEN (**phosphatase tensin homologue**) in Akt pathway
    - Cowden's, Bannayan-Riley-Revulcaba, Proteus and Lhermitte-Duclos syndromes can be united under the label PTEN hamartoma syndrome
        - "My Cow's Banana is Pro-Lific (PTEN stands for Penis is 10/10)"
- Skin: facial trichilemmomas ("trichilem-moo-mas"; yellow-tan verrucous papules), sclerotic fibromas, acral keratoses ("cows have keratotic hooves"), lipomas and IFKs
- Oral: **cobblestoning of lips, gingival/labial/buccal mucosa** due to oral papillomas
    - "Mouth is warty/bumpy like a cows"; Dariers disease also has this oral finding
- GI: hamartomatous polyps w/ low risk of malignancy ("cows make you think of ham")
- Other findings: ovarian cysts, adenoid facies, **craniomegaly** ("cows have huge heads")
- Cancers in order of likelihood ("Cows eat Beatles → BTEL)": **Breast adenocarcinoma (#1), follicular Thyroid carcinoma**, Endometrial carcinoma, Lhermitte-Duclos disease (hamartoma of cerebellum which p/w ataxia, seizures and ↑ ICP)
    - "BTEL is in the major criteria but colon and **renal** cancer are in the minor criteria"

- Workup/screening: annual thyroid US, colonoscopy, and mammogram

Genoderms with colon polyps: "Bad Genoderms Contain Colon Polpys"
Bannayan-Riley, Garners, Cowdens, Cronkite-Canada, Peutz-Jeghers

Gardner syndrome ("A-G")

- AD mutation in the **APC gene** (tumor suppressor gene that **regulates β-catenin**)
- Skin: **Epidermoid Cysts w/ pilomatricoma changes**, Fibromas, Fatty tumors (lipomas)
    - o "Planting many cysts, pilomatricomas and lipomas in the garden"
- GI: Adenocarcinomas (100% affected) and **Desmoid tumors** (locally aggressive)
    - o "Planting many GI tumors in the garden"
- Eyes: Congenital hypertrophy of retinal pigment epithelium (**CHIRP**; 70%; first sign)
    - o "Birds CHIRP'n in the garden"
- Other findings: Brain tumors (Glioblastomas), Bone tumors (osteomas), Extra teeth
    - o "Planting extra teeth, brain and bones in the garden"
- Rx: prophylactic Colectomy

Reed syndrome

- o AD mutation in fumurate hydratase (**Kreb's cycle** enzyme: catalyzes fumarate to malate)
- o p/w uterine and cutaneous leiomyomas; **Renal cell carcinoma**
- o Rx: excision or CCBs (lessens pain a/w the smooth muscle spasms in leiomyomas)
- o Screening: **annual Renal imaging (MRI) beginning at age 10**

Familial atypical multiple mole melanoma syndrome (FAMMM)

- AD mutation in tumor suppressor gene **CDKN2A** (CDK4, MITF, POT1, BAP1 are less common) whose gene product p16INK4A regulates the G1-S transition in the cell cycle
- p/w multiple atypical nevi and high risk of melanomas
- ↑ risk of several internal malignancies, most notably **pancreatic cancer** but renal and neural are also seen (mesothelioma, RCC, cholangiocarcinoma w/ BAP1 mutation)
- Workup: biopsy nevi suspicious of melanoma, abdominal imaging, and genetic testing
  - o Rule of 3s: three melanomas + family history → send to genetics
- Refer to section 6.3 for management of melanoma

Rombo syndrome

- AD mutation
- p/w BCCs, trichoepitheliomas, milia, atrophoderma vermiculatum (atrophic papules on the cheeks), hypotrichosis, telangiectasias, and peripheral cyanosis
  - o "I think of Silvester Stallon in Rambo who is a Dominant male (AD), has acne scars on his cheeks, he sweats (no hypohidrosis), shaves his jacked body (hypotrichosis) and wears little clothing so he gets cold (peripheral cyanosis)

Bazex-Dupré-Christol syndrome (BDCS)

- XLD (females)
- Like Rombo, p/w BCCs, trichoepitheliomas, milia, hypotrichosis but unlike Rombo, has hypohidrosis, facial hyperpigmentation, lacks peripheral cyanosis and has follicular atrophoderma (MC on dorsal hands) instead of atrophoderma vermiculatum on cheeks

4.6 Vascular Disorders

Vascular hemangiomas

- Infantile hemangiomas are discussed in section 6.11

PHACE syndrome

- Posterior fossa malformations: **Dandy Walker #1**, cerebellar hypoplasia → brain MRI
- Hemangiomas: p/w segmental, facial **plaque** (Ddx: PWS in Sturge-Weber is a patch)
- **Arterial anomalies: Corkscrew arteries are pathognomonic; neck is #1 location; cerebrovascular anomalies are MC extracutaneous manifestation** → head/neck MRA
- **Cardiac anomalies: Coarctation of aorta is #1 → get echo**
- **Eye anomalies** (but **not glaucoma**, this is seen in Sturge-Weber): → **send to ophtho**
- Sternal cleft or Supraumbilical abdominal raphe: indented chest/abdomen, respectively
- **XLD** (MC in females) sporadic postzygotic somatic mosaic mutation of unknown gene
    - o Somatic mutations occur in any cells besides sex cells (MC in a mosaic pattern)
        - ▪ Mosaic: 2 distinct cell lines (some cells are normal and some are altered)
- Dx: **MRI/MRA of head/neck** to evaluate for Posterior fossa and Arterial anomalies
- **ECHO before starting Propranolol (1st line Rx)** → stroke if Coarctation of aorta present
- Workup: next best step in child w/ segmental facial hemangioma is **ophtho exam**
- Rx: propranolol (titrate up to 3.4 mg/kg/day divided BID)

LUMBAR/SACRAL/PELVIS syndrome (3 acronyms that all basically say the same thing)

- Lower back/Lower body hemangioma/Lipomas
- **Urogenital anomalies**, Ulceration
- Myelopathy (tethered spinal cord or **Myelomeningocele**)
- Bone anomalies (hip dysplasia/length-width discrepancies)
- **Anorectal anomalies (imperforate anus)**
- **Renal anomalies**
- Workup: imaging for spinal dysraphism and urinary abnormalities
    - o < 4 months (vertebrae not fully formed): spinal US (MRI if abnormal) and US w/ doppler of abdomen and pelvis (urologic evaluation if abnormal)
    - o > 4 months: MRI of spine; US abdomen/pelvis (urologic evaluation if abnormal)
- Rx: propranolol

Diffuse neonatal Hemangiomatosis

- Defined as ≥ 5 hemangiomas (NF1 had ≥ 6 CALMs)
- Hemangiomas in any organ (#1 is **liver/Hepatic**) → **high output Heart failure (CHF)**
- GI hemangiomas de-iodinate thyroid Hormone → severe Hypothyroidism
- Ddx: recognize difference b/w **red hemangiomas** (diffuse neonatal Hemangiomatosis), **soft dark blue venous malformations** (Blue rubber bleb nevus syndrome) and **blue-red dome shaped paps of extramedullary/dermal hematopoiesis** (blueberry muffin baby)
- Rx: propranolol is 1st line if visceral involvement
- Workup: next step in a baby with ≥ 5 hemangiomas → **liver US**

Kasabach-Merritt ("Casaback-Merritt") syndrome

- Consumption Coagulopathy in kaposiform hemangio-endothelioma > tufted angioma
    - o Both hemangiomas are **GLUT-1 (-)** and rapidly enlarge in the first months of life
- Complications include high output Cardiac failure, CHF and DIC (20% mortality)
- Rx: Corticosteroids, vinCristine and anti-Coagulation therapy

Congenital hemangiomas

- GNAQ mutation; **GLUT-1 negative** (**vs infantile hemangiomas which are GLUT-1+**)
- Arise in utero and can be diagnosed with prenatal US
- **p/w hemangioma at birth w/ characteristic blanched and telangiectatic border**
- Categorized based on their natural history
    - o RICH: rapidly involuting congenital hemangioma
    - o NICH: non-involuting congenital hemangioma

Vascular malformations

- In contrast to infantile hemangiomas → present at birth, do not involute and GLUT-1 (-)
    - o Capillary malformations (CM) p/w red macules: activating mutations in **GNAQ**
        - ▪ Variants: nevus simplex (salmon patch), PWS, CMTC, telangiectasias
        - ▪ Dx: if in V1, get neuro (MRI) and ophtho exam to rule out Sturge-Weber
        - ▪ Rx: **PDL** > Alexandrite or Nd:YAG +/- sirolimus (rapamycin)
        - ▪ Mid-face and distal extremities are most resistant to treatment with PDL
    - o Venous malformations (VM) p/w blue compressible papules: **TEK (TIE2) > PIK3CA**

    - "TEK is a guy who wears a TIE, guys have a penis that rhymes w/ venous"
    - p/w blue, compressibe, soft papule that tends to fill w/ dependency
    - Use to be called cavernous hemangiomas (misnomer)
    - Dx: **T2 weighted MRI (best)**, US (shows slow flow lesions), D-dimer
    - Rx: Sclerotherapy + Surgery (LMWH, ASA or Rapamycin for coagulopathy)
        - Dx and Rx Venous malformations w/ "RSTUVwxyz" in alphabet
- Lymphatic malformations (LM) p/w vesicles or large cysts: PIK3CA
    - Rx: sclerotherapy (macrocystic LMs), surgical excisions (microcystic LMs)
  - Arteriovenous malformations (AVMs) p/w 4 stages: red macule → expansile mass with thrill → painful ulcer → high output cardiac failure (+ stage 2 and 3)
    - Rx: surgical excision w/ embolization (pure ethanol is best embolic agent)

PIK3CA mutations: "Mormons get to PIK 3 LOVES"

Lymphatic malformations* (e.g., CLOVE syndrome, Klippel-Trenaunay, M-CM syndrome)
Oncogene for various cancers (e.g., breast, colon, etc.)
Venous malformations (e.g., CLOVE syndrome, Klippel-Trenaunay)
Epidermal nevus
SK and variants (e.g., lentigo, DPNs, stucco keratoses)

*CLOVES, hereditary hemihyperplasia-multiple lipomatosis syndrome, Klippel-Trenaunay syndrome, isolated large lymphatic malformation syndrome and macrocephaly-capillary malformation syndrome are all considered part of the PIK3CA-related overgrowth spectrum and are potential candidates for rapamycin therapy

Syndromes w/ capillary malformations: Big Syndromes Can p/w Diffuse Kapillary Malformations

- Beckwith-Wiedemann, Sturge-Weber, CMTC, CLOVES, Proteus, Phakomatosis pigmentovascularis, -pigmentokeratotica, Diffuse capillary malformation w/ overgrowth (DCMO), Klippel-Trenaunay (KTS), Macrocephaly-Capillary Malformation (M-CM)

BECKwith-Wiedemann syndrome

- Big organs (organomegaly/omphalocele), Big tongue (macroglossia), Big baby
- **Ears (circular pits/diagonal earlobe crease),** Exophthalmos, **Endocrine (↓glucose)**
- **Capillary malformation on face, Circular depression/Creases (ears),** Cyclin- dependent kinase inhibitor gene, Cancers (**Wilms tumor** > hepatoblastoma > rhabdomyosarcoma)
- KIP 2 gene (p57) → gene is over ("Big") methylated vs undermethylated in Russel Silver
- Workup: serum glucose, AFP to screen for hepatoblastoma and abdominal/renal US

Sturge-Weber (encephalotrigeminal angiomatosis) syndrome

- **Mutation in GNAQ → stimulates MAPK signaling →** ↑cell proliferation and ↓apoptosis
- Capillary malformation on face (V1 > V2 > V3) with underlying soft tissue hypertrophy
- **MC w/ unilateral PWS in V1 and V2** > just V1
- ↑ intracranial pressure causes **glaucoma** (50%) and **seizures** (75%)
- Rx: prophylactic aspirin reduces frequency of stroke-like episodes and seizures
- Workup: ophtho exam and **MRI** w/ gadolinium (or magnetic resonance SWI) of head shows cortical calcifications (occipital region is MC) that resemble "tram-track" lines

- "Picture a seizing spider w/ a facial PWS on a web with train tracks (occipital tram track calcifications) crossing the web. The train will NAQ (GNAQ) him on his ass (Rx ASA)"

CLOVES syndrome

- Proteus-like syndrome characterized by Congenital Lipomatous Overgrowth, Vascular anomalies (VMs, LMs, and dark truncal CMs, which overly lipomatous masses), Epidermal nevi, Scoliosis/Skeletal anomalies (broad hands/feet), **Spinal AVMs**, and Seizures
  - o If it sounds like Proteus but there is no plantar collagenoma, it's probably CLOVES
- Post-zygotic mutation in **PIK3CA** (upstream of PTEN)
- Rx: mTOR inhibitor (rapamycin) helps w/ overgrowths and vascular anomalies

Cutis marmorata telangiectatica conGENITA (CMTC)

- **Glaucoma (get ophtho exam)**
- Extremities (LE > UP) w/ reticulated vascular networks Early in life (at birth) then fades
- **Neurologic symptoms (seizures, MR, macrocephaly)**
- Ipsilateral limb hypoplasia and ulceration may occur
- Transverse limb defects (TLD) in Adams Oliver syndrome
- Adams Oliver syndrome: CMTC w/ scalp ACC, cardiac issues (O = heart) and Limb defects
- Workup: same as PHACES and Sturge Weber w/ ophtho and neuro exam

Proteus (L-T; letters around P in alphabet) syndrome

- Sporadic somatic **AKTivating point mutation of AKT1 oncogene** which encodes a serine-threonine protein kinase which is involved in the mTOR signaling pathway

  - "Joseph Merrick had Proteus syndrome. The guy who played him in the movie *Elephant Man* was an AKTor"
- **Linear epidermal nevus**, Lipomas, **Lung problems (emphysema)**
- Malformations (capillary/venous/lymphatic), Macrocephaly, **Meningioma**
- Nystagmus and other eye problems
- Organomegaly, Overgrowth of extremities/digits/cranium, **Ovarian cystadenoma (B/L)**
- **Plantar collagenoma (pathognomonic), Parotid adenoma (MC tumor)**
- Retardation (MR)
- Sporadic inheritance, Scoliosis, Strabismus, Syndactyly, Subcutaneous masses
- **Thrombosis (DVT and pulmonary emboli)**
- Testicular tumors especially testicular papillary adenocarcinoma
- Rx: mTOR inhibitors (Sirolimus)
- Criteria (must meet the 1 in category A, 2 in category B and 3 in category C)
  - A: cerebriform connective tissue nevus (usually plantar)
  - B: epidermal nevi, growth/tumors (B/L ovarian cystadenoma, parotid adenoma)
  - C: dysfunctional adipose tissue (lipoma, dermal hypoplasia), vascular malformation, characteristic facies (long face, downward palpebra, open mouth)

Phakomatosis pigmentovascularis

- **GNAQ or GNA11** mutations
- Widespread capillary malformations (a/w Sturge-Weber) + other cutaneous findings
- "I remember the 5 types by saying PEN, PM, PN, PMN, CM"

- I: PWS + Epidermal Nevus
- **II (phakomatosis cesioflammea): PWS + Mongolian spot (MC form)**
- III (phakomatosis spilorosa): PWS + Nevus spilus
- IV: PWS + Mongolian spot + Nevus spilus
- V (phakomatosis cesiomarmorata): CMTC + Mongolian spot

Phakomatosis Pigmentokeratotica: "your PP is Honestly Really NaSTy"

- **HRAS** mutation (regulates cell-division through process known as signal transduction)
- **Hypophosphatemic vitamin D-resistant Rickets** can develop
- **Nevus Spilus + Nevus Sebaceous (Trichoblastoma** > SPAP > BCC may develop inside)
  - MC mutation in nevus sebaceous is HRAS (helps to remember this syndrome)

KLIPpel-Trenaunay syndrome (KTS)

- **Koagulability (DVT of legs → PE)**
- **Leg** has cap/venous/lymph malformations with underlying soft tissue/bone hypertrophy
- **Increased output cardiac failure → pulmonary HTN**
- **PIK3CA** mutation
- **Rx: prophylactic anticoagulation, periodic echo (pulmonary HTN), duplex US**

Diffuse capillary malformation with overgrowth

- Unknown gene (GNA11 in some patients)
- p/w widespread reticulated and confluent CMs (PWS) a/w soft tissue/bony hypertrophy
  - **But unlike KTS, the overgrowth and PWS is not limited to the leg, and there usually is a sharp midline demarcation of the PWS**

- Other features: syndactyly, VMs, limb length discrepancies (> 2 cm require ortho eval)

Macrocephaly (Megalencephaly)-Capillary Malformation Syndrome

- Post-zygotic mutation in PIK3CA (upstream up PTEN)
- Macrocephaly (get periodic MRIs)
- CNS dysfunction (seizures, neonatal hypotonia, MR)
- **Mid-face has a reticulated PWS with hemihypertrophy of the contralateral side**
- **Syndactyly** (especially second and third toes)
- Rx: rapamycin

<u>Vascular disorders characterized by telangiectasias ("A GASH causes broken blood vessels")</u>

- Generalized essential telangiectasia (GET): sporadic/ idiopathic disease w/ telangiectasias that starts on the **B/L legs** of girls → spreads proximally but spares face
- Angioma serpiginosum: **multiple tiny punctate (size of a pinhead) red or purple lesions** arranged in a gyrate or **serpiginous** pattern usually arise on the leg of female children
- Ataxia telangiectasia (Louis-Bar): AR defect in Ataxia Telangiectasia Mutated (ATM) gene
    - Gene encodes a protein kinase that responds to DNA Breaks by triggering accumulation of p53 tumor suppressor (but when mutated it causes cancers)
    - **p/w ataxia (1st sign)** and later w/ **telangiectasias on Bulbar conjunctiva** (age 4)
    - Other skin features: **non-infectious granulomas** and sclerodermoid changes
    - Immunodeficiency (all Ig are ↓ except IgM which is ↑) → chronic lung infections
        - "By turning the letter M 90° in a clockwise motion in looks like a B"

- **Bronchiectasis** → respiratory failure (#1 cause of death)
- Blood cancers (lymphoma/leukemia) is the MC cancer
- **Female carriers have ↑ risk of Breast cancer and Blood cancers**
- Dx: **↓ T lymphocytes** (small or absent thymus) and **↑ α-fetoprotein** in serum

- Spider angioma: usually idiopathic in children but may be a/w high estrogen states such as liver disease, pregnancy and OCPs in adults
  - p/w blanchable red lines radiating from a central red papule (MC face and hands)
- Hereditary benign telangiectasia: AD defect in TELAB1 w/ slowly progressive telangiectasias of variable morphology and no associated systemic diseases
- Hereditary hemorrhagic telangiectasia (HHT; Osler-Weber-Rendu syndrome): AD defect in endoglin (lung AVMs; "endo-lung"), ALK1 (AVMs in liver; "AVMs in Liver Kind") or SMAD4 (juvenile polyposis w/ HHT; "SMall ADenoms in GI")
  - Function of genes: **TGF-β stimulation**
  - MC p/w **epistaxis** (1st sign; age 12) and iron deficiency **anemia** (from GI bleeding)
  - Telangiectasias appear later and are MC on lips/mouth, ears, palms/soles/nails
  - Pulmonary AVMs: hypoxemia, pulmonary hemorrhage, strokes
  - Liver AVMs: portal HTN and high-output cardiac failure
  - Workup (look for AVMs): **lung (echo/CT)** > liver (US/CT) > brain (MRI)
  - Rx: nasal moisturization and tranexamic acid (nosebleeds); embolization (AVMs)

Venous malformations (VMs)

- 2 types of VMs: common and familial VMs (95%) and glomuvenous malformations (5%)
- 50% of sporadic VMs have TEK (TIE2) mutation, 25% have PIK3CA mutation
- p/w soft, blue, compressible mass that fills with dependency
- Dx: US shows slow flow lesion; best test is T2 weighted MRI, if positive get coagulation studies such as D-dimer and if positive treat with ASA (mild) or LMWH (severe)
- Rx: sclerotherapy

GLOMuvenous malformations (glomangiomas)

- Glomulin (GLMN) gene; AD
- Legs are #1 site
- Often asymptomatic
- Multiple soft, partially compressible dark blue nodules that appear in infancy
- Modified smooth muscle cells of Sucquet-Hoyer canal origin
- Treatment is difficult
    - Compare with glomuS Tumor which is Three times more common; onset is in Teenage years or later; consists of a Solitary blue nodule on the palms or Subungual areas with Tenderness and Sensitivity to cold; Treatable with excision

Blue-rubber bleb nevus syndrome (BRBNS)

- Caused by double (cis) somatic activating TEK mutations (2 mutations in same allele)
- p/w widely distributed dark blue papules/nodules and skin-colored compressible masses
- VMs also numerous in the **GI tract → hemorrhage→** iron deficiency anemia

Familial cutaneous and mucosal venous malformation syndrome

- AD mutation in TEK → hyperphosphorylation and constitutive activation of TIE-2
- p/w widespread VMs of skin, oral mucosa and muscles **w/o visceral VMs (vs BRBNS)**

Maffucci syndrome ("Massive hands")

- **Non-inherited sporadic somatic Mosaic** mutations in IDH1/IDH2 ("Increased Diameter of Hands") gene which was formerly PTHR1 gene ("Pretty Thick Hand Radius")
- p/w VMs of hands > feet (1st sign; early infancy), **hemangiomas**, enchondromas (cartilage in the bones) of hands (MC) → fractures
- 50% risk for chondrosarcoma which occurs within enchondromas (esp. in the skull)
- ↑ risk of other cancers such as ovarian and liver

Lymphatic malformation: D2-40 (podoplanin) and LYVE-1 positive ("Down 2 LYVE in lymph")

Microcystic/superficial lymPHATIC malformations (lymphangioma circumscriptum)

- Purple Papulovesicles (blood-tinged fluid) Hanging out on Abdomen, Axilla or Tongue In Clusters and Coalescing into a plaque resembling "frog spawn" and Confined to one anatomic region; Rx: CO2 laser (or PDL, sclerotherapy w/ bleomycin, surgical excision)

Macrocystic lymphatic malformation (cystic hygroma)

- Congenital lesion a/w Noonan, Turner and Down syndromes
  - o "Noone turns down large (macrocystic) lymphatic malformations"
- Presents as a large, soft bluish tumor that transilluminates w/ light on head/neck/chest

- Rx: sclerotherapy w/ doxycycline as the sclerosant

Familial lymphedema (hereditary congenital lymphedema; Milroy syndrome)

- Female > male
- AD; **FLT4 gene** (encodes **VEGFR3** required for lymphatic development) → **congenital lymphatic hypoplasia** (vs secondary lymphedema which causes lymphatic hyperplasia)
- Presents at birth (in Fetus) w/ pitting edema of the B/L Feet → Firm and Fibrotic w/ time
- a/w hydroceles (Fluid in scrotum) in males
- Compare to lymphedema praecox (Meige syndrome), lymphedema-distichiasis and lymphedema-yellow nail syndrome which have FOXC2 mutations and present at puberty
    - "Meige was a fox before she got lymphedema, yellow nails and 2 eyelash rows"
- Other rare lymphedema/lymphatic malformation syndromes
    - Gorham-Stout syndrome ("disappearing bone syndrome"): progressive boney destruction due to overlying lymphatic malformations (PIK3CA pathway)
    - Hennekam syndrome: lymphedema of the extremities, MR, abnormal facies and intestinal lymphangiectasia causing a protein-losing enteropathy
    - Aagenaes syndrome: underdevelopment of lymphatic vessels which p/w lymphedema of the legs and feet at birth (just like in Milroy syndrome)

WILD syndrome

- AD; **GATA2** mutation ("GATO is cat in Spanish so I think of a WILD cat")
- Warts (disseminated), Immunodeficiency, Lymphedema, **anogenital** Dysplasia

Arteriovenous malformations (AVMs): "PC culture is flowing-fast and is potentially dangerous"

- RASA1 mutation (tumor suppressor)
- An AVM is an abnormal communication b/w an artery and a vein causing fast-flow shunting of arterial blood to the venous circulation and is potentially dangerous
- p/w red warm Patches/nodules w/ a Painful Palpable thrill or Pulsation (**Cephalic is MC**)
  - These head/neck lesions are often misdiagnosed as PWS or infantile hemangioma at birth (quiescent; stage 1) but may later grow and have palpable thrill (expansion; stage 2) → necrosis (destruction; stage 3) → **CHF** (stage 4)
- Exacerbating factors are Puberty and Pregnancy
- **Most dangerous sequala is CHF and Consumptive Coagulopathy**
- Dx: US or MRI
- **Rx: Cutting them out (embolization + excision)**
- Syndromes w/ AVMs include Parkes-Weber, PTEN hamartoma tumor syndrome, CM-AVM, Cobb, CLOVES (spinal AVMs), HHT, Stewart-Bluefarb, and Bonnet-Duchaume-Blanc

Parkes-Weber syndrome

- Mutation in RASA1 → modulates MAPK signaling (GNAQ mutations did this also)
- Capillary/venous/lymphatic malformations and **multiple fast-flow AVMs**
- Causes soft tissue/bony hypertrophy of legs like Klippel-Trenaunay but is fast flow
- Other features include **high output cardiac failure** and **lytic bone lesions**
  - "I imagine a guy at the Park training for a race (RASA) running fast to work out his big strong legs to the point of high output cardiac failure and bone pain"

- Dx: path, duplex US or MRI showing AVMs will differentiate from Klippel-Trenaunay
- Rx: besides surgery/embolization for AVM, send to ortho for limb length discrepancy

PTEN hamartoma tumor syndrome

- AD mutations in PTEN (**tumor suppressor gene**) which encodes a phosphatase
- Includes ("CBS"): Cowden, Bannayan-Riley-Ruvalcaba and SOLAMEN syndrome
- Generally see Macrocephaly, Malignancy (breast, thyroid, endometrium), genital pigmented Macules, lipomas and fast-flow vascular Malformations in Muscles
- Rx: oral sirolimus (rapa-Mycin)

Capillary malformation- AV malformation (CM-AVM)

- AD loss of function mutation in **RASA1** (#1), EPHB4 (#2) → modulates MAPK signaling
- Multiple **CMs w/ blanched border** and overlying hypotrichosis on the extremities
- 1/3rd of patients have fast flow vascular anomalies → **CHF**
- CNS AVMS → neurologic symptoms/intracranial hemorrhage
- Workup: get MRI/MRA spine/head (even if child is asymptomatic)

Tumor syndromes and overgrowth syndromes in the RAS-MAPK pathway: "PLAN C"

Parkes-Weber syndrome: AD mutation in RASA1
Legius syndrome: AD mutation in SPRED1
Leukocyte adhesion deficiency type 3: AR mutation in KIND3
Capillary malformation-arteriovenous malformation (CM-AVM): AD mutation in RASA1
NF-1: AD mutation in neurofibromin
Noonan syndrome and Noonan syndrome w/ multiple lentigines (LEOPARD): AD; PTPN11
Cardio-facio-cutaneous syndrome: sporadic mutations in BRAF, KRAS, MAP2K1, and MAP2K2
Costello syndrome: AR mutation in HRAS

*All RASopathies have overlapping features of craniofacial, cardiac (pulmonary valve is MC), and MSK anomalies

Cobb syndrome (cutaneomeningospinal angiomatosis)

- p/w a dermatomal skin PWS (it is actually a stage 1 AVM, not a CM), a fast-flow intramedullary spinal AVM and a vertebral AVM in the same segment
- Neurologic abnormalities due to enlarging AVM compressing spinal cord → paraplegia
- Dx: MRI, US or angiography
- Rx: endovascular embolization of spinal AVM may improve prognosis
- "Imagine a kid getting stabbed in the back with a corn on the cob causing vascular lesions on the lower back and paralysis of the legs"

Stewart-Bluefarb syndrome

- Acroangiodermatitis + AVM of the lower leg ("Stewart Bluefarb has a blue foot")

Bonnet-Duchaume-Blanc syndrome (A-F)

- AVMs in the Brain's Choroid plexus, Chiasm of the Eye (p/w blindness), AVMs on Face

Tumor syndromes and overgrowth syndromes in the PIK3/MTOR pathway ("PAM")
PIK3CA gene: CLOVES, M-CMS, Klippel-Trenaunay and Gorham Stout syndrome PTEN gene ("CBS"): Cowden, Bannayan-Riley-Ruvalcaba and SOLAMEN syndrome AKT gene: Proteus syndrome MTOR gene: Tuberous sclerosis

***mTOR inhibitor (rapamycin) may help the tumors and overgrowths in all these conditions**

Angiokeratoma corporis diffusum (ACD)

- Seen in lysosomal storage diseases such as Galactosialidosis, GM1 gangliosidosis, Fabry's disease, Fucosidosis and Sialidosis ("My girlfriends/GFs have angiokeratomas")
- GM1 gangliosidosis: AR deficiency in β-galactosidase-1
    - Fatal neurodegenerative disease
- Fabry's disease (A-G): **XLR** mutation in **Alpha-Galactosidase** (GLA gene) → accumulation of **Ceramide** trihexoside (globotriaosylceramide) in multiple organs
    - p/w **Angiokeratomas in the "Bathing suit" distribution**, **whorl-like Corneal opacities**, posterior capsular Cataracts, **Cardiac** issues, CVAs, **CKD** (**UA shows birefringent lipid globules known as Maltese Crosses**) and Debilitating acral paresthesias triggered by stress (Fabry's Crisis)
    - Dx: lipid (Fat) in Epithelial cells on urinary sediment ("Mulberry cells) and lamellar bodies in Endothelial cells on EM ("Zebra bodies")
    - Rx: recombinant Enzyme therapy
    - Female carriers commonly have symptoms (**Corneal opacities** > Angiokeratomas)
        - Female carriers of X-linked ichthyosis also have corneal opacities
- Fucosidosis: AR deficiency in α-L fucosidase

- Fatal neurodegenerative disease w/ generalized ACD (age 5) and coarse facies

Birefringence on microscopy
Lipids/Fat: Fabry's (Maltese Crosses in urine) and Gaucher's disease Crystals: gout (urate; negative birefringence) and Pseudogout (Ca Pyrophosphate; Positive) Protein: amyloid (positive birefringence on polarized light w/ Congo red stain)

Gaucher's disease

- Although this is not a vascular disorder it is included here to compare to Fabry's disease
- AR deficiency in **acid β-glucocerebrocidase** (GBA gene vs GLA in Fabry's) → accumulation of the glyco-sphingolipid lactosyl **ceramide**
- Skin: acral hyperpigmentation (head/neck, hands/feet) and petechia
- Other: hepatosplenomegaly, LAD, bone pain/deformities ("Erlenmeyer flask on X-ray")
- Like Fabry's you see lipid in cells (macrophages in Gaucher's)
- Like Fabry's the treatment is enzyme replacement

4.7 Disorders of Hair and Nails

Pachyonychia congenita

- "Pachy" = thick; "onychia" = nails → patients develop thickened yellow "pincer nails"
    - Clouston (alopecia) and EB (blisters) can also have pincer-like nails and PPK
- **Painful focal PPK (100% by childhood)** w/ hyperhidrosis, secondary fissures and bullae
- Two types: in addition to thick nails and PPK they each have 1 key skin and oral finding

- Type 1: Jadassohn-Lewandowski
  - KRT6A and KRT16
  - Skin: follicular hyperkeratosis of knees, elbows, back and buttocks
  - Oral: **benign oral leukoplakia** of tongue/buccal mucosa (**vs pre-malignant in DC**)
- Type 2: Jackson-Lawler
  - KRT6B and KRT17
  - Skin: steatocystoms (with a milder palmoplantar keratoderma)
  - Oral: natal teeth ("I imagine a cystic baby smiling as he comes out of the womb")
- Rx: efforts to minimize pressure (orthotic shoes) help w/ the painful PPK

Ectodermal dysplasias

- Hypohidrotic ectodermal dysplasia (HED; Christ-Siemens-Touraine syndrome)
  - XLR mutation in ectodysplasin (ED1) or AD/AR mutations in the ectodysplasin receptor (**EDARDD, EDAR**): x-inactivation causes mild features in female carriers
  - Clinical triad: Hypo-Trichosis + abnormal Teeth + ↓ sweating → hyper-Thermia
    - Other features: frontal bossing, thin arched eyebrow, thick everted lips, **darkening of skin under eyes**, keratoconjunctivitis sicca, lung infections
    - Female carriers: more mild symptoms of "3 Ts" and breast asymmetry
    - EM of hair shows longitudinal grooves and path shows ↓ eccrine glands
    - HED w/ immunodeficiency is due to an XLR mutation in NEMO (IKBKG; NFkB pathway) → **both IP (NEMO/IKBKG) and HED have pegged teeth**

- Hidrotic ectodermal dysplasia (Clouston syndrome)
  - AD mutation in JGB6 (connexin 30)
  - Clinical triad: PPK, marked onychodystrophy, hypotrichosis, and normal sweating
  - Normal teeth and facial features but can get eye issues and tufted distal phalanx
  - "I imagine a sweaty guy at the gym who lifts so much that he gets PPK, nail dystrophy and tufted distal phalanges; gym guys shave their hair (hypotrichosis)"
- Ectodermal dysplasia due to p63 mutation
  - AD mutation in p63 (critical **transcription factor** for development)
  - Three types, all which may have ↓hair/teeth/sweating and dystrophic nails
    - Ankyloblepharon-Ectodermal dysplasia-Clefting syndr. (AEC; Hay-Wells)
      - Ankyloblepharon (congenital fusion of eyelids)
      - **Erosive scalp dermatitis at birth** w/ frequent staph infections
      - Collodion baby at birth; Cleft lip/palate
    - Ectrodactyly ectodermal dysplasia-cleft lip/palate syndrome (EED)
      - Ectrodactyly (missing digits) → lobster claw
      - Conductive hearing loss and genitourinary issues (hydronephrosis)
      - "Digits, Deafness, and Dick problems"
    - Rapp-Hodgkin syndrome
      - Clefting of lip/palate/uvula and small maxilla/nails/teeth
- Rubinstein-Taybi syndrome
  - AD mutation in CREBBP or EP300 gene
    - Congenital heart defects; Cryptorchidism; **Keloids** ("Celoids")

        - Retardation
        - Epicanthal folds; low set Ears
        - **Brachyonychia (racquet nails) w/ Broad thumbs**; Beaked nose
        - Pilomatricomas
- Schopf-Schulz-Passarge syndrome (SSPS)
    - AR mutation in **WNT10A** (signaling molecule w/ many roles in embryogenesis)
    - p/w PPK, nail dystrophy, hypodontia, hypotrichosis and **multiple periocular and eyelid apocrine hidrocystomas**
- Odonto-onycho-dermal dysplasia
    - Like SSPS it's an AR mutation in WNT10A causing ectodermal dysplasia w/ severe oligodontia, nail dystrophy, PPK and hypotrichosis but instead of periocular hidrocystomas there are erythematous lesions on the face and a smooth tongue

Pediatric hair disorders that present at the time of birth
Pili torti, Wooly hair, Marie Unna hypotrichosis ("Pili torti, wooly, Marie all rhyme with baby")

Structural hair abnormalities with increased hair fragility (T's Tear/brake easily with Trauma)

- Bubble hair from Traumatic heat styling/**ironing**: p/w localized area of fragile hair
    - Light microscopy: hair shafts w/ large, irregularly spaced bubbles
- Monilethrix ("LETHRIKS"): LPP-like changes w/ perifollicular Erythema, Thin/short/fragile hair w/ follicular Hyperkeratosis of the occipital scalp > eyebrows/ eyelashes; Regular appearing hair at birth but abnormality appears within first few months; Improves with age and during pregnancy; Koilonychia is common; Keratosis pilaris is MC association; **KRT 86** > 81, 83 (AD) > Dsg4 (AR) mutation

- Light microscopy: Sign-wave/beaded appearance due to hairs w/ uniform elliptical nodes of normal thickness and intermittent abnormal constrictions

- Pili Torti: twisted hairs → fragility: "DUMB HAIR" (DUMB H is inherited, AIR is acquired)
  - Ectodermal Dysplasias
  - Urea cycle defects
    - Argininosuccinic aciduria: AR; deficiency of argininosuccinate lyase → hyperammonemia (ammonia is neurotoxic) → vomiting, lethargy, coma
      - Rx: restricted protein diet and arginine supplementation
    - Citrullinemia (presents the same way)
  - Menke's disease (ABCD): XLR mutation in ATP7A (**defective copper transport**) → Alopecia w/ sparse lusterless hair on scalp (pili torti or trichorrhexis nodosa); Bone/Brain issues; Cupid's bow; Doughy lax skin w/ Diffuse hypopigmentation
  - Bjornstad/Crandall syndrome: pili torti w/ deafness (+ hypogonadism in Crandall)
  - Bazex-Dupré-Christol syndrome: hypotrichosis due to pili torti, hypohidrosis, follicular atrophoderma on face and extremities, milia and BCCs
  - Hypotrichosis w/ juvenile macular dystrophy
  - Anorexia nervosa (malnutrition)
  - Inflammatory hair conditions (SLE)
  - Retinoid therapy
- Trichorrhexis invaginata ("bamboo hair"): Netherton syndrome (SPINK5 gene which encodes **serine protease inhibitor** LEKT1) → p/w **ichthyosis linearis circumflexa**, atopy, **FTT**, **hypernatremia** and short, fragile hair in infancy ("I Nether turn down a vagina")
  - Light microscopy: ball-in-socket (**invaginata**) or golf tee-shaped appearance
- Trichorrhexis nodosa: MC structural hair abnormality

  - Congenital: argininosuccinic aciduria > citrullinemia
  - Acquired (three variants): Proximal (from hair straightening Practices), Distal (from cuticular Damage) and circumscribed
  - Light microscopy: **resembles two paint brushes pushed against each other**
- Trichothiodystrophy (PIBIDS)
  - AR mutation in ERCC2 (XPD) and ERCC3 (XPB) → **poor nucleotide excision repair**
  - Photosensitivity; Ichthyosis; Brittle hair due to sulfur deficiency; Intellectual impairment; Decreased fertility; Decreased immunoglobins; Short stature
  - Light microscopy: transverse fractures (trichoschisis) w/ alternating light and dark bands under **polarized light**
  - No risk of carcinogenesis (vs XP) as nucleotide excision repair is not 100% absent

Structural hair abnormalities without increased hair fragility (**normal hair strength**)

- Acquired progressive kinking of the hair: frizzy lusterless hair that is an early sign of AGA
  - "Bald men with pattern alopecia are kinky"
- Loose anagen hair syndrome: **poor cornification of IRS** → poorly anchored anagen hairs
  - **p/w short blond hair that never needs to be cut and scalp hairs that can be easily and painlessly plucked in Caucasian girls age 2–6**
  - Microscopy: "hockey stick" anagen hairs w/ ruffled cuticle and absent IRS/ORS
  - "I imagine a loose (promiscuous) blond girl who plays hockey, looks roughed up (ruffled cuticle) and is not wearing any clothing (absent sheath)"
- Pili Annulati ("ringed hair"): Alternating light and dark bands due to Air-filled spaces

  - Do not need polarized light to see (vs trichothiodystrophy)
- Pili bifurcati: individual hair shafts bifurcate in two
- Pili multigemini: multiple hair shafts come out of the same papilla; MC on the beard
  - Hairs share a common ORS, but each have their own IRS
- Pili trianguli et canaliculi ("spun glass hair/uncombable hair"): p/w blond dry unruly spun glass hair in infancy (triangular shaped hair w/ canalicular longitudinal grooves → hypohidrotic ectodermal dysplasia and Marie Unna hypotrichosis show this also)
- Wooly hair syndrome
  - Naxos: diffuse Non-epidermolytic PPK, RVH, wooly hair; Plakoglobulin mutation
  - Carvajal: Linear Epidermolytic PPK, LVH, wooly hair; Demsoplakin mutation
    - The first letter in the name is close in the alphabet to the first letter of the mutation, and the last letter reminds you of the side of heart failure

Other hair and nail disorders not discussed elsewhere

- Temporal triangular alopecia: frontotemporal scalp alopecia in 1st decade of life
  - Trichoscopy: ↓ terminal hairs and ↑ vellus hairs
- Atrichia w/ papules: should be called "trichia-atrichia w/ papules" because hair is normal at birth then is quickly shed after birth and then milia-like papules appear later
  - Mutation in hairless (HR) gene
  - a/w Vitamin-D-resistant Rickets
- Marie Unna hypotrichosis (hereditary trichodysplasia): absence of scalp, eyebrow and eyelash hair at birth; hair grows in course but then is lost beginning in adolescence

  - AD mutation in U2HR
  - Light microscopy: hair shafts w/ variable diameter w/ a twisted/bent appearance
  - EM: longitudinal grooves ("gruuves") and peeling of the cuticle
- Nevoid hypertrichosis: localized patches of terminal hairs commonly seen on the lumbosacral area, anterior neck and elbows (hypertrichosis cubiti)
- Congenital hypertrichosis
  - Ambras syndrome ("werewolf syndrome"): p/w excess vellus-like hairs on the face, ears and shoulders; due to mutation in TRPS1 gene
    - "Vellus hairs above their braws and TRAPS (face/ears/shoulders)"
  - Cornellia de Lange syndrome (NIPBL gene): p/w Congenital hair issues (hirsutism, synophrys, trichomegaly, low hairline), 5th finger Clinodactyly, simian Crease, Congenital heart defects, Cryptorchidism as well as deafness and renal issues
- Keratosis pilaris: abnormal keratinization of hair follicles which p/w small pink follicular papules on the cheeks, upper arms, thighs and butt; a/w atopy and ichthyosis vulgaris
- Keratosis pilaris atrophicans, atrophoderma vermiculatum subtype: p/w erythematous papules w/ follicular plugging and atrophic "worm-like' scarring of the **cheeks** of children
  - Seen in Loeys-Diets, Nicholau-Balus and Rombo syndromes
    - "There's already worms growing out of his face, just sign the DNR"
- Keratosis pilaris atrophicans, ulerythema ophyrogenes subtype: p/w erythematous papules w/ follicular plugging, atrophic scarring and scarring alopecia of the **eyebrows**

    - Seen in cardio-facio-cutaneous, Cornellia de Lange and Wooly hair syndromes
- Keratosis pilaris Atrophicans, Keratosis follicularis spinulosa decalvans subtype: p/w severe KP in Kids and scarring Alopecia of the scalp in Adolescence
    - XLR mutation in SSAT or mutation in MBTPS2 (allelic w/ IPAF)
- Eruptive vellus Hair Cysts: p/w small Hyperpigmented papules that favor the mid Chest
    - a/w Pachyonychia Congenita, Hidrotic and Hypohidrotic ectodermal dysplasia
- Congenital malalignment of the great toes: p/w B/L yellow, thick, ridged great toenails

4.8 Inherited Metabolic Disorders

Acrodermatitis enteropathica (ADE)

- AR mutation in **SLC39A4** (encodes intestinal zinc transporter ZIP4) → zinc deficiency
- Secondary zinc deficiency due to ↓ intake has similar clinical findings and is seen in **cystic fibrosis** patients, alcoholics, anorexia, preterm infants, any infant who breastfeeds from zinc deficient mothers and any **infant when weaned from breast milk to formula**
- p/w the triad of ADE: **Alopecia + Diarrhea + Erosive vesiculopustular Eczematous lesions** involving Acral sites, the Diaper area and the peri-oral region (where they Eat)
    - The eczematous lesions have an orange hue and spare the upper cutaneous lip and gives a classic "U-shape" when on the face (vs infantile eczema which spare the diaper area and the central face and gives a "car headlights" appearance)
- Other features: FTT, irritability, photophobia, glossitis/ stomatitis and nail dystrophy

- MCC of death is secondary infection and respiratory failure
- Path: keratinocytes with cytoplasmic pallor in an acanthotic psoriasiform epidermis
- Labs: ↓ **Alkaline phosphatase** which is a zinc-Dependent Enzyme (and ↓ zinc obviously)
- Rx: zinc supplementation

Wilson's disease

- AR mutation in ATP7B (encodes ATPase CU^{2+}-transporting peptide) → CU^{2+} accumulates
  - o ATP7A mutation was seen in Menke's and caused a copper deficiency
- p/w **blue lanula**, pretibial hyperpigmentation, Kayser-fleischer rings (yellow-brown copper deposits in Descemet's membrane of the cornea), cirrhosis, ataxia and dementia
  - o I imagine Tom Hanks yelling "Wilson" in the movie Cast Away. His fingernails are dirty (blue lanula), his legs are pigmented from being on the island without sunscreen and he becomes demented and talks to a volleyball he names Wilson.
- Labs: ↓ serum ceruloplasmin and ↑ serum/urine copper levels
- Rx: oral penicillamine, ↓ copper intake and ↑ zinc intake; liver transplant
  - o Copper is needed for elastin so penicillamine causes various disorders of elastin including EPS, PXE, cutis laxa, etc.

Hemochromatosis

- AR mutation in **HFE gene** → ↑ intestinal iron absorption → deposition in various organs
- Presents around 5th decade so really should not be in the pediatric section

- p/w Hair abnormalities (sparse/absent), generalized Hyperpigmentation ("bronze diabetes"), Hepatomegaly (cirrhosis), Hypogonadism, Heart block/failure and diabetes
- Labs: High levels of ferritin and iron
- Rx: phlebotomy; iron chelation w/ deferoxamine

Biotinidase deficiency/multiple carboxylase deficiency

- AR mutation in biotinidase or holocarboxylase synthetase → ↓ serum biotin
- Presents in early infancy with: "botox (biotinidase/carboxylase def.) the DAOs"
    - Dermatitis (periorificial or generalized)
    - Alopecia
    - Optic atrophy or other neurologic sequela (seizures, deafness)
- Labs: ↓ serum biotin and metabolic acidosis
- Rx: IV biotin replacement

Hartnup disease

- AR mutation in SLC6A19 gene (encodes the BOAT1 GI/renal neutral amino acid transporter) → ↓ **tryptophan which is required for niacin production** → pellagra-like syndrome with massive aminoaciduria from unabsorbed tryptophan derivatives
- Pellagra-like symptoms: acute photodermatitis in childhood w/ beet-red erythema, blistering, crusting and scarring in sun exposed areas after sun-exposure
    - May also see atrophic glossitis, alopecia and longitudinal nail streaks
- Neurologic symptoms from aminoaciduria: cerebellar ataxia, seizures, MR, psychosis
- Rx: sun avoidance and **oral nicotinamide** supplementation (not niacin due to flushing)

- "I imagine a turnup (hartnup) baking out all day in the sun (photosensitivity). Turnips are beet-red, acidic (acidic urine), and have no brains (neurologic issues)"

SLC mutations (solute carrier family): "Slick HAIL"
Hartnup (SLC6A19); Hemochromatosis (SLC11A3)
Acrodermatitis enteropathica (SLC39A4)
Ichthyosis prematurity syndrome (SLC27A4)
Leukocyte adhesion deficiency type 2 (SLC35C1)

Phenylketonuria

- AR mutation in phenylalanine hydroxylase → can't convert phenylalanine to tryptophan (↑ phenylalanine inhibits tyrosine in melanogenesis and has toxic effects on CNS)
- p/w "SHENylketonuria"
  - o Sclerodermoid changes (generalized)
  - o Hypopigmentation (generalized) with blue eyes and blond hair
  - o Eczematous dermatitis
  - o Neuro symptoms (MR, seizures, hypereflexia, psychomotor delay)
  - o Uria: urine has mousy odor
- Rx: low phenylalanine diet implemented early will prevent skin and CNS changes

Homocystinuria ("Sherlock HOLMES is on CBS")

- AR mutation in cystathionine β-synthase (CBS) gene → accumulation of homocysteine
- p/w (HOLMES)
  - o Hypopigmentation, **Hypercoagulability** (thrombotic and embolic phenomena)
  - o Osteoporosis
  - o **Leg Ulcers, Livedo reticularis**
  - o Malar erythema, Mental retardation, Marfanoid habitus, MVP, MI

 - Ectopia lentis (downward displacement of lens vs upwards in Marfans)
 - Sparse blonde friable hair, Seizures (and other neuro symptoms)
- Labs: ↑ homocysteine and methionine levels in blood and urine
- Rx (CBS): Cystine-rich/low methionine diet and **vitamin B (6 > 9, 12) Supplements**

Lesch-Nyhan syndrome ("LMNOPqRST")

- XLR mutation in hypoxanthine-guanine phosphoribosyl transferase (HGPRT gene)
- p/w (M-T): Megaloblastic anemia, MR, Neurodevelopmental delays, Nephropathy, **Orange uric acid crystals in diaper**, cerebral Palsy, **Red urine**, **Renal failure (MCC of death)**, Self-mutilation, Short stature, gout/gouty **Tophi**
- If you were to give azathioprine to these patients it would not work
- Rx: hypouricemic agents such as allopurinol

Prolidase deficiency

- AR defect in Peptidase D (PEPD) which encodes Prolidase involved in Protein catabolism
- p/w Progressive leg ulcerations, Photosensitivity and recurrent Pyogenic infections
- Other features: MR, hyperbilirubinemia, HSM, abnormal facies (hypertelorism, Ptosis)

Alagille syndrome

- AD mutation in Jagged 1 (JAG1) which encodes ligand for Notch receptor
- Triangular faces (broad forehead, hypertelorism, deep-set eyes, large ears, pointed chin)

- Congenital intrahepatic biliary hypoplasia ("Absent Gallbladder ducts") → cholestasis → ↑ triglycerides/ cholesterol → tuberous xanthomas
- Rx: liver transplantation and lipid lowering agents

Hunter syndrome

- XLR ("shoot at the X") mutation in IDS ("Incredible Deer Shooter") gene which encodes a lysosomal enzyme (iduronate sulfatase) → glycosaminoglycans accumulate in tissues
- **p/w pebbly ivory-colored plaque b/w the scapula on upper back (great Kodachrome)**
    - o "Aim b/w the scapula on the back when you are hunting for pebbled ivory tusks"
- Other features: Hypertrichosis/Hirsutism, coarse faces (Huge tongue/lips/nose), claw Hand, Hydrocephalus → MR, Hearing loss, umbilical/inguinal Hernia, HSM, Hoarse voice
- Path: vacuoles (Holes) and granules in fibroblasts; vacuolated cells (Holes) in eccrine glands and hair follicles ("Gargoyl cells"), ↑ mucin, Hyalinized collagen
    - o Granules are Alcian blue (+), colloidal iron (+), metachromatic w/ toluidine blue
- Labs: ↑ urinary Heparin sulfate/dermatan sulfate/ chondroitin sulfate
- Rx: enzyme replacement

Hurler syndrome

- AR mutation in IDUA which encodes α-L-iduronidase (↑ dermatan and heparin sulfate)
- Presents like Hunter except you see Mongolian spots instead of pebbly ivory colored plaque on the back and in Hurler corneal clouding is present ("Hunters need to see")

- Another mucopolysaccharidosis is Morquio syndrome B (GLB1 encodes **β-galactosidase**) which p/w skeletal deformities and motor dysfunctions

Alkaptonuria (A-I)

- Arthritis/Arthropathy of larger joints
- Blue-gray pigmentation (ochronosis) of skin (face) and cartilage (hands, nasal tip, ears)
  - Kodachrome may look similar to drug-induced pigmentation (minocycline) but **ochronosis has more texture ("caviar-like papules")**
- Cardiac issues (valvulitis/MI); Calcification of intervertebral discs
- Dark sweat, cerumen and urine at ↑ pH (commonly noticed when using alkaline cleaning products such as sodium hydroxide)
- Ears, Eyes and Face are most commonly affected by pigmentary changes
- AR mutation in Homogentisic 1,2-dioxygenase (HGO) gene → ↑ homogentisic acid
- Rx: nitisinone (reduces homogentisic acid)

4.9 Inherited Connective Tissue Disorders

Cutis laxa (generalized elastolysis; A-H)

- ATP7A mutation (XLR, known as occipital horn syndrome: wedge-shaped calcifications)
  - other ATP mutations: ATP2C1 (Hailey-Hailey), ATP2A2 (Dariers), and ATP7A (Menkes)
- Acquired cutis laxa with D-penicillamine use and systemic diseases (SLE, RA, and infections)
- Aged facial appearance due to loose, saggy, and inelastic skin
- Aortic dilation → Aneurism
- Bladder diverticula

- **Cor pulmonale**
- Copper metabolism is ↓ → ↓ lysyl oxidase → ↓ desmosine crosslinks
- Corneal Clouding/Cataracts in an AR subtype known as De Barsy syndrome (PYCR1 gene)
- Diaphragmatic hernia, Deep voice due to vocal cord laxity
- Labs: ↓ Desmosine mRNA levels, ↓ Elastin mRNA levels
- Elastin mutation (AD), **Emphysema**
- **Fibulin 5 mutation (AR) is MC form → skin and severe internal involvement**
- GI/GU diverticula
- Hound dog faces, Hip dislocations (joint laxity), Hernias (umbilical, diaphragmatic)
- Hypoplastic lungs in newborns

Pseudoxanthoma elasticuM (PXE): "P = skin (occurs first), M = internal symptoms (occurs later)"

- Acquired (Penicillamine) or AR mutation in ABCC6 → calcification of elastic tissue
- Presents during Puberty with thin, yellow Papules in flexural sites (usually appears on lateral neck first) which coalesce into Plaques resembling "Plucked chicken skin"
- Perforating PXE can occur in advanced disease
- Rupture of Bruch's Membrane of eye → **angioid streaks** (also seen in HOT APPLES: Hypophosphatemia, Osteogenesis imperfecta, Thalassemia, Age-related degeneration, Acromegaly, Paget's disease of bone, PXE, Lead poisoning, EDS and Sickle cell anemia)
- Macular degeneration
- Mottling of retinal pigment epithelium is most prevalent eye finding and first finding overall (congenital hypertrophy of retinal pigment epithelium is in Gardner's disease)

- **MVP, Myocardial infarction and atherosclerosis of Medium sized arteries** (esp. in extremities) → loss of peripheral pulses, strokes and HTN due to decreased renal flow
- Melena in stool due to **gastric artery hemorrhage** (**aspirin is CI** even though they get MI)
  - Uterine hemorrhage and aortic aneurisms also occur
- ↑ risk of first trimester Miscarriage
- Rx: Magnesium helps
- Path: fragmented, clumped and calcified elastic fibers ("bramble bush") in the dermis
  - Will stain w/ both Von-Kossa (calcium stain) and VVG (elastin stain)
  - D-penicillamine use looks like PXE on path but only stains w/ VVG, not Von-Kossa
- **Refer to cardiology and ophthalmology**

Ehlers-Danlos syndrome

Remember types of collagen: Collagen 1 (one) found in Bone → EDS and OI; Collagen 2 found in cartilage ("car-2-lage") → Relapsing polychondritis, MAGIC; Collagen 3 ("Big Gross Stinky Feet"): Blood vessels, GI tract, Scars, Fetal skin) → EDS, vascular type; Collagen 5 in skin EDS, classic

Mnemonic is Coll 1, Coll 3, Coll 5, TAL (Coll's are AD, TAL is AR except T which is AD/AR)

- COL1A (arthrochalasic form): **hypermobile joints** with moderate skin involvement
  - Most severe joint hypermobility and congenital hip dislocation (Coll one in bone)
- COL3A (vascular form): **translucent non-hypermobile skin** (underlying vessels visible)
  - Also see life-threatening **arterial/GI/uterine/intestinal rupture**, acrogyria (bird face), blue

sclera, CVAs, club feet; joint hypermobility is limited to fingers

- COL5A (classical form; A-H): **hypermobile joints and skin**
    - o **Atrophic "fish mouth" or "cigarette paper" scars**, **Blue sclera**, easy Bruising, Beighton scale assesses joint hypermobility, Calcified fat lobules presenting as SQ nodules, Cardiac manifestations (**MVP**), **Dilation of aortic root**, Double-jointed fingers, ↑ Extensibility of skin, Early rupture of fetal membranes, Extensor joints have overlying molluscoid pseudotumors, Flat Feet (pes planus), (+) Gorlin's sign (absent lingual frenulum), GI bleeding, Hiatal/ inguinal Hernias
- TNXB/Tenascin-X (hypermobility form): **hypermobile joints and skin**
    - o Classic-EDS phenotype with more severe joint subluxations
    - o Both AD and AR forms exist; AR form gets congenital adrenal hyperplasia (CAH → "tenas-CAH mutation") and AD has minimal skin involvement
- ADAMTS2/procollagen N-proteinase (**Dermatosparaxis**; "derm-adam-spraxis"): **bruised sagging skin**
    - o **Cutis laxa phenotype** with puffy eyelids and premature rupture of membranes
- Lysyl hydroxylase/PLOD1 (kyphoscoliotic form): **hypermobile joints**
    - o Severe kyphoscoliosis with marfanoid habitus, floppy baby at birth, eye issues (ruptured globe, blindness, retinal detachment, keratoconus); Rx: vytamin C

Osteogenesis imperfecta (OI; "im-Berfecta")

- AD mutation in **type 1 collagen** (COL1A1 and COL1A2) found in Bone

- AR mutation in WNT1 (regulates β-catenin) is less common

- Type 1 is mild and most common (normal life span), type 2 is most severe (fatal in perinatal period), type 3 (death in 3rd/4th decade due to respiratory failure; **can't Breath**)
- Bluish translucent teeth, **Blue sclera**, and thin translucent Bruised skin
- Joints are hypermobile like in Ehlers-Danlos but skin in OI is not hyperelastic (similar to arthrochalasic EDS w/ COL1 mutation)
- Brittle bones (fractures), Bowing of long bones, temporal and frontal Bossing, Beaded ribs (also seen in Rickets) and Bad hearing (**deafness**)
- Blood Backflows in heart from mitral and aortic valve prolapse/dilatation/regurgitation
- Neuro sequela from **macrocephaly**/hydrocephalus (Big Brain) and Basilar invagination
- Workup: PFTs, echo, neuro, and ortho consult

Know your teeth: send all these patients to dentistry
Gardner syndrome: odontomas and supernumerary teeth ("plant many teeth in the Garden")
Late congenital syphilis: notched incisors (mulberry molars)
Dyskeratosis congenita, EBD, Cockayne, Kindler: dental caries ("Dental Ckaries")
Hyper IgE (Job's) syndrome: retention of primary teeth → double row of teeth
Pachyonychia congenita type 2: natal teeth (erupted primary teeth at birth)
KID and progeria: delayed eruption of primary teeth
Congenital erythropoietic porphyria: red-brown teeth
Osteogenesis imperfecta: dentinogenesis imperfecta (blue-gray translucent teeth)
Alkaptonuria and teeth staining from tetracyclines: blue-gray teeth (not translucent)
Tuberous sclerosis, Goltz, Junctional EB: dental pits ("To Go eat Junk food rots teeth")
Letterer-Siwe: floating teeth due to resorption of alveolar ridge ("floating like seaweed")
Papillon-Levefre, EDS, LAD type 1, Naegeli-Franceschetti-Jadassohn: Periodontitis ("Poor ELF")
Incontinentia pigmenti and hypohidrotic ectodermal dysplasia: hypodontia and peg teeth
IP, hypomelanosis of Ito, various ectodermal dysplasias (EED, ADE): hypodontia/anodontia

Fibrillin mutations ("Do not be a fibber and tell on me to MS. C")
Fibrillin-1: Marfan, linear Morphea (autoantibody), Stiff skin syndrome
Fibrillin-2: Congenital contractural arachnodactyly

Marfan syndrome

- AD mutation in FBN1 (Fibrillin-1)
- To remember the clinical manifestations, I think of **"long and lax"**
  - Long extremities with kyphoscoliosis and joint laxity
  - **MC skin findings are long striae** but **EPS** is another testable skin finding

    - Fingers are long, slender and curved, like the legs of a spider (arachnodactyly)
        - Thumb sign: thumb sticks out the other side of a closed fist
        - Wrist sign: can wrap their fingers easily around their wrist
    - The **lens** is lax and is displaced upwards and **retina** is lax and frequently detaches
    - The heart is lax with MVP and **dilatation of ascending aorta** → AR → CHF/dissection/aneurysm/rupture (**cardiac complications is MCC of death**)
    - The lungs are lax resulting in spontaneous pneumothoraxes → emphysema
- Workup: send to ophtho and order an echo to monitor the aortic root

Stiff Skin Syndrome

- AD mutation in fibrillin-1 (FBN1)
- p/w **Stone-hard Skin that Spares hands/feet and inguinal folds in infancy** (sclerema neonatorum is similar but sicker) → large joint contractures, Scoliosis, Short Stature
    - Diffuse hard skin in neonates ddx ("Really Hard Skin"): Restrictive dermopathy, Hutchinson-Gilford progeria, Stiff skin syndrome, Sclerema neonatorum
        - Progeria usually presents later (12 months) than the others and the scleroderma is more localized (bathing suit distribution)
- Path: **Sclerosis of the fascia** with Sclerotic collagen bundles but unlike morphea, there is **no inflammation at the dermal/SQ junction, and it does not trap adnexal structures**
- Rx: physical therapy

Congenital Contractural arachnodactyly

- AD mutation in fibrillin 2 (FBN2) gene
- **Crumpled ears** and other characteristic facial features (high forehead, hypertelorism, down-slanting palpebral fissures, anteverted nostrils, retromicrognathia, short neck)
- **Cardiac manifestations (MVP and aortic root dilation like Marfans → get echo)**
- Arachnodactyly w/ marfanoid habitus, kyphoscoliosis and congenital joint contractures
  - o "Looks like Marfan but has more joint/bone contractures"
- Workup: echo and ortho consult

Genoderms with marfanoid features: "Give Marfan the HEIM-LICK"
Homocystinuria, Ehlers-Danlos syndrome kyphoscoliotic type, MEN2B Loeys-Dietz, Congenital contractural arachnodactyly, Klinefelter syndrome

Buschke-Ollendorf syndrome: "Ollem-Dorf"

- AD mutation in LEMD3/MAN1 → **↑TGF-β signaling**
  - o HHT (Osler-Weber-Rendu) had mutation in genes involved in TGF-β signaling
- Osteopoikilosis ("spotted bones"): asymptomatic circular densities in epiphyses and mataphyses of long bones often noted incidentally on x-ray
- Dermatofibrosis lenticularis disseminata: elastoma > collagenoma on butt, trunk > limbs which p/w symmetric, small, uniform, yellowish papules in infancy

Infantile systemic hyalinosis (ISH) and juvenile hyaline fibromatosis (JHF): "HEIGHT"

- Hyalinization of skin/internal organs d/t AR disease in CMG2 gene ("Can't Move Good")
  - o Encodes ANTXR2 which interacts w/ collagen → collagen accumulation/fibrosis

- **Ears > perinasal/perioral/perianal areas** have tiny papules to large fibrotic nodules
- Internal organ involvement: **malabsorption in ISH** and **osteolytic bone lesions in JHF**
- **Infections (pulmonary)** and GI complications are the MCC of death in ISH
    - o Death by 2 years vs 4th decade in JHF
- **Gingival Hypertrophy** and Thickening of the oral mucosa are classic oral findings
- Terrible joint contractures limit movement and shrink them in "HEIGHT"
- Path: hyalinized, homogenous, amorphous PAS-positive connective tissue stroma
- Rx: surgical excision or ILK of papules/nodules, SQ IFN-α-2b, proteasome inhibitors

Lipoid proteinosis (A-E words so I say "prot-AE-nosis")

- Alopecia and **Atrophic "ice-pick" scars on face** after initial facial bullous lesions resolve
- **Beaded eyelid papules (string of pearls)**, Big tongue, **Breathing problems (early death)**
- **Cry is hoarse at birth**; **Calcifications in the temporal lobe** (hippocampus/amygdala)
- Dental anomalies
- Extensor surfaces (Elbows, hands) develop verrucous papules
- Eversion of the lips (which are studded with tiny yellow nodules)
- Path: Amorphous BM-like material containing Collagen types II and IV are Deposited around Adnexa, Blood vessels, Connective tissue and the DEJ
    - o Material is PAS + and diastase-resistant
- Rx: Acitretin, Corticosteroids, D-penicillamine, Dimethylsulphoxide (DMSO)
- Extracellular matrix protein 1 (**ECM1**) gene is mutated (LS&A has antibodies to this gene)

Focal dermal hypoplasia (Goltz syndrome, Goltz-Gorlin syndrome): F looks like a P

- **XLD (Females)** mutation in PORCN gene which encodes a Putative O-acyltransferase involved in Palmitoylation of **Wnt** (a morphogen important in development)
- Involves all three embryonic layers: ectoderm (skin and teeth), mesoderm (dermis and bone) and endoderm (mucosa of mouth and larynx) in a mosaic pattern
- p/w Poikiloderma (**atrophy**/telangiectasias) and Fat herniations in **blaschkoid lines**
    - **Raspberry-like Papillomas that favor the lips and anogenital region (good koda)**
        - These look different than oral papillomas seen in Dariers and Cowdens
    - Dysmorphic Faces (notched nasal ala/ears), ocular findings (**coloboma,** hyper- and hypo-Pigmented retina), absent hair/nails/teeth with **dental pits**
        - TS, Goltz, Junctional EB has dental pits ("To Go eat Junk food rots teeth")
    - Finger anomalies (ectrodactyly/**lobster claw** deformity, syndactyly, polydactyly)
    - Osteopathia striata (vertical striations in long bone metaphyses on x-ray)
        - "Goltz scratches his long bones with his lobster claws"
- Path: markedly decreased or absent dermis with SQ fat abutting the epidermis
- Workup: send to ophtho, dentistry, ortho, otolaryngologist (papillomas of the larynx)

Know your pits

Palmar pits: Gorlin's syndrome, Darier's disease and reticulate acropigmentation of Kitamura
Helical (ear) pits: Beckwith-Weideman
Enamel pits: Tuberous sclerosis, Goltz, Junctional EB ("To Go eat Junk food rots teeth")
Lip pits: Van der Woude syndrome, Kabuki syndrome, popliteal pterygium syndrome
Preauricular pits (accessory tragi): Treacher-Collins syndrome, Goldenhar syndrome

- "Teachers will give you a Gold star if you listen (preauricular pits)"

Sacral dimples: Robinow, Smith-Lemli-Opitz, Carpenter syndrome

- "Rob Smith was a carpenter that sat on his ass all day causing sacral dimples"

Weird things in Blaschoid lines

Conradi-Hünermann-Happle: ichthyosiform erythroderma → follicular atrophoderma
Incontinentia pigmenti: bullous → verrucous → hyperpigmented → hypopigmented
Goltz: telangiectasias, hypopigmentation, hyperpigmentation, dermal atrophy, fat herniation
*All of these conditions are XLD (vast majority are females)

Restrictive dermopathy ("LMNOPqRST")

- AR mutation in Lamin-A (LMNA; same gene as Progeria) or zinc Metalloproteinase STE24 (ZMPSTE24) → ↑ Prelamin A → Nuclear Membrane Toxicity
- Prenatal course (MNOP): ↓ fetal Movement, No clavicle, Polyhydramnios and PROM
- Face: Micrognathia, Mouth is fixed open in an "O-shaped", Nose is Pinched and Small
- Neonate dies from Respiratory failure due to Restrictive pulmonary disease (stiff thorax)
- Joints: Severe flexion contractures
- Skin: Taut Translucent, Thin eroded skin that Tears during delivery

4.10 Autoinflammatory Disorders (Periodic Fever Syndromes)

- Hereditary syndromes characterized by recurrent fevers and multi-organ inflammation
- Pathogenesis: aberrant activation of innate immune system (vs autoimmune disease w/ altered humoral immune system) → ↑ NFkB and Inflammasome-mediated activation of inflammatory cytokines (IFN-α, IFN-γ TNF-α, **IL-1**β) via activation of caspases
- Patients present in infancy or early childhood except FMF and TRAPS (present any age)
- Path: moderately dense dermal perivascular and interstitial neutrophils (neutrophilic urticarial dermatitis) except PAPA/DIRA/DITRA (pustules) and Blau (granulomatous)
- Rx: IL-1 antagonsists like **anakinra** (colchicine is crucial in preventing amyloidosis in FMF)
- Prognosis: fatal if untreated (CAPS, TRAPS, and FMF may get secondary AA amyloidosis)

Cryopyrin-associated periodic fevers (CAPS; includes FCAS, Muckle-Wells syndrome, NOMID)

- All are AD mutations in CIAS-1/NLRP3 (which processes IL-1β via caspase-1)
    - o "Dominant Men's favorite CAPS are CIALIS which Neurochemically Lengthens Repressed Penises"
- All present in infancy w/ periodic fevers, urticaria and secondary AA amyloidosis
- Treat all with IL-1 antagonists (canakinumab, rilonacept, anakinra)
- CAPS: Familial cold autoinflammatory syndrome, Muckle-wells and NOMID
    - o "To swallow your CAPS (pills), theres nothing like a Cold Well drink to a NOMAD"

- Familial Cold Autoinflammatory Syndrome (FCAS) is the mildest form with febrile attacks usually only lasts hours, **urticaria is cold-induced,** and patients have normal hearing
- **Muckle-wells syndrome** (muckle reminds me of chuckle/laughed → "LAUF'D")
  - **Lancing Limb pain, AA Amyloid, Urticaria, Febrile attacks lasting days, and Deafness**
- Neonatal Onset Multisystem Inflammatory Disorder (NOMID; "NOMID is a NOMAD"): the most severe form with nearly continuous febrile attacks, No eyesight/hearing, high Morbidity/Mortality, Meningitis, deforming Arthropathy, Amyloid, and Dysmorphic faces

Autoinflammatory pyogenic/pustular disorders ("My PAPA has a Designated Driver for his CAR")

- Pyogenic arthritis (PAPA/PAPASH): AD ("my PAPA is a dominant man") mutation in PSTPIP1/CD2BP1 which p/w PG, Acne conglobate and sterile Pyogenic Arthritis +/- HS
  - Rx: IL-1 antagonists or TNF-α inhibitors
- Deficiency of the IL-1 Receptor Antagonist (DIRA): AR mutation in IL1RN which p/w a recurrent **pustular psoriasis-like rash** which starts in **infancy** + **osteitis** (get bone X-rays)
  - Occurs commonly in Puerto Ricans
  - Rx: IL-1 antagonists (anakinra)
- Deficiency of the IL-36 receptor antagonist (DITRA): AR mutation in IL36RN which shows DIRA-like skin findings (pustular psoriasis) but presents later (children) and lacks osteitis
  - Rx: IL-1 antagonists or psoriasis drugs (IL-36 inhibitors are on the horizon)
- CARD14-Mediated Psoriasis (CAMPS): due to **gain-of-function mutation in CARD14**, which **encodes NF-kβ**

activating scaffold protein downstream of protein kinase C
- o p/w early onset severe generalized pustulosis, plaque psoriasis, PRP-like rash
- o Rx: **inhibitors of the IL-17/23 pathway (e.g., guselkumab)**

Familial Mediterranean Fever ("He's not a maniac, he's a Mediter-RANEAC")
- AR mutation in pyrin protein (MEFV); Arthritis treated by NSAIDS; **Erysipelas-like rash on lower Extremities**; secondary **AA Amyloidosis prevented by Colchicine (TOC)**

Hyper-IgD syndrome (mevalonate kinase deficiency)
- AR mutation in **MVK (mevalonate kinase):** "The D makes me & val orgasm kind of"
- ↑ incidence in the Dutch population
- p/w **in infancy w/ Diffuse urticaria or morbilliform rash, periodic fevers lasting Days,** arthritis, **abdominal pain**, N/V/D, LAD/HSM
  - o Periodic fever, transient urticarial rash, abdominal pain = Hyper-IgD syndrome
  - o Periodic fever, transient urticarial rash, limb pain (and deafness) = Muckle-wells
  - o Periodic fever, transient salmon-colored rash, joint pain = Stills disease
- Labs: ↑ serum IgD and ↑ urinary mevalonate levels
- Rx: IL-1 antagonists or TNF-α inhibitors

TNF-Receptor Associated periodic syndrome (TRAPS)
- AD mutation in TNFRSF1A (TNF receptor superfamily 1A/p55 TNF receptor)
- p/w painful migratory red plaques on extremities w/ underlying migratory myalgias

    - "I imagine a dominant (AD) guy working out his TRAPS. The intense workout gives him migratory red painful extremities and underlying painful muscles"
- Secondary AA Amyloid: Familial Mediterranean Fever, CAPS, TRAPS get Amyloid; 20%
    - "Amy loves when Family Men in CAPS work out their TRAPS"
- Rx: corticosteroids ("guys with huge TRAPS love steroids") and TNF-α inhibitors

Blau Syndrome ("sarcoid in kids")

- AD mutation in **NOD2/CARD15** gene
- p/w sarcoidal granulomatous dermatitis, fevers and acral polyarticular arthritis in kids
    - CARD14 mutation cause psoriasis in kids, CARD15 mutation cause sarcoid in kids
        - "Sarcoidosis has more letters (and more CARDs) than psoriasis"

ADA2 deficiency ("vasculitis in kids")

- AR mutation in ADA2 (adenosine deaminase 2)
- p/w childhood onset PAN (livedo racemosa is MC skin finding), HSP, early-onset strokes

Majeed syndrome ("Sweets in kids"; "Majeed can't read because he can't' PIN down his ABC'S")

- AR mutation in LPIN2
- p/w Anemia, Bone lesions, Cryptorchidism, Congenital heart defects, and recurrent Sweet's syndrome in infancy

Type 1 interferonopathies are characterized by ↑ IFN signaling and encephalopathies ("CSF")

- Chronic Atypical Neutrophilic Dermatitis with Lipodystrophy and Elevated temperature (CANDLE syndrome): AD mutation in PSMB8 which p/w Calcification of the basal ganglia (just like Cockayne syndrome), **Annular violaceous plaques**, also known as Nakajo/Nishimura syndrome, AD inheritance, Lipodystrophy and Eyelid Edema

- Stimulator of Interferon Genes (STING)-Associated Vasculopathy with Onset in Infancy (SAVI): AD mutation in transmembrane protein 173 (TMEM173) which **p/w acral violaceous papules**/infarcts with bone resorption and loss of digits, nails, nose and ears
- Familial chilblain lupus (Aicardi-Goutieres syndrome): AD mutation in TREX1 which p/w **pernio-like lesions on hands/feet/ears** in infancy with arthritis and encephalopathy
    - "Imagine a T-REX with blue fingers/toes, joint contractures and encephalitis"

4.11 Neurocutaneous Syndromes

- RASopathies were formerly called neurocutaneous syndromes but no longer as there are RASopathies that are not neurocutaneous syndromes (e.g., CM-AVM; good chart in section 4.6) and there are neurocutaneous syndromes that are not RASopathies
- RASopathies ("PLAN C") have mutations in the RAS-MAPK pathway and have overlapping features of craniofacial, cardiac (esp pulmonary valve) and MSK anomalies
    - Parkes-Weber, Legius, LAD type 3, CM-AVM, NF-1, Noonan and Noonan w/ multiple lentigines (LEOPARD), Cardio-facio-cutaneous syndrome, Costello
    - Noonan and the "Cs" in "PLAN C" commonly have lymphatic malformations like the entities in

the PIK3CA-related overgrowth spectrum (e.g., CLOVES)

Neurocutaneous syndromes that are RASopathies

Neurofibromatosis type 1 (NF1; von Recklinghausen's disease; "LMNOPqRST")

- AD mutation in the tumor suppressor gene **Neurofibromin** (NF1), **a GTPase-activating protein which negatively regulates the RAS pathway** (turns active GTP to inactive GDP)
    - Loss of NF1 increases RAS activity → various cancers (**breast**, melanoma, etc.)
    - Loss of heterozygosity is a phenomenon seen in many conditions (esp those w/ loss of function mutations in tumor suppressor genes) in which the pt has a germline mutation in one copy of the allele and every neurofibroma or tumor you see in NF1 is due to an acquired loss of heterozygosity of the second allele
- **Diagnostic criteria** (must have **2 or more** of the following: LMNOPqRST)
    - **Lisch nodules** (2 or more): tan hamartomas of the iris (90% by 10 years of age)
    - **Café-au-lait Macules** (**6 or more** > 0.5 cm prepubertal or > 1.5 cm postpubertal)
    - **Neurofibromas** (**2 or more**) or 1 plexiform neurofibroma (bag of worms feel)
    - **Optic nerve glioma** which can cause blindness (vs NF2 which can cause deafness)
    - **Pigment in the axilla or inguinal region (Crowe's sign)**; must be bilateral
    - Relative with NF1 (new criteria changed this to parent w/ NF1)
    - Sphenoid wing dysplasia: p/w pulsating exophthalmos but often asymptomatic

- Tibial dysplasia/pseudarthrosis

- Other important features (LMNOPqRST)
    - Learning disability, Leukemias (**CML** is MC)
    - Macrocephaly (infancy), Meningiomas (prebubertal), Malignant peripheral nerve sheath tumors (rapid enlargement/pain of a plexiform neurofibroma in an adult)
    - Neurofibrosarcoma, Nevus anemicus
    - Ocular manifestations (Lisch nodules, optic glioma, glaucoma); Ovarian cancer
    - **Pheochromocytomas** (HTN); Prostate cancer
    - Pseudoatrophic macules (slightly depressed oval lesions) and blue-red macules are recently reported cutaneous findings (MC on trunk) seen in 10% of NF1 pts
        - Path: Perivascular neural tissue
    - **Pulmonic stenosis + NF1 features = Watson syndrome**
    - p53 is the MC 2nd mutation causing malignant transformation of a neurofibroma
    - Rhabdomyosarcoma
    - Seizures, Short stature, Scoliosis and other Skeletal dysplasias
- **1st sign = congenital skeletal dysplasia (tibial/sphenoid wing); 1st skin sign = CALMs**
- 25% of NF1 pts have a plexiform neurofibroma (PNF) which undergo malignant transformation to MPNST (neurofibrosarcoma) in 3–15% of pts which may p/w rapid growth, increased firmness, persistent pain within an established PNF or the development of new neurologic deficits (any of these symptoms in a PNF → **PET-CT**)
- Rx: MEK inhibitor Selumetinib is now FDA approved for associated tumors
- Workup: screen for hypertension (Renal angiography and 24-hour urine collection for catecholamines in

those w/ HTN), NCCN recommends annual breast MRI starting at age 25 to 40, Ophtho exam before age 8, brain MRI for neuro symptoms and PET-CT (above)

- Consult: ortho, ophtho, endocrine and neuro

Legius syndrome

- AD mutation in SPRED1 (interacts with Ras)
- Has cutaneous features of NF1 except the neurofibromas (CALMs, Crowe's sign)
    - "Spred your legs so I can see your intertriginous freckles"
- Patients may also have learning disabilities, but all other NF features are absent

NF2 (bilateral acoustic Schwannomas)

- AD mutation in tumor Suppressor gene SCH (encodes schwannomin/**merlin**)
- Skin findings usually absent but can get CALMs and SQ neurofibromas (vs dermal in NF1)
    - **SQ neurofibromas have overlying pigment or hair**
- Bilateral vestibular Schwannomas → deafness/tinnitus/dizziness (DO NOT Swim alone)
- Ocular finding: juvenile posterior Subcapsular lenticular cataract
- MCC of death: CNS tumors (meningiomas, astrocytomas, ependymomas)

Genoderms with CALMs: "When a MAN FARTs he stays CALM"
MEN-1, McCune-Albright, Ataxia-telangiectasia, Noonan, NF1 and legius > NF2 Fanconi, Ataxia-telangiectasia again, Russel-Silver, and Tuberous sclerosis

Costello syndrome (facio-cutaneo-skeletal syndrome)

- AR mutation in **HRAS** (RAS-MAPK pathway)

- p/w thick **loose skin on hands** w/ **deep palmoplantar Creases** and ulnar deviation of the wrist, Coarse facies w/ **nasolabial warts,** periorificial papillomas, AN, curly hair, MR
    - "Costellow" has low skin hanging on hands, low/deep hand creases and low IQ
- Cardiac: **pulmonic stenosis**, cardiomyopathy, lymphatic malformations (lymphedema)
- Cancer: rhabdomyosarcoma, transitional cell (bladder) cancer
- Phenotyping overlap w/ Cardio-facio-cutaneous syndrome (KRAS mutation)
- All RASopathies ("PLAN C," e.g., CFC, NF1) present similar; need genetic tests to distinguish

Neurocutaneous syndromes that are not RASopathies

Tuberous sclerosis complex (TSC)

- AD mutation in the tumor suppressor genes hamartin (TSC1) or tuberin (TSC2) which are GTPases that negatively regulate the **mTOR** (mammalian target of rapamycin) pathway
- Diagnostic criteria: "BOARDS CRAP"
    - **Brain stuff (MCC death)**: subependymal giant cell astrocytoma, subependymal nodules (often calcified), cortical tubers (often calcified)
    - **Seizures/infantile spasms is the MC presentation** (a/w worse prognosis)
        - Ocular hamartomas: retinal phakomas
    - Ash-leaf macules (> 2 hypopigmented macules > 5mm each): **1st cutaneous sign**
    - Renal stuff (renal failure is 2nd MCC of death): angiomyolipomas, cysts
    - Dental enamel pits (> 2)
    - Shagreen patch: collagenoma MC on the back

  - CALMs (only entity in this mnemonic that is NOT in the diagnostic criteria)
  - Rhabdomyoma (cardiac) → Wolf-Parkinson-White arrythmia
    - **First sign and can be detected on prenatal US**
  - Angiofibromas on the face (> 2; adenoma sebaceum) or fibrous cephalic plaque
    - Rx: topical rapamycin
  - Pulmonary lymphangioleiomyomatosis (p/w pneumothorax in females)
    - Dx: high resolution CT scan shows thin-walled cysts; VEGF-D blood test
  - Periungual fibromas (> 1; Koenen tumors)
- All entities in the above mnemonic are major criteria except for renal cysts (minor), dental pits (minor) and CALMS (not a criteria); other minor criteria include confetti-like macules, nonrenal hamartomas, retinal achromic patch and oral fibromas
- Dx: **2 major** or **1 major and 2 minor** is a definitive diagnosis (order **MRI brain/abdomen**)
- Rx: topical rapamycin for facial angiofibromas; systemic mTOR inhibitors (sirolimus) for renal/hepatic angiomyolipomas and subependymal giant cell astrocytoma

Incontinentia pigmenti (IP)

- **XLD loss of function mutation in nuclear factor-kB (NF-kB)** essential modulator (NEMO; IKBKG) → protein product normally **confers protection against TNF-mediated apoptosis**
  - X-inactivation results in only cutaneous findings (blaschkoid pattern)
- Cutaneous manifestations follow a blaschkoid pattern and have 4 distinct stages
  - Vesicular (weeks): inflammatory vesicles and pustules
  - Verrucous (months): warty papules
  - Hyperpigmented (years): blue to brown streaks

  - Hypopigmented (persists throughout life): atrophic hypopigmented streaks
- Other skin findings: scarring alopecia, **subungual tumors (resemble SCC)**, nail dystrophy
- Other findings: pegged teeth/anodontia (50%; **MC extracutaneous finding)**, scarring alopecia (30%), seizures/MR (30%), **eye issues** (30%), breast/nipple abnormalities (20%)
- Path
  - **Vesicular: eosinophilic spongiosis w/ dyskeratotic keratinocytes**
  - Verrucous: hyperkeratosis and papillomatosis w/ dyskeratosis in whorls/clusters
  - **Hyperpigmented: pigment incontinence (dermal melanophages)**
  - Hypopigmented: normal to decreased melanocytes +/- dermal fibrosis
- Consult: **dental, neuro, long term ophtho** f/u for retinal vascular changes/optic atrophy
- Female carriers with mild IP phenotype can bear children with hypohidrotic ectodermal dysplasia w/ immunodeficiency (both HEP and IP have teeth and breast abnormalities)

4.12 Chromosome Disorders, Premature Aging Syndromes, and DNA Repair Disorders

Skin findings in Down's syndrome ("Flat SPEECH")

- Flat nipples, Flat nasal bridge, Flat face, and Flat occiput
- Syringomas, Scrotal tongue, Single palmar crease (Simian crease), and white Brushfield Spots
- Premature wrinkling
- **EPS** (#1 cause in MAD PORES mnemonic)

- Extensive neonatal vesiculopustular Eruption (a/w congenital leukemoid reaction)
- Alopecia areata
- **Cutis marmorata (persistent)**, Calcinosis cutis of hands, Cheilitis
- Heart disease and Hypotonia in infancy (not skin findings but completes mnemonic)

Persistent cutis marmorata in infancy: "Durable Cutis Marmorata"
Downs syndrome, Cornelia de Lange syndrome, Menke's disease

Turner syndrome

- XO monosomy
- p/w ("turn a CAN") **Coartation of Aorta**, Congenital Aplasia of lymphatic channels → peripheral edema in infancy, redundant Neck folds/webbed Neck (fetal cystic hygroma remnant; macrocystic lymphangioma → **can compress airway**), multiple large Nevi, low set Nuchal hairline, wide-set Nipples, Nails are hypoplastic, hyperconvex and deep-set

Noonan syndrome

- Not a chromosomal abnormality but discussed here because of its similarity to Turner
- AD mutation in PTPN11 is MC (allelic with LEOPARD → has lentigines and CALMs)
- p/w ("PLAN on noon"): **Pulmonic stenosis**, Lymphedematous Legs, Atrial septal defects, redundant Neck folds/webbed Neck (fetal cystic hygroma remnant which can compress airway), multiple large Nevi, low set Nuchal hairline

Klinefelter syndrome

- XXY
- p/w **Leg ulcers**, **Leg veins**, Little body/pubic hair, Little penis/testes, and Long Limbs

- Labs: Low testosterone
- Rx: testosterone replacement

Progeria (LMNOP)

- **AD mutation in LMNA** (**encodes Lamin A** which is a protein which contributes to the structure and function of the Nuclear envelope)
- Cutaneous changes begin at year 1 with Localized sclerodermatous changes (in a bathing suit distribution) of Proximal Lower extremities, cyanosis of the Mouth and Nasolabial folds and Pigmentary changes
    - o Patients are normal at birth → 1st sign is growth retardation
- Other skin changes include Lipodystrophy, Onychodystrophy, and Prominent veins
- Facial features/bony changes include Large head, Micrognathia, beaked Nose, Osteoporosis/Osteolysis of distal phalanges and high-Pitched voice
- Over time patient show signs of **Premature aging** atherosclerosis → **MI/stroke**
    - o Complications of cardiac disease are the MCC of mortality (death at 13 years)
- Rx: **Lonfarnib** (farnesyltransferase inhibitor) is FDA approved (↓ mortality)

Helicase family mutations
Werner (2 vowels): RecQL2 → death by skin cancers, osteogenic sarcoma or CVAs Bloom ("Blooom"; 3 vowels): RecQL3 → death by leukemia/lymphoma Rothmund-Thomson (4 vowels): RecQL4 → death by acral SCCs or osteosarcoma

Werner (Adult progeria)

- AR mutation in RECQL2 gene (encodes a DNA helicase) → ↓ genomic stability

  - Mutation increases telomere-driven replicated senescence → **Accelerated Aging**
- Symptoms begin in 3rd or 4th decade (vs infancy in Progeria): progressive Alopecia, bird-like faces, **Acrofacial Atrophic/sclerodermatous changes**, mottled pigmentation, hyperkeratotic ulcers over pressure points, **leg ulcers**, calcinosis cutis, cataracts, osteoporosis, DM, and hypogonadism
- Mortality due to malignancy (esp. osteogenic sarcoma, fibrosarcoma) and CVA/MI
- Rx: **vitamin C (Ascorbic Acid)** may reverse aging abnormalities and lengthen lifespan

Bloom syndrome (congenital telangiectatic erythema)

- AR mutation in RECQL3/BLM (DNA helicase) → ↑ **rates of sister chromatid exchange**
  - These specific chromosomal breaks and rearrangements can be seen on chromosomal instability testing
- p/w **photosensitivity**/malar erythema ("the sun makes flowers bloom"), bird-like noses with high pitched voices ("birds love flowers in bloom"), short stature ("they fail to bloom"), hypogonadism ("testicles fail to bloom"), **MR** ("intelligence fails to bloom"), ↓ IgA and IgM → respiratory and GI infections ("immunoglobins fail to bloom")
- Café-au lait macules (CALM) and hypopigmentation are other clues
- Cancers (MCC of death) esp of blood (**leukemia/lymphoma** > SCC, GI adenocarcinoma)

Rothmund-Thomson syndrome (poikiloderma congenitale)

- AR mutation in RECQL4 (DNA helicase that repairs DNA after UV damage)
- Similar to bloom: photosensitivity/malar erythema, faces, short stature, hypogonadism

    - Cheeks are affected first in early infancy w/ red reticulated patches and edema
- Additional features: **poikiloderma**, immunoglobins and intelligence are normal, **absent thumbs/radius/ ulna**, nail dystrophy, alopecia, **juvenile cataracts**, acral keratoses → SCC
    - "RECQL4 stands for 4 vowels (Rothmund-Thomson) and 4 fingers (no thumbs)"
- Cancers: osteosarcoma (#1 cause of death in teens), SCCs (#1 cause of death in adults)
- Workup: ophtho and ortho referral; regular skin exams
- ROTHMUND'S CAP ("he wears a cap because he's so photosensitive")
    - AR, Radius absent, Osteosarcoma, Telangiectasia, absent Thumb, Hypogonadism, MSK (short stature), absent Ulna, Dystrophic nails, Normal intelligence, and SCCs
    - Cataracts (juvenile), Alopecia, Acral keratoses, and Poikiloderma

ERCC gene mutations: function in DNA repair

"Ericca does XTC"

- XPD, XPB, and XPG (ERCC2, ERCC3, and ERCC5, respectively)
- Trichothiodystrophy (ERCC2 and ERCC3)
- Cockayne syndrome (ERCC6 and ERCC8)

Xeroderma pigmentosa

- AR mutation in XPA to XPG genes which encode **nucleotide excision repair** proteins
    - Not to be confused w/ Muir-Torre which is a defect in DNA Mismatch repair
- ↑ sensitivity to UV-induced skin damage due to abnormalities in **DNA repair pathways**
    - Recognition of damaged DNA via DNA damage binding protein: XPA and XPE
    - Unwinding of DNA via DNA helicase: XPB and XPD

   - Incision/removal of damaged DNA via endonuclease: XPC, XPF and XPG
   - Abnormal post-replication repair pathway (DNA polymerase-η defect): XP variant
- High yield subtypes
   - XPA (DDB1 gene): De Santis-Cacchione syndrome (**severe neurologic deficits**)
      - "Democrats say that Ron Desantis is severely neurologically impaired"
   - XPB (ERCC3 gene), XPD (ERCC2): a/w trichothiodystrophy (neuro deficits)
   - XPG (ERCC5 gene) encode an endonuclease: overlap syndrome w/ Cockayne
   - **XPC (XPC gene): no neurologic abnormalities; MC form in USA**
   - XP Variant (POLH gene): no neurologic abnormalities; common (30% of all cases)
      - "You won't find any neurologic deficits on my CV"
- p/w erythema in infancy → poikiloderma → any skin cancer (1000x risk) by 8 years old
- **Ophthalmologic and neurodevelopmental deficits common (like in Cockayne)**
   - p/w progressive CNS degeneration w/ MR, sensorineural deafness, ataxia, etc.
- Prophylaxis: oral retinoids can reduce skin cancers by 63% in XP
- Death by skin cancer around age 20
   - **Trichothiodystrophy and Cockayne have photosensitivity but no skin cancers**

Trichothiodystrophy (Tay syndrome; PIBIDS)

- AR mutation in **ERCC2** (XPD) > ERCC3 (XPB), GTF2H (p8/TTDA) → defective DNA repair
   - "Trichothio-distrophy" → Tri = 3, di = 2"

- Photosensitivity (**no pigmentary changes or ↑ risk of skin cancers** just like in Cockayne)
- **Ichthyosis**
- **Brittle hair (due to sulfur deficiency)**: "tiger-tail" banding (alternating light and dark bands under polarized light), trichoschisis and trichorrhexis nodosa
- **Intellectual impairment**
- Decreased fertility (hypogonadism); Decreased immunoglobins (hypogammaglobinemia)
- Short stature
    - There is a form which lacks Photosensitivity and Ichthyosis ("just BIDS")

Cockayne syndrome

- AR mutation in ERCC6, -8 → **defective transcription-Coupled nucleotide excision repair**
    - "My cock is 6–8 inches, just kidding it's cm ☹"
- Like Bloom and Rothmund-Thomson there is a bird-like face with telangiectatic erythema/**photosensitivity but Cockayne lacks pigmentary changes and SCCs**
- **Neuro (#1 cause of death)**: progressive demyelination of the CNS/PNS, basal ganglia calcification, ataxia, spasticity, MR, microcephaly, sensorineural hearing loss
- MSK: short stature, thin body ("cachectic dwarfism")
- Eyes: salt and pepper retinopathy, optic atrophy
- I like the *Genoderms made ludicrously easy* illustration of a penis (cockayne) where the head is a cachectic photosensitive mouse head and the testicles are a brain and an eye

Genodermatoses with photosensitivity: "Hard Blue Opiates make Rothmund's Poor Kind Cock Hide from Trichy X-rays"
Hartnup, Bloom, Opitz, Rothmund-Thompson, Porphrias, Pellagra, Kindler, Cockayne, Hydroa vacciniforme, Trichothiodystrophy, XP

4.13 Primary Immunodeficiency Disorders

- Signs of immunodeficiency: recurrent infection and infections with opportunistic bugs
- p/w recurrent staph infections and widespread viral or fungal infections
- Rx: hematopoietic stem cell transplantation may be warranted

Immunodeficiencies with an Atopic phenotype ("vowels except u")

- Wiskott-Aldrich syndrome, IgA deficiency, hyper IgE syndrome, IPEX, Omenn syndrome

Wiskott-Aldrich ("WAITER")

- WAS gene mutation (**XLR**; **defect in CD43, aka sialophorin**)
- Actin cytoskeleton defect
- ↑IgA, IgD, IgE, **↓IgM** (M is down bc M is an upside-down W) → **lymphomas (NHL is MC)**
- **Thrombocytopenia → petechiae**/purpura/epistaxis/bloody diarrhea
- **Eczema** with food allergies/asthma/urticaria (**Kodachrome w/ eczema and petechiae**)
- Recurrent encapsulated bacterial infections (otitis media, PNA, meningitis), HSV, HPV

IgA deficiency (discussed below)

Hyper IgE syndrome (Job syndrome)

- **Mutation in STAT3 (AD)** > DOCK8 (AR) → ↓Th17 cells → poor neutrophil recruitment
- p/w recurrent **"cold abscesses"** (named due to lack of redness/warmth), **Eczema, Extra (double) row of teeth, joint hyper-Extensibility, osteopenia** (**frac-**

tures common), numerous viral infections such as HPV/HSV (AR form), coarse facial features (AD form)
  - Commonly see a neonatal papulopustular Eruption followed by severe Eczema
- Dx: high serum levels of IgE (> 2,000) and Eosinophilia

Immunodeficiency Polyendocrinopathy and X-linked (IPEX)

- XLR mutation in FOXP3
- p/w eczema ("X-zema"), diarrhea, DM, hypothyroidism, and autoimmune hemolytic anemia
- Workup: TSH, CBC, and glucose

Omenn syndrome

- AR form of SCID with mutation in RAG1 or RAG2 → non-functioning T-cell receptors
- Presents shortly after birth w/ **erythroderma**, **alopecia**, **LAD**, HSM, and features of SCID (FTT, chronic diarrhea, thrush, and recurrent infections with any organism)
  - "No men would use rags to clean up their red bloody (erythroderma) baby"
- Dx: eosinophilia, ↑IgE, ↓IgM, IgA, IgG, no B cells, **↑T-cells (but impaired function)**

Severe Combined Immunodeficiency (SCID)

- **XLR** mutation in **IL2RG** (MC), AR mutation in ADA (↑adenosine) or AR mutation in JAK3
  - "When the titanic SCID into the iceberg and sank, Jack said I'L 2 (too) get on the floating door but adding Jacks weight made it sink. Jack froze to death and Rose yelled his name 3 times (JAK3) before letting him go"
  - p/w FTT, diarrhea, recurrent infections with any organism, **no palpable LNs**

- Transplacental transfer of maternal T-cells cause neonate w/ SCID to p/w signs of **GVHD** (morbilliform, LP-like, seborrheic dermatitis-like, sclerodermatous change)
- **SCID** (w/ AR mutation in ADA) is a/w multicentric **childhood DFSP**
  - "SCID, GVHD, DFSP have 4 letters so you won't forget these associations"
- Dx: **no T-cells** (B-cells vary depending on type of SCID)
- Rx: bone marrow transplant (no concern for rejection)

Antibody deficiencies ("ABC")

- Diseases in this category have Autoimmune diseases (except Bruton's), Blood Cancers (except IgA def) and non-infectious granulomas

IgA deficiency

- IGAD1 mutation
- MC Ig deficiency: most Asymptomatic but can p/w Airway/GI infections, Autoimmunity, Atopy, **Anaphylaxis to IgA containing products (check IgA level before giving IVIG)**
- Dx: IgA < 7 mg/dL; normal IgG and IgM levels

X-linked Bruton's hypogammaglobinemia

- XLR (↑ in Boys) defect in **BTK (tyrosine kinase gene)** → no B-cell maturation
- Presents at 6 months (when moms IgG wears off) w/ recurrent Bacterial infections
- Non-infectious granulomas, absent LNs/tonsils and ↑ risk of Blood cancers
- Dx: ↓ B-cells and immunoglobins of all classes

Common variable immunodeficiency

- Defect in B-cell differentiation to plasma cells
- Presents in adults w/ Cough (bronchiectasis, recurrent upper airway infections), non-infectious granulomas of skin, ↑ risk of autoimmune diseases (AI-CTD), blood Cancers
- Dx: **normal # of B-cells; ↓ plasma cells, ↓ immunoglobins**

Phagocyte deficiencies

Chronic Granulomatous disease (CGD)

- **XLR** mutation in CYBB or CYBA (Beta or Alpha subunit of **Cytochrome B**) → **defective oxidative metabolism** (absent NADPH oxidase) → cannot kill intracellular organisms
- As name implies, there are non-infectious granulomas everywhere (skin/GI/GU/lung)
- Recurrent infections with Catalase (+) organisms (SPACE): S. aureus (pyodermas), Serratia marcescens (osteomyelitis), Pseudomonas, Aspergillus (PNA), Candida, Enterobacter → recurrent pneumonia and skin (perianal) abscesses ("butt-Crack")
- Lymphadenopathy (Cervical is #1)
- Female Carriers of x-linked CGD have ↑ risk of SCLE/ **discoid lupus**
- Dx: nitroblue tetrazolium test (tests NADPH activity) Continues to be yellow
    - Turns blue in normal patients and is half blue/half yellow in female carriers
- Rx: interferon Gamma

Leukocyte adhesion deficiency type 1 (LAD)

- AR mutation in ITBG2 (encodes **β2 integrin** subunit of LFA-1, CR-3 and p150) → neutrophils are unable

to adhere to the endothelium and migrate to sites of infection
   - "The young LAD has integrity"
- **p/w delayed separation of umbilical cord**, recurrent bacterial infections which lack pus, **gingivitis/periodontitis, poor wound healing → bacterial ulcerations which mimic PG**
   - "The young LAD has missing teeth, skin ulcers and an attached umbilical cord"
- **Dx: peripheral neutrophilia (10x normal)**

Chediak Higashi (huge PMNs in blood smear) and Griscelli were discussed in section 4.3

Disorders of the innate immune system

Hypohidrotic ectodermal dysplasia (HED) with immunodeficiency
- Mutation in NEMO (allelic to incontinentia pigmenti)
- Like HED (Christ-Siemens-Touraine syndrome) it p/w the clinical triad: Hypo-Trichosis + abnormal Teeth (conical teeth) + ↓ sweating → hyper-Thermia but patients are also susceptible to recurrent pyogenic and atypical mycobacterial infections

Chronic mucocutaneous candidiasis (CMC; familial candidiasis)
- Heterogenous group of disorders (AR inheritance) marked by chronic and recurrent candida infections (thrush, paronychia, perleche, intertrigo, tooth enamel hypoplasia)
- MC is APECED: mutation in **AIRE** gene; p/w Autoimmune Poly-Endocrinopathy (**MC is hypoparathyroidism**, Addison's disease is 2nd MC), Candidiasis, Ectodermal Dysplasia
   - Other features: autoimmune (alopecia areata, vitiligo, pernicious anemia, etc.)

- Other CMC syndromes are seen in genes remembered by this covid vaccine mnemonic
  - "I'll collect your covid card stat"
  - IL-17RA/IL17F (**IL-17 inhibitors all cause candidiasis**), CLEC7A, CARD9, **STAT1**
  - Covid also reminds me of APECED gene because w/ covid you can't breathe AIRE

WHIM syndrome

- AD mutation in **CXCR4** chemokine receptor → ↓release of mature B-, T-cells from BM
  - "WHIM and CXCR both have 4 letters"
- Warts, Hypogammaglobinemia, Infections (HPV, bacteria), Myelokathexis (**peripheral neutropenia with retention of neutrophils in the BM**)
- Rx: plerixafor ("plerixa-four") blocks CXCR4 signaling →↑cell counts and ↓infections

Leiner's disease (erythroderma desquamativum)

- Mutation in **C5 gene** ("e is the 5th letter in the alphabet) → **compliment deficiency**
- Presents in infancy with **severe seborrheic dermatitis** (often erythrodermic), recurrent infections, diarrhea, meningococcal infections (any deficiency in C5-C9 will do this), FTT
- Rx: antibiotics and infusions of FFP or whole blood

GATA2 deficiency (WILD syndrome, monoMAC syndrome)

- AD mutation in GATA2 mutation ("GATO is Spanish for cat so I imagine a WILD cat")
- Encompasses 3 related syndromes with much phenotypic overlap
  - WILD syndrome: Warts, Immunodeficiency, Lymphedema, anogenital Dysplasia
  - Monocytopenia and mycobacterial infection (monoMAC)/ Emberger syndrome

    - Familial myelodysplastic syndrome
- p/w disseminated warts and non-TB mycobacterial infections, lymphedema, EN (1/3rd)
- Myelodysplasia → AML is MC (another L in WILD should stand for Leukemia/Lymphoma)
- Labs ("WILD has ↓ WHITE BLOOD cells"): ↓ dendritic cells, monocytes, B-cells, NK cells

4.14 Disorders of Cornification

- Inherited ichthyosis are a heterogenous group of inherited disorders which all share the common phenotype of hyperkeratosis of skin
    - Some present w/ collodion membrane at birth (lamellar ichthyosis, non-bullous CIE, Netherton, neutral lipid storage disease, Sjögren-Larsen, and PIBIDS)
    - Rx: **emollients**, keratolytics and retinoids
- Palmoplantar keratodermas (PPKs) are a heterogenous group of inherited and acquired disorders which show hyperkeratosis of the palms and soles
    - Three types include focal (usually over pressure points), diffuse (PPK over entire palmar surface) and punctate (1–2 mm keratotic papules)
    - Rx: keratolytics and retinoids

Ichthyosis vulgaris ("vulgar AF")

- **Adherent dirty-brown polygonal scales on Arms/legs > trunk (spares face/flexures)**
- Accentuated palmar markings
- Atopic diathesis with keratosis pilaris
- **Absent granular layer over areas of orthohyperkeratosis on path** (unique finding!)
- Flexures and Face spared
- Furrowed heals (accentuated plantar markings)

- **Fillagrin** gene mutation (AD)
- Rx: moisturizers and topical retinoids; **disease improves w/ age but does not resolve**

Steroid Sulfatase deficiency (X-linked recessive ichthyosis): "SCEROID"

- **STS gene mutation →** Steroid sulfatase (aka arylsulfatase C) ↓ in leukocytes
- Scales that Spare flexures, palms, soles and **central face (lateral face/neck is affected)**
- Contiguous gene syndrome: Cooccurrence of Kallmann ("Callmann") syndrome (anosmia, hypogonadism) or XLR Chondrodysplasia punctata (bone dysplasia, stippled epiphyses)
- **Cryptorchidism**/testicular Cancer (**urology** referral for orchiopexy to undescended teste)
- **Carriers: Comma shaped Corneal opacities and prolonged labor ("Child Comes Slow")**
- Dx: Cholesterol sulfate ↑ in plasma, Corneodesmosomes retained in stratum Corneum
- Dx: Estriol ↓ in quad screen of pregnant mothers; ↓ Estrogens/↑ Androgens
- Dx: **Lipoprotein Electrophoresis** can diagnose (β-fraction migrates faster and further) XLR
- **Opacities in corneum that are comma shaped (in female carriers too) → Ophtho exam**
- Infancy onset (although 17% of patients may show scaling at birth)
- **Dark brown adherent scales on extremities, trunk, neck and lateral face ("dirty neck")**

Know your eyes: send all of these patients to ophtho

X-linked ichthyosis: comma shaped corneal opacities
Fabrys: spoke-like or "whorled" corneal opacities
Nail-patella: lester iris (darker zone of pigmentation around the **central/ pupil part of the iris**)
Wilsons: Kayser-Fleischer rings (golden-brown pigment in the cornea and **peripheral iris)**
Refsum and Cockayne: Retinitis pigmentosa (Colored) w/ salt and pepper retinal pigment
Sjögren-Larsson syndrome: perifoveal glistening dots
Richner-Hanhart: dendritic keratitis w/ corneal ulceration and tyrosine crystals on slit-lamp
Waardenburg syndrome: heterochromia iridis and dystopia canthorum
Sturge-Weber: glaucoma
Albinism, Hermansky-Pudlak, Chédiak-Higashi: réd reflex (also photophobia, nystagmus)
NF type 1: Lisch nodules (iris hamartomas; **yellow brown** spots in the iris) and optic gliomas
Down syndrome: Brushfield spots (**pale, milky-white** connective tissue deposits in the iris)
NF type 2: juvenile posterior subcapsular lenticular opacities
Tuberous sclerosis: retinal phakomas (retinal hamartomas)
Von Hippel Lindau: retinal hemangioblastoma
PXE and EDS: angioid streaks
Homocystinuria: downward displacement of lens ("homosexuals are always down")
Marfans: upward displacement of lens ("Mars is up in the sky")
Goltz and Gorlins: Coloboma (both also have cataracts, strabismus, nystagmus)
Gardner's: CHIRP (congenital pigmented spot on retinal exam)
PHACE syndrome: microphthalmia (small eyes), optic nerve hypoplasia, morning glory discs
Gaucher and alkaptonuria: pinguecula (alkaptonuria also has blue-gray sclera/Osler sign)
Osteogenesis imperfecta, Alkaptonuria and EDS: blue sclera ("Oz, Al and ED have blue eyes")
Incontinentia pigmenti: retinal vascular changes and optic atrophy
Niemann-Pick disease: cherry red spot on retinal exam ("Niemann picks red cherries")
Multiple carboxylase deficiency: optic atrophy

Lamellar ichthyosis "When a paper is laminated it has an exterior casing"

- TGM1 mutation: "I'D Peel → Ichthyosis (TGM1), DH (TGM3), Acral peeling skin (TGM5)
- When they are born, they are encased in a collodion membrane → ectropion, eclabium
- When this sheds, it is replaced by **large thick plates of brown scale (especially on the flexures)** which encases the patient → heat intolerance, hypohidrosis, scarring alopecia
- Palms and soles are encased too → PPK, nail dystrophy

Congenital ichthyosiform erythroderma (CIE)/ non-bullous CIE

- Grouped w/ lamellar ichthyosis under the umbrella term of AR ichthyoses
- Like lamellar ichthyosis, it is caused by a AR mutation in TGM1 (but also ALOXE3 and ALOX12B) and p/w collodion membrane at birth → thick scale with **flexural involvement** → ectropion, eclabium, heat intolerance, scarring alopecia
- Unlike lamellar ichthyosis, scale is white (like lox/cream cheese) on a red background
- MCC of collodion baby (lamellar ichthyosis is 2nd MC)

Congenital self-healing collodion baby

- AR mutation in TGM1, ALOXE3, and ALOX12B with collodion membrane at birth with complete resolution and no further abnormalities
- **The most likely result of a collodion baby is an AR ichthyosis (TGM1 or ALOX mutation)**

Harlequin ichthyosis ("HARLEY")

- Hypothermia and Hypernatremia
- ABCA12 gene mutation ("baby dies before he knows his ABCs")
- Rx: systemic Retinoids

- Lipid metabolism error → **Lipid accumulation in stratum corneum**, **defective Lamellar body formation**, **Lamellar granules absent on electron microscopy** and ↓ calpain
- Extreme Ectropion, Eclabium, Ear deformities, Early death (sepsis or respiratory failure)
- Yellow-brown plates of scales separated by red fissures which encase the neonate

Epidermolytic ichthyosis (EHK; bullous CIE): "epidermolytiCK iCKthyosis"

- AD mutation in **KRT 1 (severe PPK w/ digital contractures)** or KRT10 (no PPK)
- Somatic mosaicism results in extensive epidermal nevi
- p/w blistering at birth ("epidermolytic") with subsequent **Corrugated hyperKeratosis** ("ichthyosis") in a **Cobblestone pattern which is more prominent over the joints (anti-Cubital fossa)** that appears from 3 months of age on → skin infections and **malodor**
- **Clumped Keratin** and acantholysis in the epidermis w/ hyperkeratosis on path
- **Do not give retinoids** as they can exacerbate skin fragility in an already lysed epidermis

Other keratinopathic ichthyoses (All AD mutations in keratin with similar clinical presentations)

- Superficial epidermolytic ichthyosis (ichthyosis bullosa of Siemens)
  - AD mutation in keratin 2e (K2e)
  - Similar to EHK except skin is fragile w/ tendency to shed ("mauserung"/molting)
    - Picture a smelly molting sperm (semen) who is spitting "ktooey" (K2e)
- Ichthyosis Curth-Macklin (ichthyosis hystrix)
  - AD mutation in keratin 1

  - Similar to EHK but it has no skin fragility and since K1 is always affected, PPK is severe ("porcupine-like" verrucous scales) with severe digital contractures
- Ichthyosis en confetti
  - AD mutation in keratin 10 ("confet-ten")
  - p/w erythroderma and scaling at birth w/ white scaly confetti-like macules resulting from **revertant ("rever-ten-t") mosaicism** occurring later

Netherton syndrome (NETHER)

- Na^{+} ↑ (Neonates should be managed in the NICU for hypernatremic dehydration)
- IgE ↑ → food **allergies**/anaphylaxis/Eosinophilia
- Trichorrhexis invaginata ("bamboo hair") due to defect in keratinization of IRS
  - "I will nether take that vagina (trichorrhexis invaginata) for a spin (**SPINK5 gene mutation which encodes LEKT1, serine protease inhibitor**)"
- Toxicity w/ Topical Tacrolimus; failure **To Thrive**
- Hair is short and sparse (eyebrow hair is affected MC) but not until > 1 after birth
- HPV infection is common and extensive → SCCs
- **Eczema w/ a double-edged scale (ichthyosis linearis circumflexa) is MC > 2 years old**
- Red scaly baby (congenital ichthyosiform erythroderma) is MC in neonates
- Rx: secukinumab or ustekinumab > dupilumab

Neutral Lipid storage disease with ichthyosis (Chanarin-Dorfman syndrome)

- ABHD5 (CGI-58) gene mutation
- Neutral → **Neuro**: myopathy, developmental delay, sensorineural deafness, cataracts
- Lipid → **Liver**: hepatomegaly with liver fibrosis and ↑ LFTs

- Storage: stores globular electron-lucent inclusions in epidermis and stores cytoplasmic lipid vacuoles in leukocytes detected on peripheral smear
- Ichthyosis: clinically identical to non-bullous CIE (white scales with erythema)

Sjögren-Larsen syndrome (PqRS are contiguous in the alphabet)

- AR mutation in Fatty aldehyde dehydrogenase gene ("Patty aldehyde dehydrogenase")
- p/w Pruritis, Plate-like scale, PPK, and Photophobia with **Perifoveal glistening white dots**
- Retardation, Retinitis pigmentosa (Cockayne and refsum also have retinitis pigmentosa)
- Scissor gait, Spastic di- and tetraplegia, Seizures, and Speech impairment
- More common in Sweden (Scandanavians)
- Rx: patients are very itchy from ↑ leukotriene B4 so treat with zileuton ("Sileuton")

Refsum disease

- AR mutation in peroxin7 (PEX7) or phytanoyl coenzyme A hydroxylase (PAHX/PHYH)
- Ichthyosis usually presents in adulthood ("adult refs are scaly")
- Neuro symptoms in childhood: cerebellar ataxia, peripheral motor and sensory neuropathy, sensorineural deafness, anosmia, muscle wasting
- **Eyes: "Salt and pepper" retinitis pigmentosa (just like cockayne syndrome)**
- Heart: Cardiomyopathy, arrhythmias, heart block
- Path: lipid vacuoles in basal keratinocytes
    - Sjögren-Larsen and Neutral lipid storage disease has lipid vacuoles in leukocytes
- Labs: ↑ plasma phytanic acid
- Rx: Diet low in green vegetables, dairy and ruminant fats (from beef or lamb)

- o Imagine a ref in boxing. He first inspects (PEX7) the gloves/paws (PAHX). After a few rounds of the fight (early symptoms) the boxers get dizzy (ataxia) and have trouble seeing (salt and pepper retinitis pigmentosa) and hearing (deafness). They look weak (muscle wasting, polyneuropathy) but they have so much heart (heart block, cardiac failure) and fight (↑ serum phytanic acid). Do not give these elite athletes a vegan (green vegetables) or a keto (dairy and animal fats) diet.

Keratitis-ichthyosis deafness (KID) syndrome: "I imagine a KID playing in a sandbox"

- AD (most cases are sporadic) mutation in GJB2 (connexin 26)
- Transient neonatal erythroderma ("kid gets sunburnt playing outside in the sandbox")
- Well demarcated erythematous hyperkeratotic plaques on face and extremities ("the kid is on his hands and knees with his face in the sand")
- **Stippled PPK** ("looks like little grains of sand on the kid's hands"; great Kodachrome)
- Alopecia in scalp, eyelashes and eyebrows ("sand is covering his hair on his head")
- **Congenital deafness and vascularized keratitis → blindness ("sand in ears and eyes")**
- Recurrent mucocutaneous infections (e.g., candida) ("kids get fungal infections outside")
- ↑ risk of mucocutaneous **SCC** ("kids who play outside in the sand all day will get SCCs")
- Patients heterozygous for GJB2 can get blaschkoid porokeratotic eccrine ostial and dermal duct nevi (PEODD) from type 2 segmental mosaicism ("kid PEED in the sandbox")

Erythrokeratodermia variabilis (Mendes de Costa syndrome)

- AD mutation in GJB3 (connexin 31) and GJB4 (connexin 30.3)
- p/w well-demarcated burning erythema that changes shape and location daily (variable)
  - o Hyperkeratotic plaques are fixed and usually do not overly areas of erythema
- Rx: improves after puberty and responds exceptionally well to systemic retinoids

Progressive symmetric erythrokeratoderma (PSEK)

- AD mutation in GJB4 genes (connexin 30.3, 31) vs AD mutation in loricrin gene
- p/w hyperkeratotic plaques over areas of erythema (occur together) symmetrically distributed on the **extremities, buttocks** and face (spares trunk); PPK common

Acral peeling skin syndrome

- AR mutation in TGM5
- Separation between stratum granulosum and stratum corneum → p/w recurrent spontaneous superficial peeling on dorsal hands/feet followed by erythema

Congenital hemidysplasia with ichthyosiform erythroderma and limb defects (CHILD) syndrome

- **XLD** mutation in 3β-hydroxysteroid dehydrogenase (NSDHL; "NaS-D Hypoplastic Limbs")
  - o 11β-hydroxysteroid dehydrogenase converts steroids to active form in the liver
- p/w **unilateral** (right > left) ichthyosiform erythroderma, limbs/visceral organ hypoplasia, alopecia, stippled epiphyses (punctate Calcification), verruciform xanthomas
- Ddx: overlap w/ Conradi-Hünermann-Happle but abnormalities in CHILD are unilateral

- Rx: topical retinoids or **topical statins** (targets underlying Cholesterol pathway defects)

Conradi-Hünermann-Happle syndrome (X-linked dominant chondrodysplasia punctata)

- XLD mutation in EBP (emopamil binding protein); shares common pathway to CHILD
- p/w transient ichthyosiform erythroderma which resolves w/ hyperpigmented follicular atrophoderma by age 1, cataracts, limb/facial, asymmetry, patchy alopecia, scoliosis
- **Stippled epiphyses (punctate calcifications) are seen on x-ray but only in infancy**
- Neonatal skin biopsy shows calcium in the epidermis
- **↑ risk in children born from mothers with SLE**
- "I think of a weird girl (XLD) named Pam who is an emo (emopamil). She goes by Pam, but her real name is Conradi. She has an asymmetric face and body (scoliosis, limb asymmetry). She also has cataracts (emos put those color contacts in their eyes) and alopecia (emos commonly shave their heads). She also has a crazy hyperpigmented tattoo with swirls (blaschkoid hyperpigmented follicular atrophoderma) which she says used to be red and scaly. Since emos rarely go out in the sun they take vit D/calcium supplements (punctate calcifications and calcification in keratotic plugs in epidermis)"

Know your bones

Conradi-Hunermann: stippled epiphyses (focal bone calcification w/ a stippled look on x-ray)
McCune-Albright: polyostotic fibrous dysplasia (bone is replaced by abnormal fibrous tissue)
Goltz: osteopathia striata (vertical striations in long bones incidentally found on x-ray)
Buschke-Ollendorff: osteopoikilosis ("spotted bones" incidentally found on x-ray)
Gorlin's: bifid ribs (sternal end of the rib is cleaved into two)
Mucopolysaccharidoses: dysostosis Multiplex (chondrodystrophic skeletal changes)
Occipital horn syndrome: occipital horns (exostosis at insertion of trapezius and SCM)
Nail-patella syndrome: posterior iliac horns and absent patella
Goltz and ectrodactyly-ectodermal-dysplasia-cleft lip/palate: lobster claw deformity
Menkes: Wormian bones in sagittal and lambdoid sutures and Metaphyseal Widening
Rothmund-Thompson and Fanconi anemia: absent/hypoplastic Radius
Beckwith-Wiedemann: hemihypertrophy
Rubinstein-Taybi: broad thumbs
Hidrotic ectodermal dysplasia: tufted terminal phalanges
Gaucher disease: Erlenmeyer flask deformity

Ichthyosis follicularis-atrichia-photophobia (IFAP) syndrome

- XLR mutation in MBTPS2 gene ("Most Boys That play PS2 FAP") → encodes zinc MMP
  - Allelic with and phenotypic overlap with keratosis follicularis spinulosa decalvans
- Ichthyosis follicularis: p/w erythroderma, scaling and follicular hyperkeratosis
- Atrichia: p/w generalized alopecia including eyebrows and eyelashes
- Photophobia: p/w corneal opacities/ulcerations and vascularizing keratitis (like KID)
- Other features: KP, MR, hearing loss, seizures, skeletal anomalies and nail dystrophy

Selected hereditary PPKs with a known genetic basis

- All diseases with keratin and connexin mutations are AD and all others are AR (except Howel-Evans (AD), Vohwinkle variant (AD), and Olmsted (AD)

Diffuse non-epidermolytic PPKs ("My BEST GUN is held in my hand with diffuse PPK")

- Mutilating PPKs a/w pseudo-ainhum/autoamputations (mutilating PPKs make me VOM)
  - Vohwinkle syndrome, classic: connexin 26 mutation (GJB2); p/w diffuse **honeycombed PPK**, starfish-shaped keratotic plaques over joints and **deafness**
    - Vohwinkel, variant is AD mutation in loricrin; similar to classic but has **ichthyosis** and lacks deafness (only GJB mutations are a/w deafness)
  - Olmsted syndrome: AD mutation in TRPV3; prominent peri-Orificial plaques
  - Mal de Meleda: discussed below in transgradiens PPK section
- Bart-Pumphrey: connexin 26 mutation (GJB2); p/w knuckle pads, leukonychia, deafness
- EBS, Dowling-Meara: KRT 5,14 (EBS is usually focal PPK but Dowling-Meara is diffuse)
- Symmetric progressive erythrokeratoderma: discussed above
- Transgradiens PPKs (this diffuse PPK also goes on top of hands/feet): "If you want to graduate on top of your class, you should also get your MPH degree"
  - Mal de Maleda (SLURP-1 mutation): psoriasiform malodorous transgradiens PPK in glove and stocking distribution and dystrophic nails

  - Papillon-Lefevre (cathepsin c mutation): **Psoriasiform**, malodorous, PPK (sharply demarcated "stocking-glove" transgradiens PPK), **Periodontitis**, Pyogenic infections, Psoriasiform lesions over elbows and knees and **dural calcification**
  - Haim-Munk: allelic to Papillon-Lefevre but has onychogryphosis, acro-osteolysis
  - Hidrotic ectodermal dysplasia, aka Clouston: discussed in section 4.7
- Griether (Keratin 1 mutation): presents in infancy w/ transgradiens and progradiens PPK
- Unna-Thost (**Keratin 1 and 16 mutation**): presents in **childhood** w/ diffuse PPK
- Naxos ("NAxOs") disease: Plakoglobin mutation ("N and P are close in alphabet")
  - Diffuse Non-epidermolytic PPK in infancy, Arrythmias (RVH) in teens, wOOlly hair

Intracranial calcifications: "Watching TV (PBS or TLC) will calcify your brain"
Papillon-Lefevre syndrome: dural calcification ("P is a flipped d")
Basal cell nevus syndrome: falx cerebri calcification
Sturge-Weber syndrome: tram-track ("Web") calcifications in the temporal/ occipital cortex
Tuberous sclerosis: calcified cortical tubers and calcified subependymal nodules
Lipoid proteinosis: temporal and hippocampal calcification
Cockayne and CANDLE syndrome: Basal ganglia ("ABC")

Diffuse epidermolytic PPK (Vörner's)

- Mutation in **keratin 1 and 9 ("**öne and nine")
- Clinically identical to diffuse non-epidermolytic PPKs but **path shows epidermolysis**
  - "The umlaut over the ö looks like keratin clumps lysing"

Focal PPK: "SHARPENED Curved Keratoses"

- Schopf-Schultz-Passarge syndrome (WNT10A): similar to hidrotic ectodermal dysplasia (PPK, hypodontia, hypotrichosis and nail dystrophy) but has **eyelid hidrocystomas**
- Striate type (desmoglein 1, desmoplakin 1, keratin 1): "the 1s remind me of the straight/striate line"): p/w striate PPK presenting in adolescents
- Howel-Evans: AD mutation in TOC/IRHOM2/RHBDF2 which **inhibit EGFR signaling**
  - o p/w focal non-transgradiens PPK over pressure areas, esophageal cancer and premalignant oral leukoplakia
  - o "Imagine a wolf sitting on a TIRE howling in a raspy voice due to esophageal cancer with his white tongue out. The wolf's carpal pads of are like focal PPK"
- Areata type (mutation in Keratin 16 or 6c): p/w focal PPK presenting in adolescents
- Richner-Hanhart: mutation in tyrosine aminotransferase; "I call it Richner-Hand Eyes"
  - o Hand/feet: focal painful PPK on weight bearing-bearing areas
  - o Eyes: painful pseudo-herpetic dendritic keratitis, corneal ulcers, photophobia, blindness and **tyrosine crystals on slit-lamp exam**
- Pachyonychia congenita: discussed in section 4.7
- EBS, Weber-Cockayne: discussed in section 4.4
- Naegeli-Franschetti-Jadassohn syndrome: discussed in section 4.3
- EBS, Koebner: discussed in section 4.4
- Dyskeratosis congenita: discussed in section 4.3
- Carvajal (desmoplakin mutation): striate PPK, woolly hair and dilated left ventricular cardiomyopathy ("the L in CarvajaL reminds me its Linear PPK and Left heart failure")

- Kindler syndrome: discussed in section 4.4

Keratosis punctata palmaris et plantaris (punctate palmar keratoderma)

- AD disease
- Begins in adolescents; MC in AA patients
- p/w callus-like lesions which may have a central keratotic core and are found within palmar creases and aggravated by manual work; begins in adolescents; MC in AA pts

Acrokeratoelastoidosis

- AD disease
- Presents in childhood/puberty and is classified as a PPK
- p/w skin colored to yellowish papules over the sides of the hands and feet (good Koda)
- Path: hyperkeratosis, acanthosis, hypergranulosis and elastorrhexis

4.15 Miscellaneous Pediatric Skin Disorders

Hydroa vacciniforme, actinic prurigo, juvenile spring eruption and porphyrias discussed in 3.15

Juvenile plantar dermatosis ("Sweaty Sock Syndrome")

- Occurs in sweaty **pre-pubertal boys**
- Form of frictional ICD which p/w **Symmetric Smooth Shiny** red plaques and fissures on the plantar surfaces which have contact with the ground (**Spares the arch**)
- Rx: absorbent Socks/foot powder, **thick emollients, and med/high potency topical Steroids**

Diaper dermatitis

- See if it spares skin folds: "On InstaGram you only post pics that **spare your skin folds**"
  - ICD: erythema on convex surfaces (notice in girls there is a "W" distribution where the fatty thigh projections are outer lines and the protruding labia majora lips are inner lines of the "W") due to urine/feces contact; Rx: **frequent diaper changes**, larger sized diapers, **petrolatum/zinc** w/ every diaper change and topical steroids (ICD frequently coinfected w/ candida → add nystatin/azoles)
    - Jacquet's erosive dermatitis: severe erosive dermatitis with prominent **punched out ulcerated** papules and umbilicated nodules
    - Perianal pseudoverrucous papules and nodules: 2–8 shiny, smooth, red, moist, flat-topped **wart-like** perianal papules/nodules
      - a/w Hirschsprung's, fecal/urinary incontinence and urostomies
      - Workup: GU/GI consult
- Granuloma Gluteal infantum: unique form of ICD which represents a unique response to local inflammation, maceration and secondary infection (candida)
    - p/w **purple-red nodules**; a/w topical steroid use and fecal incontinence
    - Rx: treat initiating inflammatory process (steroids are not recommended)
- Most other causes of diaper dermatitis **do not spare the skin folds**
  - ACD: the shape and distribution of the rash are highly suggestive of the etiology
    - Nickel (in clothing snaps): linear in diaper area (and in chest/abdomen)
    - Diaper dyes: margins of diaper
    - Topically applied allergen (fragrances, MCI, neomycin): entire diaper area

- Rubber additives in elastic band (mercapto-benzothiazole, p-tertbutyl phenol): characteristic distribution on hips and outer buttocks resembling a cowboy holster

- Candidiasis: bright red erythema with **satellite** papules and pustules and scales; when it involves the genitals, lesions are more **Confluent (entire labia/scrotum)**
    - Dx: KOH (pseudohyphae and budding yeast) or fungal culture
    - Rx: topical nystatin, azoles or ciclopirox until 1 week after rash clears (will recur if other dermatoses are not treated simultaneously; treat ICD)
  - Psoriasis: bright red plaques (minimal scales due to the moisture of the diaper)
    - Ddx: candida and psoriasis are both bright red but psoriasis does not have satellite lesions and is more Patchy/localized when on genitals
    - Rx: topical steroids and emollient/barrier creams (like zinc) to ↓ irritation
  - Seborrheic dermatitis: salmon-colored (pink/red) greasy plaques w/ yellow scale and accompanied by cradle cap and more generalized intertriginous involvement
    - Rx: low potency steroids (consider azoles for candida superinfection)
    - Any pt not responding should be cultured to r/o bacterial superinfection
  - Langerhan's cell histiocytosis: rash is **petechial** w/ erosions in inguinal crease
    - Dx: CBC, ESR/CRP, skin biopsy
  - Acrodermatitis enteropathica: eczematous lesions will also be around the mouth
    - Dx: serum zinc and alk phos

  - Kawasaki: diffuse erythematous maculopapular truncal rash w/ accentuation in the groin area (desquamation would be a nice clue)

Perianal Pyramidal Protrusion

- p/w solitary, fleshy "Peanut-shaped" soft/compressible tissue Protrusion in the Perineal median raphe, **just anterior to anus in female infants**
- May be familial, related to constipation or a/w LS&A
- Rx: **reassurance** (they tend to involute over time); MiraLAX

Eosinophilic folliculitis (EF)

- Benign vesiculopustular condition of infancy
- p/w **crops** of pruritic Erythematous crusted pustules on the **scalp** or Extremity of babies
- Dx: Wright stain shows eosinophils
- Rx: lesions resolve in 2–3 years but treat w/ potent topical steroids and antihistamines

Acropustulosis of infancy

- Variant of EF that presents between birth and age 2
- p/w crops of pruritic vesicles/pustules on the **palms/soles** that recur every few weeks
- a/w scabies (**next best step is perform mineral oil prep to rule out scabies infection**)
  - Treatment for scabies in infants < 2 months is 6% sulfur w/ petrolatum
- Rx: lesions resolve in 2–3 years but treat w/ potent topical steroids +/- permethrin/sulfur

Van der Woude syndrome

- AD mutation in interferon regulatory factor 6 gene
- p/w B/L lip pits in on the lower vermillion lip spaced equidistant (0.5 cm) from midline

  - Pits represent blind sinuses or fistulas extending out from the orbicularis muscle

Mercury poisoning (acrodynia)

- Most commonly seen in infants and young children due to accidental mercury exposure
- p/w dusky, painful, edematous palms and soles w/ vesicles and then desquamation
  - Boyd termed it "Puffy, Pink, Painful, Paresthetic, Perspiring and Peeling hands"
- Non-cutaneous symptoms: irritability, poor appetite, fatigue and weight loss
- Dx: blood and urine mercury levels
- Rx: eliminate source of exposure; correct fluid/electrolytes; succimer/DMSA

Cutaneous mastocytosis

- **c-KIT mutations** (D816V activating mutations is MC) → promotes interaction of KIT (CD117) and its ligand (stem cell factor) → mast cell development and activation
- Group of disorders w/ abnormal ↑ of mast cells in organs (skin/bone marrow are MC)
- p/w Darier's sign (urticarial wheal after friction from mast cell degranulation)
- p/w tan-brown lesions in babies ("these kids look like they have been playing in MUD")
  - Mastocytoma: solitary tan peau-d'orange-textured nodule (60% present at birth)
    - Rx: no systemic workup is needed in children (reassurance/avoid triggers)
  - Urticaria pigmentosa: MC childhood presentation which p/w multiple light brown macules/papules which start on the trunk and spares the palms, soles and face; systemic symptoms (N/V/D, wheezing) and bullous lesions may be seen

        - Most have skin-limited disease and undergo resolution by adolescence
    - Diffuse cutaneous mastocytosis: diffuse red-brown leathery plaques → blisters
        - Systemic symptoms/progression to systemic mastocytosis (SM) common
- Adult forms are more likely to p/w systemic symptoms and progression to SM
    - Telangiectasia macularis eruptiva perstans (TMEP) does not have this "muddy-brown" hyperpigmentation but instead p/w telangiectatic macules
- SM (e.g., indolent systemic mastocytosis, mast cell leukemia) has a poor prognosis and may p/w skeletal lesions, BM involvement, LAD and GI symptoms
- Next step: skin biopsy (preferred site is an area you did not perform Dariers sign on)
- Path: > **20 mast cells** in dermis which stain with KIT (CD117), Leder, tryptase, toludine blue, Giemsa → "Master (mast cells) KIT Led them on a Trip to the Tall blue Gems"
    - KIT and leder stains (1st two in mnemonic) function after recent degranulation
        - KIT and leder stains are not dependent on intact mast cell granules
        - Von Leder stains mast cells red due to chloroacetate esterase activity
    - Toluidine blue and Giemsa (last 2 in mnemonic) are the metachromatic stains
- Workup: **CBC**, **tryptase** (levels c/w mast cell disease; 20–75 ng/mL = 50% has SM**;** > 75 = 100% has SM), IL6 (↑ in SM), urine methylimidazole acetic acid (histamine metabolite)
    - Performed **BM biopsy** if concern for systemic mastocytosis (tryptase > 20)
        - Not needed for TMEP or pediatric disease (unless there's evidence of SM)

  - **Can get bone survey to rule out lytic lesions**
  - **FIP1L1-PDGFRA gene rearrangement common**
- Rx
  - Any mastocytosis: UVA, **Antihistamines**, **Avoid triggers**, topical steroids
    - Triggers: ASA, NSAIDS, narcotics, anticholinergics, polymyxin B, lidocaine
  - For GI or systemic symptoms: oral **cromolyn** or cimetidine
  - For systemic mastocytosis w/ the FIP1L1-PDGFRA gene rearrangement that are D816V negative: **imatinib (c-kit D186V mutation confers resistance to imatinib)**
    - Use dasatinib, nilotinib or midostaurin for D816V-expressig mast cells
  - TMEP: PDL
  - Mastocytoma: excision
- Monitor these pts for 24 hours after general anesthesia (delayed anaphylaxis can occur)

Chapter 5: Infectious disease

5.1 Viral Diseases

DNA viruses are "HHAPPPPy"

Hepadnavirus (Hep B), Herpesvirus
Adenovirus
Poxvirus, Parvovirus, Polyomavirus, Papillomavirus
* all replicate in nucleus except Poxvirus (carries its own DNA-dependent RNA polymerase)
* all are double-stranded DNA except Parvovirus ("part of a DNA"; ssDNA)
* all are non-enveloped (**naked**) except for Poxvirus and Parvovirus (enveloped; "they have v in 3rd or 4th letter")
* all are linear except Polyomavirus and Papillomavirus (circular)
* so besides Poxvirus and Parvovirus, they are all naked, double-stranded DNA viruses that replicate in the nucleus

Human papillomavirus (HPV)

- Double stranded-DNA virus that infects skin and mucosa → warts and SCCs
- Capsid contains DNA and is composed of L1 and L2 (major and minor structural protein)
- Infection starts in basal layer keratinocytes and works its way to more superficial layers
    - Early proteins (E1-E7) → DNA replication and keratinocyte immortalization
        - E1 and E2: first genes expressed (basal layer) → replication of viral DNA
        - E4: disrupts cytokeratin network → koilocytosis ("cuatro-cytes")
        - E5, E6 and E7: allows viral DNA replication above basal layer → **amplification** ("ampli-five-seven"); **E6 and E7 are high-risk oncoproteins**

        - E6 **binds and degrades** (ubiquitin-mediated) **p53** → ↓ apoptosis
            - **P53 is a tumor suppressor gene** that **works at cell cycle G1**
        - E7 binds Rb → loss of inhibition of E2F → DNA replication
            - "#7 looks like a straw to drink Root beer and Eat 2 Fries"
    - Late proteins (L1-L2) → encodes structural proteins required for virion formation
        - L1-L2: superficial epidermis; complete virus in granular layer and above
- HPV are from genus α (most HPV types) or β (epidermodysplasia verruciformis-types)
- Cutaneous manifestations of HPV infections
    - HPV-1, 2, 4, 27, 57 (HPV 57 can cause 10-nail dystrophy)
        - Verruca vulgaris (HPV 2 is MC; "you are 2 vulgar"): exophytic papules
        - Palmoplantar warts: thick endophytic papules on palms/soles
            - Myrmecial (HPV 1 is MC): plantar warts w/ a sloping anthill look
            - Mosaic: plantar warts that coalesce into large plaques
            - Subungual warts: HPV 2 and 4
    - HPV-3, 10 (Three, Ten): Flat warts → soft smooth papules on dorsal hands/face
    - HPV-2, 7: Butcher's warts → warts on hands of meat handler
        - There are 2 syllables and 7 letters in "Butcher"
    - HPV-23b (Stucco keratosis; "S" backwards looks like a 2 and a "K" backwards is a 3)
    - HPV-42: a/w digital papillary adenocarcinoma
    - HPV-60: ridged warts (plantar warts that keep dermatoglyphs); verrucous cysts

        - Both have same path: warts w/ **eosinophilic** inclusions in keratinocytes
    - HPV-73: periungual SCC
    - HPV-5, 8 (genus β HPV types): warts and SCCs in organ transplant patients and in Epidermodysplasia verruciformis → **p/w pityriasis versicolor-like lesions (scaly, pink/hypopigmented macules)** and generalized flat warts → SCCs
        - AR mutation in EVER1 (TMC6)/EVER2 (TMC8) or acquired in HIV patients
            - EVER1 who eats Three McDonalds Cheeseburgers is a warty mess
        - Acquired form presents later and is preceded by HIV/immunodeficiency
        - Rx: retinoids, zinc, cimetidine (avoid radiotherapy in all genoderms)
    - WHIM syndrome: AD mutation in CXCR4 → Warts, Hypogammaglobinemia, Infections (bacterial and viral) and neutropenia (2° to Myelokathexis)
    - WILD syndrome: Warts, Immunodeficiency, Lymphedema, anogenital Dysplasia
- Mucosal/genital manifestations of HPV infections
    - HPV-6, 11 (low-risk types)
        - Condyloma acuminata ("condy-low-ma"): MC STD; sessile genital papules
        - Verrucous carcinomas (low-risk types): slow-growing locally destructive (Rx: excision; do NOT treat these with ionizing radiation)
            - Buschke-Lowenstein: arises on genitalia
            - Oral florid papillomatosis ("papil-low-matosis"): arises in mouth
                - Don't confuse w/ florid cutaneous papillomatosis (paraneoplastic disease a/w GI adenocarcinoma)
            - Epithelioma caniculatum (HPV-2, 16 in addition to 6, 11): on soles

        - Oral warts (low-risk types): more common in HIV
            - Heck's disease (HPV-13, 32): South American child w/ oral warts
                - "Why the Heck does this Spanish child have oral warts?"
        - Recurrent respiratory papillomatosis (low-risk types): MC tumor of larynx
    - HPV-16, 18, 31, 33, 45 (high-risk types)
        - High-grade intraepithelial neoplasia
            - Flat cervical warts (condyloma plana): whitening w/ acetic acid
            - Bowenoid papulosis: Brown genital papules; no invasive SCC risk
            - Erythroplasia of Queyrat: red penile plaque; ↑ risk of invasive SCC
- Path
    - Verruca vulgaris: papillomatous exophytic lesion w/ hypergranulosis and koilocytes (keratinocytes w/ clear cytoplasm and shriveled "raisin-like" nuclei)
    - Myrmecia: endophytic lesion w/ course red cytoplasmic inclusions
    - Verruca plana: flatter lesion w/ rounded koilocytes without the shriveled nuclei
    - Epidermodysplasia verruciformis (β HPV types): verruca plana w/ **βlue cytoplasm**
        - The truncal tinea versicolor-like macules also look like this on path
    - Condyloma acuminatum (CA): **path looks like an SK in the genitals** w/ vacuolated keratinocytes, round parakeratosis and course hypergranulosis
    - **Bowenoid papulosis: can look like CA but w/ Bowenoid full thickness atypia**
    - Verrucous cyst: cyst with wart-like lining

    - o Heck's disease: rounded parakeratosis (red) atop epithelial pallor (white)
- Rx: destruction (cryotherapy, ED&C, scissors/shave removal, PDL/CO_2 laser), topical imiquimod, IL immunotherapy with Candida, IL cidofovir, and PO retinoids
    - o Only for Cutaneous warts (early letters in alphabet): topical salicylic Acid, Adapalene and other retinoids, IL Bleomycin, Cantharidin (in-office), and 5-FU
    - o Only for genital warts: podophyllin, topical sinecatechins, TCA (in office)
- HPV vaccines: contain **L1 major structural capsid protein** so it assembles into virion particles but do not do any harm since they do not contain DNA
    - o Three types: bivalent (Cervarix; HPV-16, 18), quadrivalent (Gardasil; HPV-6, 11, 16, and 18) and 9-valent (HPV-6, 11, 16, 18, 31, 33, 45, 52, and 58)
    - o Originally approved from ages 9 to 26 (21 in males), now it is FDA approved to 45
- Athletes can return to competition as long as verruca are covered or curetted off

Human Herpes viruses

- 8 viruses all w/ icosahedral capsid containing linear DS-DNA which replicate in nucleus
- Pathogenesis involves primary infection→ latency → reactivation

Herpes simplex virus (HHV-1/HSV-1 and HHV-2/HSV-2)

- Recurrent vesicular eruption on orolabial (HSV-1 MC) and genital (HSV-2 MC) regions
- Pathogenesis: spread by saliva (HSV-1) or genital contact (HSV-2) → retrograde flow to site of latency in the dorsal root ganglia (neurons) → subsequent reactivation

    - "Tripple Ds": spread by Droplet or Direct contact; latent in Dorsal root ganglia
    - Reactivation triggers ("PUFFS"): Peels, UV light, Fever, Fractionated lasers, Stress
- Clinical presentation: clustered vesicles on red base → erosions w/ **scalloped borders**
    - Orolabial infection
        - Primary infection: prodromal symptoms of gingivostomatitis (children) or pharyngitis/ mononucleosis-like (adults) → lesions on lips and **keratinized oral mucosa** of the **anterior** mouth (hard palate, gums and dorsal tongue)
            - Ddx: aphthous ulcers (non-keratinized mucosa such as soft palate, inner lips/ cheeks, ventral tongue); and herpangina (posterior mouth)
        - Recurrent infection: **prodrome of pain →** lesions on vermillion border
    - Genital infection
        - Primary infection: asymptomatic or painful genital erosions
            - Worse in women → LAD, dysuria, urinary retention, meningitis
        - Recurrent infection: mild symptoms w/ few vesicles lasting about 1 week
        - **MC infectious cause of chronic genital/buttock ulcers in the immunocompromised population and MC infectious cause of genital ulcers in sexually active teens/adults**
- Other HSV presentations
    - Eczema herpeticum: life-threatening infection which p/w monomorphic punched out erosions and systemic symptoms in children w/ atopic dermatitis (HSV-1)
        - **Dx: obtain viral PCR for HSV**
        - **Rx: hospitalize and initiate IV acyclovir**

- Herpetic whitlow: painful grouped vesicles on digits/hands of children or adults
  - Bimodal peaks: < 10 years old (HSV-1) and 20–40 years old (HSV-2)
  - Ddx: coxsackie virus (also produces vesicles on the hands but instead of being grouped they are discrete and follow dermatoglyphics), blistering distal dactylitis (purpura precedes bullae on digit palmar fat pad)
- Herpes gladiatorum: vesicles on **lateral neck/face** due to athletic contact (HSV-1)
- HSV folliculitis (herpes sycosis): vesicles/pustules in the beard area (HSV-1)
- Ocular HSV: keratoconjunctivitis w/ LAD and branching dendritic corneal ulcers → possible blindness (HSV-2 in newborns; otherwise HSV-1)
- HSV encephalitis: MC fatal viral encephalitis in the US; a/w UNC-93B or TLR-3 mutations; p/w fever and AMS; temporal lobe #1 site (HSV-1)
  - "3 UNC TaR heel students have herpes on their brain after the frat party"
- Congenital (intrauterine) herpes simplex: ascending infection (HSV-2) infects fetus → at birth baby p/w widespread vesicles/pustules/erosions/scars, **aplasia-Cutis** on the scalp, micro-Cephaly, Chorioretinitis; 50–75% mortality if untreated
- Neonatal herpes Simplex: perinatal infection → 1–2 weeks post-partum baby p/w **CNS infection** and vesicles commonly on the scalp (presenting part) > trunk

- Dx: viral culture, DFA, serology, **PCR (most sensitive)**, and Tzanck smear
- Path: **Multinucleated keratinocytes w/ nuclear Molding and Margination of chromatin to the periphery** ("looks like a cluster of grapes to me") +/- Cowdry A inclusions ("I can't believe I got herpes from

that dry cow" → intranuclear eosinophilic inclusion bodies)

  - HSV-1, 2, 3, 5 have intranuclear inclusions; smallpox has perinuclear inclusions (Poxvirus is the only DNA virus that does not replicate in the nucleus)
- Rx: orolabial → topical or PO antivirals; genital→ PO antivirals
  - neonatal HSV/eczema herpeticum/HSV in immunocompromised → IV acyclovir
  - Acyclovir-resistant HSV **foscarnet** or cidofovir
  - Ppx before resurfacing laser: antiviral 1 day before to **10 days after** procedure
- Athletes need 5 days of antivirals w/ no new lesions for 3 days before returning to play

Varicella zoster (HSV-3/HHV-3)

- Varicella (chickenpox) is the primary infection and zoster (shingles) is the reactivation
- Pathogenesis (DDD): transmitted via Droplets and Direct contact w/ lesional fluid (pts contagious 2 days before rash until all lesions crust over) → after varicella, VZV travels to Dorsal root ganglia (site of latency) → subsequent reactivation (presents as zoster)
- Clinical presentation
  - Primary varicella: prodromal symptoms → cephalocaudal spread of vesicles on an erythematous base (dew drops on a rose pedal) → pustules → crust over
    - Crops of lesions in various stages (vesicles, pustules and crust all at once)
    - More severe disease in adolescents and adults
  - Primary varicella in pregnancy
    - Congenital varicella syndrome: infection in first 20 weeks of gestation

        - Limb (hypoplasia), ocular anomalies (Chorioretinitis, Cataracts), CNS anomalies (hydrocephalus) and Cutaneous scarring
            - "Chickenpox in pregnancy: arms look like a Chicken's wing; chickens have poor eye-site and low IQs (MR)"
        - Exposed fetus may develop reactivation (zoster) in infancy
    - Neonatal varicella: perinatal infection (5 days pre-delivery to 2 days post)
        - Widespread vesicles (vesicles in neonatal HSV is more localized to the scalp) on a red base in the same stage of development
        - Severe disease (up to 30% mortality)
- Sequelae of primary varicella
    - Reyes syndrome (brain/liver disease w/ 30% mortality) a/w aspirin intake
    - **Pneumonia (MC in older patients),** encephalitis, ataxia and hepatitis
- Herpes zoster: prodrome (dysesthesia) → painful grouped vesicles on red base in a dermatomal pattern (**trunk MC; thoracic** > trigeminal > lumbar > sacral nerve)
    - Disseminated disease: > 20 lesions outside of the original dermatome
        - ↑ risk of life-threatening pneumonitis and encephalitis
        - Almost exclusively seen in the **immunocompromised**
        - a/w **SIADH** ("Syndrome of In-Appropriate Disseminated Herpes")
    - Chronic verrucous herpes zoster is seen in AIDS patients
    - Postherpetic neuralgia: potentially chronic pain after lesions clear

- More common, severe and chronic in the **elderly**
- **Vasculopathies/vasculitis**: delayed complication of Varicella zoster
- Dermatomal-specific herpes zoster findings
    - Ramsay-Hunt syndrome: affects **geniculate ganglia** of facial nerve
        - p/w **Deafness/tinnitus** + Ear (EAM) **pain**/vesicles + **Bell's** palsy + loss of **Taste** on anterior 2/3rds of Tongue
            - "Ramsay-Hunts generic degree left him in DEBT"
    - Bell's palsy (unilateral facial nerve paralysis) if CN-VII affected
    - Herpes zoster ophthalmicus ("Uphthalmicus"): CN-II, CN-III, or CN-V
        - Hutchinson's sign (nasal tip vesicles): external division of V1 nasociliary branch affected → Uveitis → blindness
        - **Uveitis** is #1 form of ocular involvement; keratitis is #2
    - Cervical dermatome: motor neuropathy of arm; weak diaphragm
    - Thoracic dermatome: weakness/ pseudohernia of abdominal wall
    - Lumbar dermatome: motor neuropathy/ weakness of leg
    - Sacral dermatome: possible **urinary retention**/hesitancy

- Dx (same as HSV-1): viral culture, DFA, serology, PCR, Tzanck smear, skin biopsy
- Rx
    - Varicella: PO or IV acyclovir (immunocompromised) within 3 days of lesion onset
        - Postexposure ppx: **live vaccine** may be given **within 3 days of exposure**

- If Immunocompromised, pregnant or < 1 y/o give VZIg or IVIg
- Primary prevention: live vaccine given at 12–15 months and 4–6 years
  - Live vaccines CI in immunocompromised, pregnancy and neonates
- Herpes zoster: antiviral treatment (↓duration/pain of lesions, ↓PHN rate) +/- prednisone (no effect on course or development of PHN but ↓acute pain)
  - PHN: TCAs, gabapentin, pregabalin, opioids, lidocaine patch
  - Primary prevention: shingrix vaccine → ↓incidence of shingles and PHN

Epstein-Barr virus (EBV/HSV-4/HHV-4)

- Diseases a/w Epstein-Barr virus: "Epstein did NOT HANG HIMself Bro"
  - **Nasopharyngeal carcinoma**
  - **Oral hairy leukoplakia**
  - **Post-Transplant lymphoproliferative disorder**
  - **Hydroa vacciniforme**
  - **Angiodestructive B-cell lymphoma**
  - **NK/T-cell lymphoma (Nasal type)**
  - **Gianotti-Crostii syndrome (MCC in US is EBV)**
  - **Genital ulcers** in non-sexually active immunocompetent adolescents (aka reactive acute genital ulcers or Lipshültz ulcers): MC on labia minora
    - CMV: recalcitrant genital ulcers in immunocompromised patients
    - HSV: MCC of sexually related genital ulcers
  - **Various Hematologic disorders/malignancies**
  - **Infectious Mononucleosis**
  - **Burkitt's lymphoma**
  - Bug bite reactions that are chronic, exaggerated and a/w systemic symptoms

- Pathogenesis: transmitted via saliva → infects **B-cells (latency)** by binding to CR2
  - "The jail had A & B cells; before Epstein killed himself he was in the B cell"
  - EBV evades detection in B-cells by EBNA-1 and LMP-2 proteins
    - "Epstein's Body Naturally went LIMP too after he hung himself"
  - In patients with ↓ cell-mediated immunity (more important than humoral), infected B-cells continue to replicate → lymphoproliferative disorders
- Clinical features of select EBV diseases
  - Mononucleosis: young adults w/ pharyngitis, cervical LAD, splenomegaly, atypical lymphocytes, petechia on eyelids/palate, genital ulcers (females)
    - "Hanging yourself causes painful swollen neck (cervical LAD and pharyngitis) and petechia; Epstein already had the genital ulcers"
  - Oral Hairy leukoplakia: white plaque on lateral tongue; strongly a/w HIV
  - Gianotti-Crostii syndrome (papular acrodermatitis of childhood): p/w acute eruption of monomorphic papules on the face, butt and extensor extremities
- Dx
  - Monospot test: asses IgM heterophilic Abs; inaccurate in young children
  - EBV-specific Abs: accurate in young kids; can determine current vs prior infection
  - CBC: lymphocytosis w/ atypical lymphocytes and thrombocytopenia
    - Positive heterophilic Ab + > 10% atypical lymphs = acute infection
  - PCR from blood/tissue or RT-PCR from lymphoid cells may be done
- Rx: supportive; avoid contact sports until splenomegaly resolves (spleen rupture)

Cytomegalovirus (CMV/HSV-5/HHV-5)

- Transmitted by my FIST: Fomites, body Fluids, Intrauterine, **Stem cell/organ Transplants**
- Infects monocytes (sites of latency) → disseminates to various organs
- In-utero TORCH infection which is the MC infectious cause of "MR DICS"
    - Mental Retardation (#1 infectious cause of congenital MR)
    - Deafness, Intracranial calcifications, Cutaneous blueberry muffin rash, Seizures
- Most infections are asymptomatic and reactivation only occurs if immunocompromised
    - Cutaneous features: "MR"
        - Mononucleosis-like presentation in healthy adults
        - Recalcitrant **Rectal ulcers** and **Retinitis**/blindness in transplant patients
- Diagnosed by "my FIST"
    - human Fibroblast culture (gold standard but slow)
    - **Intranuclear inclusions surrounded by clear halo ("owl's eye") → large swollen endothelial cells of superficial vessels on path** of ulcers
    - Shell vial assay allows for the detection of CMV in tissue cultures within 1–2 days
    - Standard Tests such as serology and PCR may be employed
- Rx: ganciclovir

Exanthem Subitum (HHV-6/HSV-6, roseola infantum, "Sixth disease")

- Six to twenty-Six months of age; occurs mostly in Spring
- Caused by **HHV-6** (Six) > HHV-7 (Seven) and transmitted by oral Secretions

- High fever up to 5 days (common cause of febrile Seizures); fever resolves as rash starts
    - Subtle maculopapular rash with truncal predominance which lasts 2–3 days
    - **Nagayama's Spots**: red macules on Soft palate/uvula
- Virus remains **latent in monocytes** → reactivation a/w **pityriasis rosea, oral LP, DRESS**
    - EBV, CMV, HHV-6, HHV-7 a/w DRESS ("Herpes 4, 5, 6 & 7 are under the DRESS")

HHV-7

- Shares significant homology with HHV-6; co-infection with HHV-6 in exanthem subitum
- Reactivation a/w pityriasis rosea and DRESS (like HHV-6)

HHV-8 (Kaposi sarcoma-associated herpes virus)

- Virus remains latent in B and T-cells; remember these associations: "8th PICK"
    - **Paraneoplastic Pemphigus**, **Primary effusion lymphoma**
    - Immunocompromised pts get a primary infection (rash, fever, LAD, and BM failure)
    - **Castleman disease** (multicentric)
    - **Kaposi sarcoma**: discussed in section 6.11 on vascular proliferations

Types of herpes viruses

- HSV-1, -2, -3 are α, herpesviruses and lie dormant in nerves (dorsal root ganglia)
- HSV-5, -6, -7 are β herpesviruses and lie dormant in monocytes/macrophage precursors
- HSV-4, -8 are γ herpesviruses and lie dormant in B or T lymphocytes

Other viruses not covered elsewhere

Kawasaki disease

- Likely immunologic response to unidentified virus which infects young children
- Diagnostic criteria ("CRASH and burn"; must have burning fever and 4 of CRASH)
    - Conjunctivitis: B/L non-exudative injection w/ rim of sparring around iris
    - Rash: polymorphous and nonspecific (scarlatiniform/EM-like/urticarial)
        - The rash tends to be acral and **perineal** ("I call it cock-asaki")
    - Adenopathy: U/L cervical, non-fluctuant adenopathy > 1.5 cm in size
    - Strawberry tongue: also fissured lips and non-exudative red pharynx
    - Hands/feet with edema/desquamation/EM-like lesions
    - Burning fever (> 39° C) of at least 5 days
- Ddx: acute adenovirus infection (adenovirus conjunctivitis and pharyngitis is more purulent, and rash is more vesicular without any perineal desquamation); post-covid multi-system inflammatory syndrome (discussed below), Scarlet fever (pt is slightly older w/ sandpaper rash, Pastia's lines, strawberry tongue, perioral pallor)
- Most severe systemic side effect is coronary artery aneurism (workup: get **serial echo**)
- WATCH labs: White count, Anemia, Thrombocytosis, CRP, and Hypoalbuminemia
- Rx: **high dose aspirin + IVIG** (↓ coronary issues and death)

Post-covid multi-system inflammatory syndrome (MISC)

- Both Kawasaki's and MISC share the **upregulation of IL-1β** → proinflammatory cascade

- p/w fever (97%), GI symptoms (80%), skin rash (60%), shock (55%), conjunctivitis (54%), respiratory symptoms (39%), neurologic problems (33%) and skin desquamation (30%)
- Like Kawasaki, it p/w persistent fever (> 38° C x 5 days), rash (polymorphous/vasculitic), non-exudative conjunctival injection, oropharyngeal erythema, lip swelling/redness, N/V
- In contrast to Kawasaki's, post-covid MISC presents more frequently w/ septic shock, more often is a/w myocarditis (low EF on echo), more often spares coronary arteries and **more likely to show periorbital redness/swelling**
- MISC also simulates staph/strept TSS which also p/w fever, rash w/ desquamation, hypotension and multisystem organ involvement
- Dx: EKG, CXR, COVID-19 serologies, rule out other infections (blood culture, ASO)

Poxviruses "these Pox viruses are going to make me want to VOMM"

- Smallpox (Variola virus; **Orthopox** genus): spread by inhalation; p/w febrile prodrome → eruption (macule papule → vesicle → pustule → scarring; **all lesions in same stage**) that **starts on palms/soles and spreads inwards with oral lesions and toxic appearance → encephalitis**, blindness, pneumonitis
    - o Path: epidermal necrosis w/ **reticular degeneration** and eosinophilic cytoplasmic inclusions, aka Guarnieri bodies (appear black w/ Gispen's modified silver stain)
    - o Dx/Rx: PCR or viral culture to diagnose and treatment is supportive
- Monkeypox (Monkeypox virus; **Orthopox** genus): spread by inhalation or cutaneous contact with infected animals; presents similar to smallpox with

febrile prodrome small-pox-like lesions which also favor the palms/soles and systemic symptoms
  - o Spread by monkeys (Africa), prairie dogs (US) and close physical contact (MSM)
  - o Path: epidermal necrosis, ballooning degeneration, multinucleated keratinocytes
- Cowpox (Cowpox virus; **Orthopox** genus): spread by cutaneous contact with infected animals (**cat**;"cow and cat have 3 letters and start with C"); p/w solitary lesion on hand (vesicle → hemorrhagic pustule → ulcer with **eschar** → large depressed scar)
- Vaccinia (vaccinia virus; **Orthopox** genus): **live attenuated** smallpox Vaccine; **MC SE is autoinoculation** (MC sites are face, eyelids, nose, mouth, genitalia and rectum), but others include LAD, ocular vaccinia, generalized vaccinia, and eczema vaccinatum in AD
- Orf (ecthyma contagiosum; Orf virus; **Parapox** genus): spread by contact with **sheep, goats or reindeer** utters; commonly an Occupational exposure (shepherds, butchers or veterinarians); p/w solitary lesion on hands with a 6-stage evolution
  - o Umbilicated maculopapular → targetoid (rim of white "milk") → acute (weeping nodule) → regenerative (nodule w/ black dots) → papillomatous → regressive
  - o Path for parapox infections like Orf and Milker's nodule ("ENBREL")
    - ▪ Epidermal Necrosis (late lesions)
    - ▪ Bodies (eosinophilic cytoplasmic viral inclusion bodies in keratinocytes)
    - ▪ Reticular degeneration (intraepidermal vesiculation)
    - ▪ Eosinophilic viral inclusions are characteristic of parapox virus infection
    - ▪ Long slender epidermal acanthosis

- Milker's nodule (Paravaccinia virus; **Parapox** genus): spread through contact w/ infected calve/cow Muzzles; presents similar to orf and cowpox but w/ Multiple small nodules on the hand that are less likely to ulcerate than Orf
    - Parapox Rx: self-resolves in weeks
- Molluscum Contagiosum (Molluscum virus; Molluscipox genus): spread by direct Contact or fomites; p/w umbilicated papules in young Children
    - Path: Cup-shaped lesion with Henderson-Paterson bodies
    - Rx: **self-limited**, Cryo, Cantharidin, Curettage, Cimetidine, and Candida antigen
    - Athletes can return to Competition as long as lesions are Covered or Curetted off

Viruses transmitted by Aedes Eagypti mosquito: "Z dang yellow chicken has AIDS (Aedes)"
Zika, Dengue, Yellow fever, Chikungunya *All are Flaviviridae (Hep C is also a flavivirus) family except Chikungunya which is Togaviridae family (like Rubella) *Aedes mosquito can be identified by its unique red belly, black top and white dots *Anopheles mosquito (red belly, brown top) transmits malaria *Culex mosquito (brown) transmits West Nile

Zika virus (A-F)

- Aedes mosquito; Arthritis/Arthralgias
- Bleeding gums (avoid aspirin), a/w Guillain-Barré syndrome
- **Cephalocaudal spread** (spares palms/soles) of non-specific rash w/ **Conjunctivitis**
- DEET is preventative (also can use picardin, IR3535, oil of lemon eucalyptus and others)
- ELISA/RT-PCR to diagnose; Edema on hands and feet
    - CDC recommends serum and urine PCR and IgM serologies for all symptomatic pts and asymptom-

atic pregnant pts w/ a possible exposure to Zika virus

- Face affected first by rash with Follicular accentuation; **Fetal microcephaly**; Flaviviridae

Dengue virus

- Wide range of symptomatology
    - Asymptomatic infection: MC presentation ("Dang, you have no symptoms?")
    - Classic Dengue fever: rash w/ islands of sparring ("Dang that looks like PRP"), flu-like sx, **severe HA/ myalgias/arthralgias/retroorbital pain** ("Dang that's painful")
    - Dengue hemorrhagic fever develops in **children** who were vaccinated (vaccine trials were halted) or naturally infected by Dengue and subsequently get infected with a different serotype; p/w circumoral cyanosis, severe bleeding, shock, death
        - This is a result of pathogenic priming (antibody dependent enhancement)
- Dx: ELISA or RT-PCR in acute infection; IgM serologies later
- Rx: supportive (avoid platelet inhibitors like aspirin)

Yellow fever

- p/w flu-like symptoms 3–6 days after bite by Aedes mosquito in Africa or Brazil
- 15% get severe disease: bleeding, shock, organ failure (liver failure → jaundice), death
- Dx: Councilmann bodies: eosinophilic globules in dying hepatocytes

Chikungunya virus (A-F)

- Aedes; marked Arthritis/Arthralgias; seen in Africa and Asia; Acral edema/neuropathy

- Back pain; Bent joints (Chikungunya means "bent" in Africa); Bullous eruption in infants
    - o "I imagine a chicken in a small coop who is bent down and its joints hurt"
- Chikungunya
- "Dogaviridae" (Togaviridae; only Aedes-born illness not in the Flaviviridae)
- Ecchymosis; Edema (acro-facial)
- Freckle-like macules (exacerbation of melasma) and pigmented Flagellate streaks

Cutaneous manifestations of viral Hepatitis B or C

- Hep B > C: Gianotti-Crosti syndrome, erythema nodosum, polyarteritis nodosum
- Hep C > B: Cryglobulinemia, **necrolytic acral erythema,** lichen planus, sarcoid, **PCT**
- Hep B = C: small vessel vasculitis, urticarial vasculitis, serum-sickness-like reaction, EM

Viral-associated trichodysplasia spinulosa of immunosuppression (SPINULosa)

- Solid organ transplant recipient
- **Polyomavirus** (same virus seen in Merkel cell and "peacock plumage" discussed below)
- **Inclusions (eosinophilic trichohyaline granules) in hair follicles**; **IRS dysmaturation**
- **Nose has numerous papules with long spiny projections**
- Ugly faces (alopecia of eyebrows and eyelashes; thickening of facial skin)
- Leonine faces

Ddx of trichodysplasia spinulosa

- Trichodysplasia spinulosa: flesh-colored papules and **long** keratin spines on the nose
- Paraneoplastic sign of multiple myeloma: **small** hyperkeratotic spicules on the nose
- Trichostasis spinulosa: retention of multiple vellus hairs in a hyperkeratotic dilated hair follicle which **resembles blackheads** on the nose

Pruritic and dyskeratotic dermatoses w/ "Peacock Plumage" Parakeratosis

- Like Viral-associated trichodysplasia spinulosa, this entity is caused by the **Polyomavirus** and affects immunocompromised people w/ solid organ transplants
- p/w severely Pruritic erythematous to brown slightly scaly Papules and Plaques
- Path: Parakeratotic cells in a thickened stratum corneum that look like **Peacock feathers**

Cutaneous manifestations of COVID-19

- MC skin findings: **maculopapular**, pseudo-chilblains/covid toes (happens late), urticarial
  - May also see livedo reticularis/retiform purpura, vesicular eruption w/ all lesions in the same stage (vs varicella) and oral lesions (ulcers, glossitis, mucositis)
- MC hair finding: telogen effluvium
- MC nail findings: lanula w/ red border ("red half-moon sign"), green fluorescence of proximal nails w/ favipiravir and Beau's lines/onychomadesis (happens late)

5.2 HIV/AIDS Dermatology

AIDS pathogenesis is best understood by understanding drug therapies: "C FRIP"

- Caused by ssRNA lentiviruses in the Retroviridae family (HIV-1 > HIV-2)
- Viral envelope proteins **gp120** and gp41 bind to **CCR5** or CXCR4 (CCR5 inhibitors)
- Following binding, viral envelope fuses w/ plasma membrane (Fusion inhibitors)
- HIV RNA is transcribed into a dsDNA copy by **reverse transcriptase** (RT inhibitors)
- This viral DNA copy is integrated into the host DNA via integrase (Integrase inhibitors)
- Viral DNA is translated into HIV proteins (Protease inhibitors)
- Causes ↓ $CD4^+$ T cells and **↑ in $CD8^+$ T cells** to fight the infection

HIV-associated inflammatory dermatoses (APES)

- Acute retroviral syndrome (primary HIV exanthem): p/w mononucleosis-like syndrome 2–6 weeks after HIV exposure with an ill-defined erythematous maculopapular rash
- Aphthous stomatitis: major aphthae p/w large painful destructive oral lesions in HIV pts
- Pruritic papular eruption: aberrant immunologic response to insect bites leads to an intensely Pruritic condition with hyperPigmented excoriated Papules symmetrically distributed (spares mucous membranes, palms, soles and digital web spaces)
- Photodermatitis in HIV: group of photodistributed rashes (lichenoid is MC) from photosensitizing drug exposure (TMP-SMX is MC), PCT or chronic actinic dermatitis

- Primary cutaneous mucinoses esp. localized papular variants of lichen myxedematosis
- Eosinophilic folliculitis (EF): intensely pruritic follicular papules on the upper trunk, neck, face and scalp that are persistent vs cyclic and circinate in classic EF (Ofuji's disease)
- Erythema elevated diutinum: often a/w β-hemolytic strep infection in HIV
- Seborrheic dermatitis/psoriasis: more severe presentations; resistant to treatment

Immune reconstitution inflammatory syndrome (IRIS)

- Paradoxical exacerbations of the clinical manifestations of infectious, neoplastic and inflammatory diseases following antiretroviral therapy (ART)-induced rise in CD4 count
- **p/w worsening of infections even though the correct anti-microbial regimen is used**
- Rx: supportive/symptomatic; may use prednisone in severe disease

HIV-associated infectious dermatoses (1st five herpes infections + BDSM)

- HSV-1/HSV-2: p/w large exophytic verrucous acyclovir-resistant ulcerative lesions
    - o "HSV-1/2 infections in HIV patients are Hypertrophic and Hard to treat"
- HSV-3 (herpes zoster): atypical presentations (e.g., **disseminated or verrucous zoster**)
- HSV-4 (EBV): causes oral hairy leukoplakia which p/w white plaque on lateral tongue
- HSV-5 (CMV): colonize areas of HSV ulceration if CD4 < 50 cells/mm^3; p/w ("CURE") Colitis, mucosal Ulcers, Retinitis and Esophagitis in HIV pts; Rx: valganciclovir/ganciclovir

- Bacillary angiomatosis ("bacillary angioma-2-sis"): **p/w friable dome-shaped vascular papulonodules when CD4 < 200** cells/mm^3; only 20% recall cat bite/scratch
- Disseminated mycoses: **umbilicated, molluscum-like paps** (HIV Can Cause Pox-like paps)
    - o Histoplasmosis, Cryptococcus, Coccidioides, Penicillium
- Disseminated candida: candida is the MC fungal disease in HIV (and in non-HIV pts too)
- Demodicosis: D. folliculorum/brevis infestation p/w "burning" facial erythema
- Proximal white Subungual onychomycosis: proximal nail plate is white due to T. rubrum
    - o Sub (submissive) is a BDSM term so associate this w/ HIV and don't confuse w/ white superficial onychomycosis (p/w diffuse white color) which is caused MC by T. interdigitales var mentogrophytes in adults (T. rubrum is MC in kids or HIV pts)
    - o Proximal white subungual is specific to HIV; distal subungual is MC form in HIV
- S. aureus (MC bacterial pathogen in HIV pts)
- Strongyloidiasis: 2x risk in HIV pts
- Scabies: more likely to be the crusted (Norwegian) variant than non-HIV pts
- Syphilis: HIV pts commonly p/w multiple chancres → lues maligna → neurosyphilis
- Molluscum contagiosum in HIV: atypical and **giant molluscum** commonly on the face
- Mycobacterium: discussed in section 5.3
- MRSA is more common in HIV

HIV and cutaneous malignancies

- HIV pts have an ↑ risk of NMSC (BCC > SCC > melanoma)
- Kaposi's sarcoma: etiologic agent is HSV-8; p/w red-purplish papules/plaques/nodules w/ a predilec-

tion for the face, upper body, hard palate of mouth and genitalia

- EBV causes oral hairy leukoplakia and non-Hodgkin B-cell lymphomas in HIV pts

HIV-associated dermatoses by CD4+ count: "Get UPP, California (CA) MEN BIKE & SHOP & SAVE"

- **< 50 cells/mm^3 (Get UPP): Giant molluscum, large non-healing herpes Ulcers, Pruritic papular eruption, and HIV Photodermatitis**
- **< 100 cells/mm^3** (CA): **Cryptococcus, CMV**, and major Aphthae
- **< 200 cells/mm^3** (MEN BIKE): Molluscum, Eosinophilic folliculitis, Norwegian scabies, Bacillary angiomatosis, Ichthyosis, Kaposi sarcoma, EED (and other vasculitides), and Eczema
- < 500 cells/mm^3 (SHOP): Skin cancer, Staph, HPV, HSV, Oropharyngeal candida, and Psoriasis
- > 500 cells/mm^3 (SAVE): Seborrheic dermatitis, Acute exanthema of primary HIV infection, Vaginal candidiasis, and EBV (oral hairy leukoplakia)

HIV treatment-associated dermatoses

- Immune reconstitution inflammatory syndrome: rapid improvement in immunologic status **(↓ viral load, ↑ CD4+ cells**) weeks-months after ART can paradoxically result in clinical exacerbations of inflammatory, infectious and neoplastic diseases
- Cutaneous SEs of ART: "PHIL commonly gets rashes from his ART therapy"
    - Paronychia/Periungual PG: Protease inhibitors (**indinavir**), lamivudine
        - "SCREAM": Sirolimus, Capecitabine, Retinoids, EGFR inhibitors (e.g., gefitinib, erlotinib, cetuximab), Antiretrovirals (indinavir), MTX

- HyperPigmentation: **zidovudine (AZT)** > emtricitabine (esp. nails/palmoplantar)
- Hypersensitivity syndrome (DIHS/DRESS): **Abacavir** (NRTI) > **TMP-SMX, dapsone**
  - Screen pts for HLA-B*5701 before starting abacavir ("abacavir is 100 back from the Han Chinese HLA (5801-100=5701) which is common in DRESS")
- Hypersensitivity rashes (less severe): NRTIs are the MCC of morbilliform rashes
- Injection-site reactions: fusion inhibitors (enfuvirtide; "needle fuses into arm")
- Lipodystrophy: discussed below

HIV lipodystrophy

- SQ fat is wasted while visceral fat is accumulated
  - Central lipohypertrophy (**accumulation of visceral fat**): MC from protease inhibitors → abdominal protrusion ("protease paunch"), gynecomastia and buffalo hump
  - Peripheral fat wasting/lipoatrophy: MC from NRTIs (esp stavudine, zidovudine)
    - Rx: poly-L-lactic acid and calcium hydroxyapatite are FDA approved fillers

HIV Preexposure prophylaxis (PrEP)

- Tenofovir and emtricitabine taken in a single pill reduces risk of acquiring HIV by 90%
  - "You want these meds on your Teem to prevent HIV"
- CDC recommends that any MSM adult male without HIV who is not in a monogamous relationship w/ an HIV-negative man take it if one of the following are met…
  - Any anal sex without condoms in the last 6 months
  - Any STIs diagnosed or reported in the last 6 months

- o In an ongoing sexual relationship w/ an HIV-positive male partner

5.3 Bacterial Infections

Gram-positive skin infections

Staphylococcal skin infections

Impetigo (staph → "f-sound")

- MC bacterial skin infection in **children**
- Two forms (bullous vs non-bullous) both forms are most commonly due to **Staph aureus**
  - o S. pyogenes impetigo rarely causes poststreptococcal glomerulonephritis (PSGN) (antibiotics do not alter risk); no risk of rheumatic fever from strept impetigo
- Non-bullous impetigo (70%): p/w honey-colored crusts on Face of child > adult
- Bullous impetigo (30%): p/w Flaccid bullae w/ collarettes of scale and yellow crust
  - o Phage group II (type 55 and 71) S. aureus release exfoliatoxins A (chromosomally encoded) and B (plasmid encoded) which cleaves desmoglein 1 → acantholysis
  - o Bullous impetigo in renal Failure pts → SSSS from dissemination of exfoliatoxin
- Desmoglein mnemonic: "PISS ARF Vulgar ALARM"
  - o Desmoglein 1 (PISS): Pemphigus Foliaceus, Impetigo (bullous), SSSS, Striate PPK
- Path: "PISS" all have similar histology with a **subcorneal split** but whereas SSSS and P. foliaceous are pauci-inflammatory, bullous impetigo has bacteria and leukocytes

- Dx: gram stain reveals gram positive cocci; culture and sensitivities
- Rx: First gen cephalosporin (cephalexin) or oral β-lactamase resistant PNC x 5 day
    - If localized → topical mupirocin or Fusidic acid x 5 days
    - If complicated → IV ceftriaxone
    - Recurrent disease: mupirocin to nares, chlorhexidine washes, bleach baths
- Staph infection is the MC sports-related infection; can prevent infection by showering after exercise; athletes must be on antibiotics for 3 days before returning to competition

Staphylococcal scalded skin syndrome (SSSS) → (staph → "f-sound")

- MC in infants (low mortality, < 5%) and adults with renal Failure (high mortality, > 50%)
    - Usually occurs in the First weeks of life
- Phage group II (type 55 and 71) S. aureus → exfoliatoxins A and B disseminate via bloodstream → widespread cleavage of desmoglein 1 → acantholysis
- p/w Febrile prodrome, rhinorrhea, conjunctivitis and generalized skin tenderness
    - Eruption starts on Face (**periorificial radial Fissuring; "sad-clown" appearance**) and skin Folds (**no mucosal involvement**) → generalizes as wrinkled appearing skin w/ Flaccid bullae (Nikolsky +) → desquamation → heals without scarring
- MC primary site of infection in children is the nasopharynx or conjunctiva (Face mucosa)
- Path: superficial subcorneal split without staph colonies or inflammation
- Dx: cultures (nasopharynx, nostrils, conjunctiva, blood); frozen section of sloughed skin will reveal superficial acantholysis (vs full-thickness necrosis in TEN)

  - o Cultures from bullae and blood are negative (blood cultures positive in adults)
- Rx: manage fluids/electrolytes, emollients (petrolatum), contact precautions
  - o Mild: oral dicloxacillin, cephalexin, clindamycin (follow closely outpatient)
  - o Moderate/severe: IV nafcillin or methicillin (hospitalize)

Bacterial folliculitis

- MC form is staph folliculitis: MC on Face (beard area) → Rx: First gen cephalosporin
  - o Superficial form (Bockhart's impetigo): small papulopustules on a red base
  - o Deep form (sycosis barbae): large red papulopustules +/- plaques
- Gram Negative folliculitis: acne patients on long-term antibiotics later p/w pustules in the facial T-zone and peri-Nasal distribution → Rx: ciprofloxacin or isotretinoin
- Pseudomonal folliculitis: a/w poorly chlorinated hot tubs; p/w pruritic papulopustules at sites covered by bathing suits → Rx: self-resolves (ciprofloxacin if immunocompromised)

Abscesses, furuncles and carbuncles

- Walled off collection of pus from S. aureus (often **MRSA**) +/- cellulitis and/or phlebitis
- Abscess: inflamed nodules arising at Any site
- Furuncle: only occurs in a/w hair Follicles ("furuncles at fury sites"); MC on head/Face
- Carbuncle: Collection of furuncles, often w/ deeper multiple draining sinuses; MC on thick skin (posterior neck, back and thighs); a/w systemic symptoms and scarring
- Management for Abscesses (BCD)

- Simple: warm Compresses and Incision and Drainage w/ Culture and sensitivities
- Complex: Bactrim (TMP-SMX), Clindamycin or Doxycycline
- Recurrent infection: Bleach Bath or Chlorhexidine wash to Decolonize skin/nares

Methicillin resistant staphylococcal aureus (MRSA)

- p/w **furunculosis**; often mistaken for spider bite
- Resistance is due to **mecA** gene which encodes penicillin-binding protein (**PBP2a**)
  - "If you change Penicillin in PBP2a to Methicillin, then MRSA, mecA and now MBP2a all start with M and ends with A"
- Community acquired MRSA has Panton-Valentine leucocidin (**PVL**) virulence factor
  - "When you're in the community, you must wear your Pants on Valentine's day"
- Rx: same as complex abscesses/furuncles/carbuncles; vancomycin if severe

Staphylococcal toxic shock syndrome (S-TSS)

- Pathogenesis: S. aureus strains produce TSS Toxin-1 (TSST-1) which act as Superantigen binding to **Vβ region** on T cells → Nonspecific T-cell activation (↑TNF-α, TLR2/4)
- Severe multisystem disease with skin and internal organ involvement (**renal** is MC)
- Affects young healthy adults (Teenagers) with an **occult** primary site of infection
  - Stept-TSS is not occult as it presents with severe pain in an extremity
- Two forms: Menstrual TSS vs nonmenstrual TSS (a/w nasal packing)
- CDC diagnostic criteria (6/6 is definite): fever > 102 °F, diffuse macular erythroderma, desquamation, hypo-

tension, involvement of ≥ 3 organs and rule out other causes
    - o "They look like an erythrodermic patient (rash/ desquamation) in Septic Shock"
- Rash is **Scarlatiniform**: mucocutaneous macular red rash **starting on the Trunk**; red Strawberry Tongue and red conjunctiva; Swelling of palms/Soles; resolves w/ desquamation; onychomadesis (nail Shedding) and Telogen effluvium occur late
    - o Erythema is difficult to see in skin of color: acral Swelling may be the sole finding
- Dx: blood cultures negative in 85% of cases, **hypocalcemia** is prominent, ↑ LFTs
- Rx: **IV clindamycin** (treats staph and suppresses toxin production), vancomycin, IV fluids

PyoMyositis (pyo = pus; myositis = muscle inflammation)

- Infection of skeletal Muscle with **S. aureus**
- Predisposing factors: immunosuppression, diabetes Mellites, trauma (esp IVDU or IV steroids), hematologic Malignancies, chemotherapy and alcoholic liver disease
- p/w fever, Myalgias, Muscle pain, indurated soft tissue Mass → Muscle abscess
    - o Pus can be aspirated from muscle 2–3 weeks after initial symptoms
- Dx: MRI; culture of blood and drainage
- Rx: I&D and IV antibiotics (usually vancomycin)

Botryomycosis (Botryo means "cluster of GRAPES") → yellow GRAPES

- Named for its characteristic groups of granules that resembles yellow grapes
- Risk factors are the same as in pyomyositis
- p/w (GRAPES) Yellow Granules and Pus that drain from Plaques (Eroded or vegetating) on Extremities and

from draining Sinuses caused by **S. Aureus (#1)** or Pseudomonas (#2)

- Skin limited but organ involvement (**Pulmonary** MC) is seen in the immunocompromised
- Labs: Penias (↓T-cell counts)
- Path (GRAPES): Granules w/ central basophilic zone comprised of bacteria w/ Peripheral Eosinophilic zone comprised of IgG and C3 deposits → Splendore-Hoeppli phenomenon
    - Granules are Gram (+), Giemsa (+) and PAS (+)
- Rx: antibiotic therapy should be directed by culture and sensitivity

<u>Streptococcal skin infections</u>

- GAS ("ABC pyogENES"): peri-Anal dermatitis (children), Blistering distal dactylitis (children), Cellulitis (adults; cellulitis in children is more commonly s. aureus), Erysipelas (adults), Necrotizing fasciitis (children; in adults polymicrobial infection is more common), Echthyma (children), Scarlet fever (children), Streptococcal TSS (adults)
- GBS: impetigo (newborn) and perianal dermatitis (post-partum women)
- Streptococcal iniae: cellulitis of hands in fish handlers (tilapia is MC fish)

Peri-Anal streptococcal skin infection

- p/w sharply demarcated perianal red plaque in **young boys**; anal pain and hematochezia
- Can trigger classic/inverse/**guttate psoriasis** (also sharply demarcated)
- Dx: rapid strept antigen test or perianal skin culture
- Rx: cefuroxime ("fury anus"), penicillin, amoxicillin, clindamycin or erythromycin
- Complications: like strept impetigo, may cause PSGN (**monitor with UA**)

Blistering distal dactylitis

- p/w indurated Blue-red distal digit volar fat pad in **child** → purulent Bullae on red base
- Infection caused by **S. pyogenes** (Group A strept) > s. aureus
- Dx: gram stain and culture of blister fluid reveals multiple gram-positive cocci in chains
- Rx: I&D and oral β-lactam x 10 days (cephalexin if organism is unknown, penicillin V if stept is the cause, amoxicillin/clavulanic acid if staph is the cause)

Cellulitis

- Infection of deep dermis/SQ in adults (**GAS** is MC) > children (S. aureus is MC)
- p/w tender, red, warm, swollen **ill-defined** plaques on the legs (adults), head/neck (children) or arms (IVDA) +/- fever, chills, lymphangitis
- Orbital cellulitis: p/w painful red eyelids and proptosis → vision loss (ophtho referal)
- Dx: Clinical diagnosis (blood cultures negative except in the immunocompromised)
- Rx: oral Cephalexin, Clindamycin or dicloxacillin
  - o Suspected MRSA: Bactrim, Clindamycin or Doxycycline
  - o Cellulitis a/w diabetic or decubitus ulcer: piperacillin/tazobactam

Erysipelas ("St. Anthony's Fire")

- More superficial (upper-mid dermis) variant of cellulitis caused by GAS
- Risk factors: **lymphedema** (major RF), DM, HIV, nephrotic syndrome, and alcohol abuse
- p/w **burning** pain w/ **sharply defined** (ridge-like) borders w/ a fiery-red color; **legs** > face ("erysipe-legs"; like cellulitis, it is usually preceded by abrupt onset fever, chills, malaise)

- Whereas orbital cellulitis is a unique and worrisome presentation of cellulitis, penile erysipelas is progressive, chronic and can lead to permanent swelling (elephantiasis)
- Dx: like cellulitis is it is a clinical diagnosis (cultures are negative)
- Rx: penicillin (clindamycin if PCN-allergic)
- ERYSIPelas: Extremity (lower) > face, Red Ridge-like border, lYmphatic involvement (lYmphedema risk factor), Strept, Sharply defined, Increased DNAase/ASO; Rx: Penicillin

Necrotizing Fasciitis (NF; ABCDEFG)

- Caused by **GAS M types 1 and 3** (children) or **polymicrobial** (adults) via portal of entry
- **Rapidly progressing** necrosis of skin, SQ and fascia with high mortality (50%)
- p/w **pain out of proportion to skin findings** → Erythema/Edema → Dusky Blue/Gray skin with hemorrhagic Bullae, Crepitus, Foul-smelling watery Discharge and induration
  - MC site: Extremities (looks like cellulitis but it does not respond to antibiotics)
  - **Edema extends beyond areas of Erythema** (despite antibiotics the edema progresses and can be a/w Bullae, necrosis and Ecchymosis)
  - Patient is severely toxic (fever, tachycardia, AMS, renal failure, septic shock)
  - Late in course skin becomes Anesthetic
- Fornier's Gangrene: necrotizing fasciitis involving Genitalia/perineum (MC in diabetics)
- Dx: Gas in tissue on CT/MRI (but it is a clinical diagnosis so don't delay treatment for CT)
  - White count, Cr, CRP can aid in diagnosis; ↑ **CPK can differentiate from cellulitis**

  - Only surgeons can confirm diagnosis: thin, brown exudate + swollen gray fascia
- Rx: **Fasciotomy (Extensive Debridement)** + IV Broad-spectrum ABX (vancomycin + pipercillin-tazobactam or carbapenem or ceftriaxone + metronidazole)
  - NSAIDS masks symptoms and delay diagnosis (avoid if considering this diagnosis)
- Prognostic factors a/w ↑ mortality (also A-G): old Age, ↑ lactic acid ("Blactic acid"), ↑ Creatinine, ↑ time to first Debridement, ↑ Extent of infection, Female Gender

Ecthyma

- Don't confuse w/ ecthyma gangrenosum (pseudomonas) or ecthyma contagiosum (orf)
- Deep variant of impetigo; MC in children; caused by S. pyogenes
- p/w vesiculopustules on the legs → crust or **punched-out ulcers w/ raised edge → scars**
- Dx: gram stain or wound culture is confirmatory (blood cultures negative)
- Rx: β-lactamase resistant PCN (dicloxacillin) or first generation CSN (cephalexin) x 7 days
  - Impetigo was same treatment but for 5 days
- ECTHyma: Extremity (lower), Child, Culture of wound Confirmatory, Cephalexin, Thin punched-out ulcers with raised border and Hemorrhagic crust

Scarlet fever

- GAS → produces Streptococcal Pyrogenic Toxins A, B and C
- Child with a Strept pharyngitis/tonsillitis (Sore throat and high fever) → mucocutaneous rash starting on the **trunk** which has a papular Sandpaper appearance which spreads to the extremities w/ characteristic Pastia's lines (**linear petechia in folds**), perioral pallor, **red Strawberry tongue (enlarged papillae)**, red

conjunctiva, Swelling of palms/Soles which resolves w/ desquamation; onychomadesis telogen effluvium occur later

- Ddx: Staph-TSS (similar rash but no preceding Stept throat and is more toxic), Kawasaki (rash is perineal and acral and less papular and there are no Pastia's lines)
- Dx: throat/nasal culture; ASO, anti-DNase B, anti-hyaluronidase or anti-fibrinolysin Abs
- Rx: penicillin for 10–14 days (clindamycin if PNC-allergic)
- Complications: PSGN and rheumatic fever (treating scarlets prevents RF but not PSGN)
  - o PSGN can also result from S. pyogenes impetigo (regardless of treatment status)

Streptococcal toxic shock syndrome

- Similar clinical features as staph-TSS but affects adults (vs children), more severe with higher mortality (50%), a/w florid skin/soft-tissue infection (vs occult), rare rash (derm won't be consulted) and far more frequent blood culture positivity (>50%)
- Primary infection p/w severe pain in extremity (like necrotizing fasciitis) → septic shock
- Pathogenesis: GAS M types 1 and 3 produce various toxins (strept pyrogenic toxins, strept mitogenic toxin or steptolysin O) which bind to Vβ region to act as superantigens
- Dx: blood cultures, hypocalcemia is prominent (staph-TSS also), ↑ PT/PTT, ↑ LFTs
- Rx: surgical debridement + clindamycin + penicillin; vancomycin and IVIG are options
- Emerging pathogen is Streptococcus suis which is transmitted from pigs to humans (eating undercooked pork is main RF) and is causing outbreaks of TSS in Asia

Toxin mediated rashes (fever + rash)

- SSSS (staph): Infant (or adult with CRF) p/w erythema of **face and folds (spares mucosa)**
  - o Exfoliatoxins A and B; Rx: dicloxacillin or clindamycin (mild); IV nafcillin (severe)
- Kawasaki disease (CRASH and burn): young Child w/ Conjunctivitis, Rash (perineal/acral), Adenopathy, Strawberry tongue, Hands/feet w/edema/erythema/ desquamation; fever
  - o Unknown toxin; **Rx: ASA and IVIG**
- Scarlet fever: Child w/ Sore throat → **truncal rash** which becomes papular (Sandpaper), Pastia's lines, Strawberry tongue, Swelling of palms/Soles and conjunctival hyperemia
  - o Streptococcal Pyrogenic Toxins A, B and C; Rx: Penicillin
- Staph-TSS: Teenager w/ Scarlatiniform rash and Septic Shock (fever and **hypo-Tension)**
  - o TSST-1 acts as Superantigen, binding to Vβ region of TCR; Rx: clindamycin + Vanc

<u>Corynebacterial skin infections</u> ("Cory is a teacher's PET"; Rx all w/ erythromycin)

- Pitted keratolysis
  - o Caused by Kytococcus sedentarius > corynobacterium
  - o p/w small crater-like pits on weight-bearing soles of feet with **foul odor**
    - ▪ "Stop being sedentary and get on your feet"
  - o Rx: topical **erythromycin**, 20% aluminum chloride
- Erythrasma
  - o Caused by C. minitissimum (G+ filamentous rod)
  - o p/w brown, minimally scaly plaques in the folds, whereas in the toe webs (4th web space MC) it p/w macerated white plaques with surrounding yellowish color

        - "C. minitissimum is minute enough to get b/w the folds and the toes"
    - Dx: fluoresces coral red w/ Woods lamp due to **coproporphyrin III**
    - Rx: treat erythrasma with topical (1st line) or oral erythromycin
- Trichomycosis axillaris > pubis >> capitis (infants)
    - Caused by C. Tenuis (trichomycosis is a misnomer because C. tenuis is a bacteria)
    - **Adherent Tan yellow concretions on axillary hair that fluoresce w/ Woods lamp**
        - Ddx: nits (head lice eggs), Piedra (fungus) and hair casts are on the scalp; also these others p/w small nodes on hair **vs trichomycosis which has concretions along Total length of the hair shaft** (much more noticeable)
    - Rx: shaving (TOC) or **topical erythromycin**/benzoyl peroxide

<u>Clostridium skin infections</u>

Clostridial myonecrosis (gas gangrene; xxx)

- **Rapidly progressive**, fatal soft-tissue infection with gas-production (like in NF)
- Due to **traumatic inoculation** of C. perfringes (Gram+ spore forming anaerobic rod)
    - **α-toxin** (vascular obstruction → tissue necrosis); **theta-toxin/perfringolysin O**
- p/w **Crepitus**, pain **and foul-smelling exudate** (dirty brown color vs watery in NF)
    - Differentiate from cellulitis based on crepitus, tissue necrosis and bullae
- Dx: gram stain and Culture of exudate or a tissue sample; blood culture; CT shows gas
- Rx: like NF we treat with extensive Sx debridement and ABX but also **hyperbaric oxygen**

Filamentous bacteria

- Mycetoma is a chronic suppurative infection of the skin/SQ characterized by the triad of swelling of the affected area, sinus formation and purulent discharge containing grains
- Mycetomas can be caused by fungus (eumycetoma) or bacteria (actinomycetoma)
- 2 causes of actinomycetomas are the filamentous bacteria Actinomyces and Nocardia
- Path: Splendore-Hoeppli phenomenon (immunoglobin deposit next to grains)
- Compare bacterial mycetomas to Botryomycosis: both are caused by traumatic inoculation of G+ bacteria leading to deep granulomatous/suppurative infections with draining sinuses that drain yellow granules; Splendore-Hoeppli phenomenon on path

Actinomycosis

- Caused by Actinomyces israelii (**G+ nonacid fast anaerobic** filamentous bacteria)
- Part of **normal flora of mouth** → infection arises after **trauma (dental procedures)**
- Granulomatous infection with suppurating abscesses and sinus tracts
- Forms
    - Cervicofacial (MC; 70%): p/w abscesses and sinus tracts draining yellow sulfur granules in **jaw** ("lumpy jaw"); a/w poor dental hygiene and dental procedures
    - Pulmonary/thoracic (2nd MC): aspiration leads to pulmonary cavities in lung base
    - GI: p/w granulomatous lesions of bowel
- Path: central basophilic granules w/ peripheral eosinophilic zone (Splendore-Hoeppli)
- Rx: IM penicillin daily x 3 weeks

Nocardiosis

- Nocardia is a **Gram+ weakly acid-fast filamentous bacteria** ubiquitous in soil (foot!)
  - Weakly acid-fast bacteria stain with Fite (know what this stain looks like)
    - "Fite for your LANd" → Leprosy, Atypical mycobacteria and Nocardia
- Forms
  - Actinomycotic mycetoma, aka actinomycetoma (**N. brasiliensis**): traumatic inoculation into foot → painless nodule that drains sulfur granules
  - Lymphocutaneous: p/w sporotrichoid pattern of papulonodules after trauma
  - Pulmonary/systemic (N. asteroids): SQ abscess in chest wall; fatal if untreated
    - Disseminated disease only occurs in the immunocompromised
- Path: dermal/SQ neutrophilic infiltrate w/ abscesses and granulomatous inflammation
- Rx: sulfonamides ("SNAP your fingers to treat the filamentous bacterial mycetomas")
  - SNAP: Sulfonamides treat Nocardia; Actinomyces requires Penicillin

<u>Other Gram-positive infections</u>

Anthrax (ABCDE'S)

- Caused by Bacillus anthracis (**G+ Spore forming rod**)
- Virulence factors: poly-D-glutamic acid **Capsule** (resists phagocytosis), **Edema toxin** (↑ cAMP → edema) and **lethal toxin** (↑TNF-α and IL-1β → septic shock, death)
- Three forms: cutaneous (MC and least fatal), pulmonary and GI anthrax
- Cutaneous anthrax arises via occupational exposure from direct contact to Animals

- p/w Blue Blisters that drains Blood → **Eschar** (black crust) which is **surrounded by a zone of Erythema and Edema; the necrotic ulcer is usually painless (vs spider bite)**
- Dx: gram stain; use Dacron or rayon swabs for culture and culture on Sheep's Blood Agar
- Rx: Ciprofloxacin or Doxycycline (even for young children)
    - Treatment does not alter cutaneous lesions but they do ↓ mortality
    - Vaccine (BioThrax) for adults 18–65 w/ suspected or confirmed exposure

Erysipeloid (ERySiPeloid)

- Occupational disease of **fisherman** caused by Erysipelothrix Rhusiopathiae (**Gram + Rod**)
- p/w Red-violaceous well-defined plaques w/ edema and raised borders (cellulitis)
- Classically affects back of hands and fingers w/ **Sparring of terminal Phalanges**
- Dx: gram stain/culture from aspirate, skin scrapings or skin biopsy
- Rx: Self-limited (resolves in 3–4 weeks); **Penicillin or cephalosporins** hastens resolution

Gram-negative skin infections

Mycoplasma-induced rash and mucositis (MIRM)

- Occurs 1–2 weeks after mycoplasma pneumonia
- Pathogenesis: cloning of B cells w/ subsequent cutaneous Immune complex deposition and formation of compliment (vs Fas ligand-mediated toxicity in SJS/TEN)
- p/w ulcerative Mucosal eruption (**94% oral, 82% ocular**, 63% urogenital) and targetoid acral cutaneous

vesiculobullous rash (47%) in adolescents (median age is 12)

- Path: similar to EM/SJS/TEN
- Dx: M. pneumoniae serum IgM level and CXR
- Rx: symptomatic care (Magic Mouthwash, pain control) and antibiotics (TCN/Macrolide)

Pseudomonas ("GEOFF has Pseudomonas")

- Green nail syndrome: green nail discoloration from P. aeruginosa pyocyanin pigment
  - Rx: topical quinolones or aminoglycosides
- Ecthyma gangrenosum: P. aeruginosa septicemia in pt. with severe **neutropenia** p/w purpuric macules → hemorrhagic bullae → **Eschar** (genital region or Extremities MC)
  - Rx: IV aminoglycosides + antipseudomonal PCN
- Otitis externa: p/w edema, green exudate and severe pain ("Ouch") when touching ear
  - Rx: topical antipseudomonal agents
  - Malignant otitis externa is seen in diabetics and immunosuppressed; p/w granulation tissue down to bony portion of ear; Rx: IV antipseudomonal agents
- Pseudomonas Folliculitis (hot tub folliculitis): p/w perifollicular papulopustules in the bathing suit distribution 2 days after hot tub exposure
  - Rx: none required; self-resolves (consider ciprofloxacin if immunosuppressed)
- Pseudomonas hot Foot syndrome: a/w wading pools; p/w acute onset, exquisitely tender, red violaceous plaques on weight bearing areas of soles of children
  - Rx: none required; self-resolves (supportive care w/ acetaminophen)
- Pseudomonal Pyoderma: p/w superficial erosions w/ blue-green Purulent exudate and macerated moth-

eaten borders with a Pungent grapey odor in Previous burns/wounds
    - Rx: topical and oral anti-Pseudomonal agents
- Pseudomonal infection of the toe webs: p/w sharply demarcated greenish maceration of the skin of the tightly compressed, non-aerated toe webs ("trench foot")
    - Rx: counsel that lack of aeration leads to over-hydration of the skin (avoid heavy boots); Potassium Permanganate soaks w/ drying of feet +/- ciprofloxacin

Bartonella

- Intracellular **Gram-negative aerobic bacilli** (bartonella)
- Three species
    - B. Henselae (cat flea vector): **cat scratch** ("hens and cats") and peliosis hepatitis
    - B. Quintana (human body louse vector): **Trench fever**
    - B. henselae and B. quintana both cause bacillary angiomatosis, chronic afebrile bacteremia and endocarditis in addition to the above diseases
        - TB Epidemic don't Quit (Quintana): Trench fever, Bacillary angiomatosis, Bacteremia/ endocarditis, Body louse (Epidemic typhus has this vector)
    - B. Bacilliformis: Bartonellosis (Carrion's disease/ Oroya fever/verruga peruana)
- Cat scratch disease: self-limited disease; p/w papule at inoculation site (lasts weeks) and tender LAD (axilla MC) starting in weeks and lasting for weeks-months; oculoglandular syndrome of Parinaud (**U/L conjunctivitis and ipsilateral preauricular LAD**) occur in 5%
    - Vector: Cat flea (Ctenocephalides felis)

  - Dx: IFA for B. henselae; PCR on tissue or blood; may see ↑ eos, ↑ LFTs, ↑ ESR
  - Path: stellate abscesses surrounded by palisading histiocytes w/ G (-) bacilli on Warthin-Starry ("Barthin-Starhi" → Bartonella, Spirochette, Rhinoscleroma)
  - Rx: supportive (analgesics, "just make cats comfy"); azithromycin/doxy (optional)
- Bacillary angiomatosis ("angioma-2-sis"): occurs in HIV patients w/ CD4 counts < 200; only 20% recall cat bite/scratch; p/w dome-shaped vascular (PG-like) papulonodules
  - Vectors: cat flea (carries B. henselae) and human body louse (carries B. quintana)
  - Dx: skin biopsy w/ Warthin-Starry stain; culture on chocolate agar
  - Path: resembles PG (capillary proliferation) but has a dense **neutrophilic** infiltrate and **organisms within endothelial cells** seen with Warthin-Starry stain
  - Rx: **erythromycin (1st line)**; doxycycline, azithromycin or clarithromycin (2nd line)
    - Jarisch-Herxheimer-like reaction: worsening fever w/ onset of treatment
- Trench fever "five-day fever": a/w homelessness and poor hygiene
  - Vector: human body louse
  - Rx: gentamicin plus doxycycline
    - "Homeless people in the trenches need Gentlemanly Dox on their side"
- Bartonellosis (Carrion's disease): onset of Oroya fever is sudden ("arroyo in Spanish means fast flowing stream") with severe flu-like symptoms and massive **hemolysis**; when death occurs, it is due to Salmonella infection ("salmon swim in the stream"); those who recover may develop verruga peruana lesions composed of

bright red papules/nodules within small erythematous patches on the head and extremities

- Vector: phlebotomine sand fly (**Lutzomyia**; same as New World Leishmaniasis)
- Dx (arroyo fever): Giemsa stain of a peripheral smear shows organisms in RBCs
- Path (verruga peruana): bacilli in verrucous lesions
- Rx (Oroya fever): **Ciprofloxacin** (preferred) or Chloramphenicol + Ceftriaxone
    - Pregnancy: amoxicillin-Clavulanic acid
- Rx (verruga peruana): Azithromycin (in pregnancy too)
    - "First letter in Carrion's disease is C, second is A" → this also helps you remember we culture bartonella on **Chocolate Agar**

Rickettsial diseases

- Obligately intracellular gram-negative bacteria transmitted by arthropods
- Labs: thrombocytopenia, leukopenia, transaminitis
- Dx: PCR, IHC or culture of biopsy specimen
- Rx: **doxycycline** (kids too) except Scrub typhus in pregnancy (azithromycin), non-life threatening RMSF in pregnancy (chloramphenicol) and Rickettsialpox (self-resolves)
- Mnemonic: "RAM MEC'S is a human" (see below)
    - RAM: spotted fever group which p/w fevers, **petechial rash (MC on wrists and ankles)** in > 85% of patients and an **eschar** (**except RMSF which has no eschar**)
    - MEC: typhus group which is similar to spotted fever group except that the rash starts in the **axilla** and is only present in 50–80% of pts and there is **no eschar**
    - S: scrub typhus group which p/w rash (**axilla**) in 50% of pts plus **eschar** ("S-char")

- Human: Rickettsia-like bacteria (human monocytic/granulocytic Ehrlichiosis)

- Rocky Mountain Spotted Fever
  - Agent: Rickettsia rickettsii
  - Vector: **Dermacentor variabilis** (MC; Eastern US); D. andersoni (#2; Western US)
  - p/w fever, HA, myalgias and GI symptoms 1–2 weeks after tick bite → 90% develop rash days after these initial symptoms which starts as red macules on the wrists/ankles and later spreads to the trunk and becomes **petechial**/purpuric
  - 25% mortality w/o Abx (< 5% if treated early); most severe Rickettsial disease
  - Major pathophysiologic effect of Rickettsial infection is ↑ vascular permeability
    - Two similar diseases but which do not cause death are R. parkeri rickettsiosis (southern US) and African tick bite fever (Africa) which p/w mild systemic symptoms, tender LAD and rash on trunk and extremities
- Rickettsialpox ("I imagine an urban city")
  - Agent: Rickettsia akari ("There are many Kars in an urban city")
  - Vector: Liponyssoides sanguineus (house mouse mite); only one caused by **mites**
    - "Women get Lipo and there are houses, mice and mites in urban cities"
  - p/w fever, HA and papulovesicle eschar at bite site and widespread erythematous macules and papulovesicles w/ hemorrhagic crust **(varicella-like)**
  - Only Rickettsial disease which self-resolves but still can treat w/ doxycycline
    - "Infections are less severe in urban cities"
  - Negative Weil-Felix test ("You don't need wheels in the city, you just walk")
- African tick bite fever

    - Agent: Rickettsia Africae (has leopard/giraffe skin pattern)
    - Vector: Amblyomma genus
    - p/w **multiple eschars** at tick bite site → maculo-papular rash, flu-like symptoms
- Mediterranean spotted fever
    - Agent: Rickettsia conorii ("I imagine a Mediterranean guy named Conor")
    - Vector: Rhipicephalus sanguineus (brown dog tick)
        - "Conor has a brown dog that barks (roof-icephalus)"
    - p/w necrotic papule at tick bite site (Tache noir) → maculopapular rash on legs
        - "Conor's brown dog attacks (Tache noir) people's legs"
- Murine/endemic Typhus
    - Agent: Rickettsia typhi
    - Vector: Xenopsylla cheopis (oriental rat flea; same vector as the bubonic plague)
    - p/w fever, systemic symptoms (HA, myalgias) and rash that starts in the **axilla**
- Epidemic Typhus
    - Agent: Rickettsia prowazekii
    - Vector: Pediculus humanus (human body louse; same as B. Quintana infections)
        - TB Epidemic don't Quit (Quintana): Trench fever, Bacillary angiomatosis, Bacteremia/endocarditis, Body louse (Epidemic typhus has this vector)
    - Presents like murine typhus
    - May see recurrence of latent infection decades later (Brill-Zinsser disease)
    - Flying squirrel typhus is a variant caused by contact w/ flying squirrels
- Cat flea Typhus
    - Agent: Rickettsia felis

    - Vector: Ctenocephalides felis (cat flea; same vector as in Cat scratch disease)
    - Presents like murine typhus
- Scrub Typhus
    - Agent: Orientia tsutsugamushi (formerly Rickettsia tsutsugamushi)
    - Vector: larval trombiculid mites (chiggers; "Shiggers")
    - Presents like typhus group (MEC) but **has eschar** at bite site and rash in only 50%
    - MC in Asia, particularly in areas of dense Scrub vegetation
- Rickettsia-like bacteria
    - Human Monocytic Ehrlichiosis (HME)
        - Agent: Ehrlichia chaffeensis
        - Vector: Amblyomma Americanum and Dermacentor variabilis
            - White-tailed deer is the major reservoir
        - p/w fevers, myalgias, and maculopapular rash MC on the trunk; no eschar
        - Dx: smear shows morulae (intracytoplasmic microcolonies)
    - Human Granulocytic Anaplasmosis/ehrlichiosis
        - Agent: Anaplasma phagocytophilum (Ehrlichia phagocytophilum)
        - Vector: Ixodes scapularis and I. pacificus (same vector as Lyme disease)
        - Presents like HME

Other Gram-negative skin infections

Neisseria Meningitidis

- Gram negative diplococcus which tests positive for the enzyme cytochrome c Oxidase
- Pathogenesis/virulence

    - Lipoligosaccharide acts as an endotoxin and is responsible for septic shock
    - Factor H binding protein inhibits complement-mediated death
    - Polysaccharide capsule prevents phagocytosis by immune cells
    - Uses iron to resist oxidative killing by producing catalase/superoxide dismutase
- Causes purpura fulminans (dermatologic emergency)
    - p/w multiple violaceous, non-blanching, retiform macules and skin necrosis
    - **MC seen in young adults (esp. MSM w/ HIV) by N. meningitidis** (S. pneumoniae and VZV are less common) but can be seen in neonates (protein C/S deficiency)
- Dx: gram stain, blood (chocolate or Thayer-Martin agar) or CSF culture, PCR
- Rx: IV penicillin or 3rd gen cephalosporin (ceftriaxone)
- Prevention: vaccination or rifampin for recent contacts

Brucellosis (Malta fever; undulant fever): "unDDDulant"

- Caused by Gram (-) coccobacillus, Brucella spp.
- MC zoonosis worldwide; acquired through the consumption of contaminated goat milk (developing world) or from Direct contact w/ animals (occupational disease in the US)
- p/w undulating fevers, arthralgias, LAD, hepatosplenomegaly, malodorous perspiration and skin disease in 10% of pts. (Disseminated violaceous papules and erythema nodosa)
- Rx: multidrug regimen (**Doxycycline** + either streptomycin/gentamycin or rifampin)
    - Politely recommend they use Deodorant for their bromhidrosis

Glanders

- Caused by gram (-) bacillus, **Burkholderia mallei** due to contact w/ **horses or donkeys**
- It is an ulceroglandular disease; the "ulcero" refers to the localized form w/ an ulcerative papulopustule at inoculation site; the "glandular" refers to the chronic form w/ multiple soft tissue nodules ("**farcy buds**") on skin overlying lymphatics
    - There is also a septicemic and a pulmonary form both with > 95% mortality
- Rx: amoxicillin/clavulanate (Augmentin), doxycycline or TMP/SMX (Bactrim)
    - "To communicate across the land (Glanders), you need to send Burkholder's mail via horses/donkeys far (farcy buds) distances to Augment the Dox to come Back"

Melioidosis

- Caused by gram (-) bacillus, **Burkholderia pseudomallei** due to contact with **water/soil**
- RFs: diabetes and chronic kidney disease
- Clinical presentation, mortality rates and treatment are same as Glanders
    - "I think of a chamelion (melioidoses) that copies ("pseudoglanders"/B. pseudomallei) other colors and lives in the water/soil"

Malacoplakia

- Chronic infection resulting from the inability of macrophages to kill phagocytosed **E. coli**
- Affects immune-compromised patients (**bone marrow transplant** > HIV/AIDS)
- Because E. coli is found in the **GI tract**, we see ulcerations, abscesses with draining sinuses, soft yellow/pink papules and hard red nodules on the **perianal/genital skin**

- Path: dense granulomatous infiltrate composed of **von Hansemann cells** (large eosinophilic macrophages) which contain **Michaelis-Gutmann bodies** (intracytoplasmic laminated concretions representing incompletely killed bacteria within calcified, iron containing phagolysosomes, so they stain w/ von Kossa ("Cossa"), Perls, PAS and Giemsa)
    - "Big red histiocytes w/ small blue Bull's eye-shaped calcium deposits"
- Rx: surgical correction (ciprofloxacin, TMP/SMX, clofazimine for nonsurgical candidates)

Tularemia (rabbit fever; deer fly fever)

- Gram (-) non-motile coccobacillus, Francisella Tularensis
- Tick bites or deer fly are the MC routes of transmission in the US; ↑ risk in hunters
- p/w **Ulceroglandular** disease (80%): punched-out ulcer at bite site → suppurative LAD
- Rx: Aminoglycosides like Streptomycin
- Rabbit carcasses was the classic mode of transmission but less common now

H. influenzae (Hib) cellulitis

- Gram (-) coccobacillus; incidence has ↓ significantly since Hib vaccine
- p/w **Blue-violaceous cellulitis (MC on peri-orbital or Buccal region) of Babies** s/p URI
- Dx: **Blood cultures** usually positive (vs other forms of cellulitis)
- Rx: third generation cephalosporin

Rhinoscleroma

- Chronic granulomatous infection of the nose
- Caused by inhalation of Klebsiella rhinoscleromatis; occurs in adults in tropical locations

    - "I imagine adults in a tropical place inhaling cocaine in their nose at a club (kleb)"
- Mechanism similar to malakoplakia: cellular immune defects cause an inability of macrophages to kill phagocytosed bacteria → **Mikulicz cells**
    - "Mike licks (Mikulicz cells) the residual cocaine off his nose"
- Three phases
    - Catarrhal phase: nasal obstruction/rhinitis
        - "cocaine 1st obstructs and inflames the nose"
    - Granulomatous/infiltrative phase: epistaxis, anesthesia of soft palate, dysphonia and Hebra's nose (deformation and expansion of anterior nares)
        - "Later cocaine causes nose bleeds, anesthesia and nasal deformity"
    - Sclerotic phase: extensive scarring
        - "Cocaine will scar your nose, do NOT do cocaine at the club (klebsiella)"
- Path: dense plasma cell infiltrate w/ **Mikulicz cells** (large foam cells w/ vacuolated cytoplasm which contain causative bacilli seen w/ Warthin-Starry and Giemsa) and **Russel bodies** (plasma cells "pregnant" w/ immunoglobin)
    - "Mike and Russel did the cocaine at the kleb"
- Rx: **ciprofloxacin** ("sip makes me think of mouth/ nose") and **TCNs** like doxycycline ("Mike and Russel will need to see a doc after doing all this cocaine") are first line

Salmonellosis (typhoid fever): "S-sounds"

- Infection with Salmonella typhi spread by direct contact with infected individuals
- p/w fever, abdominal pain, N/V/**D** and **rose Spots on trunk** (small grouped pink papules)
- Rx: Ciprofloxacin (use third gen cephalosporin like Cefdinir in children)

Rat-bite fever ("Haverhill fever")

- Caused by **Streptobacillus moniliformis** (US) or Spirillum minus (Asia)
- Results from rat bite or ingestion of contaminated food/water/milk ("Haverhill fever")
- Child (50%) p/w erythema, edema, abscess, ulceration at bite site → **paroxysms of fever** and regional LAD → **migratory polyarthritis** and acral eruption (**palms/ soles**)
    - In addition to rat bite fever (Streptobacillus) other diseases to consider with the triad of fever, rash and arthritis are Spotted fevers, Secondary Syphilis, Still's disease, SLE, Serum Sickness, Sweets, Schnitzler's and periodic fever Syndromes
- Occurs in urban areas (w/ rats); up to 15% mortality
- Tx: penicillin ("strepto")

Differential diagnosis of ulceroglandular disease (ulcer at inoculation site → LAD):
"Mel's Tall Aunt Rarely Permits Glandular diseases To-be-chanced"

Melioidosis, Tularemia, Anthrax, Rat-bite fever, Plague, Glanders, TB-chancre

Plague

- Caused by G (-) bipolar bacillus, Yersinia Pestis; "safety Pin" look on Gram/Giemsa stain
- Live on **rodents** and transmitted to humans by oriental rat flea (Xenopsylla cheopis) bite
- Forms
    - **Bubonic** (MC): Pustule or ulcer at inoculation site → Painful Purulent regional LAD (**buboes**; groin and axilla MC)
    - Septicemic: vesiculopustular eruption with Petechiae and Purpura; GI and nasopharyngeal necrosis; 100% mortality if untreated

  - Pneumonic: acute pneumonitis; 100% mortality if untreated
- Rx: streptomycin → "strept and Pest (Y. Pestis) have the same letters"

Vibrio vulnificans

- RFs: old males, HIV, **liver** disease (hemochromatosis, cirrhosis), CKD or DM
- Reservoir: **shellfish** ("shell-vish")
- Two modes of infection
  - Cutaneous exposure to contaminated seawater/ shellfish → primary skin infection → necrotizing fasciitis, myositis or septicemia
  - Consumption of undercooked shellfish (raw oysters MC) → abdominal cramps, septic shock, purple macules/vesicles → hemorrhagic bullae w/ necrotic plaques
- Rx: doxycycline (oral or IV) plus IV third generation cephalosporin (ceftriaxone)

Bite-induced infections

- Dog bites are most common; human bites are most likely to get infected
- Mouths contain a lot of bacteria
  - **Pasteurella multocida**: dog bites and cat bites ("multiple animals")
  - Pasteurella canis and Pasteurella canimorsus: dog bites ("think k-9 police dogs")
  - Eikenella corrodens: human bites ("Eik, Ken, and Cory are human names")
- Rx: amoxicillin/clavulanate

Nonvenereal spirochete infections

Borrelia (Lyme disease)

- Europe: Borrelia garinii and Borrelia afzelii reside on the Ixodes Ricinus tick
- USA: B. burgdorferi lives on I. scapularis/I. dammini (NE US) or I. pacificus (West US) tick
- Ixodes tick looks like it has a BAL on its back → Babesiosis, Anaplasmosis, Lyme disease
    - Frequent co-infection with all three; doxycycline treats all three infections
- In european Lyme disease there is ↑ incidence of neurologic sequelae and ↓ arthritis
- Three clinical stages of Lyme disease
    - Early localized
        - **Erythema migrans (EM): p/w expanding annular plaque w/central clearing** on trunk (children) or legs (adults) which self-resolves in 1 month
        - Disseminated erythema migrans: multiple smaller lesions arise after EM
    - Early disseminated
        - Borrelia lymphocytoma (rare; Europe only; **Afzelii** > B. garinii/): p/w firm red-blue tender nodule on **Earlobe** (children) or **Areola** (adults)
            - "When you are Bored (Borrelia) AF, European kids play w/ their earlobes and European adults play with their areolas"
        - Arthritis (60%): mono/oligo-articular (**knee** MC) arising months after bite
        - Neurologic abnormalities (10%): **Bell's palsy** MC
        - Cardiac complications: **A-V block** MC
    - Chronic

        - Acrodermatitis chronica atrophicans (10%; Europe only): two phases
            - Early edematous phase: edematous erythematous plaques acrally
            - Late atrophic phase: "cigarette paper" skin w/ telangiectasias
                - "B. afzelli > garini: Atropic Fixed Zones comes after Edema"
- Dx: C6 peptide antibody assay (best 1st test) or two-tier serology (ELISA + Western blot)
- Rx: doxycycline (amoxicillin if < 8 years old or pregnant) x 3 weeks
    - IV or IM ceftriaxone if cardiac or neurologic symptoms x 2 weeks

Non-Lyme borrelia infections

- Louse-borne relapsing fever (Africa): 3–4 relapses of paroxysmal fevers; more severe
    - Agent: Borrelia recurrentis
    - Vector: Pediculus humanus var. corporis (human body louse)
    - Rx: doxycycline
- Tick-borne relapsing fever (Western US): 1–2 relapses of paroxysmal fevers; less severe
    - Agents: Borellia duttonii and B. hermsii
    - Vector: Ornithodoros (Hodor mnemonic at end of section 5.5 on Arachnids)
    - Rx: doxycycline

Leptospirosis (Weil's disease)

- Agent: leptospira (commonly transmitted by rodents who excrete the organism in urine)
- p/w fever, muscle pains, HA, conjunctival injection and **jaundice w/ purpura/petechia**
- Dx: isolating organism from the blood; serology titers
- Rx: penicillin or doxycycline

Nonvenereal (endemic) treponematoses

- "YEP, you've got nonvenereal T. pallidum" (the Y and P are on the ends of the mnemonic and begin by affecting the ends of the body (**legs**); the mnemonic goes in chronological order so the Y and E affect children whereas the P effects people of any age)
  - Yaws (T. pallidum pertenue): affects children in tropical climates
    - Stage 1: indurated red papule on leg → ulcerates ("Mother Yaws")
    - Stage 2: multiple smaller widespread ulcers ("Daughter Yaws")
    - Stage 3: necrotic and ulcerative abscesses that heal with deforming scars
      - Yaws = Jaws = bites out of skin which hurt which rhymes w/ pert
  - Endemic syphilis (T. pallidum endemicum): affects children in hot dry climates
    - Stage 1: inconspicuous papule in mouth or mammary areas of mothers
    - Stage 2: mucous membrane lesion (mucosal patches, condyloma lata)
    - Stage 3: gumma formation of mucous membranes, skin and bones
- Pinta (T. pallidum carateum): affects all ages in Latin America
    - Stage 1: enlarging papules surrounded by red halos on the leg
    - Stage 2: psoriasiform papules/plaques ("pintids") change color from **red** → **blue** → **brown** → **gray/black**
    - Stage 3: symmetric vitiligo-like lesions (**white**) over bony prominences
      - "Pintar la cara colores" means to paint the face colors in Spanish

- Labs: the serologic tests in syphilis are used here but cannot differentiate b/w them
    - o Treponemal tests (**FTA-ABS**, MHA-TP, TPHA, TPPA): specific; **best tests for late stages as it remains positive for life (Forever)**
    - o Nontreponemal tests (RPR, VDRL, USR, RST, TRUST): less specific; useful for identifying Recent infections and monitoring Response to treatment (four-fold ↓ in titers = successful treatment; four-fold ↑ in titers = Reinfection/Relapse)
- Rx: Benzathine Penicillin (azithromycin now is TOC for yaws; "Z-pack for yawz")

<u>Sexually transmitted bacterial infections</u>

Syphilis

- Gram (-) spirochete Treponema pallidum
- Early congenital Syphilis (< 2 years old): Similar Skin findings as Secondary Syphilis (copper-colored acral papules), but there is also Split/fissured oral commissures, Snuffles, acral Scale/blisters/erosions, Skeletal involvement → pseudoparalysis
- Late congenital syph (> 2 years): Hutchinson's triad (interstitial keratitis, Hutchinson's teeth, 8th nerve deafness), Hyperplastic first molar (Mulberry's molar), **Higoumenakis sign (U/L thickening of the dominant sides clavicle)**, rhagades (linear scars at oral commissures that replaced fissures), High-arched palate, saber shins, Clutton's joints
- Primary syphilis (weeks post exposure): painless **indurated** well-defined chancre
- Secondary syphilis (months post-primary syphilis): p/w **non-pruritic papulosquamous copper-colored rash** that begins on the trunk but generalizes and effects **palms/soles**, genitals and face; other presentations include macular (erythematous macules), follic-

ular (↑ risk of neurosyphilis), annular, condyloma lata (soft exophytic papules in the genitals), condyloma lata-like papules in the mouth, **non-scarring "moth-eaten" alopecia, split papules at oral commissures**, hypopigmented macules on neck (Necklace of Venus), Rupoid syphilis/Leus maligna (rare ulcerative nodular form a/w HIV)

- **Two presentations in the mouth (tongue, mucosal lips and soft palate are MC)**
    - **Multiple oval aphthous-like ulcers w/ raised white pseudomembrane**
    - **White serpiginous "snail-track"** ulcers (contiguous version of other one)

- Latent syphilis: early latent (< 1 year) and late latent (> 1 year or unknown duration)
    - In late latent, 1/3rd are asymptomatic w/ negative RPR but positive treponemal test (always stay +), 1/3rd are asymptomatic w/ both tests positive, 1/3rd progress to tertiary syphilis w/ RPR usually positive and treponemal tests positive
- Tertiary syphilis (months to years' post-secondary syphillis): MC and hallmark lesion is the gumma (non-infectious firm brownish-red granulomatous papulonodule which heal w/ scarring), cardiovascular syphilis (proximal aortitis), neurosyphilis (paresis, meningitis, optic atrophy, tabes dorsalis, Argyll-Robertson pupil)
- Path
    - Primary syphilis: non-specific ulcer w/ necrosis, fibrin, neuts and plasma cells
    - Secondary syphilis: looks like LP and psoriasis had a messy baby → vacuolar interface w/ long slender sexy rete ridges, neuts in the horn, plasma cells in the dermis and endothelial swelling obliterating the lumen of small vessels
    - Condyloma lata: pseudoepitheliomatous hyperplasia w/ ballooning degeneration and numerous

neutrophils in the epidermis and plasma cells in the dermis

- Dx (see lab section on nonvenereal treponematoses above)
    - o Primary: **darkfield-microscopy** or multiplex > serology (non-treponemal tests)
    - o Secondary: cardiolipin (RPR), treponemal tests, multiplex IgG test (see below)
    - o Latent: patients are asymptomatic w/ positive serologies (RPR may be negative)
    - o Tertiary: patients are symptomatic w/ positive serologies/CSF antibodies
    - o RPR and VDRL have more false Positives: Virsuses (EBV, HIV, hepatitis) and Vaccines, Drugs (e.g., narcotics), RA, Lupus, Leprosy, Lyme disease, Lymphoma, Pregnancy, Pinta/Yaws/Endemic; false negatives are seen in the setting of HIV
    - o Treponemal test (FTA-ABS) false positives are only Autoimmune diseases (e.g., RA, lupus), AIDS infection and other Spirochete infections (Lyme, pinta, yaws, etc.)
- Rx
    - o Primary/secondary/early latent syphilis: IM PCN x 1 dose (**doxycycline if allergic**)
    - o Syphilis in pregnancy: IM PCN x 2 weekly doses (desensitization if allergic)
    - o Late latent, CV or gummatous syphilis or retreatment: IM PCN x 3 weekly doses
    - o Symptomatic congenital syphilis, neurosyphilis or ocular syphilis: IV PNC
        - ▪ Congenital syphilis in babies older than 6 months: IM PNC x 1 dose
- Jarisch-Herxheimer reaction: fever, chills, HA, tachycardia 8 hours after post-treatment
    - o Seen in all spirochete diseases (Lyme, leptospirosis, louse-borne relapsing fever)

- **Workup**: get HIV test, report all cases of syphilis to the health department (does not require patient consent), all sexual partners in the last 3 months (primary), 6 months (secondary) or 1 year (tertiary) should be notified, patient should abstain from sexual activity for at least 1 week off treatment and until all symptoms resolve

Gonorrhea

- Gram (-) diplococci Neisseria gonorrhea
- Women are more likely to be asymptomatic but both sexes p/w dysuria and discharge
- Disseminated gonococcemia: "Don't let females w/ gonorrhea FART on you"
  - Fever, Arthritis (large joints), Rash (acral pustules, esp fingers), Tenosynovitis
- Interesting facts (FARTS): F > M; Antibiotic Resistance testing recommended; Thayer-Martin culture media is gold standard for dx; Smears show G (-) diplococci in neutrophils
- Dx: gram stain and culture of urethral, anal and vaginal **discharge** show G (-) diplococci in neutrophils (swab from lesions themselves are negative)
  - DNA hybridization tests are efficient but do not permit antibiotic sensitivity
- Rx: dual therapy w/ ceftriaxone and azithromycin (chlamydia co-infection) both x 1 dose

Chancroid

- Gram (-) coccobacilli Hemophilus ducreyi ("do cry")
- "Do cry" p/w PG-like ulcer (painful ulcer w/ undermined borders) and a **yellow fibrinous base** ("yell and cry") on parts of the penis w/ the most pain/sense receptors (**prepuce, coronal sulcus, frenulum**) and painful inguinal LAD (buboes) which may ulcerate

    - **Ulcer(s) occur within the 1st two weeks of sexual intercourse**
- MC in males and prostitutes
    - "Because only those 2 demographics would still have sex w/ this painful ulcer"
- Dx: "school of fish/train-tracks" of organisms on Giemsa stain; culture
- Path (ulcer): 3 zones of change → superficial zone of necrosis w/ fibrin and neutrophils, granulation tissue underneath, and lymphocytes/plasma cells even deeper in the dermis
- Rx: azithromycin (azithro-"cry"-cin) > ceftriaxone, ciprofloxacin, erythromycin

Lymphogranuloma venereum (LGV)

- Chlamydia trachomatis (serotypes L1-L3)
- Stage 1 (L; days after exposure): pain-Less transient genital ulcer +/- Lymphangitis
    - Ulcer is MC on the coronal sulcus (men) or posterior vaginal wall (women)
- Stage 2 (G; weeks after stage 1): painful inguinal buboes w/ **Groove sign** (enlarged LNs above and below Poupart ligament) that rupture → fistulas, sinus tracts and strictures
- Stage 3 (V; months-years after stage 2): **lesions on the anal Verge** (ano-genito-rectal syndrome: proctocolitis w/ peri-rectal abscesses/fistulas/strictures and "lymphoroids")
- Dx (G): Gamna-Favre bodies (intracytoplasmic basophilic inclusions) in macrophages on Giemsa stain or in endothelial cells on path; PCR or serology for chlamydia
    - Malakoplakia also had intracytoplasmic Michaelis Gutmann bodies in macrophages and p/w anogenital lesions similar to stage 3 LGV
- Rx: **doxycycline** 100 mg BID x 3 weeks > erythromycin

Granuloma inguinale

- Gram (-) bacillus Klebsiella granulamatis
- p/w (GRAN): painless **ulcer w/ hypertrophic Granulation tissue that is Red/beefy**; Autoinoculation results in extragenital lesions; smelly Necrotic "psuedobuboe" Nodules
- Dx: "safety-pin" Donovan bodies (Yersinia pestis also have a safety-pin appearance)
- Rx (A-E): **Azithromycin** 1 g weekly x 3 weeks > Bactrim, Cipro, Doxycycline, Erythromycin

Mycobacterial infections

Leprosy (Hansen's disease)

- Mycobacterium leprae: intracytoplasmic parasite of **macrophages** and **Schwann cells**
  - o Weakly acid-fast bacillus so Fite stain is positive (**Fite is a modified Ziehl-Neelsen stain; both stain organisms bright red w/ a blue background**)
    - "Fite for you LANd" (**Leprosy, Atypical mycobacterium**, Nocardia)
  - o Requires Low temperatures for growth so affects cooler skin (ear-Lobes, nose)
  - o Transmitted by nasal/oral droplets and contact w/ armadillos (SE USA)
  - o **Must be cultured in mouse foot-pads (cannot be cultured in vitro)**
    - "Hand-sen's must be cultured in foot pads"
- Chronic granulomatous and neurotropic disease affecting skin and peripheral nerves
- Long incubation period (avg 4–10 years) with bimodal age range (10–15 and 30–60 y/o)
- **Large peripheral nerves are seen in acral sites (Low temp; 35°C is best for growth)**
  - o Causes claw hand, stocking glove anesthesia, neuropathic ulcers, ocular damage

- Ridley-Jopling scale divides leprosy into two polar forms (Tuberculoid/TT which is Th1 driven or Lepromatous/LL which is Th2 driven) and 3 borderline forms (BT, BB, BL)
    - o Polar forms are stable and do not change while borderline forms may change their minds on what they want to do ("just like borderline people in politics")
- TT (cell mediated/Th1 response) p/w one or few localized (asymmetric) well-defined scaly hypopigmented (Light-colored) anesthetic lesions w/ raised erythematous borders
    - o Path: sarcoidal granulomas tracking East to West along nerves (no globi present)
- Borderline (BT > BB) has many asymmetric annular anesthetic hypopigmented macules
    - o Path: perineural fibrosis w/ lamellar or onion skin pattern
- LL (humoral/Th2 response) p/w numerous widespread symmetric ill-defined erythematous macules/papules/nodules/plaques on the face, buttock and legs
    - o Late findings: Loss of eyebrows, Long earLobes, Lagophthalmos, Leonine faces
    - o Plantar lesions are at ↑ risk to develop SCC
    - o Path: Grenz zone w/ diffuse infiltrate of parasitized histiocytes (Virchow cells) with free floating clumps of bacilli (globi) in large masses in the dermis
- There is also **intermediate leprosy** (earliest stage) which p/w a solitary hypopigmented (Light) macule and is the only form of leprosy lacking peripheral nerve enlargement
    - o May self-resolve or turn into one of the 5 later forms (TT, BT, BB, BL, LL)
- **Vitamin D** can change TH1/TH2 ratio and influence which pole of leprosy is expressed

- Dx: Lepromin (Mitsuda) or pilocarpine skin test; 16S ribosomal RNA gene PCR assay
- **Rx (WHO updated guidelines in 2018; "DR Clof"): Dapsone, Rifampin and Clofazimine** (x 6 months for tuberculoid/paucibacillary; x 12 months for lepromatous/multibacillary)
- Reactional states: acute inflammation that appears suddenly after initiation of therapy
  - Type 1 (reversal) reaction: delayed type-hypersensitivity
    - p/w **nerve pain** and ulceration of existing lesions
    - MC in **borderline forms** and causes upgrading to TT or downgrading to LL
    - Rx: prednisone
      - Prednisone, borderline and neuro all have the letters "one"
- Type 2 reaction (erythema nodosum leprosum; dos is #2 in Spanish): formation of immune complexes w/ excessive humoral reaction (Th2) → **vasculitis**, fever, joint pain and **erythema nodosum-like lesions** in previously unaffected sites
    - MC in lepromatous ("leproma-dos") leprosy
    - Rx: thalidomide ("thali-dos-mide")
  - Lucio phenomenon: severe vasculitis which p/w hemorrhagic infarcts on the Lower Legs and occurs in patients w/ diffuse and untreated LL from Mexico
    - Path: LCV and epidermal infarction
    - Rx: prednisone

Cutaneous tuberculosis

- Mycobacterium tuberculosis: acid- and alcohol-fast, aerobic bacillus; ↑ risk in HIV pts.
- Inoculation-induced (exogenous exposure)

- Tuberculous Chancre: patients w/o previous infection (no immunity against TB)
  - p/w painless red indurated papule that ulcerates → self-resolves in a year
- Tuberculosis verruca Cutis: reinfection in pts. w/ prior infection (high immunity)
  - p/w enlarging warty/verrucous nodule → self-resolves over years
  - MC form of cutaneous TB

- Spread from endogenous site ("TB spreading from endogenous sites have big GOALS")
  - Tuberculous Gumma: hematogenous spread in immunosuppressed patients
    - p/w firm SQ nodule that ulcerates and drains (extremities > trunk)
  - Orificial tuberculosis: autoinoculation of skin/mucosa close to an orifice draining active TB infection seen in pts w/ advanced TB and poor cell-mediated immunity
    - p/w edematous red papule that ulcerates (MC in the mouth esp. tongue)
  - Acute miliary TB: hematogenous spread (lung MC) in immunosuppressed pts
    - p/w pinpoint blue-red papules capped with vesicles → crust → scars
  - Lupus vulgaris: reinfection in pts w/ prior infection (high immunity; "**lupus Vulgaris and tuberculosis Verruca cutis have Very high immunity to TB** meaning they are not immunosuppressed and have already been exposed → + skin test)
    - p/w red-brown plaque w/ central scarring; apple-jelly color on diascopy
    - MC on the head/neck region especially the nose, cheeks and earlobes
  - Scrofuloderma: contiguous spread of underlying infection (cervical LNs is MC)

        - p/w Suppurative SQ nodule w/ ulceration and Sinus tract formation
        - Pts are immuneSuppressed (low immunity) → **likely to find organisms**
- Tuberculids: immune-reactions of the skin due to hematogenous spread of M. Tuberculosis in pts w/ strong antituberculosis cell-mediated immunity; a/w systemic TB (tuberculids look like miliary TB but has strong immunity vs poor immunity in miliary TB)
    - Papulonecrotic tuberculid: p/w symmetric, dusky-red papules or papulopustules widely distributed favoring extensor surfaces → self-resolves w/ scarring
    - Lichen scrufulosorum: p/w perifollicular, pink or yellow-brown, tiny flat-topped papules w/ scale grouped in clusters on the trunk → self-resolves w/o scarring
    - Erythema induratum of Bazin: SQ nodule on the calves of women; a/w vasculitis
- Dx: tuberculin skin test, IFN-γ release assay, staining for acid-fast bacilli, PCR, and culture
- Rx (RIPE): Rifampin, Isoniazid, Pyrazinamide, and Ethambutol

Atypical mycobacterial skin infections (non-tuberculous mycobacteria)

- All transmitted to the skin via exogenous inoculation producing cutaneous disease
- Predisposition in individuals w/ innate defects of the IL-12/IFN-γ axis (STAT1, GATA2)
- Until diagnosis, empirically treat w/ **clarithromycin**
- Over a dozen forms: "atypical mycobacteria is A SHMUCK"
    - M. Avium Complex (MAC): common opportunistic infection in AIDS pts

    - p/w chronic pulmonary symptoms, β-symptoms, rarely Abscesses on legs
    - Labs: ↑ Alkaline phosphatase levels
    - Rx: Azithromycin/clarithromycin + ethambutol
- M. Scrufulaceum: formerly grouped w/ MAC but has distinct clinical features
    - Self-limited lymphadenitis (vs chronic lung disease in MAC)
    - p/w Slowly enlarging, painful LAD in Submandibular and Submaxillary LNs
        - May also produce skin lesions in a Sporotrichoid pattern
    - Dx: culture of sputum, skin or involved LNs
    - Rx: Surgical excision of involved LNs
- M. Haemophilum: opportunistic infection but causes cervical lymphadenitis in healthy children and cutaneous infections following **tattooing** or acupuncture
    - p/w single blue-red tender papule → pustule → abscess
    - Dx: culture of tissue or synovial fluid (grows only in cold temps: 30–32° C)
    - Rx: rifampin/rifabutin ("rhifampin")+ clarithromycin
- M. Marinum: acquired by direct contact (usually hands) w/ aquatic environments
    - p/w **blue-red ulcerating nodules in a sporotrichoid pattern**
    - Dx: culture (grows best at **31° C** vs 37° C for most other mycobacteria)
        - "Water is cold"
    - Rx: Minocycline + Macrolide (clarithromycin)
- M. Ulcerans (Buruli ulcer): MC in Africa; MC atypical mycobacteria worldwide
    - p/w single SQ nodule → huge painless Ulcer w/ Undermined borders

    - Dx: PCR, culture, Ziehl-Neelsen stain shows acid-fast bacilli
    - Rx (ulcers): **Excision** (TOC); Rifampin + Streptomycin if too large to excise
- M. Chelonae (M. Fortuitum, M. Abscessus): these saprophytic organisms are grouped together due to similar clinical features
    - Occurs following trauma, surgery or other procedures w/ **Contaminated medical instruments** (tattoos, acupuncture, breast implants, **botox**, filler)
        - M. fortuitum is a/w pedicures
    - p/w multiple red SQ nodules in a sporotrichoid pattern
    - Dx: culture on routine bacterial culture agar (e.g., Chocolate agar)
    - Rx: Clarithromycin
- M. Kansasii: **yellow** bacillus due to deposition of β-carotene after light exposure
    - Closely related to M. tuberculosis and like TB the primary infection is the lungs w/ cutaneous infection acquired via trauma or endogenous spread
    - p/w verrucous plaques, ulcers or nodules in a sporotrichoid pattern
    - Dx: PCR > culture
    - Rx: same as for TB (RIPE but clarithromycin may be used instead of INH)

5.4 Fungal Diseases

Superficial mycoses

Dermatophytes

- Pathogenesis: hydrolases and keratinases are virulence factors which permit penetration into the stratum corneum inducing a Th1 response in the host
- Species: Microsporum, Epidermophyton, and Trichophyton ("He MET dermatophyte fungi")
- T. rubrum is the MCC of many tinea infections and they can be remembered by the T. rubrum song: "Rub my yocki, my body, hands/feet/nails and secret spotty"
    - T. rubrum #1: Majocchi granuloma, tinea corporis/manus/pedis/unguium/cruris
    - Exceptions to this rule are vesicular variant of T. pedis and white superficial variant of T. unguium in adult patients in which MCC is T. interdigitale
        - Tinea pedis variants with MC associated organisms
            - Mocassin: T. rubrum > E. floccosum
            - Interdigital: T. rubrum > T. interdigitale
            - Bullous: **T. interdigitale**
        - Onychomycosis (T. unguium)
            - Distal lateral subungual (MCC): T. rubrum
            - Proximal white subungual (HIV pts.): T. rubrum (refer to section 5.2)
            - White superficial: T. mentogrophytes or T. rubrum (kids/HIV pts)
            - Other species include C. albicans (massive hyperkeratosis of nails w/ chronic paronychia), Fusarium and Scopulariopsis (p/w large quantities of cheesy debri; Dx: grows in chains: "cops put people in chains"), Scytalidium (black onychomycosis; also T. rubrum)

- Tinea capitis: **T. tonsurans is MC** ("Tinea on top of your head"), M. canis #2 (pt has pets)
  - Endothrix (**black dot**; arthroconidia within hair shaft so it never fluoresces)
    - T. schoenleinii, T. soudanense, T. gourvilli, T. violaceum, T. yaounde, T. tonsurans (These have O in the 1st syllable and are "Twithin" the hairshaft)
  - Ectothrix (KOH shows arthroconidia on the outside of the hair shaft)
    - Flourescent: fluoresce greenish-yellow under Woods lamp from **pteridine**
      - M. canis, M. audouinii, M. distortum, M. ferrugineum, M. gypseum, T. schoenleinii (Just know that all M's fluoresce except M. nanum and that T. schoenleinii is both endothrix and fluorescent ectothrix)
    - Nonflourescent: M. nanum, T. gypseum, T. rubrum, T. mentagrophytes, T. verrucosum, T. megninii ("Just remember that non-fluorescent ectothrix are the T's [except M. nanum] that don't have an 'o' in the first syllable")
  - Favus: yellow crusting on the scalp w/ hair loss; a/w **T. schoenleinii** > M. gypseum, T. violaceum ("My Fav show is a gypsy violinist who has yellow hair")
    - Hair shafts infected with T. schoenleinii demonstrates air-filled spaces
  - Kerion: inflamed tender pus-filled area on scalp a/w T. mentagrophytes, M. canis, T. verrucosum, T. tonsurans → "Caring (kerion) Men Can be Very Tolerant"
- Tinea barbae: same species as seen in kerion ("Bearded Men Can be Very Tolerant")
- Tinea faceii: T. mentagrophytes, T. rubrum, T. tonsurans, M. canis

- Tinea imbricatum: T. concentricum ("fascinating concentric polycyclic rings of scales")
- Geography: zoophilic (primarily affect animals; massive inflammation), geophilic (found in soil) and anthropophilic (restricted to humans; mild inflammation)
    - Zoophilic: T. Mentagrophytes (rodents esp Mice), M. canis (cats), T. verrucosum (cows; "verru-cow-sum"), T. nanum (pigs) → "Men Can be Very Nasty animals"
    - Geophilic: M. Gypseum
    - Anthropophilic: all other species
- **p/w annular, erythematous scaling plaques w/ active border and central clearing**
    - Majocchi granuloma: fluctuant red dermal nodules w/ hair follicle invasion
    - Tinea incognito: patches w/ less erythema and more subtle scale
    - Tinea capitus: numerous scaly patches w/ broken hairs ("black dots") and LAD
        - M. canis is more inflammatory w/ papules and pustules
        - Kerion: severely inflamed w/ boggy, suppurating and crusted plaques
    - Tinea cruris: pruritic red scaly annular rash on inner thighs that spares scrotum
        - Ddx: candida burns more than itches, is redder and involves scrotum
    - Tinea manuum: non-inflammatory and often unilateral ("2 feet and 1 hand syndrome") w/ **scaly accentuation of palmar creases** +/- onychomycosis
        - Variants: interdigital, hyperkeratotic, vesicular, exfoliative, papular
    - Tinea pedis: presentation varies but usually p/w interdigital maceration (esp. lateral toe webs), red-scaly moccasin-like plaque on the sole (T. rubrum)

or bullous lesions (T. interdigitale formerly T. mentogrophytes var interdigitale)
    - T. pedis commonly results in an id reaction that presents differently than normal → **p/w vesicles on lateral fingers (mimics dyshidrotic dermatitis)**
  - o Tinea unguium
    - Distal lateral subungual (T. rubrum): p/w thick, yellow nails
    - Proximal subungual: p/w **beige-white opacity under proximal nail plate**
    - Superficial: entire nail is white (T. mentogrophytes) > black (T. rubrum)
- Dx: biopsy (horizontal septate hyphae in stratum corneum), KOH or culture (Wood's lamp is of no help in tinea skin infections but it will fluoresce in ectothrix T. capitis)
  - o KOH: scrape scale onto a slide, apply 10% KOH and then heat up
    - Dimethyl sulfoxide can be added which does not require heating
    - Staining with chlorazol/black E or Parker blue-black can identify tinea
  - o Dermatophyte Test Media (DTM) and Sabouraud media: culture is (+) if after 3 weeks a white fluffy colony grows AND the media has turned from yellow to red
  - o Trichophyton produces elongated, cigar-shaped macroconidia w/ parallel sides
  - o Microsporum species have **spindled** or boat/football shaped macroconidia
    - M. nanum is unique in being round
  - o Scopulariopsis brevis grows in chains (must culture without cycloheximide)
  - o For onychomycosis, nail clipping w/ PAS stain or PCR testing can be performed

- Rx: **topical or systemic** (better for hairy sites) **terbinafine** > azoles or naftin
  - o Terbinafine (250mg) is now the preferred oral agent due to ↑ resistance and prolonged treatment course w/ griseofulvin **(20 mg/kg/day; take w/ fatty meal)**
    - ▪ Tinea skin infection: 2 weeks w/ terbinafine or 4 weeks w/ griseofulvin
    - ▪ T. capitis: 6 weeks w/ terbinafine and 8 weeks w/ griseofulvin
      - 2/4/6/8 who do we appreciate, terbinafine & griseo for skin & scalp
    - ▪ T. pedis: is notoriously refractile to therapy (esp if nails involved)
      - Terbinafine for 4 weeks for tinea pedis, 6 weeks for onychomycosis of the fingernails and 12 weeks for onychomycosis of the toenails
- Tinea infections are the 2nd MC sport-related infection (s. aureus/bacteria is #1)
  - o T. capitus: athletes must be treated for 2 weeks before returning to competition, but students can return to school as soon as they start therapy
  - o T. corporis: athletes must be treated for 3 days and lesions must be covered

Tinea versicolor (pityriasis versicolor)

- Species: Malassezia globosa and M. furfur
  - o Unicellular yeast (skin flora) turns to multicellular mold (hyphae) in disease state
- Pathogenesis: overgrowth of normal flora; hypopigmentation due to tyrosinase inhibition by azelaic acid (byproduct of Malassezia)
- p/w hyper or hypo-pigmented scaly macules in seborrheic areas (trunk/upper arms)

  - In skin of color, the hypopigmented spots are more obvious, and it can present in an inverse pattern (**face**, knees, elbows, groin, armpits, hands, and feet)
- Diagnosis: biopsy, KOH, culture (requires **olive oil** for growth; shows "**ziti and meatballs**")
- Rx: topical or systemic antifungals, selenium sulfide shampoo, and topical ciclopirox

Piedra

- Species
  - Black Piedra: Piedra hortae ("honorable black people")
  - White Piedra: Trichosporon asahii can cause disseminated disease in the immunocompromised ("Tricky Ass white people are very opportunistic"), T. inkum, T. ovoides, T. cutaneum ("Incredibly Overprivileged Cute white people")
- Microscopy: soft mobile nodules (white) or hard non-mobile nodules (black) along hair ("white people are soft and easy to move while black people are hard and immovable")
  - Ddx for nodes on scalp hair: hair casts (freely mobile), lice/pediculosis capitis (nits usually live close to scalp), trichorrhexis nodosa, monilethrix
    - Trichomycosis axillaris: presents in the axilla (not scalp) and p/w broad Tan concretions that encircle the Total length of hair shaft (vs nodes)
- p/w asymptomatic hair breakage on the **scalp** (MC)
- Dx: trichoscopy (multiple oval nodules), KOH, culture
- Rx: hair shaving/cutting or anti-fungals

Tinea Nigra

- Species: Hortaea werneckii
- p/w expanding homogenous brown macule/patch on the palms/soles
    - Ddx: **acral lentiginous melanoma** is multicolored and **talon noir** (calcaneal petechiae) is a homogenous dark brown plantar macule that arises after exercise
- Microscopy/pathology: dark brown septate hyphae
- Rx: topical azoles, Whitfield ointment (keratolytic w/ benzoic and salicylic acid)

Subcutaneous mycoses

- SCLE: Sporotrichosis, Chromoblastomycosis, Lobomycosis, Eumycetoma
    - All are due to traumatic inoculation in tropical areas (e.g., South America)
    - Organisms can be highlighted w/ PAS or GMS stain on path
    - All should be treated with **itraconazole** except lobomycosis (Rx: excision)

Sporotrichosis

- Species: Sporothrix Schenckii (dimorphic fungus)
- Geography: Saprophyte (fungus found on dying organic matter); MC in South America
- Pathogenesis: traumatic inoculation from Soil, wood Splinters or Sphagnum moss
- p/w multiple ascending SQ abscess/nodules (Sporotrichoid Spread)
- Path: **organisms usually absent** but when present are cigar ("Sigar")-Shaped yeast
- Dx: culture on Sabouraud agar (shows black and white rings of mold/hyphal colonies)
- Rx: SSKI or itraconazole

Chromoblastomycosis: "Pedro, Phil and Claud collect Copper pennies"

- Species: **Fonsecaea pedrosoi** > Phialophora, Exophiala, Cladophialophora, Rhinocladiella
- Pathology: PEH + puss differential w/ Copper pennies (pigmented medlar bodies)
- p/w pruritic papules expanding into **verrucous plaques w/ black dots + Central scarring**
- Chronic lesions can progress into SCC

Lobomycosis

- Species: Lacazia (loboa loboi) infects freshwater **dolphins** in South American rivers
    - o "Lobo means wolf in Spanish and dolphins are the wolves of the water"
- p/w **keloid-like nodules** ("Wolves can scar you up")
- Pathology: **yeast in chains which look like "pop-beads"** ("Wolves hunt in packs/chains")
- Rx: surgical excision of keloids ("If you get attacked by a wolf you will need surgery")

Eumycetoma

- Species: **Pseudallescheria boydii** > Madurella, Exophialia jeanselmei, Acremonium
- p/w sinus tracks w/ draining grains MC on the feet (or any site of traumatic inoculation)
- Grains are black or white: "You (Eu-mycetoma) look at everything in black or white"
    - o Black grain eumycetoma organisms: "My Lousy Greasy Jeans are black" (Madurella mycetomatis, Leptosphaeria, M. grisea, Exophiala jeanselmei)
    - o White (non-pigmented) grain organisms: P. boydi is MC ("white boy")
- Rx: surgical debridement and several months of azole antifungals

Actinomycetoma (this is a bacteria, but it is listed here to compare to eumycetoma)

- Mycetoma caused by bacteria such as Nocardia brasiliensis (white grains: "white note cards") > Actinomadura pelletieri (red grains), A. madurae (cream-pink grains), Streptomyces Somaliensis (yellow-brown grains; "Yellow like the Simpsons")
    - These colors (besides white) are specific to actinomycetoma
- Same presentation as eumycetoma (white grains are MC in both; know the other colors)
- Rx: sulfonamides (TMP-SMX)

Systemic dimorphic mycoses

- Dimorphic mycoses: "multicellular mold in cold (in culture), unicellular yeast in beast"
    - Sporotrichosis is also a dimorphic fungus but it is SQ, not systemic
- Consists of blastomycoses, histoplasmosis, coccidioidomycoses, paracoccidioidomycoses
- Pathogenesis: **inhalation (lungs)** and **hematogenous spread** to organs including skin
    - Only in blastomycoses it is common (> 75% of cases) to see spread to the skin
    - Only in paracoccidioidomycosis it is common (70%) to see spread to the mouth
- **Ddx: deep fungal infections are exophytic whereas cutaneous leishmaniasis p/w ulcers**
- Rx: itraconazole or amphotericin B depending on severity
    - "Blast his cocc and paracocc away with itraconazole or amphotericin"

Blastomycosis ("North American blastomycoses")

- Species: Blastomyces dermatitidis
- Geography: Eastern US (e.g., **Mississippi River valleys, Great Lakes, Ohio**)
- Pathogenesis: inhalation and hematogenous spread to skin and Bones
- p/w Bumpy ("heaped up") verrucous nodules w/ Black crust and sharp/irregular Borders
- **Skin disease is MC extrapulmonary manifestation** (Lung is MC organ affected)
- Culture (mold in cold): filamentous moldlike structures w/ short conidia ("**Lollipops**")
    - We also saw "lollipops" on path of nephrogenic systemic fibrosis
- Path (yeast in beast): PEH + puss ddx w/ Broad-Based Budding yeasts ("Snowmen")
    - If no budding is present, yeast can still be recognized by its thick refractile wall

Histoplasmosis

- Species: Histoplasma capsulatum var. capsulatum (var. duboisii in Africa)
- Geography similar to Blastomycosis (Ohio and Mississippi River valley)
- Pathogenesis: inhalation of bird and bat feces ("Histo Hides in bat caves")
- Skin lesions are more common in HIV and p/w umbilicated molluscoid pox-like papules
    - "HIV Can Cause Pox-like lesions": Histo, Coccidio, Crypto, Penicillium
- Culture: mold w/ tuberculate macroconidia and smooth-walled spherical microconidia
- Path (yeast): parasitized histiocytes w/ 2–4 μm yeasts evenly distributed in the histiocyte
    - Ddx: leishmaniasis (parasites rim the border of the histiocyte)

Coccidioidomycosis

- Species: Coccidioides immitis (US) or C. posadasii (South/Central America)
- Geography: desert Southwest US (Central Valley/San Joaquin Valley, California), Mexico
- Pathogenesis: inhalation → spreads to CNS, bones and sometimes skin
- p/w blastomycosis-like verrucous nodules +/- **erythema nodosum (good prognosis)**
  - In HIV, papules may be umbilicated ("molluscoid")
- Pathology: PEH + pus differential w/ large (100 μm) spherules containing endospores

Paracoccidioidomycosis ("Mexican/South American blastomycoses")

- Species: Paracoccidioides brasiliensis
- Geography: Mexico/South America > Southern US
- p/w verrucous ulcerative lesions in and around the Mouth w/ Massive LAD in **Men**
- Path: yeast w/ the characteristic "Mariner's wheel" configuration may be found

Opportunistic systemic mycoses

- CAP: Candidiasis, Cryptococcus, Aspergillosis/fusarium, Penicilliosis, Pheohyphomycosis
- Rx: antifungals (also excision of pheohyphomycosis/phaeohyphomycotic cysts)

Candidiasis

- Species: **C. albicans > C. tropicalis** (systemic), C. parapsilosis (chronic paronychia), C. glabrata and C. krusei (fluconazole resistance), C. dubliniensis (oropharyngeal in HIV)
- Pathogenesis: normal skin/GI/GU flora w/ pathologic state in the immunosuppressed and in microbiome

imbalance → chitin, mannoprotein and glucan allow for adhesion whereas secretory aspartyl proteinases and phospholipases allow for tissue invasion

- Clinical presentations: "I MET AN Opportunistic Candidiasis"
    - Intertrigo: beefy red color w/ satellite lesions
    - Median rhomboid glossitis: smooth (loss of papillae) red patch on the tongue
    - Erosio interdigitalis blastomycetica: red plaque in the 3rd web space of fingers
    - Thrush: non-adherent "cottage cheese-like" lesions in the mouth
    - Angular cheilitis: erythematous plaques at the oral commissures
    - Neutropenic disseminated candidiasis: recalcitrant candidiasis in neutropenic pts w/ scattered ecthyma gangrenosum-like nodules and internal organ involvement
    - Neonatal candidiasis: monomorphic paps in diaper area +/- thrush at 2 weeks
    - Onychomycosis: thickened discolored nail plates
    - Congenital candidiasis: widespread eruption of monomorphic papules at birth
    - Chronic paronychia: inflammation of the nail fold lasting > 6 weeks
- Risk factors: diabetes and immunosuppression
- Microscopy: KOH shows yeast and pseudohyphae
- Rx: azoles (C. glabrata, C. krusei >> C. albicans are becoming resistant to azoles)

Cryptococcus: "Crypto is a Massive PIG"

- Species: C. neoformans (ubiquitous) and C. Gattii (tropics)
- Pathogenesis: similar to systemic dimorphic mycoses (inhalation of **pigeon** feces → primary pulmonary

infection → hematogenous spread to CNS, bones and skin)
  - "PIG": more common in Pregnancy and in the Immunocompromised (HIV/AIDS); **Glucuronoxylomannan polysaccharide capsule is the virulence factor**
- p/w (Massive): Mulluscoid papules around Mouth (face, nose) +/- Meningoencephalitis
- Microscopy/path: single yeast cells w/ a thick capsule; collections of organisms look like soap bubbles ("this massive pig needs a bubble bath")
  - Stains w/ ("Massive PIG"): **Mucicarmine**, **Fontana-Masson**, PAS, India ink, GMS
- Rx: oral fluconazole (amphotericin B + flucytosine if CNS involvement)

Aspergillosis and fusarium (hyalohyphomycosis)
- Aspergillosis species: **A. fumigatus** (disseminated disease in the immunocompromised from inhalation; "fumigate makes you think of inhalation") > A. flavus (direct inoculation)
- Fusarium species: Fusarium solani (direct inoculation in toes of **burn patients**)
  - "Solani should make you think soles of the foot/ toes"
- Geography: ubiquitous in soil (saprophytic)
- 2nd MC opportunistic fungal disease (candida #1) in leukemic/solid organ transplant pts.
- Pathogenesis: hematogenous spread → vascular invasion thrombosis and necrosis
- p/w red edematous plaques w/ necrotic centers (**sites of IV cannulas are MC locations**)
- Microscopy/path: **non-pigmented septate hyphae in tissue branching in Acute Angles**
- Rx: Azole antifungals, Amphotericin B (fusarium is difficult to treat)

Penicilliosis

- Species: Penicillium marneffei (caused by bamboo rat exposure in SE Asia)
- Pathogenesis (inhalation), presentation (pulmonary symptoms w/ molluscum-like lesions), path (parasitized histiocytes), Rx (itraconazole) are identical to histoplasmosis

Phaeohyphomycosis: "I think of Lizzo"

- Group of dematiaceous (pigmented) fungal infections
    - o **Exophiala jeanselmei:** MCC of phaeohyphomycotic cyst; immunocompetent pts
        - "Lizzo always wears jeans"
        - E. jeanselmei also causes black grain eumycetoma/chromoblastomycosis
    - o **Bipolaris** spicifera: MCC of invasive phaeohyphomycosis; immunocompromised
        - "Lizzo is bipolar because she yells at her staff for being overweight"
- p/w subcutaneous inflammatory abscess/cysts that may drain (may mimic Baker cyst)
- Path: **pigmented hyphae** in tissue w/ bubbly cytoplasm ("Lizzo is pigmented and bubbly")
- Rx: excision of cyst and itraconazole

Uncommon fungal, algae, and protozoal pathogens

Zygomycosis (Rhinocerebral mucormycosis)

- Species: Rhizopus (order Mucorales)
- Geography: ubiquitous in soil and decaying vegetation
- Pathogenesis: enters via Respiratory tract → vascular invasion → thrombosis/necrosis
- A known virulence factor is its ability to sequester iron from host so **iron ("Rhino") overload syndromes**

(pt w/ multiple blood transfusions) is a **major RF for infection**

- MC subtype is Rhinocerebral (a/w diabetics w/ DKA) but primary cutaneous (from surgery, burns), GI, pulmonary and disseminated types also exist
  - o All forms are Rapidly progressive and commonly fatal
- p/w **necrotic eschars on face** (nose, mouth) w/ **periorbital cellulitis** and **epistaxis**
- Path: broad Ribbon-like non-septate hyphae which branch at Right angles
- Rx: **Resection** of necrotic tissue, **amphotericin B (1st line), isavuconazole** (2nd line)

Protothecosis: "Protothecosis reminds me of hyperthecosis in a WOMAN"

- Due to contact w/ **Water** that is contaminated w/ the algae Prototheca Wickerhamii
- p/w **Olecranon bursitis**
- Path: Morula (soccer ball-like) vs non-murulating form (looks like an eyeball)
  - o "O's in protothecosis remind me of the round soccer balls or eyeballs on path"
- Rx: we treat this **Algae** w/ Antifungals (**Azoles** or Amphotericin B)
- Other clinical presentations include Nodules, ulcers, or plaques

Rhinosporidiosis

- Species: Rhinosporidium seeberi (a protozoa)
- Geography: India, Sri Lanka
- Pathogenesis: like protothecosis it is caused by contact w/ contaminated water
- p/w slow growing red-purple lobulated nasal polyps in young men

- Path: huge (300 μm; 3x the size of coccidioides) sporangia w/ many endospores
- Rx: excision

5.5 Parasites and Other Creatures

Parasitic infections

Scabies ("Oh Scabies")

- Species: Sarcoptes scabies var. hominis
- Overcrowding is the most consistent factor a/w scabies
- One-month life cycle in the stratum corneum; One-week survival off human host
- p/w intensely pruritic erythematous papules and burrows that classically effects the axilla, finger web spaces, wrists and **genitals (nodular scabies)**
    - o **Classic pediatric Kodachrome is a baby with blisters on the hands**
- Crusted scabies is seen in the immunosuppressed and p/w marked hyperkeratosis
- Dx: mineral Oil scraping shows mites, ovum (small round eggs) and scabala (dark feces)
- Path: mites and egg case remnants **("pig-tails")** in the corneum; dermal infiltrate w/ eos
    - o Crusted scabies will show massive ortho and parakeratosis w/ many mites
- Rx: permethrin 5% cream (TOC in pregnant patients and infants 2 months and up), ivermectin and sulfur ointment 5%–10% (infants less than 2 months)

Lice

- Head louse (Pediculus humanus capitis: "CAPItis")
    - o Close (< 5 mm) to scalp skin (Dx: direct examination of lice/nits on hair shaft)
    - o Adheres strong and tight to hair shaft

- Postauricular and occipital areas of the scalp are the MC locations
- Ivermectin or other antiparasitics are effective (permethrin resistance common)
  - Malathion and Spinosad are ovicidal → may not require repeat treatment
    - "MS. Are you sure you want to kill your eggs?"
  - Children can return to school immediately after beginning treatment

- Body louse (Pediculus humanus corporis: "QORPoris")
  - B. Quintana can transmit and cause trench fever ("Qench fever") among others
    - TB Epidemic don't Quit (Quintana): Trench fever, Bacillary angiomatosis, Bacteremia/ endocarditis, Body louse (Epidemic typhus has this vector)
  - On clothes of homeless people (who never wash them)
  - B. Recurrentis can be transmitted which can cause Relapsing fever
  - R. Prowazekii can be transmitted which can cause **epidemic typhus**
  - Dx: "clothing biopsy" (carefully examen all clothing seems)
  - Rx: topical steroids can be used but the TOC is addressing issues of poor hygiene
- Pubic louse (Pthirus pubis: "PUBIS")
  - Permethrin (topical 1%) is 1st line therapy
  - Under clothes
  - **Blue-gray macules due to Bites (maculae ceruleae)**
  - **Broad Body** and crab-like appendages give it the nickname "crabs"
  - Ivermectin (topical 0.5%) lotion is FDA approved
  - Screen for other STDs; Shaving is therapeutic

Tungiasis (Tunga penetrans, burrowing flea)
- The flea is endemic in sub-Saharan Africa, India, Caribbean, Central/South America
- Acquired by walking barefoot (or w/ open-Toed shoes) near rotting vegetation
- The flea cannot jump high so involved sites are limited to the **foot (esp peri-ungually)**
- p/w asymptomatic **papules w/ dark central puncta,** which enlarges and becomes painful
- Path: Trippy looking organism (Tubules, guts, striated muscle) embedded in acral skin
- Rx: self-limited; sterile surgical removal and Tetanus prophylaxis
- Other diseases involving fleas: "The flea is a G"
    - Tungiasis, plague, bacillary angiomatosis, and guinea worm (draculunciasis)

Myiasis (human botfly)
- Myiasis represents infection/infestation with fly larvae (maggots)
- Human Botfly (Dermatobia hominis) can be transmitted by mosquitos to exposed skin
- p/w single or multiple 1–3 cm (larger than tungiasis) nodules w/ central punctum
- Path: organism w/ an undulating chitinis wall and pigmented (yellow) setae
- Rx: surgical removal of larvae, ivermectin, and tetanus prophylaxis

Protozoa

Leishmaniasis
- Chronic infection due to obligate intracellular protozoan (Leishmania spp.)
- Exists in 2 forms: promastigote and amastigote

  - Sandfly bites human and transfers promastigotes → macrophages engulf promastigotes which then transform into amastigotes
    - "In a Macrophage it Matures into a Mastigote (amastigote)"
- Vectors are sandflies (LmNOP): **Lutzomyia** (New world) or Phlebotomus (Old world)
- Classified clinically and geographically
  - Cutaneous: limited to skin (Th1 cytokine profile); old world > new world
    - Old world cutaneous
      - **L. tropica and L. major** ("the troop's major had old skin")
      - Solitary nodule at bite site (exposed skin) that ulcerates → **sporotrichoid spread** → heals with **scarring** over months
        - **Classically p/w ulcer with raised borders**
          - Ddx: deep fungal infections are usually exophytic
      - L. recidivans: soft red papules form at margins of an old healed ulcer/scar w/ "apple jelly" color on diascopy (**L. tropica is MC**)
    - New world cutaneous
      - **L. Mexicana** > L. braziliensis ("Mexicans have beautiful new skin")
      - Presents similar to old world cutaneous leishmaniasis but a high yield presentation is **ear ulcers** (Chiclero ulcer) in workers
  - Diffuse cutaneous: more widespread skin lesions in immunocompromised pts w/ multiple **keloidal lesions** (esp. on nose/face; not ulcers like in cutaneous form)
    - Old world diffuse cutaneous (**L. aethiopica**) is seen in Africa

    - New world diffuse cutaneous (**L. amazonensis**) is seen in the Americas
        - "The Amazon and Ethiopian forest are diffuse/widespread"
        - Nose keloids: rhinoscleroma and diffuse cutaneous leishmaniasis
        - Ear keloids: lobomycosis and juvenile hyaline fibromatosis
  - Mucocutaneous **(L. braziliensis is MC)**: affects mucous membranes; New world
    - p/w lip, nose or oropharyngeal ulceration/destruction → airway obstruction and perforation of nasal septum ("tapir face"/**espundia**)
    - "Braziliensis bugs always effect feet or mucosa"
        - Feet: Ancylostoma braziliense is MCC of cutaneous larva migrans and Nocardia braziliensis is MCC of actinomycosis
        - Mucosa: Paracoccidoides braziliensis is MC oral deep fungal infection and L. braziliensis is MCC of mucocutaneous leishmania)
  - Visceral (Kala-azar, "black fever"; Th2 cytokine profile): parasites in organ; Old > New world; p/w fever, emaciation/wasting, HSM, LAD and pancytopenia
    - Most common agents: DIC ("DIC's go inside/visceral")
        - L. Donovani (adults in India, Sudan and Bangledesh)
        - L. Infantum (Infants in China, Africa, Middle East; a/w HIV)
        - L. Chagasi (Children; Americas esp Central America)
    - Post-kala-azar dermal leishmaniasis p/w hypopigmented macules (Asia) or papules (Africa) years after recovery from visceral leishmaniasis
- Diagnosis of "Leish-Maniasis"

  - Marquee sign on histology (organisms around periphery of Macrophages)
    - Helpful stains include Giemsa and CD1a
  - Montenegro delayed skin reaction test: (+) in cutaneous leishmaniasis and remains (+) after cure; negative in visceral and diffuse cutaneous leishmaniasis
  - Novy-McNeal-Nicolle medium is how we culture
  - Can also use PCR or ELISA +/- recombinant kinesin antigen (rK39)
- Rx: old world cutaneous and new world cutaneous leish 2° to L. Mexicana self-resolve
  - Most cutaneous and all mucocutaneous Leish ("leish-Maniasis"): oral Miltefosine or IV Pentavalent antimony (Sodium Stibogluconate, Meglumine antimonate)
    - SEs of Pentavalent antimony: **QT Prolongation → cardiac arrythmias**
    - There is ↑ resistance to antimonials; if no improvement, try Amphotericin
  - Visceral leishmaniasis: treat with Amphotericin B or other drugs above

Trypanosomiasis

- American trypanosomiasis (Chagas disease)
  - Species is T. cruzi; vector is triatomine bug (Reduviidae) in central/south America
    - "Tri getting on a Red Cruz to Central and South America"
  - Days: swollen inflammatory lesion (usually on face) at site of entry (chagoma)
  - Weeks: Romana's sign (unilateral eyelid edema/ conjunctivitis at site of inoculation) is accompanied by Parinaud sign (preauricular LAD)
  - Months/years: heart, esophagus and intestinal enlargement (megacolon)

        - First big face, then big eye, then big organs: "everything is big in America"
    - Dx: peripheral blood smear shows parasites (best in 1st 4–8 weeks), ELISA, IFA
    - Rx: **Benznidazole** (1st line) and nifurtimox (2nd line)
        - "Driving a Mercedes Benz in my American tryp"
- African trypanosomiasis (sleeping sickness)
    - Species: T. brucei gambiense (W. Africa); T. brucei Rhodesiense (E./Right Africa)
    - Vector: Tsetse fly (Glossina): Bruce's tryp is set to Fly to Africa on Glossina airline
    - p/w chancre (1st sign) at bite site → ulcer → eschar ("take a chance on a tryp")
        - Eschar ddx: EZCAR (Echthyma gangrenosa, Zygomycosis, Cowpox, African trypanosomiasis, Anthrax, Rickettsial diseases, Recluse spider bite)
    - West African trypanosomiasis (gambiense)
        - Days: chancre → ulcer → eschar (Dead skin at bite site)
        - Weeks: Winterbottom's sign (post. cervical LAD): "take a tryp in winter"
        - Months: trypanids (Macular diffuse erythematous or urticarial eruption)
        - Years: Kerandel's deep delayed hyperesthesia and sleepiness ("Yawns")
    - East African trypanosomiasis is more "eacute" with earlier CNS involvement
    - Dx: smear (chancre fluid/blood) can be stained w/ Giemsa to look for parasites
    - Rx ("SPErM"): Suramin or **Pentamide** (early infection), Eflornithine (CNS involvement West African Tryp), Melarsoprol (CNS involvement East Africa Tryp)

Toxoplasmosis

- Species is toxoplasma gondii and vector is intestinal parasites of cats > dogs and rabbits
- p/w hemorrhagic papules ("bloody like plasma") occurring in pregnant (congenital disease discussed in pediatric section) and immunocompromised patients
- Rx ("PLAS"): Pyrimethamine and Sulfadiazine

Helminths (worms)

- Classified by phyla or life cycle
    - Phyla: Nematoda (roundworms) vs Platyhelminthes (flatworms)
    - Life cycle
        - Soil-transmitted (all are hookworms): "Don't step on a SAC of worms"
            - Strongyloidiasis, Ancylostomiasis, Cutaneous larva migrans
        - Insect-transmitted (all are roundworms): "Worms FOL out of insects"
            - Filariasis, Onchocerciasis, Loiasis
        - Acquired via ingestion: "Chew The EG" (in parentheses is what's ingested)
            - Cystercercosis (ova), Trichinosis (larval cyst), Toxocariasis (larva), Echinococcosis (ova), Enterobiasis (ova), Gnathostomiasis (larva)
        - Life-cycle involves snails (trematodes/flukes): Fascioliasis, Schistosomiasis

Migrating rashes: "Gotta Love Creeping Eruptions"

- Gnathostomiasis (20 cm/day): deep migratory swellings w/ tracking purpura
- Larva currens (10 cm/day): perianal rash → thumbprint purpura

- Cutaneous larva migrans (2 cm/day): superficial serpinginous tracts on feet
- Erythema gyratum repens (1 cm/day) and Erythema annulare centrifugum (2 mm/day)

Gnathostomiasis

- Species: G. spinigerum
- Acquired from ingestion of raw freshwater fish
- p/w migratory panniculitis which disappears then reappears days later a few cm away along w/ purpura along the larva's migratory tract
- CBC: eosinophilia
- Rx: ivermectin or albendazole/thiabendazole

Larva currens

- Currens is latin for running (correr means "to run" in Spanish) → runs 10 cm/day
- Tanscutaneous infection of larvae (larva currens) → travels to lungs and GI → skin
- Species: **Strongyloides stercoralis** (nematode; "run strong and run stern")
- Forms: "runs straight towards the anus (localized) or umbilicus (disseminated)"
    - Localized: **pruritic** traveling serpiginous wheals that are **perianal** or on trunk
        - Resolves when larva enters circulation and heads towards the lungs
    - Disseminated: **periumbilical petechiae (thumbprint purpura)** in HIV-patients
    - Chronic: Loeffler's syndrome (affects Lungs, Eosinophilia)
        - Original description was infection w/ Ascaris lumbricoides (roundworm) but now includes any parasitic infection resulting in lung eosinophilia

        - Do not confuse with LOFGRENS syndrome (sarcoidosis): LAD, Ocular sx, Fever, Good prognosis, R-thritis, Erythema Nodosa, Scandinavians)
- Dx: **ova and parasite stool study**
- Rx: **ivermectin or albendazole/thiabendazole**

Cutaneous larva migrans
- Species: **Ancylostoma braziliensis** > A. caninum (**larvae of hookworms**)
- p/w erythematous pruritic serpiginous "creeping" tracks on feet
    - Unable to penetrate the BMZ and cause systemic disease
- Moves **2 cm/day** (2–10 mm/hour)
- Rx: **ivermectin or albendazole/thiabendazole**

Insect-transmitted ("Round worms FOL out of insects"): Filariasis, Onchocerciasis, Loiasis

Filariasis (elephantiasis)
- Species: Wuchereria bancrofti ("Fil goes to the bank")
- Vector: various mosquitos ("Fil goes to a mosque")
- Acute phase: lymphangitis and orchitis ("Fil's testicles hurt")
- Chronic phase: lymphatic obstruction/**lymphedema → elephantiasis (gross enlargement of legs)**, chyluria, hydrocele ("Fil's legs and testicles are really big")
- Path: round worm w/ **thick muscular layer** ("Fil goes to the gym to work out his thick legs") interrupted by lateral cords w/ surrounding dense infiltrate w/ eosinophils
- Rx: diethylcarbamazine

Onchocerciasis ("River blindness"; LMNO)
- Species: Onchocerca volvulus
- Vector: Simulium (black fly): "Black flies smoke POT"

    - Pemphigus foliaceous (Fogo selvagem), Onchocerciasis, Tularemia
- Geography: **sub-Saharan (equatorial) Africa** near fast flowing (well-oxygenated) rivers
- Clinical manifestations (LMNO) are due to Microfilariae in the skin
    - Acute: Microfilariae in cornea (seen with slit lamp), SQ Nodules over bony prominences (fibrous tissue surrounding worms), acute papular Onchodermatitis
    - Chronic: Lichenified dermatitis (legs), **Leopard skin** (atrophy and depigmentation with perifollicular sparring) of legs, Lymphatic obstruction → "hanging groin"
    - Mazzotti reaction: hypersensitivity reaction with diethylcarbamazine or suramin
- Path: male and female worms w/ thin muscle layer mating together ("worm Orgy")
    - "Whereas filariasis is a solitary worm w/ a thick muscular layer (single guys go to the gym), onchocerciasis is a male/female couple who don't go (thin muscles)"
- Rx: Ivermectin ("River blindness") and surgical excision of onchocercomas (only insect-transmitted nematode infection where TOC isn't diethylcarbamazine)

Loiasis ("Lo-eye-asis")

- Species: Loa loa
- Vector: Chrysops (ops reminds me of eye) aka Mango/deer fly ("fl-eye")
- p/w recurrent migratory focal angioedema of the joints of the limbs ("calabar swellings") and visible migration of adult worms across the eye
- Rx: diethylcarbamazine ("d-eye-ethylcarbamazine")

Swimmer's itch and Seabather's eruption

- Swimmer's itch (cercarial dermatitis)
  - Species: Schistosoma (snails are vectors)
  - Freshwater (lake)
  - p/w papules and papulovesicles on **uncovered** skin
  - Rx: supportive (antihistamines, topical steroids)
- Seabather's eruption (not a helminth but discussed here to compare to Swimmers itch)
  - Species: Edwardsiella lineata (sea anemone) and Linuche unguiculate (jellyfish)
  - Saltwater
  - p/w pruritic papules and wheals in **covered** areas
    - "Seabathers occurs at sea (saltwater) in the bathing suite distribution"
  - Rx: immediately after contact deactivate nematocysts w/ **vinegar**

Trichinosis (PqRST)

- Species: Trichinella spiralis
- Vectors: Humans eat undercooked wild Pigs (MC) or bears which eat infected Rodents
- p/w Periorbital edema (type 1 allergic reaction) and Petechiae (Splinter hemorrhages)
- Dx: muscle biopsy is diagnostic
- Rx: Systemic Steroids and Thiabendazole/albendazole

Dracunculiasis (Guinea worm; CDEFG)

- Species: Dracunculus medinensis
- Vector: Cyclops water Flea
- p/w lower Extremity nodules and ulcers (ingested cyclops travels from GI to SQ tissue)
  - You will physically see the shape of the worm underneath the skin
- Prevent with water **Filters**

- Rx: wound Care, Excision of worm and Flagyl (metronidazole)

Cutaneous amebiasis: "Ameba's will be the BANE of my existence"

- Balamuthia: painless red granulomatous plaques on **central face** near the mouth ("bala-mouth-ia") and fatal encephalitis (interestingly, immunocompromised pts do better)
- Acanthomoeba: subacute granulomatous amebic encephalitis and **chronic skin ulcers**
- Naegleria: fatal acute Necrotizing meningoencephalitis after swimming in fresh water
- Entamoeba histolytica: amebic colitis → cutaneous **perianal** lesions
  - o Sexual transmission → painful ulcerative plaques at inoculation site
- Path (amoebas): size of a histiocyte w/ a central karyosome and a vacuolized cytoplasm
- Rx: metronidazole

Bites and stings

Biting and stinging insects

- Fire ants (Solenopsis): initial urticarial papule → sterile inflammatory **pustules** MC on the legs (Ddx: blister beetle bites p/w blisters; chigger/fleas p/w red papules on legs)
  - o Toxin: solenopsin D ("In Spanish Sol means sun and sun reminds me of fire")
- Hornets/bees/wasps (Hymenoptera): common cause of **anaphylaxis**
  - o Toxin: **phospholipase A**

- Bed bugs: p/w "breakfast, lunch and dinner" urticarial papules on exposed areas like face, neck, arms, and hands ("breakfast in bed")
    - Species: Cimex lectularius ("cimex looks like cama which is Spanish for bed")
- Lytta vesicatoria (Spanish fly; blister beetle): secretes **cantharidin** vesicles/blisters
- Paederus beetles: herpetiform lesions +/- "kiss sign" (venom also contacts skin on the other side of a skin flexure)
- Fleas: vectors for endemic typhus ("endemic ty-flea"), bubonic plague, guinea worm (dracunculiasis), bacillary angiomatosis and infectious agent in tungiasis ("fleas are Gs")
    - Rat flea (xenopsylla): vector for R. typhi (endemic typhus) and Y. pestis (plague)
    - Cyclops water flea: vector for dracunculiasis (guinea worm)
    - Cat flea (Ctenocephalides): vector for Bartonella henselae (cat scratch disease and bacillary angiomatosis (BA)) and Bartonella Quintana (BA and trench fever)
    - Human flea (pulex irritans)
    - Flea bites (FLEA): small Flat papules surrounded by Erythematous Annular halo
- Lepidopterism (caterpillar dermatitis): p/w train-track appearance of urticaria and hemorrhage; ophthalmia nodosa is an ocular reaction to caterpillar hairs
    - Specific types of caterpillars: "caterpillars look like BIG PILS"
        - Buck moth caterpillar (Hemileuca maia): Brown or Black body w/ white-yellow dots and **radiating spines** → p/w edema, erythema, **radiating pain**
        - Io (Automeris io): green with longitudinal white strip ("long like letter I")

        - Gypsy (Lymantria dispar): has 5 pairs of blue dots and 6 pairs of red dots
        - Puss (Megalopyge opercularis): brown whooly ("hairy puss") appearance
            - p/w **Proximally radiating Pain, linear grid-like Pattern of Petechia**
            - **Most dangerous caterpillar in the US (p/w systemic symptoms)**
        - Io: see above
        - Lonomia South American moth caterpillar: brown or green w/ twig-like spines → may p/w life-threatening consumptive coagulopathy
        - Saddleback (Sibine Stimulea): green Saddle-like area on the back
    - Dx: CBC, Cr/BUN, platelets, fibrinogen and clotting workup
    - Ppx: DEET, picardin, oil of lemon eucalyptus (p-menthane 3,8-diol; plant-based)
    - Rx: remove hairs w/ adhesive tape; supportive therapy (steroids, antihistamines)

Arachnids (ticks, mites, spiders, and scorpions)

- Ticks: bites initially p/w firm papule and intense pruritis (toxins in saliva) but later can p/w chronic edematous nodule similar to a foreign body granuloma (mouth-parts); "comet tail" sign describes multiple bites on legs from larvae contact on plants
    - Ornithodorus: soft-bodied tick; soft grayish appearance; transmits Borrellia duttonii (tick-borne relapsing fever; Western US → non-specific rash)
        - "Hodor (Game of Thrones reference) is a soft-bodied (fat) man who is always dressed in gray clothes and has relapsing spells of saying Hodor. Hodor is a borring dude (Borrellia duttonii)"

- Dermacentor variabilis (dog tick): has alternating (variable) light and dark spots (tick w/ spotted scutum and transmits RMSF → petechial rash)
  - "Dogs are variable in appearance in the Rocky Mountains"
- Dermacentor andersonii (**wood tick**): looks like dog tick and also transmits RMSF
- Rhicephalus sanguineus (brown dog tick): red brown tick → Mediterranean fever
- Amblyomma (lone star tick): lone white dot (star) on back; "lone-STER" (Southern tick-associated rash illness, Tularemia, Ehrlichiosis and Richettsial infections including African tick bite fever and Brazil spotted fever)
  - **Pts w/ α-gal allergy get acute urticaria after eating pork/beef due to cross-reactivity between α-gal epitope in the saliva of the lone star tick**
- Ixodes tick: has a black BAL on its brown back: Babesiosis, Anaplasmosis, Lyme

- Mites (CDeFGH)
  - Chiggers/harvest mite (Trombicula alfreddugesi): red mite which result in grouped red pruritic papules/vesicles on the waistband, ankles or penis (summer penile syndrome); vector for R. tsutsugamushi which causes scrub typhus
    - "Tsutsugamushi scrubs his trombone of chiggers so his penis doesn't itch"
  - Cheese mite (Glyciphages): "everyone loves to eat (phage) cheese"
  - Demodex (Demodicidae): lives in human hair follicles; a/w rosacea/perioral derm
  - Dust mite (Dermatophagoides): involved in allergies in AD patients
  - Walking Dandruff (Cheyletiella): **mite with bull horns on head**; **p/w itchy truncal eruption** (older

lesions have central necrosis) in patients with dog or cat contact
    - "When you walk your dog or cat they say hey to everyone, even bulls"
- Fowl mite (Dermanyssus, Ornithonyssus): vector for western equine encephalitis
- Grain mite (Acarus siro): white body and **pink legs**
    - "I imagine a car in the rain with white body and pink tires"
- House mouse mite (Liponyssoides sanguineus): vector for R. akari (rickettsialpox)
    - I call rickettsialpox "rick city pox" because in cities there are houses with mice and mites; people in cities get liposuction and drive kars"

- Spiders
    - Black widow spider (Lactrodectus mactans, ABC): red hourglass on black body
        - p/w pain → **Abdominal pain/rigidity**, pain/edema at Bite site, Chest pain
        - Toxin: α- Lactotoxin depolarizes neurons
        - Rx: Antivenom, Benzodiazepine, and IV Calcium gluconate
    - Brown reclussss (Loxosceles reclusa): dark brown violin/fiddle shaped markings
        - p/w characteristic **marble plaque (1st)** then **necrosis/eschar** ("S-char")
        - May see hemolytic anemia, renal insufficiency, **Shock** and death
        - Toxin: **Sphingomyelinase D**; hyaluronidase plays a less important role
            - "He plays the brown violin w/ his sphinger"
        - Rx: **Supportive** (do not debride; RICE); anti-Loxosceles Fab Ab fragments
    - Jumping spider (Phidippus formosus): dark and hairy w/ 4 eyes (2 large/2 small)
        - Toxin: Hyaluronidase

        - "Phidip is in form, jumps hy and has his 4 hairy eyes on the prize"
- Wolf spider (Lycosidae): brown w/ black pattern, 8 eyes and large wolf-like fangs
    - Toxin: Histamine
        - "Wolfs lyc and his"
- Sac spider (Chiracanthium): yellow spider
    - Toxin: lipase
        - "Sac rac, low lip"
- Hobo spider (Tegenaria agrestis): Brown recluse-like but w/ Herringbone pattern
    - Toxin: agatoxin
        - "Hobos can be very aggressive if you don't throw them a bone"
    - Painless bite → local necrosis/eschar
    - Web is funnel-shaped ("looks like a black Hole")
- Green lynx spider (Peucetia viridans): neon-green color with red spots
    - Painful bite without systemic symptoms
        - "Viridans sounds like verde which means green in Spanish"
- Tarantula (Theraphosidae): ejects urticating hairs on skin (dermatitis) or eyes (ophthalmia nodosa → chronic granulomatous reaction → blindness)

Scorpions (centruroides sculpturatus and gertschi)
- Pain and paresthesia out of proportion to skin lesions with systemic symptoms

Millipedes and centipedes
- Centipedes (Chilopoda class; Scolopendra spp); one pair of legs per segment
    - p/w pain and paresthesia at bite site (**two puncture wounds**: "one pair")
- Millipedes (Diplopoda): two pairs of legs per segment

- p/w chemical ICD (inflammation → hyperpigmentation; "M for Melanin")
  - C is before M in alphabet, so centipedes have one pair of legs and one pair of bites whereas millipedes have 2 pairs of legs

Snake bites

- Copperhead and rattlesnake (Viperidae/Crotalidae): triangular head w/ deep nostril pits
  - p/w thrombocytopenia and DIC (multiple toxins e.g., thrombin-like glycoproteins)
- Coral snake (Elapidae): round eyes with red, yellow and black banding
  - "Red touches yellow, kills a fellow"
  - Toxins: A-Neurotoxin (CNS symptoms) and Phospholipase A2 (wound effects)

Marine injuries

- Cnidarians (jellyfish, Portuguese man of war, coral, and anemones, AbCDEF)
  - Causes Flagellate Erythema/hyperpigmentation
  - Rx: vinegar (Dilute Acetic Acid) which Denatures nematocysts
    - Pacific box jellyfish (Chironex Fleckeri): stings cause shock → Fatal
      - "The X in Box and in Chironex reminds me of shock and death"
    - Portuguese man of war (Physalia spp.): p/w intense pain followed by linear Purpuric/Petechial lesions → Paralysis & cardiac symptoms
- Echinoderms
  - Sea urchins: spines break off into wounds → foreign body reaction
  - Sea Cucumbers: eject an irritating liquid (holothurin) → Conjunctivitis

Chapter 6: Neoplastic dermatology

6.1 Keratinocytic Neoplasms

Benign keratinocytic neoplasms

Seborrheic keratosis (SK)

- Very common benign neoplasm w/ AD inheritance but incomplete penetrance
- PIK3CA and FGFR3 activating mutations ("PIK 3 Full Grown FReckles")
    - Do not confuse w/ FGFR2 in Apert, Beare-Stevens, Crouzon, nevus comedonicus
- p/w well-demarcated waxy-brown "Stuck on" papules on hair-bearing sites
- Hyperpigmentation due to endothelin-1 (primary keratinocyte melanogen)
    - Dermoscopy: milia-like cysts, fissures/ridges and gyri (cerebriform surface)
- Path: acanthosis, hyperkeratosis (loose lamellar "Shredded wheat" keratin) w/ pseudo-horn cysts and a completely flat base ("String Sign") composed of bland keratinocytes
- Sign of Leser-Trelat: eruptive SKs due to underlying adenocarcinoma (GI is MC)

Seborrheic keratosis clinical variants ("Sebastian, would you Ker to do LSD in CALI In MARCH?")

- Lichenoid keratosis: inflamed/regressing lentigo or SK that clinically mimics BCC or SCCIS
    - Path: resembles LP (also known as lichen planus-like keratosis)

- Stucco Keratosis: white scaly variant of SK found on B/L lower legs of adults (M > F)
    - a/w HPV-23b ("S" backwards looks like a 2 and a "K" backwards looks like a 3)
    - Path: "church Spire" pattern (hyperkeratosis and papillomatosis)
- Dermatosis papulosa nigra: hyperpigmented keratosis papules on face of AA patients
    - Path: identical to SKs except lacks pseudo-horn cysts
- Clear cell acanthoma: solitary red papule on the lower **legs**
    - Dermoscopy: Coiled vessels (like in SCCIS) but in a string of pearls configuration
    - Path: resembles psoriasis (w/ sharply demarcated zone of pale keratinocytes)
        - **Phosphorylase deficiency → glycogen accumulation** → PAS+ pale cells
- Acrokeratosis verruciformis of Hopf: tan warty papules on the dorsal hands/feet (Acral)
    - a/w ATP2A2 mutations (thus seen commonly in Dariers disease)
    - Path: identical to stucco keratosis ("church-spire")
- Large cell acanthoma: represents a flat SK w/ large cells on path
    - Path: SK w/ large and slightly atypical keratinocytes
- Inverted follicular keratosis: endophytic SK variant that p/w a pink papule on the face
    - Path: endophytic SK with many **squamous eddies**

Seborrheic keratosis histologic variants (Sebastian, would you Ker to do LSD in CALI In MARCH)

- Inflamed: lymphocytes and spongiosis are present in the epidermis
- Irritated: whorls of pink keratinocytes (squamous eddies)

- Melanoacanthoma: heavily pigmented (mostly in dendritic melanocytes > keratinocytes) acanthoma w/ parakeratosis instead of the typical loose lamellar keratin
- Acanthotic: MC and most typical (acanthosis, horn cysts and lamellar hyperkeratosis)
- Reticulated: thin pigmented interlacing downward proliferation of epidermis; horn cysts
- **Clonal**: clonal islands of small keratinocytes with bland nuclei (vs clonal Bowens) and no ducts in the clones (vs hydroacanthoma simplex type of poroma)
- Hyperkeratotic: prominent hyperkeratosis and papillomatosis ("church-spire")

Porokeratosis ("BDSM Porn")

- All lesions on path display a cornoid lamella (angled column of parakeratosis overlying dyskeratotic cells) which correspond to a **slightly raised peripheral rim of scale clinically**
    - Blaschkoid/linear porokeratosis: linear lesions MC on the legs in infancy
        - Highest risk of SCC (since develops in kids cancers have a lifetime to form)
    - Disseminated Superficial Actinic porokeratosis: numerous brown-red scaly macules on sun exposed areas (MC on the legs) in middle-aged adults
        - 2nd lowest risk of SCC (punctate form has no risk)
        - Mutation in **SART3** gene
        - a/w SLE
    - Porokeratosis of Mibelli: classic large circinate plaque MC on the legs of children
        - "Porokeratosis (and angiokeratoma) of Mibelli is far from the belly"

- o Punctate porokeratosis: 1–2 mm "seed-like" papules on the palms and soles of adolescence; no risk of SCC
  - ▪ Ddx: punctate keratosis of palmar creases
- o Porokeratosis Palmaris Plantaris et disseminate (PPPD): seed-like keratotic papules start on the palms/soles but then disseminate; MC in adolescence
  - ▪ Ddx: arsenic keratosis but look for the raised rim of scale in porokeratosis and **age of pt is a good clue** (arsenic keratosis develops 20–30 years after exposure whereas PPPD presents in the first 20 years of life)
- o Porokeratosis Ptychotropica: scaly verrucous gluteal/peri-anal lesions in adults
  - ▪ Path: cornoid lamella are multiple w/ surrounding orthohyperkeratosis
- o Porokeratotic eccrine ostial and dermal duct nevus (PEODD): type of epidermal nevus w/ **keratotic**/ comedo-like papules/plaques (MC on an extremity) of infants
  - ▪ Represents a **mosaic form of KID syndrome** (GJB2 encoding connexin 26)
    - "The KID PEED (PEODD) in the sandbox"
  - ▪ **Path: cornoid lamella centered exclusively over acrosyringia**

- Dermoscopy: diffuse vessels as dots and well-defined peripheral thickened rim
- Rx: cholesterol/lovastatin cream; monitor for malignant transformation (rare)

Epidermal nevus

- Hamartoma of the epidermis or papillary dermis which occurs in the first year of life
- Same activating mutations seen in SKs (**PIK3CA and FGFR3**); also **HRAS** > KRAS, NRAS

- **p/w hyperkeratotic papillomatous linear plaques in Blaschko's lines**
- Variants
  - Nevus comedonicus: linear comedones on face (MC); path shows horn cysts
  - Ichthyosis hystrix: hyperkeratotic spiny scales mainly over extensor limbs w/ PPK
  - Nevus Sebaceous: in infants it usually presents as a **yellow-tan plaque on the scalp** (subtle, may just look like alopecia) which gets thick and bumpy at puberty
    - a/w **HRAS** > KRAS mutations and CNS abnormalities (seizures, MR)
  - Inflammatory linear verrucous epidermal nevus (ILVEN): p/w itchy, red, warty plaques in a Blaschkoid pattern that presents at birth or shortly after
    - Ddx: red/itchy (vs epidermal nevus), does not respond to topical steroids (vs linear psoriasis) and does not regress (vs lichen striatus)
  - Epidermal nevus syndrome (Shimmelpenning): a/w CNS, eye, MSK abnormalities
    - a/w vitamin D-resistant rickets and postzygotic mosaic HRAS mutations
- Path: "church-spire" (epidermal papillomatosis and orthohyperkeratosis)
  - May see epidermolytic hyperkeratosis (EHK) due to mosaicism (**offspring have a risk of full blown bullous congenital ichthyosiform erythroderma**)
- Workup: eye and developmental assessment; biopsy after childhood to rule out EHK

Flegel disease (hyperkeratosis lenticularis perstans)

- AD inheritance with adult-onset hyperkeratotic papules on the distal extremities

- Path: thick orthohyperkeratosis overlying thin epidermis; lichenoid dermal infiltrate
- Electron microscopy: absent/altered Odland bodies (lamellar granules)

Warty dyskeratoma

- p/w solitary verrucous papule w/ central keratotic plug on the head/neck in adults
- Path: acantholytic dyskeratosis (corp ronds/grains) in a cup-like configuration

Borderline or malignant keratinocytic neoplasms

Actinic keratosis (AK)

- RFs: Caucasian, immune-Compromise, old males (more Time in sun), UVR/Tanning (#1)
- Pathogenesis: **UVB** damages DNA by formation of photoproducts such as **Cyclobutene pyrimidine dimers (MC)** which forms Thymine dimers (covalent bonds between two thymines) which are mutagenic (**C → T is MC mutation**; "aC→Tinic keratosis")
- Mutations in the tumor suppressor gene **p53** are highly a/w actinic keratosis and SCCs
    - o "p53 puts a freeze on the cell cycle"
- p/w red scaly plaques on sun-exposed sites
- Dermoscopy: strawberry pattern (red pseudo-network around follicular openings)
- Path: keratinocyte atypia in the lower 1/3rd of epidermis w/ overlying parakeratosis (pink) which alternates w/ orthokeratosis (blue) → "Flag sign"
- Rx: Cryo, ED&C, CO_2 ablation, 5-FU, imiquimod, PDT, diclofenac, Tirbanibulin, and TCA peel
- Prophylaxis: oral niacinamide/nicotinamide (vitamin B-Three) and Tretinoin (retinoids)
- Erosive pustular dermatosis occurs on the scalp of elderly patients and presents w/ sterile pustules and

chronic crusted erosions on a severely actinically damaged scalp
   - Rx: potent topical corticosteroids

Bowen's disease (Squamous cell carcinoma in situ)

- Risk factors: similar to AK but also include HPV and arsenic exposure
- Pathogenesis: AK, Bowen's and SCC have the same pathogenesis
- p/w hyperkeratotic erythematous plaque in sun-exposed site (but may occur anywhere)
- Dermoscopy: glomerular vessels (most specific) or vessels as red dots
- Path: full-thickness keratinocyte atypia w/ a disorganized "wind-blown" architecture
- Variants
   - Bowenoid papulosis: Brown penile papules (a/w HPV); low risk of invasive SCC
   - Erythroplasia of Queyrat: red erosive plaques on glans penis: high risk of invasion
- Rx: ED&C, excision or MOHs (consider AK treatments in non-surgical candidates)
- Prognosis: 3–5% Bowen's disease progress to invasive SCC

Squamous cell carcinoma ("ABC's of SCCs")

- Risk factors: similar to AK and Bowen's but also include
   - Genetic syndromes: helicase family mutations (XP, Werner, Bloom, Rothmund-Thompson), albinism, DEB, EDV, dyskeratosis congenita, and KID syndrome)
   - Chronic inflammation/ulcers (**MC RF in AAs**): leg ulcers, hypertrophic LE/LP
   - Drugs (ABC): Azoles (voriconazole), Azathioprine, Biologics (TNF inhibitors), BRAF inhibitors (vemu-

    - rafenib), Corticosteroids, Calcineurin inhibitors, and Cyclosporine
  - Chemical exposures (ABC): **Arsenic**, Bromide, and Cigarettes (tobacco)
- Mutations: p53 > CDKN2A, NOTCH1/2, deregulation of EGFR pathway
- MC malignant tumor of **nail** unit (a/w HPV 16, 31 and 73; melanoma is #2)
  - BCC and aggressive digital papillary adenocarcinoma are less common
- MC skin cancer in AAs, Asian Indians and in organ transplant recipients
  - Transplant recipients: **SCC (65x risk)**, Merkel (25x), BCC (10x), melanoma (3.4x)
    - SCCs are more aggressive in transplant pts (vs BCCs → usually superficial)
  - Treatment of multiple SCCs in organ transplant recipients: add **oral acitretin** (most effective); change CNI to the mTOR inhibitor sirolimus (2nd most effective)
- p/w red scaly papulonodule MC on the head/neck or dorsal extremities
- Dermoscopy: same vessels as in Bowens (glomerular or dots) which may be in a linear distribution, brown circles in a linear distribution (pigmented SCC), scale, tan-orange structures (keratin), white scale, blood spots and crystalline (white reflective) structures
- Path: dermal invasion of atypical keratinocytes which are often more differentiated (more eosinophilic/keratinizing) than surrounding keratinocytes
  - Variants: acantholytic, spindled, pseudoglandular, KA and verrucous carcinoma
- IHC: **AE1/AE3** cytokeratin stains, p63, MN116, S100 can highlight PNI of SCC
- Staging systems

- Brigham and Women's Hospital: the 4 risk factors are the 4 Ds (Diameter ≥ **2 cm**, perineural invasion in a nerve ≥ 0.1 mm in Diameter, poor Differentiation, Deep invasion (beyond fat but excluding bone which automatically upgrades to T3)
  - **T1 = 0 risk factors (0.1% 10-year nodal metastasis)**
  - **T2a = 1 RFs (3% 10-year risk of nodal metastasis)**
  - **T2b = 2–3 RFs** (20% 10-year risk of nodal metastasis **get CT head/neck**)
    - "T2B, 2 to 3 (RFs), twenty, get CT" (it all rhymes)
  - **T3 = 4 RFs or any bony invasion (67% 10-year risk of nodal metastasis)**
- AJCC8: stage 0 (in situ), stage 1 (T1), stage 2 (T2), stage 3 (T3 even w/o nodal disease or N_{any}), stage 4 (T4 w/ N_{any}, T3 w/ ≥ 2 nodes of ≥ 3 cm, or M_{any})
  - T1: ≤ 2 cm in greatest diameter
  - T2: 2.01 cm to 4 cm in greatest diameter
  - T3 (ABCD): tumor invasion After Adipose (or > 6 mm deep), minor Bone erosion, PNI of ≥ 0.1mm Caliber (or subdermal) nerve, Diameter > 4 cm
  - T4: extensive bone invasion (T4a) or invasion of the base of the cranium or invasion through the skull foramen of the base of the cranium (T4b)
    - "4A is A-xtensive bone invasion, 4B is to Base or through 4men"
  - BWH is a better predictor of SCC metastasis than AJCC8 (perhaps because **AJCC8 does not include poor differentiation** as a risk factor for staging)

        - Hint: AJCC8 staging always has the "point-zero" round down (e.g., 2.0 cm SCC is AJCC8 T1; for BWH however, a 2.0 counts as a risk factor)
- **NCCN management guidelines (HIGH YIELD)**
    - ED&C should only be used to treat local low risk SCCs and w/ 3 caveats…
        - Do not use in areas w/ terminal hairs (scalp, axilla, pubis, beard in males)
        - If SQ later is reached during ED&C then excision must be performed next
        - If high risk path features are identified then perform additional treatment
    - WLE: usually 0.4 cm margins; 0.6 – 1 cm margins if SCC is high risk (see below)
        - Positive margins → consider MOHs or re-excise
        - Negative margins but extensive PNI (> 0.1 mm) → consider adjuvant RT
    - MOHs: most effective treatment option for high-risk local disease (see below)
        - Positive margins or extensive PNI → consider adjuvant RT
    - RT: pts w/ unresectable, inoperable or incompletely resected disease (combine w/ cisplatin) or combine w/ PD-1 for pts w/ regional recurrence or distant mets
        - **CI: genetic syndromes like Gorlin's or XP;** (relative CI w/ scleroderma)
    - Guidelines for SLNB for SCC is not established, but publications (Tejera et al. Derm surg 2020) endorse SLNB for AJCC8 T3 and BWH T2b and greater SCCs
    - Bone invasion is suspected → order CT w/ contrast ("B next to C in alphabet")
    - Perineural invasion is suspected → order MRI w/ contrast ("P next to M")
    - Local recurrence is suspected → biopsy (MRI can assess extent of local disease)

- PET-CT is best for assessing metastases
- Pembrolizumab and cemiplimab are TOC for locally advanced/metastatic disease
    - 2nd line is chemo (cisplastin) or cetuximab (EGFR inh that is FDA approved for mucosal laSCC of head/neck but used off label for cutaneous SCC)
- LN dissection for regional disease (ipsilateral dissection +/- RT for solitary or multiple ipsilateral LNs; B/L neck dissection + RT for B/L nodal involvement)
- **Stepwise process of evaluating aggressive SCCs of ≥ T2 ("ABC")**
    - **Assess LNs** (clinically or with imaging) → if nodal disease then…
    - **Biopsy (US guided FNA** or **core needle**) involved LNs, and if positive get…
    - **CT scan w/ IV Contrast of involved nodal basin** and get a **PET-CT** or **CT Chest/abdomen/pelvis** to rule out distant metastases
    - Ppx ("I'm a FAN of SCC prophylaxis"): 5-FU cream, Acitretin, Nicotinamide 500mg

- Follow-up
    - Local disease: at least annually but more frequent if pt/lesion are high risk
        - Node negative: 3–12 months x 2 years and 6–12 months x 3 years
        - Node negative but high risk: 3–6 months x 2 yrs then 6–12 months for life
    - Regional disease: q 2–3 months x 1 year; then q 2–4 months x 1 year; then q 4–6 months x 3 year; then q 6–12 months for life
- ↑ risk of mets/death (ABCDE): Breslow depth > 2mm, arising in Burns/scars, immune-Compromised, **Diameter > 2cm** (#1 risk), poorly Differentiated/ Desmoplastic, Ear/lip

- Management for nail SCC: currently no guidelines exist for proper use of imaging but since many nail SCCs involve the bone which may change management (from MOHs to distal digital amputation), imaging may be warranted (CT w/ contrast > X-ray)
- In a recent JAAD article, **hydrochlorothiazide** was significantly a/w NMSC, especially SCC

VerrucouS carcinoma

- Low grade but locally destructive SCC a/w low risk HPV types (6 and 11)
- Large verrucous nodule w/ three clinical variants: epithelioma caniculatum (plantar foot), Buschke-Lowenstein tumor (anogenital) and oral florid papillomatosis (mouth)
    - o MC location is in **mouth** and also a/w chewing tobacco ("Snuff dipper's cancer")
- **Risk factors: HPV 6 (Six) > 11, Sexual activity, history of STDs, Smoking, immuno-Suppression, male gender (boys have more Sex), age > 60 (Sixty)**
- Path: cytologically bland (no atypia) but is massive with a bulbous/pushing border
- Rx: **Surgical excision** (also diagnostic because must see architecture); **do NOT irradiate!**

Keratoacanthoma

- Unique variant of SCC w/ initial rapid growth (weeks) → resolves/involutes (months)
    - o Subungual KAs never involute
- RFs: UV, immunosuppression, HPV, drugs (vemurafenib, vismodegib, sorafenib)
- Genetic syndromes with KAs
    - o Ferguson-Smith: AD mutation in **TGFBR1** ("Fergie parties, TGIF") which p/w rapid-onset of multiple KAs in adolescents → resolves → may reappear later

- Gryzbowski: sporadic inheritance w/ numerous milia-like KAs in later adulthood which affect the airway ("Old Grizzlies Growl") and cause scarring → ectropion
  - Rx: surgery and/or oral retinoids
- Muir-Torre ("more SICK"): Sebaceous tumors, Internal Cancers (Colon MC), KAs

- Path: crateriform nodule composed of well-differentiated keratinocytes, central keratin plug, neutrophilic micro-abscesses, eosinophils and elastic trapping peripherally
- Subungual and mucosal KAs are unlikely to regress spontaneously
- Rx: IL MTX/5-FU, excision or MOHs (may observe if it is already involuting)
  - 66/69 KAs were successfully treated with IL MTX (25 mg/mL) in one study

Basal cell carcinoma

- RFs (similar to SCC): intermittent/intense UV exposure (vs cumulative for SCC), sunburns at any age (vs sunburns in childhood for SCC), arsenic exposure (produces superficial BCCs), immunosuppression, radiation, fair skin, old age
- Mutations in the tumor suppressor genes PTCH (MC; 66%) and p53 (#2; 50% of BCCs)
  - Patched normally inhibits smoothened (sonic hedgehog molecule is in the unbound state) but when mutated, it activates GL1/2 transcription factors to promote transcription of genes involved in cell growth
- Essentially no metastatic potential (depends on stroma for growth)
- BCC variants
  - Nodular: MC variant; pearly pink papule which favors the head/neck

        - Path: large dermal nodules w/ peripheral palisade and stromal retraction
    - Superficial: MC type in younger patients; red scaly plaque on trunk or extremities
        - MC subtype in those who have received an organ transplant (in this setting even superficial BCCs should be considered high risk)
        - Path: multiple epidermal buds in the papillary dermis
    - Morpheaform: scar-like pink-white plaque
        - Path: small angulated nests in a **sclerotic stroma** w/ minimal retraction
    - Infiltrative: path term referring to an aggressive BCC with jagged angulated nests
    - Micronodular: best thought of as an intermediate tumor between nodular (not aggressive) and infiltrative (aggressive) composed of small round nests
    - Fibroepithelioma of Pinkus: pedunculated lesion MC on the lower back
        - Path: thin anastomosing pink epithelial strands w/ embedded blue basaloid buds and **eccrine ducts**
    - Infundibulocystic: resembles benign follicular tumors; not aggressive
        - SUFU mutations are commonly seen
        - Path: pink epithelial strands w/ blue buds and horn cysts
    - Adenoid: histologic variant w/ blue islands in an adenoid pattern (clear spaces)
    - Basosquamous: aggressive tumor w/ features of BCC and SCC (MC perinasal)
- Genoderms with BCCs ("Bad X-Rays Synthesize Basals"): Brooke-Spiegler, XP, Rombo, Schöpf-Schulz-Passarge, Basal cell nevus syndrome, Basex-Dupré-Christol
- Dermoscopy: arborizing vessels, leaf-like structures, large blue-gray ovoid nests

- Path: basaloid nests w/ ↑N:C ratio, peripheral palisading w/ disorganized pattern centrally, retraction between stroma and tumor, myxoid stroma, ↑ mitoses
    - IHC: **Ber-EP4, strong diffuse BCL-2 staining, AR**, AE1/AE3, CD10, MN116
- Rx: excision, MOHs, ED&C, radiation (NCCN: adjuvant therapy if PNI ≥ 1mm or invasion of nerve below dermis) or vismodegib/sondegib/cemiplimab (inoperable)
    - "The Vegetarian PAs bind and inhibit the smooth doctor (inhibit smoothened)"
        - Erivedge, Patched, cyclopamine (itraconazole also treats BCCs but not by binding to smoothened, rather it inhibits smoothened accumulation)
    - SUFU mutations are downstream of PATCH (would not respond to vismodegib)
- NCCN management guidelines
    - ED&C should only be used to treat local low risk BCCs and w/ 3 caveats…
        - Do not use in areas w/ terminal hairs (scalp, axilla, pubis, beard in males)
        - If SQ later is reached during ED&C then excision must be performed next
        - If high risk path features are identified then perform additional treatment
    - WLE: usually 0.4 cm margins; 0.6 – 1 cm margins if BCC is high risk (see below)
    - MOHs: most effective treatment option for BCCs that are high risk (see below)
    - Topical therapies can be considered for superficial BCC if surgery or RT is CI
        - 5-year tumor-free survival is 80% w/ imiquimod and 70% w/ 5-FU
        - Cryo (poor cosmesis) and PDT can be considered but have poorer efficacy

- Radiotherapy (RT) can be considered as a primary therapy in those w/ limited metastatic BCC (mBCC), locally advanced BCC (laBCC) that have recurred following surgery and those patients who cannot tolerate surgery
    - RT is recommended for BCCs w/ positive margins or significant PNI
    - RT as a primary treatment for BCC had higher recurrence (7.5% vs < 1%), poorer cosmetic outcomes and more complications than excision
    - Consider post-op RT for T3/T4 lesions, recurrent lesions, desmoplastic lesions in setting of immunosuppression or for close/positive margins
    - RT is CI in genetic syndromes (Gorlins) and relative CI in scleroderma
- Hedgehog inhibitors (HHI) are approved in those w/ metastatic, locally advanced and inoperable BCCs and those w/ genoderms such as Gorlin's syndrome
    - Sonidegib is only approved for locally advanced BCC (not metastatic)
- Cemiplimab is approved for mBCC or laBCC in those previously treated w/ HHIs or in whom HHI are not appropriate (cannot tolerate their SEs)
- Bone invasion is suspected → order CT w/ contrast ("B next to C in alphabet")
- Perineural invasion is suspected → order MRI w/ contrast ("P next to M")
- Local recurrence is suspected → biopsy (MRI can assess extent of local disease)
- Nodal metastasis is suspected → histologic analysis (e.g., FNA or core biopsy)
- Metastasis is suspected → CT or PET-CT can be used to gauge extent of disease

    - Ppx: 20% decrease in BCCs after 1-year w/ nicotinamide (acitretin, celecoxib, acitretin, capecitabine and tazarotene are also effective prophylactic agents)
- **Less than 0.1%** of BCCs develop metastasis (MC to **lymph nodes and lungs**)
- Follow-up (NCCN): complete skin exam every 6–12 months x 5 years and then annually
- Boards factoid: 2018 JAAD article showed higher risk of BCCs in men who take statins

NCCN guidelines high risk factors of NMSC: "HIGH RISK NMSC"

- **High risk locations (H or M; esp ears/lips for SCC)**; Huge tumor (> 2 cm)
    - > 1 cm on M area is high risk (any size in H is high risk; SCC-KA on central face)
    - > 4 cm wide and > 6 mm deep or invasion beyond fat is very high risk in SCC
        - Any of these would automatically result in SCC being AJCC8 stage T3
- Immunosuppressed patient (transplant/lymphoma/iatrogenic/HIV)
- Growth is fast (this feature is specific for SCC)
- **High risk Histo**
    - BCC: infiltrative, sclerosing, morpheaform, micronodular, metatypical
    - SCC: spindle cell/desmoplastic or adenoid subtype or poorly differentiated tumor
        - Notice desmoplasia is higher risk in NMSC but lower risk in melanoma
- Radiation previously done at site of cancer; Recurrence
- Ill-defined borders; Invasion of nerves > 0.1mm, lymphatics or vessels on path
- Scars (Marjolin's ulcers; this high-risk feature is specific for SCCs)

- Key patient characteristics (genetic syndromes or immunocompromised)
- Neuro symptoms (SCC only): pain/paresthesia/anesthesia/diplopia (suggests PNI)

Recommended WLE margins for malignant neoplasms ("SLAM'D Angi Extra")
• SCC/Sebaceous carcinoma: 0.4–1 cm (melanoma in-Situ is 0.6–1 cm) • Leiomyosarcoma/AFX/Merkel cell carcinoma/invasive Melanoma: 1–2 cm • DFSP: 2–5 cm (2 cm → 40% recurrence rate; 3 cm → 15%; 5 cm → 5%) • Angiosarcoma/Extramammary Paget's disease: 5 cm

6.2 Cysts

"A DUMB Cystic VEST": VEST is AD inheritance (**Rx for cysts, even pseudocyst such as mucocele, is excision**; for congenital defects like dermoid cysts, infected urachal cyst or omphalomesenteric duct cyst, get imaging and refer to a pediatric surgeon; if it is midline, like a dermoid cyst, we have to rule out intracranial extension w/ MRI but if this is not a concern, like branchial cleft cyst, your next step can be an US but MRI is still best; for classic dermoid cysts in the Eyebrow when you can palpate the posterior aspect you proceed w/ Excision)

- Apocrine/eccrine hydrocystoma: translucent bluish cyst on the face (eyelids are MC)
    - Path: lined by 2 layers of flat cuboidal epithelium w/ large empty cystic space
    - a/w Schopf-Schulz-Passarge: multiple hydrocystomas, PPK, hypodontia
- Apocrine cystadenoma: has been used interchangeably w/ apocrine hydrocystoma but inside the cyst there are papillary projections ("mix between HPAP and hydrocystoma")

  - o Ddx: tubular apocrine adenoma has many small cyst-like spaces w/ these papilla
- Auricular pseudocyst: erythematous firm nodule on ear (ddx: relapsing polychondritis)
  - o Path: cystic space in cartilage w/ no epithelial lining; no inflammation in cartilage
  - o a/w trauma (cell phones and wrestling)
- Dermoid cyst: nodule on lateral eyebrow of infants (**occur along embryonic fusion lines**)
  - o Path: stratified squamous epithelium (SSE) w/ granular layer and adnexal structures (sebaceous/ eccrine/apocrine glands and **hair follicles**); may contain red shark-tooth lining like steatocystomas; lamellar keratin is inside cyst cavity
  - o **Workup: image before excising midline lesions** (may communicate w/ the CNS)
  - o Nasal dermoid sinus cyst p/w midline nasal papule w/ tuft of hairs
    - ▪ Workup: imaging (MRI > CT) before surgical excision (ENT/neurosurgery)
- Digital mucus cyst/ganglion cyst: nodules on distal phalanx/dorsal wrist, respectively
  - o Path: mucin inside pseudocyst (no epithelial lining)
- Urachal cyst: collection of tissue/fluid b/w bladder and Umbilicus (infra-Umbilical mass)
  - o Path: ectopic bladder epithelium (cuboidal or flat, atrophic epithelia)
  - o Ddx: omphalomesenteric duct remnant (p/w umbilical mass w/ persistent drainage; GI mucosa w/ goblet cells on path) vs umbilical granuloma (umbilical mass w/ persistent drainage; vascular proliferation on path; Rx silver nitrate)
- Median raphe cyst: cyst on the ventral penis
  - o Path: dirty debris ("dirty penis") in cyst; genital skin features (smooth muscle)

- Rx: most are asymptomatic → observation is appropriate
- Mucocele: dome-shaped skin colored to bluish **translucent papule on lower mucosal lip**
  - Path: mucin inside pseudocyst (no epithelial lining) +/- adjacent salivary glands
- Branchial cleft ("claft") cyst: lateral neck
  - Path: variable lining w/ surrounding **Lymphoid Aggregates (germinal centers)**
  - May communicate w/ the auditory canal or pharynx (not the CNS)
- Bronchogenic cyst: midline inferior neck mass at birth (**suprasternal notch**)
  - Path: ciliated columnar epithelium w/ cartilage, smooth muscle and goblet cells
  - May communicate w/ the trachea/bronchioles
- Cutaneous Ciliated Cyst (lower legs) and Ciliated Cysts of vulva: mullerian duct origin
  - Path: Columnar Ciliated epithelium +/- dirty debris in cyst ("dirty vulva")
- Cutaneous endometriosis: bloody cyst-like lesion in lower abdomen of females
  - Slow-growing, tender nodules that cause cyclical pain during menses
  - Path (GIRL): Glandular spaces, Iron, RBCs, Loose concentric fibromyxoid stroma
- Verrucous cyst (HPV-60)
  - Path: looks like a pilar cyst but has papillomatosis, hypergranulosis +/- koilocytes
- Vellus hair cyst: multiple eruptive domed-shaped skin colored or **hyperpigmented** papules on trunk (inherited AD; keratin 17 mutation; may be seen in PC type 2)
  - Path: looks like epidermoid cyst but w/ multiple vellus hairs in cyst cavity
- Ear pits: branchial arch defect (AD) which p/w cyst/invagination in the preauricular area

  - Path: lined by stratified squamous epithelium (SSE) w/ a granular layer
- Epidermoid cyst: MC cyst; face or upper trunk; derived from the follicular infundibulum ("infundibular cyst") or traumatically implanted ("epidermal inclusion cyst")
  - Variants: proliferating epidermoid cyst, milia and scrotal cysts
  - Path: cystic cavity filled w/ **laminated keratin** lined by SSE w/ a granular layer
  - a/w Gardner syndrome, Gorlin's syndrome and BRAF inhibitors
- Steatocystoma: single or multiple (AD; KRT17: PC type 2) lesions that drain oily fluid
  - Path: lined by SSE w/ no granular layer and thin bright pink corrugated ("Shark-tooth") cuticle w/ Sebaceous glands in wall (no hair follicles in cyst wall or lamellar keratin in cyst cavity like in dermoid cyst)
- Trichilemmal (pilar cyst): firm nodule on scalp; no punctum; usually multiple and AD
  - Path: SSE w/ **no granular layer and dense pink homogenized keratin** +/- calcium
- Thyroglossal duct cyst: midline superior neck mass in children; moves w/ swallowing
  - Variable lining w/ bright pink thyroid follicles in the wall

6.3 Melanocytic Neoplasms

Ephelides (freckles)

- Pigmented macules on sun-exposed skin from ↑ melanogenesis and melanin transfer
- Path: ↑ basilar keratinocyte hyperpigmentation without ↑ melanocyte density

CALM (café-au lait macule)

- Larger pigmented macules/patches; isolated finding in 10–20% of people
- a/w genodermatoses: "when a MAN FARTs, he stays CALM"
    - o MEN-1, McCune Albright, Ataxia telangiectasia, Noonan, NF1 > 2 (RASopathies)
    - o Fanconi syndrome, Ataxia telangiectasia, Russel-Silver, Tuberous sclerosis
- Path: ↑ basilar keratinocyte hyperpigmentation without ↑ melanocyte density

Solar lentigo

- Pigmented macules on sun exposed areas ubiquitous in Caucasians over 60 years old
- Path: elongated rete ridges with basilar keratinocyte hyperpigmentation ("dirty socks")

Lentigo simplex

- Well demarcated, evenly pigmented brown to black macule at any age and any site
    - o Think of a solar lentigo as a flat SK, and a lentigo simplex as a flat nevus
- a/w with genodermatoses: "Big Lentigo Problems need TLC"
    - o Bannayan-Riley-Ruvalcaba (penile), LEOPARD (diffuse), Puetz-Jeghers (perioral)
    - o Touraine's (centrofacial), Laugier-Hunziker (perioral/genitals), Carney (perioral, sclera, oral), Cronkhite-Canada (hands, feet, buccal mucosa)
- Path: ↑ basilar keratinocyte hyperpigmentation **with mild ↑ melanocyte density**

Addison's hyperpigmentation

- Pathogenesis: ↑ ACTH causes melanocytes to produce more melanin

- Path: ↑ basilar keratinocyte hyperpigmentation w/ dermal melanophages

Mucosal melanotic macule

- Type of lentigo on mucosal surfaces; may appear slightly irregular/mottled
- MC in adults > 40; MC on the vermillion border of the lip and the labia minora
- Path: acanthosis with mild basilar hyperpigmentation and mild ↑ in melanocyte density

Dermal melanocytosis

- Mongolian spot: blue-gray patch (due to the Tyndall effect) on the lumbosacral region that is present at birth in most Asians and AAs; resolves in childhood
    - o Path: dendritic melanocytes in lower 2/3rd of dermis lying parallel to epidermis
- Nevus of ota ("Ota has GUTS"): presents in first year of life or around puberty
    - o GNAQ mutation in some; Glaucoma in 10%
    - o Uveal melanoma is possible; Unilateral (90%) blue-gray plaque > bilateral
    - o Upper dermis is where the elongated dendritic melanocytes lie on pathology
    - o Trigeminal (V1/V2) distribution
    - o Scleral involvement (60%)
- Nevus of Ito: blue-gray patch on the shoulder, supraclavicular and scapular regions which has no risk of progression to melanoma
- Hori's nevus: acquired nevus of Ota-like macules bilaterally on the zygoma
- Sun's nevus: acquired unilateral variant of Hori's nevus
- Rx: QS-RAN lasers (Ruby is best; Nd:YAG is safest in POC)

Blue nevus ("that's So blue")

- Homogenous blue papule MC on the Scalp, Sacral region and Sun-exposed extremities
- Due to GNAQ and GNA11 mutations ("Get GiNA's NUMBER") → activates MAPK pathway
  - Nevi (blue/spitz), Nevus of Ota, **Uveal mel**, **Mesothelioma**, **Malignant blue nevi**, BCC, clear cell **RCC** (concomitant BAP-1 loss in UMR cancers will ↑ risk of mets)
- Genoderm: multiple blue nevi and epithelioid blue nevi are seen in Carney complex
- Dermoscopy: homogenous blue color throughout lesion
- Variants
  - Common blue nevus: small (< 1 cm) blue papule
    - Path: wedge-shaped lesion in upper 2/3rd of dermis composed entirely of long dendritic melanocytes embedded in a Sclerotic stroma
  - Cellular blue nevus: blue nodule (1–3 cm) that favors the Scalp and Sacral region
    - Path: proliferation of both epithelioid (plump) and dendritic melanocytes in a Sclerotic stroma that bulges into the SQ ("big black ball in the fat")
  - Epithelioid blue nevus: heavily pigmented papule/nodule; a/w Carney complex
    - Path: proliferation composed entirely of epithelioid (plump) melanocytes but no sclerotic stroma (looks like animal-type melanoma w/ no atypia)
  - Malignant blue nevus (melanoma): often arises within a cellular blue nevus most commonly on the Scalp; concomitant GNAQ/GN11 mutation w/ BAP-1 loss

Deep penetrating nevus (DPN)

- Most harbor mutation in β-catenin and MAPK pathway
  - o Distinct from blue nevus due to a lack of GNAQ/ GNA11 mutation
- p/w blue/black papule (< 1 cm) on the upper body in young women (MC)
- Path: very similar to cellular blue nevus (both have epithelioid melanocytes diving deep into SQ) but **DPN'S Dive Down (more wedge-shape; classically tracking down adnexa/nerves), more Pigmented, more Nested and are more Spitzoid (cells have more abundant cytoplasm) compared to a CBN**

Spitz nevus ("shpitz")

- **HRAS** mutation w/ **11p gains** ("sp11tz") → gain of chromosome 11p never seen in mel
- p/w pigmented (75%) or pink-red (25%) papule MC on Head/neck in children
  - o "You learn how to spit from your head/neck when you're a child"
- Dermoscopy: atypical features can be seen such as crystalline structures and a negative pigment network but would be symmetrically located (vs focally located in melanoma)
- Path: symmetric and circumscribed lesion w/ large junctional nests of epithelioid melanocytes Hanging down from a Hyperplastic epidermis w/ overlying Hyperkeratosis and Hypergranulosis; **kamino bodies** (pink clumps of BMZ material) within epidermis
- Immunohistochemistry
  - o Spitz nevi: p16$^+$, Melan-A$^+$, S100$^+$, S100A6$^+$ ("when a girl PMS'S she spitz at you")
    - ▪ p16 is positive in Spitz but lost in atypical Spitz/spitzoid melanomas
    - ▪ S100A6 is strong and diffuse in Spitz (weaker in spitzoid melanoma)

            - HMB45 and Ki-67 (MIB-1) shows zonal staining (+ in Spitz up High)
                - Diffuse (superficial and deep) staining in melanoma
        - Atypical spitz/spitzoid melanoma: Melan-A+, S100+, S100A6+ (**p16 is lost**)
            - Notice how **p16 and S100A6 stain spitz** but are lost or weaker in spitzoid melanoma ("6 rhymes w/ Spitz better than it rhymes w/ spitzoid mel")
    - **Homozygous loss of 9p21** (corresponds to p16/CDKN2a gene) → **metastasis/death**
        - "If you lose both your parents (both alleles) when you are between the ages of 9 and 21, even someone spitting on you can kill you"

Pigmented spindle cell nevus of Reed

- Heavily pigmented and spindled (vs epithelioid) variant of a spitz nevus
- p/w dark macule/papule on the thighs of young females
- Dermoscopy: starburst pattern of peripheral pseudopods w/ central structureless area
- Path: like spitz but more superficial (confined to junction/superficial dermis), more pigmented (numerous melanophages) and melanocytes are spindled (vs epithelioid)

BAP-1 inactivated spitzoid nevus (BAPoma; Wiesner nevus)

- BAP-1 is a tumor suppressor gene; just like in many tumor suppressor gene mutations (e.g., NF-1), tumors are due to loss of heterozygosity (defective germline copy of BAP-1 and an acquired mutation knocks out the other copy → loss of BAP-1 staining on IHC)
    - For sporadic BAP-1 nevi to form, both copies must undergo somatic inactivation

  - In addition to BAP-1 loss, they often carry BRAF V600E mutations
- p/w flesh-colored to pink-red dome-shaped papule/papules (similar to Spitz nevi)
- Path: intradermal melanocytic proliferations composed of melanocytes w/ ample pink "glassy" cytoplasm w/ very sharp cell borders; there may be an adjacent banal nevus
- A/w lethal tumors in "get GINAs NUMBER" mnemonic (uveal mel, mesothelioma, RCC)
- Workup: send to **ophtho** (uveal melanoma) and get imaging for internal cancers

Recurrent melanocytic nevus

- Incomplete removal of nevi → pigment confined to the scar that arises within 6 months
  - Melanoma: pigment extending beyond the biopsy site
- Path: atypical junctional melanocytic proliferation (resembling MIS) located above a dermal scar; a benign dermal nevus is usually seen below or next to the dermal scar

Balloon cell nevus

- p/w papule indistinguishable from a normal benign melanocytic nevus
- Path: > 50% dermal melanocytes are "balloon cells" (large pale melanocytes w/ vacuolated cytoplasm); always can find conventional nevus somewhere
  - Balloon cell change is due to melanosome degeneration

Halo nevus

- p/w pigmented nevus w/ white halo around it, usually located on the back

- a/w **vitiligo (MC association)** and melanoma elsewhere (perform a good full body check)
- May be multiple due to treatment w/ infliximab
- Path: bland nevus w/ lymphocytes intertwined with melanocytes
    - o Lymphocytes mingle next to melanocytes in benign halo nevi ("cocktail party") whereas in melanoma they wall off the malignant melanocytes ("riot police")

Congenital melanocytic nevus

- **NRAS** >> BRAF mutations
- Subclassified into small (< 1.5 cm), medium (1.5 cm-19.9 cm) and large (> 20 cm) lesions
    - o Large congenital nevi (esp if multiple smaller satellites) have ↑ risk of melanoma
        - ▪ 5–10% of pts w/ large congenital nevi will develop melanoma in childhood
        - ▪ It is recommended to excise large congenital nevi after 6 months of age
    - o Large congenital nevi (LCN) in axial locations + melanocytic proliferation within brain parenchyma/leptomeninges = **Neurocutaneous melanosis** (high mortality)
        - ▪ 10–20% of pts w/ LCN will develop neurocutaneous melanosis (NCM) and 65% of these pts will have symptoms such as seizures and hydrocephalus
        - ▪ Workup: MRI of brain before 6 months of age if large congenital nevi is in posterior axial location or if there are numerous medium-sized satellites
            - RFs: > 40 cm (giant), ≥ 20 satellites but no giant (highest risk of NCM), posterior axial location → consider MRI if any RFs met

    - Do 6 month follow ups: if MRI or history/physical is positive for CNS symptoms, send to pediatric neurologist
- May display "proliferative Nodules," which mimic melanoma clinically and histologically
- May display **erosions/ulcerations** (do not biopsy unless other melanoma features exist)
- Dermoscopy: globular pattern (MC), hypertrichosis, perifollicular hypopigmentation, and diffuse monomorphous curved vessels (focal polymorphous vessels in melanoma)
- **Path: symmetrical broad proliferation of melanocytes in papillary and reticular dermis w/ maturation, splaying between collagen bundles and permeation of erector pili muscles, blood vessels, adnexal structures and nerves (this is not worrisome)**
- Rx: none (except for giant congenital nevi → excise to prevent melanoma)

Eclipse and cockade nevi

- 2 types of scalp nevi seen in children that may appear worrisome to the untrained eye
    - Eclipse nevi: tan center with a brown rim
    - Cockade nevi: pigmented center surrounded by a hypopigmented ring surrounded by a pigmented border ("bulls-eye")
- Rx: **observation** (biopsy is not indicated)

Nevus spilus

- p/w multiple pigmented macules/papules in a large tan patch in the first year of life
- a/w phakomatosis pigmentovascularis and phakomatosis pigmentokeratotica
- Ddx: agminated nevus appears in 2nd decade and lacks the homogenous tan background

Common Acquired melanocytic nevus

- **BRAF** (B next to A in alphabet) >> NRAS mutations
- Abtropfung hypothesis: nevus cells start at DEJ (junctional nevus) then descend into the dermis (compound nevus) until they are wholly intradermal (intradermal nevus)
- p/w small symmetric evenly pigmented papule (new lesions common in first 3 decades)
- Dermoscopy (helpful to compare to melanoma): typical reticular network w/ hypopigmented holes and brown lines that thin at the periphery (network is accentuated at the periphery in melanoma) w/ dots, globules and tan/dark structureless areas that are symmetrically distributed (vs asymmetric/focal in melanoma)
- Path: symmetrical and circumscribed junctional (at DEJ), compound (DEJ and dermis) or intradermal proliferations of nested nevoid cells which show maturation w/ depth
    - Type A nevus cells: epithelioid cells (large/pale) located at DEJ/superficial dermis
    - Type B nevus cells: lymphocyte-like cells (small/dark) located in the mid dermis
    - Type C nevus cells: spindled cells w/ pink cytoplasm located in the deep dermis
        - **IDN: round and well-nested epithelioid cells in superficial dermis; cells are more spindled (neuroid) and singly spaced in the deep dermis**

Acral nevi

- Dermoscopy is important while evaluating pigmented lesions on volar skin
- Melanin collects in the furrows in benign lesions as it represents preferential transfer of melanin from normal nevus cells to keratinocytes that reside in the crista limitans

- "Furrows are Fine"
- Malignant melanocytes inhabit the skin around the acrosyringium (found in the ridges)
  - "Ridges are Risky"

Dysplastic (Clark's) nevus

- Controversial term originally described in familial atypical multiple mole melanoma syndrome (AD mutation in CDKN2A tumor suppressor gene → **encodes p16 and p14**)
- While there is an ↑ risk of melanoma in individuals w/ multiple dysplastic nevi, current evidence does not support dysplastic nevus as a premalignant lesion
  - Melanoma arises de novo (MC) or from common nevi (2nd MC) or dysplastic nevi
- p/w large asymmetric nevi ("Ugly Duckling" when compared to the "signature nevi")
- Dermoscopy: asymmetric melanocytic network but not as atypical as melanoma
- Path: asymmetry, atypical nests at the junction extend > 2 rete ridges beyond dermal component, "bridging" of junctional nests, papillary dermal fibrosis, cytologic atypia
  - Graded based on degree (mild/mod/severe) of architectural and cytologic atypia
- Rx: excise lesions w/ severe atypia and observe lesions w/ mild or moderate atypia

Becker's nevus ("ABC'S")

- **Androgen (testosterone)**-mediated process
- Mutation in ACTB which encodes **β-actin**
- p/w hyperpigmented plaque w/ hypertrichosis and ipsilateral **Breast hypoplasia** in Boys
- MC on the Chest (upper torso)
- Path: ↑ basal melanocytes w/ a **Smooth muscle hamartoma** in the dermis

Melanoma (VERY HIGH YIELD!)

- Malignant tumor arising from melanocytes that leads to > 90% of all skin cancer deaths
- **Initiating oncogenic events** frequently affect genes involved in the mitogen-activated protein kinase (MAPK) and phosphoinositide 3-kinase (PI3K) pathways (BRAF, NRAS, KIT)
    - C-KIT, BRAF, MEK, ERK, NRAS: MAPK pathway: ("Crazy Brash MEN love maps k")
        - C-KIT: 2nd MC mutation overall; MC in **CSD** (LMM), acral and mucosal sites
        - BRAF (V600E > V600K): MC mutation overall and MC mutation in non-CSD sites (BRAF = "brief" sun damage); MC in **superficial spreading melanoma**
        - NRAS: 3rd MC mutation overall; a/w **Nodular mel** and CSD skin mel (LMM)
        - GNAQ/GNA11 (activates MAPK; "get GiNAs NUMBER"): Nevi (blue/spitz), Uveal mel, Mesothelioma, Malignant blue nevus, BCC, clear cell RCC
            - Concomitant BAP-1 loss in Uveal melanoma, Mesothelioma, Malignant blue nevus and clear cell RCC increases risk of death
    - PI3K-AKT pathway activates mTOR ("PAM pathway")
        - This pathway is inhibited by the PTEN tumor suppressor gene
            - "The fact that PAM's a TEN inhibits you from making a move"
- Secondary mutations include TERT promoter mutation, amplification of CCND1 (encodes cyclin D1), mutation of CDKN2A (encodes p16/p14) and mutation of TP53 (encodes p53)
    - TERT promoter mutation ↑ telomerase and are seen in > 60% of melanomas, especially in nodular

and superficial spreading variants (rare in acral lentiginous melanoma)

- CCND1/CDK4: amplifications seen in CSD sites, acral and mucosal melanomas

- A major risk factor includes genetic mutation in CDKN2A which encodes p14 and p16 (p16 is an important tumor suppressor; by binding to CDK4/6, p16 prevents the cyclin D1- CDK4/6 complex and as a result prevents RB activation and E2F release)
  - Other RFs include lightly pigmented skin, UVR, large # of nevi/ephelids/lentigos
- Subtypes
  - Superficial spreading (MC): peak onset 40–60 years; favors trunk (M) and legs (F)
    - p/w irregular dark macule (horizontal growth) → papule (vertical growth)
  - Nodular: onset around 6th decade; favors sites Near Neck (head, neck, back)
    - p/w rapidly growing dark nodule that lacks the horizontal growth phase
  - Lentigo maligna: onset 7th decade and older; favors CSD sites such as head/neck
    - p/w irregular macule (long horizontal growth phase precedes invasion)
  - Acral lentiginous: overall rare but MC type in POC (RIP Bob Marley)
    - p/w longitudinal melanonychia w/ Hutchinson sign (pigment on nail fold)
    - **Ddx: talon noir represents hemorrhage (hemoglobin) in the s. corneum**
      - **Dx/Rx: scrape or pare the hemorrhagic crust off**
  - Other subtypes (H): desmoplastic melanoma (MC on Head/neck; **S100⁺, SOX10⁺**, Melan-A⁻, HMB-45), **subungual melanoma (90% on thumb/big toe → Halux)**, mucosal melanoma (MC on the Hard

palate), spitzoid melanoma (Homozygous loss of 9p21 detected by FISH), uveal melanoma (GNAQ mutation often w/ BAP-1 loss), clear cell sarcoma (melanoma of the soft parts; HMB-45$^+$, S100$^+$, vimentin$^+$)

- Dermoscopy: blue-gray veil, pigment network abnormalities (asymmetric pseudopods, globules or structureless areas), focal polymorphous vessels and evidence of regression (> 25% of lesion has gray dots and granules which are asymmetrically located)
- Dermoscopy of lentigo maligna: annular granular structures, slate gray dots/globules, rhomboidal structures (thick pigmented lines around asymmetric follicular openings)
- Non-invasive melanoma detection techniques
  - Total body photography: high resolution images taken to compare to prior visit
    - Time-consuming so only use in high-risk pts (FAMM) or children w/ spitz
    - New images should be obtained at every FBSE and at least once a year
  - Sequential digital dermoscopic imaging: serial (q **3 months**) dermoscopic images
    - Recommended for pts w/ < 5 atypical nevi, monitoring ugly duckling, medium to giant congenital nevi or large or growing lentigo-like lesion
  - Reflectance confocal microscopy: uses probe to obtain horizontal sections at various locations from the epidermis to the papillary dermis; in melanoma we see dendritic/round pagetoid cells and atypical honeycomb/cobblestone pattern
    - Advantage: can be used to forgo a biopsy and move straight to treatment
    - Disadvanatages: expensive, slow, not widely available, cannot be used in lesions w/ exten-

sive crusting or ulceration or those on the palms/soles

- o Pigmented lesion assay (PLA): molecular diagnostic test done in office that samples skin for melanoma-specific genes (results returned in a week)
  - ▪ PLA uses PRAME and LINK genes (2-GEP); PLAplus adds TERT (3-GEP)
    - • Adding TERT ↑ sensitivity from 91% to 97% and keeps NPP > 99%
  - ▪ Advantage: can be used to forgo a biopsy and move straight to treatment
- o Myriad MyPath melanoma (23-GEP) and DecisionDx melanoma (35-GEP) are other gene expression tests but are invasive as they require a biopsy sample

- Path (**excisional biopsy** w/ 2 mm margins; shave is acceptable for superficial lesions; full-thickness incisional or punch biopsy may be acceptable on palm/sole/digit/face): asymmetry, poor circumscription, irregular nests w/ discohesion, confluent melanocytes along DEJ, pagetoid growth, epidermal consumption w/ extension down adnexa, lack of maturation of dermal component (large nests at base) w/ marked cytologic atypia
  - o Refer to pathology section for melanoma variants
- Breslow depth: **measured from the top of granular layer** to deepest point of invasion (not counting adnexal structures) rounded to the nearest 0.1 mm (vs 0.01 mm in AJCC7)
  - o Ulcerated lesions: measured from base of the ulcer to deepest point of invasion
- AJCC8 staging: AJCC always rounds down on the .0 (e.g., 1.0 mm is a T1 and 2.0 is a T2)
  - o Tumor depth (ulceration matters → add "a" if no ulceration or "b" w/ ulceration)

        - T1a/b: **≤1 mm** (T1a is ≤1 mm w/o ulceration; T1b is ≤ 1 mm w/ ulceration)
            - However, if tumor is 0.8–1 mm, even w/o ulceration it is still T1b
                - "T1a is < 0.8 ("point a-t cm") and absent ulceration"
        - T2a/b: 1.01–2 mm (T2a is w/o ulceration, T2b is w/ ulceration)
        - T3a/b: 2.01–4 mm (T3a is w/o ulceration, T3b is w/ ulceration)
        - T4a/b: > 4 mm (T4a is w/o ulceration, T4b is w/ ulceration)
    - Nodes: add "a" if clinically "accult" w/ micrometastases found on SLN; add "b" if macrometastases found clinically; add "c" if satellite lesions (< 2 cm from primary; called microsatellites if detected on path) or in-transit metastases (lesions > 2 cm from primary tumor but do not pass the draining nodal basin) are found
        - N1a/b/c: 1 node (N1c has no LNs affected but has in-transits/satellites)
        - N2a/b/c: 2–3 nodes (N2c has only 1 LN but also has in-transits/satellites)
        - N3a/b/c: ≥ 4 nodes (N3c has ≥ 2 nodes but also has in-transits/satellites)
    - Mets to "SLIC" (add "a" if **serum lactate dehydrogenase** is normal, add "b" if ↑)
        - M1a/b: distant **Skin** or SQ tissue that is further than the draining LN basin
        - M2a/b: **Lung metastasis (MC visceral metastasis)**
        - M3a/b: Internal organ excluding lung and CNS (liver is the 2nd MC)
        - M4a/b: CNS (3rd MC)
- 10-year survival based on stage (last number always ends in 7 except for stage 1B)

  - Stage 1: **1A = T1a = 97%**; **1B = T1b or T2a = 93%**
  - Stage 2: **2A = T2b or T3a = 67%**; **2B = T3b or T4a = 57%**; **2C = T4b = 47%**
  - Stage 3 is positive nodes and stage 4 is any mets
- Lymphatic metastases in melanoma (SNL+) is a/w ("Bad Young HUMAN"): Breslow depth, **Young age (< 60 y/o)**, Head/neck/acral locations, **Ulceration, Male gender**, Mitotic rate, Angiolymphatic invasion and Nodular subtype
- **S100B** is the most widely used serum marker for the detection of melanoma metastases
- Surgical margins (depth of excision is down to fascia for invasive mel and SQ for in-situ)
  - In situ: excise w/ **0.5–1 cm** margins
    - For lentigo maligna (LM) on face: MOHs and staged excision >> WLE
      - 12 mm margins needed to achieve 97% cure rate for LM on head
    - Only use MOHs for in-situ melanomas (LM) in cosmetically sensitive areas
    - Can use imiquimod or radiation for facial LMs not amenable to surgery
      - Imiquimod daily x 4 months (for BCC it is 5x a week for 6 weeks)
  - T1a/b: invasive melanoma ≤ 1.0 mm: 1 cm margins
  - T2a/b: invasive melanoma 1.1–2.0 mm: 1–2 cm ("1.1–2.0") margins
  - T3-4: invasive melanoma > 2 mm: 2 cm margins
- Workup: **consider (T1b) or offer (≥ T2a) SLNB** (no SNLB if purely desmoplastic type)
  - Local disease (stage 1/2): excision (consider RT or PD-1 for high-risk local disease)
    - Only image for specific symptoms (except stage 2B or higher where we will use imaging to screen for recurrences → see below under follow-up)

        - Pembrolizumab is FDA-approved for adjuvant treatment for stage 2B/2C
    - Regional disease (stage 3): **confirm clinically positive node w/ FNA**, **imaging** (US for lymph node mets and PET-CT for distant mets), **BRAF V600 testing**
        - Rx: **LN dissection before WLE** + systemic Rx (IL T-VEC, PD-1 or BRAF/MEK)
    - Metastatic disease (stage 4): confirm mets w/ biopsy, **LDH,** imaging, BRAF testing
        - Rx: IL T-VEC, PD-1 (alone or w/ ipilimumab or relatnimab) or BRAF/MEK
            - BRAF inh work fast (use if BRAF+ mel has symptoms/organ failure)
        - Useful in certain circumstances: entrectinib/ larotrectinib (NTRK+ tumors), binimetinib (NRAS+ tumors), imatinib (KIT+ tumors)
    - NCCN recommends using adjuvant radiation (RT) for **desmoplastic melanoma** w/ high risk features (e.g., head/neck, PNI) but not in other melanoma types
        - RT for definitive therapy is reserved for MIS in non-surgical candidates
- Rx and workup of melanoma is similar to Merkel cell (both get **surgery w/ 1–2 cm margins, SLNB and PD-1 inhibitors** for advanced disease; but Merkel cell gets radiation)
    - For both MIS and Merkel, MOHs AUC allows you to do MOHs on H and M areas
    - MOHs is not recommended for invasive melanomas
- Follow-up w/ emphasis on skin (FBSE) and LNs
    - Stage 0 (in situ): annual
    - Stage 1A-2A: q 6–12 months x 5 years; then annual (no blood work or imaging)
    - Stage 2B-4: q 3–6 months x 2 yrs; then q 3–12 months x 3 yrs; then annual

        - No routine blood tests
        - Consider imaging q 3–12 months x 2 years; then q 6–12 months x 3 years to screen for asymptomatic recurrence (as clinically indicated thereafter)
    - Palpable nodes → **FNA** w/ IHC (can consider nodal basin US first)
- Send to genetics (p16/CDKN2A/BAP-1 testing) if any of the following are met (rule of 3s)
    - Personal history of ≥ 3 invasive melanomas (one at a young age: < 45 y/o)
    - Melanoma, pancreatic cancer or astrocytoma in 3 family members on same side
    - ≥ 1 atypical BAP-1 tumors and family history of mesothelioma/uveal melanoma/meningioma or ≥ 2 atypical BAP-1 tumors
- MC site of metastasis in cutaneous melanoma is **skin** (lung is MC visceral site)

RAS-MAPK pathway

- **BRAF** (**phosphorylating** intracellular serine/threonine kinase) that with the GTPase activity of **NRAS** (**protooncogene;** GDP bound = off; GTP bound = on) leads to the phosphorylation of MEK and ERK → phosphorylated ERK activates **nuclear cyclin D1** which complexes w/ CDK4 and phosphorylates Rb → phosphorylated Rb releases the transcription factor E2F which leads to progression through the S phase of the cell-cycle
    - P16 (encoded by CDKN2A) is necessary for cell cycle arrest
    - P14 (also encoded by CDKN2A) binds to MDM2 and prevents p53 destruction

6.4 Adnexal Neoplasms and Hamartomas

Eccrine Poromas

- p/w solitary vascular-appearing papule that bleeds
- MC location is on **palms/soles** ("distal Ecc-tremities") due to highest # of eccrine glands
- Path: endophytic proliferation of epidermal "poroid cells" (**small red cuboidal cells**) with variably spaced sweat ducts throughout the epidermis and a highly vascularized stroma
    - "Looks like an SK but poroid cells are smaller than keratinocytes and it has ducts"
- Immunostains: EMA, CEA, PAS
- Poroma variants
    - Hidroacanthoma simplex (wholly intraepidermal poroma): clinically resembles SK
        - Path: nests of small poroid cells only in the epidermis
    - Dermal duct tumor (wholly dermal poroma)
        - Path: balls of poroid cells within the dermis with no epidermal connection
    - Porocarcinoma: MC sweat gland malignancy; MC on the lower extremities
        - Frequent metastasis (20% to regional LN) w/ 10% mortality
        - Path: resembles poroma but has cytologic atypia and infiltrative growth

Hidradenoma

- Benign sweat gland (apocrine MC) neoplasm that presents as a solitary cystic nodule
- MC on the upper half of the body ("hidradenoma is up high")
- **Path** ("SPoCK means your eyebrows are up high"): Squamoid cells + Poroid cells + Clear cells (any of these

3 cell types may dominate) + Cystic degeneration + Keloidal collagen

- Hidradenoma variants
  - Clear cell hidradenoma: has t(11;19) translocation; mimics metastatic RCC
  - Poroid hidradenoma and solid-cystic hidradenoma are others
  - Hidradenocarcinoma: high mortality; head/neck is MC site ("up high")
    - Path: hidradenoma but w/ cytologic atypia and lymphovascular invasion
    - Rx: MOHs > WLE

Syringoma ("syringomas are just a FAD")

- ↑ incidence in Females, Asians and in Down syndrome
- Benign sweat gland tumor which p/w skin-colored papules on **eyelids** > **cheeks** (Face)
- Eruptive syringomas: 100s of hyperpigmented papules on the **Anterior chest/neck** in AAs, Asians and in Down syndrome
- Clear cell syringoma: histologic variant with clear cells seen in patient with **Diabetes**
- Path: in paisley tie mnemonic (tie makes you think of BDSM: BCC, DTE, Syringoma, MAC)
  - Tadpole or comma-shaped sweat ducts (amorphous sweat within lumen) in a sclerotic stroma confined to the upper half of dermis (benign superficial tumor)
- Syringomatous carcinoma (rare malignant counterpart): always arises De novo

Mixed tumor (chondroid syringoma)

- p/w solitary nodule seen on the Mid-face (nose, cheek and upper lip) > other facial sites
- Middle-aged adults; M > F

- Comprised of a Mixture of epithelial (ectodermal) and stromal (mesodermal) cells
  - Epithelial component is usually eccrine/apocrine; stromal component is Myxoid
- Path: circumscribed tumor consisting of **glandular structures/ducts in a Myxoid stroma**
  - Branching (apocrine origin) and small tubular (eccrine origin) types
- **Pleo-Morphic adenoma** (Mouth variant): may see Malignant degeneration w/ Mets
  - MC salivary and parotid gland tumor
- Rx: benign; excision if nodule irritates patient
- Malignant mixed tumor arises de novo on foot; 50% metastatic rate w/ 25% mortality

Spiradenoma ("eccrine spiradenoma")

- Benign **apocrine** (despite historical name) sweat gland neoplasm
- p/w **painful** purple dermal/SQ nodule on the upper half of body (e.g., head)
- Path: large "blue ball" in the dermis w/ cystically dilated ducts and PAS+ hyaline droplets
  - 3 types of cells on high power: large pale cells + small blue cells + lymphocytes
- Brooke-Spiegler syndrome: "B and S and then following letters in alphabet (C and T)"
  - BCCs + Cylindroms + Spiradenoma + Trichoblastomas/Trichoepitheliomas
    - Ddx: more nodular than the tiny facial papules in TS, BHD and Cowden's
  - AD defect in CYLD tumor suppressor gene (normally binds NEMO of IKK complex)
    - In absence of CYLD you get ↑ NFkB signaling → resistance to apoptosis
- Spiradenocarcinoma: arises within benign spiradenoma; resembles spiradenoma but see cytologic

atypia and it loses its biphasic nature and intratumoral lymphocytes

Cylindroma

- Benign apocrine sweat gland neoplasm existing on a spectrum with spiradenoma
- p/w solitary red-purple nodule with telangiectasias on the head/neck (**scalp** is MC)
    - o May coalesce to form multinodular plaques on scalp ("turban tumor")
- Path: easily recognized by the **jigsaw pattern** of tumor lobules with ducts and biphasic cells encircled by thick hyalinized BMZ material (type 4 collagen)
- Cylindrocarcinoma (malignant counterpart): arises within a benign cylindroma (scalp)

Syringocystadenoma papilliferum (SPAP)

- Solitary warty papule/plaque on the Scalp (MC) presenting Soon after birth
- Oozes Serosanguinous fluid
- Commonly a/w a nevus Sebaceous
- Path: papillary glandular proliferation w/ decapitation secretions which opens to the Skin Surface ("looks like you can Slide in"); many plasma cells

Hidradenoma papilliferum (HPAP)

- Painless skin-colored nodule on the vulva (labia majora #1) in young adult women
    - o "Hides in the vulva because it is painless and skin colored so hard to find"
- Path: papillary glandular proliferation w/ decapitation secretions "hiding" in the dermis (lacks epidermal connection vs SPAP) w/ a "maze-like" architecture ("hide in the maze")
    - o Ddx: nipple adenoma (looks like an HPAP but it is on the nipple), apocrine cystadenoma (mix b/w

hidrocystoma and HPAP w/ papillary fronds budding into the lumen of the cyst), tubular apocrine adenoma (small cystic mazes) and aggressive digital papillary adenocarcinoma (consider if HPAP-like lesion on digit)

Papillary eccrine adenoma (PEA)

- Benign eccrine tumor on the legs ("Don't PEA on your legs") of black women ("POC")
- Path: proliferation of small round sweat ducts w/ Papillary projections in lumen
  - "Whereas HPAP is one huge maze, PEA/TAA is many tiny mazes"
- Tubular apocrine adenoma (TAA) is the apocrine variant which occurs on the scalp (a/w nevus sebaceous) and has more decapitation secretions

Syringofibroadenoma

- Sweat gland proliferation most commonly found on the legs
- Path: long thin strands of sweat duct-containing epithelium that hang down from epi
  - "Legs are also long, thin and hang down from hips"

Hidrocystoma

- p/w bluish translucent papules on the cheeks or eyelids (seen in Shopf-Schulz-Passarge)
- Path: simple cyst lined by cuboidal or columnar cells +/- decapitation secretions

Aggressive and Malignant adnexal neoplasms

- Aggressive digital papillary adenocarcinoma: aggressive malignant eccrine sweat gland tumor of the **volar digits** of middle-aged males (14% metastasize even w/ amputation)
  - Lung and LNs are MC sites of metastasis

  - o Path: looks like SPAP/HPAP due to numerous papillary projections but it is deeply infiltrative w/ ↑ mitoses and atypia (does not always look overtly malignant!)
  - o Rx: refer to surgical oncology for WLE/amputation
- Adenoid cystic carcinoma: may be primary (Scalp) or metastasize from the Salivary gland
  - o Path: "Swiss-cheese" appearance of basaloid nodules w/ mucin in the cribriform lumens extending deep into the SQ fat; 95% have **PNI/perineural Spread**
  - o IHC: c-KIT$^+$; ductal (CK7, CAM5.2) and myoepithelial (p63$^+$, SMA$^+$) components
  - o "Cystic, Scalp, Salivary gland, Swiss-cheese, and SQ all have an *S* sound"
  - o Rx: MOHs/WLE, radiation is usually given (chemo for distant metastases)
- Mucinous carcinoma: may be primary (**eyelids**; "mucin-eyes") or metastasize to the trunk
  - o Sebaceous carcinoma is also on the eyelid but are MC on the upper eyelid and in Asian populations (vs lower eyelid and AA populations in mucinous carcinoma)
  - o Path: blue tumor cells surrounded by mucin ("blue islands floating in sea of snot")
  - o Primary and metastatic look the same histologically so differentiate with stains
    - ▪ Primary Carcinomas are all Surrounded by a thin Myoepithelial layer **(p63$^+$, Calponin$^+$, SMA$^+$)**: this layer is never present in metastatic tumors
    - ▪ Primary is **CK7+**/CK20- whereas metastasis from GI tract is CK20+/CK7-
      - Breast seems to be the MC place of metastasis

        - Primary has sialomucin → alcian blue only positive at high (2.5) pH
            - "Pri has si and so only stains with alcian blue at high pH"
        - Metastatic has sulfomucin: alcian blue positive low (0.5) and high (2.5) pH
    - Rx: **MOHs** > WLE; up to 43% recur after resection; responds poorly to radiation
    - Workup: endoscopy/PET-CT of chest/abdomen/pelvis to look for visceral cancer
- Microcystic adnexal carcinoma (MAC): locally aggressive (but does not metastasize) adnexal carcinoma w/ bi-lineage differentiation (follicular and sweat gland)
    - p/w firm indurated plaque on Mid-face esp. the lip, chin or cheek ("where sauce gets when you are eating a big MAC") of Middle-aged women
    - Path: deeply infiltrative basaloid proliferation w/ **Multi-lineage differentiation** (horn cysts and sweat ducts), **peri-neural invasion and lymphoid aggregates**
    - IHC: CK7+, pan-keratin+, CEA+ (non-specific; stains do not help)
    - Rx: **MOHs** is TOC

6.5 Hair Follicle Neoplasms/Hamartomas

- "There is hair on my Filthy Toilet Paper" → Fibrofolliculoma, Trichofolliculoma, Trichoepithelioma, Trichilemmoma, Trichoadenoma, Tumor of the follicular infundibulum, Pilar sheath acanthoma, Pilomatricoma, Proliferating pilar tumor

Fibrofolliculoma

- Benign follicular hamartoma that p/w small skin-colored papules on the head/neck

- Path: central follicle w/ numerous thin strands of immature (no mature follicle/hair shafts) follicular epithelium radiating from it, embedded in a loose fibromyxoid stroma
- Acrochordons and trichodiscomas are variants
- Ddx: trichofolliculoma has the same central follicle but w/ fully formed vellus hairs (w/ fully formed hair shafts) radiating from it
- Birt-Hogg-Dubé ("FAT PORC"): AD mutation in folliculin
    - Skin: Fibrofolliculomas, Acrochordons, Trichodiscomas
    - Internal: Pneumothorax, Oncolytic renal tumors, RCC, pulmonary Cysts

Trichofolliculoma

- Benign follicular hamartoma
- p/w skin-colored papules w/ central follicular puncta from which vellus hairs emerge
- Path: dilated central follicle w/ smaller but still **fully formed vellus follicles** radiating from it ("mother and her babies")
- Ddx: fibrofolliculoma (discussed above) and pilar sheath acanthoma (**acanthotic epithelium w/o hair shafts which radiates from the dilated cystic follicle**)

Trichoepithelioma (TE)

- Benign neoplasm w/ follicular germinative differentiation
- p/w solitary or multiple dome-shaped papules w/ telangiectasias on the Central face
- Path: well-Circumscribed tumor of basaloid Cribriform nodules, **horn Cysts**, **Calcification** and papillary mesenchymal bodies in pink **Collagenous stroma** w/ stromal Clefting
- IHC: tumor is PHLDA1^{+} and CK20^{+}; stroma is CD10^{+} (vs BCC which has CD10 staining the tumor) and CD34^{+};

BCL-2 only stains periphery of tumor (vs diffuse staining in BCC)

- TrichoBlastoma is a variant that is Bigger/deeper (deep dermal/SQ vs superficial dermis)
- Ddx: BCC → basaloid nodules shows atypia, lacks cribriform/leaf-like architecture, clefs between tumor and stroma (vs stroma to stroma clefting in TE) and stroma is myxoid

Desmoplastic trichoepithelioma (DTE)

- p/w firm annular plaque w/ Central dell on the Cheek (MC) of a young adult female
- Path: well-Circumscribed superficial proliferation of thin Cords of basaloid cells in a pink Collagenous stroma w/ numerous horn Cysts and dystrophic Calcification
- IHC: same as trichoepithelioma
- Ddx (paisley tie mnemonic is BDSM): morpheaform BCC, DTE, Syringoma, and MAC

Trichilemmoma ("trichilem-mooo-ma")

- Benign neoplasm w/ follicular sheath (trichilemmal) differentiation
- p/w verrucous papules on the central face ("cows have warty upper lips and noses")
- Path: circumscribed proliferation of clear outer root sheath cells (contains glycogen) that hangs down from the epidermis (broad connection to epi) and has a peripheral palisade w/ hyalinized BMZ (PAS+) and a warty surface
- IHC: keratin^{+} and CD34^{+} (marker for ORS differentiation)
- Cowden syndrome has multiple trichilemmomas ("trichilem-mooo-mas")

Desmoplastic trichilemmoma

- p/w solitary (always) flesh-colored papule on the face

- Path: **often mistaken for invasive SCC** due to pseudo-infiltrative epithelial strands but you will see a classic trichilemmoma embedded in a sclerotic stroma off to the periphery
- IHC: same as trichilemmoma

Trichoadenoma

- Benign neoplasm of superficial (isthmus/infundibular) differentiation
- Non-specific clinical presentation
- Path: superficial dermal proliferation of keratinizing **milia-like cysts in a sclerotic stroma**

Tumor of the follicular infundibulum

- Benign neoplasm of superficial (isthmus/infundibular) differentiation
- p/w scaly plaque (resembles BCC) on the head/neck
- Path: downward epidermal proliferation of clear cells that run parallel to the epidermis

Pilar sheath acanthoma

- Commonly seen on the upper cutaneous lip
- Path: similar to a dilated pore of Winer but with thick epithelial fingers radiating from it

Pilomatricoma

- Benign neoplasm w/ follicular matrix differentiation
- Caused by mutation in CTNNB1 gene (encodes β-catenin) as is Myotonic dystrophy, Gardner's syndrome, Turners and Rubinstein-Taybi (all which get pilomatricomas)
    - o Deep penetrating nevi also have CTNNB1 mutation
- p/w solitary, firm, white-colored nodule on the cheek (MC) of a child
- Path: cystic architecture w/ "rolls and scrolls", blue matrical cells which have an abrupt transition to anucle-

ate shadow cells, granulomatous inflammation and calcification

Proliferating pilar tumor

- Benign neoplasm of superficial (isthmus/infundibular) differentiation
- Path: same "rolls and scrolls" architecture as pilomatricoma but has dense keratin instead of shadow cells and lacks basaloid matrical cells

6.6 Sebaceous Proliferations

Sebaceous hyperplasia

- p/w yellow papules w/ central dell on face (esp forehead) > upper trunk; very common
- Path: enlarged sebaceous glands w/ normal architecture (central mature white sebocytes w/ thin peripheral rim of immature basaloid seboblasts)
    - o "Almost entirely white but surrounded by thin rim of blue"
- **Fordyce spots** are large sebaceous glands on the lips or prepuce
- **Juxtaclavicular beaded lines** are large sebaceous glands in linear array on clavicle/neck

Sebaceous adenoma

- p/w small yellow papule on the head/neck
- Path: **superficial** endophytic proliferation w/ central mature sebocytes (less white and more pink/granular than in sebaceous hyperplasia) w/ thicker rim of basaloid seboblasts
    - o "In sebaceous adenoma we add some blue seboblasts to the periphery"
- MC sebaceous neoplasm a/w Muir-Torre ("Muire-Torre is more SICK"): Sebaceous neoplasms, Internal

cancer (MC is Colon) and KAs (some w/ sebaceous differentiation)

Sebaceous epithelioma (sebaceoma)

- p/w larger and deeply seated yellow papulonodule on the head/neck
- Path: purely intradermal mass comprised of **more blue seboblasts than white sebocytes**
    - "Se-blue-ceoma"

Sebaceous carcinoma (SC)

- Malignant (metastases common) sebaceous neoplasms w/ ocular and extraocular types
- Both ocular and extraocular SC p/w yellow–brown, painless, slowly enlarging nodules
- Ocular SC are located on the **eyelids** (most arise from Meibomian glands; 2–3x more common on the **upper eyelid** than lower); most extraocular SC are located on the head/neck but may arise anywhere sebaceous glands exist
- Ocular SC are more aggressive but éxtraocular SC are more a/w Muir–Torré
- Path
    - Ocular: intraepithelial spread of malignant cells in a **pagetoid pattern** w/ minimal sebaceous differentiation (need stains to identify)
        - IHC (Seb-A-ceous): **AR, Adipophilin**, CK7 > EMA, Factor XIIIa (AC-1A1)
            - "To remember CK7 I say seven in Spanish like si-A-tA not siete"
    - Extraocular: infiltrative sebaceous basaloid proliferation ("may have more white than blue or more blue than white") w/ atypia, mitoses and tumor necrosis
- Rx: MOHS w/ IHC >> WLE (0.4–1 cm) +/- radiation, exenteration, enucleation

- Prognosis: 70% 5-year survival (50% in those w/ metastatic disease)

6.7 Neural Neoplasms

- Anatomy of a nerve: Schwann cell (S100+) surrounds axon (neurofilament+) which both are surrounded by perineural cells (EMA+; "EMA is a groupie b/c she surrounds nerves")
- Neural neoplasms (M-T): Merkel cell carcinoma, MPNST, Neuroblastoma, Neurofibroma, Neurothekeoma, Nasal glioma, Perineuroma, PEN, "Qutaneous" ganglioneuroma, gRanular cell tumor, Shwannoma, Suppernumary digit, Tramatic neuroma

Merkel cell carcinoma (MCC; "Merkel will merk your Pretty ARMS")

- **Gene mutations** ("pretty ARMS"): **p63 expression (worse prognosis)**, p53 inactivation, ATOH1 transcription factor expression, RB inactivation, MYC/L-MYC expression, MDM2/MDM4 inactivation, Survivin expression (worse prognosis)
    - o **Polyomavirus Large T antigen** is integrated into genome in a truncated fashion
- Pathogenesis: Polyomavirus (**less deadly**), Age >70, UVR, Malfunctioned immune System
- Presentation ("Pretty ARMS"): Presents w/ Asymptomatic, Red nodule w/ Regional LAD (Metastasis in 40% at time of diagnosis) on Sun-exposed skin (MC on head/neck)
- Path ("Pretty ARMS"): tightly Packed and Atypical small blue cells w/ ↑N:C Ratio which exhibit nuclear Molding, numerous Mitoses and Speckled Salt and pepper chromatin

- IHC ("Merkel will merk your CNS"): **CK20 (perinuclear dot pattern; better prognosis)**, CD56, CAM5.2 and neuroendocrine markers Chromogranin, NSE and Synaptophysin
    - IHC can also detect the Merkel cell polyomavirus T antigen (CM2B4)
- DDx of malignant tumor w/ small blue cells ("MR LEMON"): Merkel cell carcinoma, Rhabdomyosarcoma, Lymphoma, Ewing sarcoma, Melanoma, Oat cell, Neuroblastoma
    - Merkel will be negative for TTF-1 (vs oat cell/small cell) and S100 (vs melanoma)
- AJCC8 staging (stage 1 is T1; stage 2A is T2-3; stage 2B is T4; stage 3 is N_{any}; stage 4 is M)
    - T1 (≤2cm), T2 (2.01–5cm), T3 (>5cm), T4 (invades fascia/muscle/cartilage/bone)
    - N1 (microscopic LN mets), N2 (in transit w/o LN mets), N3 (in transit w/ LN mets)
    - M1a (mets to distant skin/SQ/LN), M1b (met to lung), M1c (mets anywhere else)
        - Melanoma was SLIC (Skin/SQ = M1; Lung = M2; Internal = M3; CNS = M4)
- RFs: ("HILS"): Head/neck location, chronic T-cell Immunosuppression (HIV/CLL), Lympho-vascular invasion, **> 1 cm tumor (Size is the most important predictor of LN mets)**
- Labs: CBC, HIV (RFs such as immunosuppression help determine management) and quantitative baseline Merkel cell polyomavirus oncoprotein antibody serology (useful for monitoring recurrence and has been used in lieu of imaging in seropositive patients)
- Workup: imaging, FNA (clinically node+) vs SLNB (clinically node-), WLE (1–2 cm margins)
    - Local disease (stage 1 or 2): radiotherapy (RT) to excision site if any RFs are met

    - Regional disease (stage 3): RT to excision site/LN basin w/ LN dissection +/- PD1
    - Metastatic disease: **pembrolizumab/avelumab/nivolumab (PD1) + radiation** to lesion and LN basin (radiation is still used even if SLN-, as long there are ≥ 1 RFs)
- Rx ("Pretty ARMS"): Pembrolizumab/Avelumab/Retifanlimab (mets), Radiation (SNL+ or ≥1 RF), MOHs/WLE (always), **SNLB** (always perform as 30% of MCC will have +SLN)
    - The only way they do not get SLNB is if LAD is detected clinically → CT + FNA
    - Pembrolizumab is also approved for recurrent locally advanced disease
- **NCCN guidelines**: adjuvant radiation is recommended postoperatively to the excision site, in-transit tissue and draining LN basin (the only way they do not get radiation is if they have 0/4 RFs ("HILS"), SNLB was negative and margins were clear after excision)
- Follow-up: FBSE w/ LN exam every **3–6 months x 3 years** and then every 6–12 months
    - Palpable nodes → FNA w/ IHC (treat recurrence like stage 4 → surg, RT +/- PD1)
    - Imaging studies performed if clinically indicated (e.g., hepatosplenomegaly)
    - Routine imaging for high-risk patients (immunosuppressed or those w/ mets)
- Prognosis: 5-year survival is 15–55% depending on stage
    - Local disease (55%), nodal disease (35%), metastatic disease (15%)
    - Pts w/ MCC metastatic to lymph nodes w/ unknown primary tumor have 50% improved survival compared to similar staged pts w/ a known primary tumor

Malignant Peripheral Nerve Sheath Tumor (MPNST; neurofibrosarcoma)

- p/w rapidly growing nodule in a Plexiform Neurofibroma (Malignant Transformation)
- Lesions on Trunk and lesions in a/w NF1 or radiation (RT) have a worse prognosis
- Path: densely cellular (hypercellularity is more characteristic than atypia) proliferation of atypical intersecting spindle cells ("Herringbone pattern") w/ large areas of Necrosis
  - o Low power: "Marbling" due to alternating hypo- and hypercellular areas
- Rx: Surgical resection and radiation

Neuroblastoma ("NEURoB")

- N-MYC mutation on FISH is a/w a worse prognosis
- Eyes: classic presentation is raccoon eyes (periorbital darkening/purpura) from orbital metastases (75% of patients have metastasis at time of diagnosis)
- Urinary catecholamines are increased
- Retroperitoneum (adrenal glands) is MC 1° site (occurs where neural crest cells migrate)
- p/w Blue nodules on trunk and extremities (MC presentation) on a child
- Blue small cells which form a dermal/SQ nodule on path (in MR LEMON mnemonic)
- Boys > girls (2nd MC solid tumor of childhood)
- Blanches while stroked (due to catecholamine release)
  - o Color changes when stroked (LMN): Leiomyoma (pseudo-Darier's sign → red), Mastocytoma (Darier's sign → red) and Neuroblastoma (white)

Neurofibroma (NF)

- Benign proliferation of Schwann cells and other nerve components

- p/w flesh-colored soft nodule w/ "buttonhole sign" (lesion invaginates when pressed)
- Path: loose arrangement of haphazard small wavy (S-shaped) spindle cells in pale myxoid stroma; numerous mast cells
    - IHC: S100+, neurofilament+ (it is non-encapsulated/no perineurium so it's EMA-)
- When multiple, must work up for NF-1
- Plexiform neurofibroma (p/w grossly enlarged nerve growth w/ "bag of worms" feel) is pathognomonic for NF-1 and carries a 10% risk of malignant transformation into MPNST
    - Path: large fascicles of NF surrounded by perineurium; diffuse NF in background
    - IHC: S100 staining is more scattered (diffuse in NF) and EMA+ (negative in NF)
    - Rx: prevent malignant transformation to MPNST w/ selumetinib

Neurothekeoma (nerve sheath myxoma is the preferred name; myxoid neurothekeoma)

- p/w soft skin colored nodule MC on the hands/fingers of adults (think tendon sheaths)
- Path: multiple (plexiform) myxoid lobules containing bland spindle cells
    - IHC: **S100+** (unlike cellular neurothekeoma)

Cellular neurothekeoma

- Benign neoplasm which looks similar to neurothekeoma on path but is unrelated
- p/w firm pink papule on the face of young adults (F > M)
    - "Call it a cellular neuro-freak-eoma b/c it's on the face of horny young females"
- Path: multiple nests/lobules of epithelioid or spindled cells (looks like dermal Spitz)

- **IHC**: S100A6+, PGP9.5+, NK1/C3+; S100-
  - "Sell 100 A-quality Pegs to a Nice Kinky cellular neuro-freak-eoma"

Nasal glioma (Glial heterotopia)

- **Congenital nodule which presents around the nasal bridge**
- Connection w/ frontal lobe must be excluded w/ **neuroimaging studies preoperatively**
- Path: astrocytes w/ round vesicular nuclei in a loose neurofibrillary stroma
  - IHC: S100+, GFAP+

Perineuroma

- Intraneural, soft-tissue, sclerosing and cutaneous variants exist
- Path: circumscribed tumor of spindle cells w/ onion skin-like whorls
  - IHC: claudin-1+, EMA+, GLUT-1+
    - "I call it perineum to remind me that Claud is next to EMA's Glutes"
    - "The onion-skin whorls also remind me of nice round glutes"

Palisaded encapsulated neuroma (PEN)

- p/w solitary painless flesh-colored firm papule MC on the lower central **face** of adults
- Path: **superficial** dermal tumor w/ a **thin delicate capsule surrounding fascicles of spindle cells separated by clefts** (recapitulates normal nerve; Schwann cells:axons = 1:1)
  - May see **adjacent sebaceous glands and vellus hair follicles** typical of facial skin
  - Misnomer b/c it is not palisaded and there is no true capsule (vs Schwannoma)

- IHC: S100+ (stains Schwann cells), neurofilament+ (stains axons)
    - It does not have a true capsule (perineurium) so EMA is negative
- Ddx: schwannoma (deeper, palisaded and has EMA+ capsule), neurofibroma (individual cells are similar but neurofibromas are not organized into fascicles)
- **Mucosal neuromas of MEN2b look identical histologically** ("PEN rhymes w/ MEN")

Cutaneous Ganglioneuroma

- Path: localized collection of wavy Schwann cells admixed w/ large polygonal ganglion cells w/ large round nuclei (big cells hanging out in the superficial dermis in "gangs")
    - IHC: S100+ (Schwann cells), GFAP+ (ganglion cells)

Granular cell tumor ("grand-Ma")

- Neural crest (Schwann cell)-derived tumor that is MC on the anterior tongue (Mouth)
    - Mouth: presents as a firm yellow or pink, non-painful solitary nodule
    - Skin (MC head/neck): skin colored to brown-red painless slow-growing nodule
- 2% are Malignant: clinical findings a/w malignancy are rapid growth, ulceration, invasion of adjacent structures by imaging and diameter > 5 cm (5-year survival is 74%)
- Multiple granular cell tumors are seen in NF-1, Noonan and LEOPARD (MAPK pathway)
- Path: sheets of large polygonal cells w/ granular cytoplasm due to pink cytoplasmic inclusions (**Pustulo-Ovoid bodies of Milian → aggregated phagolysosomes**); overlying pseudoepitheliomatous hyperplasia (misdiagnosed as SCC on superficial shave biopsy)
    - **IHC: S100+**

- Rx: surgical excision to negative margins w/ close follow-up

Schwannoma (neurilemmoma)

- Large but benign proliferation of Schwann cells within a perineurial capsule (EMA+)
- p/w **solitary painful pink nodule MC on the flexural extremities** > head/neck
- Path: deep (arises from large SQ nerves) encapsulated proliferation of plump wavy Schwann cells w/ hypercellular (Antoni A) areas containing Verocay bodies (palisaded nuclei around acellular pink material) and hypocellular (Antoni B) myxoid areas
  - o "The Verocay bodies look like someone raked leaves (nuclei) into discrete piles"
  - o IHC: $S100^{+}$, EMA^{+}; $neurofilament^{-}$ (lacks axons vs NF, PEN, traumatic neuroma)
- Varients: bilateral vestibular schwannomas (seen in NF-2 patients) and psammomatous melanotic schwannoma (has psammoma bodies and melanin; seen in Carney's complex)

Supernumerary digit (rudimentary polydactyly)

- **Congenital papule MC on the base of the ulnar side of the 5th digit**
- Path: acral (thick stratum corneum) papule w/ nerve bundles
- Ddx: acquired digital fibrokeratoma (acral papule w/ collagen bundles on path)

Traumatic neuroma

- Reactive proliferation of nerve fibers after trauma (arise from attempted nerve revival)
- p/w painful flesh-colored firm papule or nodule MC on the extremities (trauma-prone)

- Path: like PEN, there is a haphazard proliferation of small nerve fascicles (resembles normal nerve in that Schwann cells and axons are in 1:1 ratio) separated by clefts however traumatic neuroma also has a background of scar and is not on the face
    - IHC: Like PEN and NF, traumatic neuroma is S100+ and neurofilament+

6.8 Tumors of Fat, Muscle, and Cartilage

Types of lipomas ("fatty FLAPS")

- Fibrolipoma: large collagen bundles ("fibro") + mature fat ("lipoma")
- Lipoma (ABC's): well-circumscribed tumor of mature lipocytes
    - p/w SQ nodule on the proximal Arms/legs, upper Back, Chest
    - Syndromes: Adiposis dolorosa (Dercum's), Bannayan-Riley-Revalcaba, **Benign symmetric lipomatosis (Madelung's; shows classic "horse collar" pattern of lipomas on neck)**, CLOVES syndrome, Diffuse lipomatosis, PTEN hamartoma syndrome, Familial multiple lipomatosis, Gardner's syndrome
- Angiolipoma: thrombosed capillary sized blood vessels ("angio") + mature fat ("lipoma")
    - p/w painful small SQ nodules on the Arms (forearms MC) of young adults
- Angiomyolipoma: smooth muscle coming off vessel walls ("angiomyo") + fat ("lipoma")
- Pleomorphic lipoma: **multinucleate floret cells** (overlapping nuclei arranged at the periphery like petals of a flower) + myxoid areas + ropey collagen bundles + mature fat

  - p/w firm, SQ nodule on the Posterior neck of adult males
- Spindle cell lipoma (like pleomorphic lipoma w/o the floret cells): myxoid areas + ropey collagen bundles + mature fat ("I call it a ropey myxoid spindle cell lipoma to remind me of the ropey collagen in a myxoid stroma with surrounding spindle cells and lipocytes")
  - p/w firm, SQ nodule on the **Shoulder and upper back** of adult males
  - Spindle cells stain positive for CD34

Hibernoma
- Shows differentiation towards brown (fetal) fat
- Occur anywhere in a fetus; arise MC on shoulder girdle, posterior neck or axilla in adults
- Path: multivacuolated "mulberry cells" admixed w/ normal appearing lipocytes

Well-differentiated liposarcoma (atypical lipomatous tumor)
- **MDM2 amplification**; rare in skin (usually involves deep soft tissue/retroperitoneum)
- Path: mix of mature fat and fibrous bands w/ atypical stromal cells +/- lipoblasts
- Myxoid/round cell liposarcoma is a rare variant w/ "chicken-wire" vessels on path

Smooth muscle neoplasms

Pilar leiomyoma (piloleiomyoma)
- Benign proliferation of smooth muscle arising from erector Pili
- p/w multiple **Painful**, firm, red-brown Papules on the **legs** (MC) in young adults
- Pseudo-Darier's sign: stroking → becomes red/painful from smooth muscle contraction

- Path: circumscribed but non-encapsulated (ill-defined) dermal nodule of intersecting bundles of smooth muscle cells (spindle cells w/ bright Pink cytoplasm and cigar-shaped nuclei w/ Perinuclear vacuole containing glycogen which muscle cell uses as energy)
    - IHC for smooth muscle: Caldesmon+, Calponin+, Desmin+, SMA+
        - "When you lie down (leiomyoma) you want to listen to smooth CD'S"
- Rx (CD'S): CO_2 laser for removal; CCB (nifedipine), anti-Depressants/gabapentin and Dysport (intralesional botulinum toxin) for pain; Surgical removal if solitary
- a/w Reed syndrome: AD mutation in fumarate hydratase which p/w multiple cutaneous and uterine leiomyomas; patients are at risk for **RCCs (workup: abdominal CT)**

Genital leiomyoma

- Benign proliferation of smooth muscle arising from smooth muscle in the genital region
- p/w painless solitary lesion on the vulva, scrotum or areola
- Path: similar to pilar leiomyoma but often larger and even less circumscribed

Angio-leiomyoma

- Benign proliferation of smooth muscle arising from muscular walls of SQ vessels
- p/w **painful** slowly enlarging papule or nodule on the **leg** of a middle-aged women
- Path: deep (SQ) nodule of smooth muscle containing slit-like vascular spaces
- IHC: same as leiomyoma ("CD'S") except desmin is often negative

  - DESMIN: Doesn't Emphasize Smooth Muscle that is Intra- or perivascular
- Rx: local excision

Painful tumors ("BLEND AN EGG")
Blue rubber blebs, Leiomyoma, Eccrine spiradenoma, Neuroma, Dermatofibroma, Angiolipoma, Neurilemoma, Endometrioma, Glomus tumor, Granular cell tumor

Leiomyosarcoma

- Malignant neoplasm arising from erector pili or genital smooth muscle; good prognosis
- Divided into dermal (10% risk of metastasis) and SQ (30% risk of metastasis) variants
- p/w red-brown nodules or plaques MC on the extremities of middle-aged males
- Path: resembles leiomyoma but w/ ↑ cellularity, atypia, pleomorphism and mitoses
  - IHC (CD'S): Desmin+, SMA+
- Rx: MOHs vs excision w/ 1–2 cm margins

Smooth muscle hamartoma

- Most are congenital plaques of the lumbosacral area or proximal extremity
- Becker's nevus has smooth muscle hamartoma + hypertrichosis + hyperpigmentation
- Path: numerous haphazard bundles of smooth muscle in the dermis

Chondroma

- Most commonly present on fingers of middle-aged adults
- Path: circumscribed mass of mature cartilage (w/ many lacunae)

Chordoma

- Tumors originating from a remnant of the notochord and are thus typically seen along the axial spine (especially the sacrococcygeal area)
- Path: physaliphorus cells (abundant pale bubbly cytoplasm) making up large nodules which are separated by fibrous bands
    - o IHC: triple positivity w/ vimentin, S100, and keratin

6.9 Hematolymphoid Neoplasms

- Workup for CTCL and CBCL includes PE (%BSA and LN exam), skin biopsy (immunostains w/ CD3 -4, 5, -7, -8, -30, -20, -79a and T-cell receptor rearrangement), CBC, BNP w/ LDH, flow cytometry for Sézary cells, PET/CT and excisional LN biopsy for LNs > 1.5 cm
    - o Preferred biopsy is a broad shave for CTCL and a deep incisional biopsy for CBCL
- Molecular assays (Southern blot/PCR), MicroRNA or qRT-PCR determines T-cell subtype
- Analysis of T-cell receptor by PCR or **high-throughput sequencing** determines clonality

Mycosis fungoides

- Malignancy of skin resident memory T-cells
- Accounts for half of all primary cutaneous lymphomas
- Progresses through patch (annular papulosquamous lesions in **non-sun-exposed skin**), plaque (violaceous plaques) and tumor (enlarging nodules w/ ulceration) stages
    - o **Lesions exhibit various shades of pigment in black skin, but the asymmetry of lesions (vs psoriasis) and sharply angulated shapes are very characteristic**

- Path (broad shave): lichenoid band w/ epidermotropism of lymphocytes (absent in tumor stage) in clusters (Pautrier's microabscesses) and lined up at the DEJ
  - In tumor stage may see large cell transformation w/ $CD30^+$ cells (poor prognosis)
- Immunophenotyping can detect abnormal phenotypes
  - **$CD3^+/CD4^+/CD8^-$ with loss of CD7 is MC** (CD5 and CD2 loss is more specific)
  - Ratio of CD4 to CD8 cells ↑ as MF progresses (about 4:1; normal skin is 1:1)
- T-cell gene rearrangement is used to determine clonality (normally there is a diverse population of T-cells which enables the adaptive immune system to respond to a broad variety of antigens but in MF there is generally a single malignant T-cell clone)
- MF can undergo large cell transformation (bad prognostic sign) defined as > 25% of cells are neoplastic T-cells that are at least 4 times the size of a normal lymphocyte
- Clinical variants ("Granny's Foll Paralyzed her Hyp")
  - Granulomatous slack skin: p/w sagging skin in the Groin/axilla w/ multinucleate giant cells and elastophagocytosis on path; indolent course/good prognosis; 30% develop **Hodgkin's lymphoma** ("clinically they really do resemble a Giant Hog")
  - Folliculotropic MF: MC MF variant; p/w KP-like lesions on the trunk/extremity (better prognosis) or alopecia on the head/neck area (worse prognosis); **path shows follicular mucinosis and atypical lymphocytes in the follicular epithelium** (typical MF phenotype); **worse prognosis** due to ↑ depth of atypical cells
    - Alopecia mucinosa p/w pink or hypopigmented plaques w/ follicular prominence and

alopecia on the face/scalp and is a/w folliculotropic MF

- Pagetoid reticulosis: p/w solitary **Psoriasiform Plaques on the distal extremities**; Prominent epidermotropism in a Pagetoid pattern on path; great prognosis; may express an atypical phenotype ($CD3^+/CD4^-/CD8^+/CD30^+$) or typical MF phenotype
- Hypopigmented MF: MC variant in kids and AAs; p/w hypopigmented plaques in AA patients; cellular phenotype is $CD3^+$/**$CD4^-/CD8^+$** (atypical MF phenotype)
- Less common variants include poikilodermic MF, hyperpigmented MF, Pustular MF (MC on Palms), bullous MF, hyperkeratotic/vegetating MF (resembles AN)

- **Staging of cutaneous T-cell lymphoma**
  - Stage 1A: < 10% of skin is covered; no blood, LN or internal organ involvement
  - Stage 1B: **≥ 10%** of skin is covered; no blood, LN or internal organ involvement
    - Notice how 10% is the cutoff for stage 1 (10% or more of BSA is stage 1B)
  - Stage 2A: **LNs are clinically enlarged** ("2A clinically has LAD")
  - Stage 2B: **tumors** on skin ≥ 1 cm in depth ("2B clinically has tumors/2-mors")
  - Stage 3: nearly all of skin is reddened ("ery-three-derma")
  - Stage 4A1: cancer is found in the blood (Sézary syndrome)
  - Stage 4A2: cancer is found in the LNs
  - Stage 4B: cancer has spread to internal organs (histologically proven lymphoma)
- Rx (close to MF in alphabet): **Mogamulizumab** (Ab against **CCR4** → SE is head/neck rash that looks like worsening of disease), topical Nitrogen mustard, NFkB

inhibitor (bortezomib), Nemolizumab (IL-31; for pruritis), Pentostatin (IL-12; adenosine deaminase inhibitor), Phototherapy, Retinoids (bexarotene), Romidepsin, Radiotherapy, topical/IL Steroids, Total skin electron beam, **Vorinostat** (histone deacetylase inhibitor)

- Stage 1A-2A (patches/plaques): topicals (CS, mechlorethamine, retinoids), PUVA, radiation w/ total dose of 10–36 grays in fractions of 1.5–2 grays over 8–10 weeks
    - NCCN: **total skin electron beam** is radiation of choice (use TSEB for CTCL)
- Stage 3 (Erythroderma): Extracorporeal photopheresis
- Systemic disease: multiagent therapy including biologics or CHOP chemotherapy
- Relapsed/refractory: histone deacetylase inhibitors (vorinostat, romidepsin, depsipeptide, panobinostat), IFN-α injections, oral bexarotene, mogamulizumab
    - Multimodality therapy: we add new therapies on, we do not take away

- Prognosis: 5-year disease specific survival for stage 1A is 99%, 1B is > 90%, 2A is 80%, 2B (tumors) is 60%, 4A is 50%; follicular MF has a 5-year survival of 70 to 80% (better than tumor but worse than patch/plaque); pagetoid reticulosis has a normal 5-year survival

Sézary syndrome

- p/w triad of Sézary cells in the skin/blood/LNs, pruritic érythroderma and adenopathy
    - Must demonstrate T-cell clone in the blood and Sézary cell count > 1000 cells/mcl or immunophenotypical abnormalities (e.g., **CD4:CD8 ratio > 10:1**)
- Cellular phenotype: MF phenotype w/ Programmed Death-1 (PD-1/CD279) gain

- Workup: CBC, skin biopsy w/TCR gene analysis (peripheral blood can also be sent for TCR gene analysis) and buffy coat smear w/ Sézary cell count, LN biopsy if pt has LAD
- Immunophenotype of circulating atypical lymphocytes: $CD4^+$, $CCR4^+$, $CCR7^+$, L-$Selectin^+$
  - CCR7: used by circulating T-cells to hone to organs (so + in Sezary but not in MF)
- Rx: Same as MF, éxtracorporeal photopheresis, alemtuzumab (depletes $CD52^+$ central memory B- and T-cells from blood; does not work in MF because that is a disease of skin resident memory T cells, not central memory T-cells like in Sézary/leukemic CTCL)
- Prognosis: 5-year survival is 25% (most die from infection 2° to immunosuppression)

Adult T-cell leukemia/lymphoma (ATLL)

- a/w HTLV-1 virus (endemic in Japan, Caribbean and central Africa)
- p/w leukemia, LAD, organomegaly, osteolytic bone lesions, skin lesions, **hypercalcemia**
  - Hypercalcemic ASS: ATLL, Sarcoidosis, Subcutaneous fat necrosis of the newborn
- Path: resembles MF but with "floret" malignant T-cells (multi-lobed nuclei)
- Cellular phenotype: MF phenotype w/ **$CD25^+$ cells** ("You are an adult when you are 25")

Lymphomatoid papulosis (LyP)

- $CD30^+$ indolent lymphoma which p/w recurrent crops of papulonecrotic lesions in various stages of evolution that resolve and heals w/ atrophic varioliform scars
  - Similar presentation as PLEVA but occurs in adults in 40s instead of children
- Path ("My Ana is aggressive and a little Extra")

- Type A (typical LyP): wedge-shaped dermal infiltrate w/ lymphocytes, neutrophils, **eosinophils** and large CD30$^+$ (Ki-1) Reed-Sternberg-like cells
  - Resembles PLEVA but PLEVA never has large CD30$^+$ cells or eosinophils
- Type B (Mycosis fungoides-like): epidermotropic infiltrate of CD30 negative cells
- Type C (Anaplastic large cell lymphoma-like): diffuse sheets of large, atypical CD30+ Reed-Sternberg-like cells in dermis
- Type D (primary cutaneous aggressive epidermotropic CD8$^+$ cytotoxic T-cell lymphoma-like): markedly epidermotropic CD8$^+$/CD30$^+$/TIA-1$^+$/granzyme B$^+$ cells
- Type E (extranodal NK/T-cell lymphoma-like): angioinvasive CD30$^+$/β F-1$^+$ cells

- 50% demonstrate clonality via T-cell gene rearrangement (clonality not a/w severity)
- Rx: **MTX** (improves ulcers and scars but does not prevent secondary lymphomas)
- Mnemonic (Lymphomatoid papulosis): Large CD30 cells on path; MC associated lymphoma is MF (ATLL is 2nd MC; Hodgkin lymphoma is MC systemic lymphoma); **MTX is TOC**; p/w Papulonecrotic PLEVA-like lesions
- Prognosis: > 98% survival but 20% have an associated lymphoma (**MF** is MC)

Dermatologic conditions with CD30$^+$ (Ki-1; Ber H2) cells: "30-year-old MALE"
MF tumor stage (some), Anaplastic large cell lymphoma, LyP, Exaggerated bug bite reaction

*Brentuximab vedotin: selectively targets tumor cells expressing CD30 ("Brent is a 30-year-old Male")

Primary cutaneous anaplastic large cell lymphoma (ALCL)

- Large ulcerated tumor (solitary > multiple) in adults which do not come and go like LyP

- Path: diffuse sheets of large, atypical $CD4^+$ > $CD30^+$ cells in the dermis +/- Hallmark (horseshoe) cells → large atypical T-cells w/ a horseshoe-shaped nucleus
- Primary cutaneous ALCL: no chromosomal translocation t(2;5) → **(-) ALK expression**
    - Primary cutaneous Anaplastic large cell lymphoma: ALK Negative
- Systemic anaplastic large cell: chromosomal translocation t(2;5) → (+) ALK expression
    - "Ana is systemically large, she weighs 2 to 5 tuns, that's A Lot of Kilos"
- Rx:
    - Solitary or localized: surgery or radiotherapy
    - Multifocal/refractory: **brentuximab vedotin** ("Ana loves Brent")
- Good prognosis (> **90% 5-year survival**)

Primary cutaneous aggressive epidermotropic CD8+ cytotoxic T-cell lymphoma

- p/w rapidly progressive papules, plaques and nodules that **ulcerate** → usually fatal
- Path (looks like MF): markedly epidermotropic $CD8^+$/β F-1^+/TIA-1^+/granzyme B^+ cells
- Prognosis: median survival is 32 months (metastases common)

Extranodal NK/T-cell lymphoma

- p/w eruptive ulcerated tumors in the nose
- Path: angioinvasive/angiodestructive **EBV^+ ($EBER^+$)**, $CD2^+$, $CD3^+$, **$CD56^+$** cells
- Rx: combined/sequential chemotherapy and radiation

Subcutaneous panniculitis-like T-cell lymphoma (SPLTCL)

- Can occur in children or adults (20% occur in those under 20 years of age)

- p/w SQ nodules **legs** (MC), arms and trunk +/- β-symptoms (fever/night sweats)
    - o 20% can p/w hemophagocytic syndrome: macrophage activation → fever, splenomegaly, cytophagocytosis, cytopenias, ↑ ferritin, ↑ IL-2 receptor
- Path: lobular panniculitis-like (**SQ**) infiltrate of neoplastic **CD8**$^{+}$, β F-1^{+}, TIA1^{+}/Granzyme B^{+} (cytotoxic phenotype) T-cells w/ an **α/β phenotype**; cytophagocytosis (beanbag cells)
    - o "Sharing a bean-bag with 8 βest Friends is toxic (cytotoxic phenotype)"
- Rx: **prednisone**, cyclosporine or other immunosuppressives (chemotherapy if severe)
- Prognosis: **80–90% 5-year survival**

Primary cutaneous γ/δ T-cell lymphoma

- p/w multiple eroded/ulcerated nodules and plaques → rapidly fatal
- Path: **SQ, dermal and epidermotropic CD56**$^{+}$, CD4^{-}/CD8^{-} (double negative), TIA-1^{+}/granzyme B^{+}/perforin^{+} (cytotoxic) T-cells w/ a **γ/δ T-cell phenotype** (TCRγ1^{+})
    - o Lichenoid interface change is a major histologic clue
        - ▪ "56 doubly negative and toxic people is something I do not like"
    - o Atypical cells are in the SQ, dermis and epidermis (vs SQ only in SPLTCL)
- Rx: **chemotherapy w/ CHOP**
- **Poor prognosis: < 20% 5-year survival**

Primary cutaneous CD4-positive small/medium pleomorphic T-cell lymphoproliferative disorder

- p/w solitary plaque or nodule on the head/neck
- Path: dense dermal/SQ infiltrate of small/medium lymphocytes w/ Grenz zone and no epidermotropism

(looks like a B-cell lymphoma on path but with T-cell phenotype)

- Rx: skin directed therapies such as surgical excision or topical/IL steroids
- Excellent prognosis

Leukemia cutis

- Myelomonocytic and Monocytic types of leukemia most commonly produce skin lesions
    - o Skin lesions are firm red-brown papules/nodules MC on the head, neck and trunk
        - ▪ Skin lesions in ALL, CLL or AML just p/w ecchymosis due to ↓ platelets
- Myeloperoxidase (**MPO**), **CD43** and Mast cell stains (**CD117/c-KIT**, **Leder**) are positive
    - o Negative for T (CD3) and B (CD20) cell markers
    - o **MPO activity is what gives chloromas their green color**
- **Indian filing** (infiltrative cords) of myeloid blasts with a Grenz zone is seen on path
- Rx: address underlying systemic leukemia (chemotherapy)

c-KIT positive tumors: "bad kitty" → MAL means bad in Spanish
Melanoma, Mastocytosis, Adenoid cystic carcinoma, Leukemia cutis

Primary cutaneous B-cell neoplasms

- **CD20**$^+$**/CD79a**$^+$ tumors w/ Grenz zones (vs epidermotropic in T-cell lymphomas)
- The high-yield ones can be remembered by the mnemonic "Full MIL" (as the mnemonic progresses, the entities go from more common to less common, the MC location goes from superior to inferior and the prognosis gets worse; interestingly, even when the indolent Follicle cell lymphoma presents on the leg, it portends a worse prognosis)

- Follicle center cell lymphoma: p/w solitary violaceous nodule on scalp/forehead
  - Path: irregular neoplastic follicles which lack follicle polarity, lacks a well-defined mantle zone, lacks tingible body macrophages and lacks t(14;18) translocation (vs systemic follicular lymphoma); **BCL-6$^+$**/BCL-2$^-$
    - Secondary cutaneous involvement by nodal (systemic) follicle center cell lymphoma is usually **BCL-6$^+$/BCL-2$^+$** but this is not reliable and the only way to rule out systemic lymphoma is PET-CT
  - **Excellent prognosis (5-year survival close to 100%)**
  - Rx: solitary (excision or **radiation**), disseminated (rituximab)
- Marginal zone lymphoma: p/w purple nodule on the upper extremity/trunk
  - Path: "inverse" pattern of central darker benign reactive lymphocytes w/ surrounding neoplastic Monocytoid B-cells (marginal zone cells) and numerous plasma cells, some w/ Dutcher bodies (internuclear immunoglobin deposits); BCL-6$^-$/**BCL-2$^+$**
    - Mantle cell lymphoma is also BCL-6$^-$/**BCL-2$^+$** but is **cyclin D1$^+$** also
  - **Excellent prognosis (5-year survival close to 100%)**
  - Rx: may self-resolve; radiotherapy, excision and rituximab are options
- Intravascular B-cell lymphoma: p/w purple patches/plaques on the trunk/thighs
  - CNS involvement common ("In the brain")
  - Path: large, atypical B-cells within vessels; CD20$^+$, CD79a$^+$
  - Poor prognosis

    - Rx: rituximab + chemo (intrathecally if CNS involved)
  - Diffuse Large B-cell lymphoma: p/w red/brown nodule on Leg of elderly female
    - Path: dense infiltrate of Large atypical cells; **MUM**$^+$/BCL2$^+$/BCL6$^+$/FOXP1$^+$
      - "Your MUM (mom) is quite large"
    - Poor prognosis (50% 5-year survival)
    - Rx: **rituximab** + anthracycline-based chemo is usually helpful

Pseudo-lymphoma

- Environmental trigger results in an aberrant proliferation of polyclonal B-/T-cells
- p/w solitary/multiple grouped plum-colored plaques/nodules on upper half of body
- Path
  - T-cell pseudo-lymphoma: resembles MF but cells are polyclonal
  - B-cell pseudo-lymphoma ("My B"): polyclonal Mixed dermal infiltrate w/ Grenz zone; dermal infiltrate organized into large follicles w/ pale germinal centers containing tingible body Macrophages and a Mantel zone
    - Mixture of kappa and lamda seen on IHC
- Common triggers: TALTZ and methotrexate
  - Tattoo reaction, Arthropod bite, Anticonvulsants, ARBs, ...azines, Antibiotics, Lyme disease, TMP-SMX, Zoster
  - MTX: can occur due to EBV in RA patients taking methotrexate
- Rx: self-resolves w/ discontinuation of drug

6.10 Fibrohistiocytc Neoplasms

"JACK F***ING DIES and the Police Department is PAGED Fast"

- Benign (JACK F***ING DIES): Juvenile hyaline fibromatosis, Angiofibroma, multinucleate cell Angiohistiocytoma, Adult myofibroma, Acquired digital fibrokeratoma, Calcifying aponeurotic fibroma, Keloid/scar, Fibromatosis, Fibrous hamartoma of infancy, pleomorphic Fibroma, Infantile myofibromatosis, Nodular fasciitis, Giant cell tumor of the tendon sheath, Dermatofibroma, Dermatomyofibroma, Infantile digital fibroma, Elastofibroma dorsi, Epithelioid cell histiocytoma, and Sclerotic fibroma
- Borderline (Police Department): Plexiform fibrohistiocytic tumor, and Desmoid tumor
- Malignant (PAGED Fast): Pleomorphic undifferentiated sarcoma, AFX, Giant cell fibroblastoma, Epithelioid sarcoma, DFSP, and Fibrosarcoma

Benign fibrohistiocytic neoplasms:
(JACK F***ING DIES)

Juvenile hyaline fibromatosis

- AR mutation in CMG2 ("Can't Move Good") or ANTRX2
- p/w nodular lesions on the head/neck/hands, gingival hypertrophy, joint contractures, and osteolytic lesions on terminal phalanges and long bones in early childhood
- Path: abundant pink amorphous PAS+ and Alcian blue+ hyaline material in the dermis
- Rx: no treatment; patients become bedridden and die young

Angiofibroma (fibrous papule)

- Variants

  - o Fibrous papule: solitary dome-shaped papule on the face (esp nose) of adults
  - o Pearly penile papules: aggregated pearly papules on the glans penis
  - o Multiple facial (adenoma sebaceum) and periungual fibromas (Koenen's periungual fibroma) are seen in tuberous sclerosis
  - o Multiple facial angiofibromas are also seen in MEN-1, Birt-Hogg-Dubé and NF-2
- Path: dermal proliferation of stellate factor 13a+ fibroblasts w/ concentric perivascular fibrosis and ectatic thin-walled vessels

Multinucleate cell angiohistiocytoma

- p/w Multiple **grouped violaceous papules on acral surfaces**
- Path: proliferation of small vessels surrounded by fibroblast-like spindle cells in a collagenous stroma (just like angiofibroma) but unlike angiofibroma it also contains **bizarre, angulated Multinucleated giant cells**

Adult myofibroma

- p/w solitary nodule MC on the head/neck
- Path: peripheral fibrovascular proliferation w/ myofibroblasts, staghorn vessels and **large nodules w/ a blue hue ("Adult myofi-blue-ma")**
  - o IHC: SMA+

Acquired digital fibrokeratoma (acral fibrokeratoma)

- p/w asymptomatic exophytic keratotic papule w/ surrounding collarette on the digit (finger or toe), nail bed or periungual area of a middle-aged adult (M > F)
- Path: compact hyperkeratosis and acanthosis w/ vertical collagen bundles in the dermis; no nerves (vs supernumerary digit)

- Rx: tumor is benign but if treatment is requested shave removal is TOC

Ddx for fibrotic tumor on the finger: "Jen Psaki's (GEN PSAKI) finger"
Giant cell tumor of the tendon sheath: firm SQ nodule on the finger of adult females
Epithelioid sarcoma: firm SQ nodule on the fingers > hands of a young adult
Nerve sheath myxoma (myxoid neurothekeoma): skin colored nodule on the fingers of adults
Palmar fibromatosis (Dupuytren's): firm fibrotic mass on base of finger of adult men
Supernumerary digit: fibrotic papule on the ulnar side of the 5th digit of a newborn
Acquired digital fibrokeratoma: keratotic papule w/ surrounding collarette on finger of adults
Keonen tumor (periungual fibroma): fibrotic papule next to toenails > fingernails of children
Infantile digital fibroma (inclusion body fibromatosis): firm papules on dorsal digit of infants

Calcifying aponeurotic fibroma

- Soft tissue tumor that occurs on the distal extremities (esp. palms/soles) of teenagers
- Path: plump epithelioid fibroblasts palisading around foci of **cartilage or calcification** w/ or w/o osteoclast-like giant cells

Keloid/hypertrophic scar/scar

- Discussed in section 3.5

Fibromatosis

- Superficial variants (Ps)
  - o Palmar (Dupuytren's): thickened fibrotic band (MC on the MCP of 4th finger)
    - Occurs in middle-aged men w/ a history of alcohol and tobacco use

  - Plantar (Ledderhose): overgrowth of fascia on the sole of the foot (arch MC)
  - Penile (Peyronie's): abnormal upward curvature of the penis
- Deep variants such as desmoid tumor (discussed later) have ↑ morbidity and mortality
- Path: deep proliferation of extremely long fascicles of corkscrew-shaped myofibroblasts
  - IHC: vimentin+, SMA+
- Rx: collagenase clostridium histolyticum injection; excision + fasciotomy is TOC

Fibrous hamartoma of infancy

- p/w painless solitary nodule/plaque MC on the trunk or proximal arms in infants (M > F)
- Path: triphasic proliferation of 3 tissue types
  - Fibroblast cells consisting of plump spindle cells in Fascicles: Actin+
  - Myxoid Mesenchymal cells (immature): Vimentin+
  - Adipose cells (mature): S100+
- Rx: surgical excision is TOC

Pleomorphic fibroma

- p/w pedunculated papules on extremities of adults; clinically resembles skin tags
- Path: looks similar to skin tags but w/ hyperchromatic, bizarre, multinucleated cells

Infantile myofibromatosis

- p/w solitary (70%) pink-violaceous dermal/SQ nodules on the head/neck (50%) occurring in the first 2 years of life (60% at birth); F > M; MC fibromatosis in children
  - Superficial disease has a great prognosis but visceral involvement may be fatal
- Path: same path as in fibromatosis (SMA+ "tram track" due to myofibroblasts)

- Rx: tends to regress spontaneously; surgery if vital organs are affected

Nodular fasciitis ("Nodu-LARR")

- Self-Limited lesion that presents MC on the Arms (upper extremities MC site overall; head/neck MC site in kids); Rapidly growing (1–5 cm); Reactive condition
- MYH9-USP6 fusion gene which can be confirmed by FISH, PCR or RNA sequencing
- Path: **Large pleomorphic fibroblasts in a Loose myxoid stroma ("tissue culture look"), Aggregates of lymphs, RBC extravasation**; late lesions show Red thick collagen bundles
    - o Spindle cells show frequent mitoses ("pseudo-sarcoma") but none are atypical
- Rx: surgical excision

Giant cell tumor of the tendon sheath (F next to G in alphabet)

- Soft tissue tumor MC found attached to the Flexor surface of the tendons of the **Fingers** (esp DIP) > hands, wrists, ankle, foot
- p/w Firm, painless, gradually enlarging soft-tissue swelling in middle-aged adults (F > M)
- Path: well-circumscribed deep tumor composed of plump Fibroblasts, Foamy macrophages, hemosiderin (Fe) in a Fibrous pseudo-capsule; **osteoclast-like Giant cells**
    - o Only testable neoplasm w/ osteoclast-like giant cells
- Fibroma of the tendon sheath is a variant without the giant cells
- Rx: surgical excision is TOC but recurrences are common

Dermatofibroma (DF; histiocytoma)

- Common benign neoplasm composed of collagen, histiocytes, capillaries and fibroblasts

- p/w firm skin-colored or pigmented papules (MC on the legs of females) w/ positive "dimple sign" (moves downward when pinched as lesion is attached to underlying fat)
- Multiple eruptive DFs occur in the setting of HIV, AICTD (esp SLE) and neoplastic disease
  - Get ANA and HIV test
- Path (DF'S): Dermal spindle cell proliferation w/ collagen trapping towards the periphery under a thickened epidermis w/ Folliculo-sebaceous induction and basal hyperpigmentation; when present, ringed lipidized Siderophages are pathognomonic (Touton giant cells w/ lipid and hemosiderin peripheral to the ring of nuclei)
  - IHC (DF'S): D2-40, Factor 13a, Stromelysin-3
- To compare w/ DFSP, DFSP are not just Dermal but they infiltrate the SQ (DF only flirts w/ upper part of fat but never penetrates deeply), they rarely show Folliculo-sebaceous induction or collagen trapping and they do not have lipidized Siderophages
  - IHC: DFSPs are (-) for D2-40, Factor 13a and Stromelysin-3 but (+) for CD34
- Histologic DF variants ("We see a dimple sign b/c DFs CLAMP Hard onto Fat")
  - Cellular DF: ↑ cellularity (confused w/ DFSP)
  - Lipidized (xanthomatous) DF: ↑ lipidized siderophages (confused w/ xanthoma)
  - Aneurismal DF: large cavernous vascular spaces (confused w/ vascular lesions)
  - Multinucleate cell angiohistiocytoma: multinucleated giant cells w/ multiple dilated vessels in the dermis (unclear histo-etiology but stains like DF)
    - p/w grouped violaceous papules/plaques on dorsal hands of old females
  - DF w/ Monster cells: large, pleomorphic cells w/ prominent nucleoli (benign)

  - Hemosiderotic DF: prominent hemosiderin and small blood vessels
  - Fibrous histiocytoma: ↑ histiocytic cells but lacks typical DF architecture
- Rx: treatment is not necessary unless symptomatic but excision is curative

Dermatomyofibroma

- p/w solitary 1–2 cm plaque MC on the upper trunk/neck of young adults (F > M)
- **Path: spindle cell proliferation w/ east-west orientation which respects adnexa**
  - IHC: SMA+ tram track (derived from myofibroblasts); CD34 (-) distinguishes from DPSP, S100 (-) from NF, factor 13a (-) from DF, desmin (-) from leiomyoma

Infantile digital fibroma (Inclusion body fibromatosis; aggressive digital fibromatosis)

- p/w **multiple firm, smooth, skin-colored papules on the dorsolateral fingers** > toes (spares thumb and first toe) in infants < 1 year of age
- Path: entire ("intire") dermis is filled w/ intersecting fascicles of plump spindle cells which contain pink-red inclusion bodies which stain **red w/ trichrome, purple w/ PTAH** (phosphotungstic acid hematoxillin) and bright red w/ lendrum phloxine tartrazine
  - IHC: inclusions have **actin** filaments (Smooth Muscle Actin$^+$, calponin$^+$, desmin$^+$)
- Rx: **observe** as spontaneous regression is typical and 50% recurrence rate after excision

Elastofibroma dorsi

- p/w pain and prominence of the **periscapular region** in middle-aged adult females

- **Path: large fibrous tumor w/ beaded elastic fibers visible on Verhoeff-van Gieson**

Epithelioid cell histiocytoma (epithelioid fibrous histiocytoma)

- p/w solitary pyogenic-granuloma-like papule MC on the **thighs** of adult women
- Path: well-circumscribed dermal proliferation of epithelioid cells (resembles spitz nevus) w/ epidermal collarette and dermal sclerosis
    - IHC: stains like DF'S (D2-40, Factor 13a, Stromelysin-3) but w/ **ALK-1 translocation** (like metastatic anaplastic large cell lymphoma)

Sclerotic fibroma

- p/w firm pearly papule
- a/w **Cowden's** syndrome
- **Path**: sclerotic collagen bundles in a plywood pattern resembling van Gogh's Starry night
    - IHC: CD34+, vimentin+ (fibroblasts), SMA+

Borderline tumors/intermediate malignancy: (Police Department)

Plexiform fibrohistiocytic tumor

- p/w slow growing painless mass MC on upper limbs of children
- Path: poorly demarcated dermal or SQ mass w/ multinodular plexiform fascicles of fibrohistiocytic spindle cells
    - IHC: vimentin+, CD68+
- Rx: excision; nodal or pulmonary metastases are rare

Desmoid tumor (aggressive fibromatosis; A-G)

- Aggressive fibromatosis
- Bland wavy nuclei on path
- β-**Catenin** mutations

- Deep infiltration
- Fibroblastic proliferation
- a/w **Gardner's syndrome**

Malignant tumors: (is PAGED Fast)

Pleomorphic undifferentiated sarcoma (Undifferentiated pleomorphic sarcoma)

- Heterogenous group of soft tissue sarcomas including malignant fibrous histiocytoma
- p/w deep soft tissue mass MC on the **thighs** of middle-aged adults
- MC sarcoma to develop at sites of prior radiation and MC soft tissue tumor in the elderly
- Path: similar ugly cells as AFX (see below) but deeply located w/ a high chance of mets
- Workup: **MRI** prior to surgery (3 cm margins); refer these patients to surgical oncology
- Prognosis: 5-year mortality = 50% (MC site of metastasis is lung)
- **Depth of invasion** distinguishes UPS (fascia) from PDS (fat) and from AFX (dermis)
- "I call it UPS even though malignant cells are much lower/deeper (fascia), it occurs on lower parts of the body (thighs) and has a much lower rate of survival than AFX or PDS"

Pleomorphic dermal sarcoma (PDS)

- Best thought of as a deeper and deadlier variant of AFX
- p/w nodule on the head/neck (like AFX) but has deeper SQ invasion and necrosis
- Path: similar to AFX but is deeper and has lymphovascular and/or perineural invasion
- Workup: probably best to refer out to surgical oncology for WLE

- Prognosis: higher risk of recurrences (28%) and metastasis (10%) than AFX

Atypical fibroxanthoma (AFX; now called superficial pleomorphic sarcoma)

- Relatively common low-grade superficial (dermally based; SLAM'd against epi) sarcoma
- Pathogenesis: UV light → p53 mutations
- p/w rapidly growing ulcerated red nodule on sun-damaged skin (**head/neck**) of **elderly**
- Path: fairly well-circumscribed but overtly malignant dermal proliferation of anaplastic, pleomorphic cells w/ high mitotic rate and wildly atypical mitoses which fills the dermis but does not invade into the fat (if it does then call it a PDS or superficial UPS); composed of 4 cell types ("call it atypical fibro-histiocytic xanthoma") → bizarre atypical multinucleated giant cells, spindle cells, histiocyte-like cells, xanthomatous cells
    - IHC (non-specific but highly testable; "CASH VAN"): **CD10**, **CD68**, CD74, CD99, Cathepsin-B, A1AT, Stromelysin-3, SMA (tram-track staining vs diffuse staining in leiomysarcoma), HAM56, Vimentin, Alpha$_1$-antitrypsin, NK1/C3
- AFX is a diagnosis of exclusion: first rule out other entities in the malignant dermal spindle cell tumors "SLAM'd" against the epidermis
    - SCC (Sarcomatoid/Spindle cell variant): keratin stains (CK903, CK5/6, p63, p40)
    - Leiomyosarcoma: stains for desmin and SMA (diffuse cytoplasmic staining)
    - AFX: negative for high molecular weight keratins, p63, p40, desmin, S100, SOX10
    - Melanoma (spindle cell/desmoplastic variant): stains for S100 and SOX10
- Rx: **excision** (1–2 cm margins; 95% of AFX can be cleared w/ 2 cm margins) or **MOHs**

- Prognosis: recurs after excision (5%) but almost never metastasizes

Giant cell fibroblastoma (GCFB)

- Juvenile variant of DFSP occurring on the head/neck and posterior thigh of kids (M > F)
- Same translocation as DFSP (COL1A1-PDGFB)
- Path: multinucleated giant cells lining pseudovascular spaces
    - IHC: CD34+
- "Both DFSP and GCFB have four letters"

Epithelioid sarcoma

- Slow growing soft-tissue neoplasm with poor long-term prognosis
- Loss of INI1 in 90% of cases
- p/w firm nodule on the finger > hand/wrist of young adults
- Path: transition from epithelioid to plump pleomorphic spindle cells **w/ central necrosis** and a surrounding lymphohistiocytic infiltrate (**looks like a palisaded granuloma**)
    - IHC ("KEV has an epithelioid sarcoma on his hands"): **Keratin+, EMA+, Vimentin+**
- Metastasis develop in 50%, usually to lymph nodes and lung

Dermatofibromasarcoma protuberans (DFSP)

- Pathogenesis: nearly 90% of DFSPs are genetically characterized by the translocation **t(17;22)** resulting in the **COL1A1-PDGFB** Fusion gene detected by FISH and **Supernumerary ring chromosomes** containing sequences from chromosomes 22 > 17
- p/w slow growing firm skin-colored plaque on the **trunk** (50%) > proximal extremities

  - o Lesions often demonstrate red/blue margins w/ surrounding telangiectasias
- Path (DFSP; Deep incisional bx): Densely hypercellular Dermal proliferation infiltrating **Fat (creates a "honeycomb" pattern)** consisting of Spindled cells w/ a **Storiform Pattern**
  - o IHC: **CD34+** (D2-40, Factor 13a, and Stromelysin-3 negative; "13A you're A OK")
- Variants: Bednar tumor (pigmented variant) and giant cell fibroblastoma (peds variant)
- ↑ COL1A1-PDGFB fusion gene → ↑ chance of **FibroSarcomatous Degeneration (15%)**
  - o Clinically: ↑ recurrence rate, ↑ metastasis (18% vs < 1% in conventional DFSP)
  - o Path: ↑ cellularity, ↑ atypia, ↑ mitoses w/ **"herringbone" pattern**
    - ▪ IHC: CD34 staining is weak or lost in DFSPs w/ fibrosarcomatous change
    - ▪ If path is equivocal you can do FISH, PCR or cytogenetics
  - o Workup: routine chest imaging to screen for mets (lung is MC site of mets)
- Rx: **MOHs** (1% recurrence) > WLE (**15% recurrence**); **imatinib** for unresectable disease
  - o WLE (DFSP): 3 cm margins and down to Deep Fascia (on Scalp go to Periosteum)
  - o Radiation for unresectable DFSP or positive margins/recurrence after resection
- Follow-up: skin and physical exam every 6–12 months
- Prognosis: does not commonly metastasize but when it does it is MC to go to the **lung**
  - o Most sarcomas metastasizes to the lung (see below)

MC site of metastasis is the lung/MC associated cancer is the lung ("BAD Pulmonary METS")
BCC (LNs and lungs)
Adenoid cystic carcinoma, IgA vasculitis (esp in adults) is a/w solid organ cancer (MC lung)
DFSP, Digital papillary adenocarcinoma, Dermatomyositis in men (ovary is MC in women)
Pleomorphic dermal sarcoma/undifferentiated pleomorphic sarcoma (and most sarcomas)
Melanoma (skin is #1), Multicentric reticulohistiocytosis is a/w solid organ cancer (MC lung)
Erythema gyratum repens (MC associated cancer is lung)
Tripe palms not a/w acanthosis nigricans (gastric cancer is MC if tripe palms is a/w AN)
Stewart-Treves syndrome (lymphangiosarcoma)

Fibrosarcoma

- Tumor of mesenchymal origin made of malignant fibroblasts in a collagen background
- Congenital cases have t(12;15) translocation ("fibulas grow when you are 12–15 y/o")
- Path: densely hypercellular proliferation → herringbone (fir tree) pattern

High yield dermatologic translocations
Chronic myelogenous leukemia: t(9;22)
Ewing sarcoma: t(11;22) → "11 x 2 = 22, Eww I hate math"
Clear cell sarcoma: t(12;22) → "You are a clear sex/sarc-aholic when you are 12–22 years old"
DFSP: t(17;22) → "17–22 are college years when you Ditch Family to go to School to Party"
Systemic anaplastic large cell: t(2;5) → "Ana is systemically large, she weighs 2 to 5 tuns"
Fibrosarcoma: t(12;15) → "Fibulas grow when you go through puberty around 12–15 y/o"
Systemic follicular cell lymphoma: t(14;18) → "Pubic hairs (follicle cell) grow from 14–18 y/o"
Clear cell variant of nodular hidradenoma: t(11;19)

6.11 Vascular Proliferations

Benign vascular lesions

Infantile Hemangioma

- Not obvious at birth → rapid growth from month 2 to month 6 of life → slow involution
  - Most rapid growth is between week 5 and 8
  - "30% will resolve in 3 years, 50% in 5 years, 70% in 7 years and 90% in 9 years"
- RFs ("things that make the baby small"): white race, premature, low-birth weight, female babies, AMA mother w/ placental insufficiency or multiple gestation pregnancy)
- Infantile hemangiomas are thought to be related to the placenta as both are GLUT-1+
- Pathogenesis: **Hypoxia** and **renin-angiotensin system** activation play an important role
  - **↑ PIK3 (mTOR pathway)** → ↑ Hypoxia inducible factor-1α → ↑ VEGF
- Hemangiomas can be superficial (50–60%; bright red), deep (15%; light blue) or mixed
- They can be focal, segmental (broad/plaque-like; PHACES/LUMBAR) or intermediate
- MC complication is cutaneous **ulceration** ("Hole in skin"; 20%) which is more common on the lips and in skin folds and is MC in large segmental hemangiomas
- The most vulnerable locations are next to Holes (**eyes → permanent amblyopia**; ears → infection/conductive hearing loss; nose → fibrofatty residua and cartilage destruction; **lower lip, chin, neck** ("beard lesions") → **airway obstruction** → **Horse cry**; mouth → difficulty feeding, delay in tooth eruption, enamel hypoplasia; anogenital → ulceration)
  - **Refer to ophtho (eye lesions) or ENT (ear or beard lesions)**

- Consider extracutaneous involvement w/ lesions on face (PHACES), lower back (LUMBAR), beard (airway hemangiomas), multifocal lesions (visceral hemangiomatosis)
- Dx (clinical): **evaluate for Hypothyroidism** (↑ iodothyronine deiodinase in proliferating hemangiomas deactivates thyroid hormone) and get **Hepatic US** (MC visceral site)
  - Get imaging when **5 or more** hemangiomas present
- Path (rarely indicated): lobular proliferations of GLUT-1 (+) dermal capillaries lined by plump endothelium (transiently positive for LYVE-1 lack other lymphatic markers)
- Rx: indications for medical therapy include locations likely to ulcerate (folds/flexures), impair function (beard area or T-zone of face), or cause disfigurement (breast, genitals, face), as well as hepatic hemangiomas and PHACES/LUMBAR syndromes
  - 1st line: Hemangeol (propranolol) 0.5 mg/kg BID and ↑ to 1 mg/kg in 1 week
    - SE: Hypotension, Hypoglycemia, bradycardia, bronchospasm
    - CI: 2nd or 3rd degree Heart block
  - Atenolol and nadolol have comparable efficacy and have ↓ SEs (don't cross BBB)
  - Can try topical timolol if lesion is small, superficial and < 1 mm in thickness
  - Lasers: PDL (best for superficial lesions) and long-pulsed Nd: YAG (deep lesions)
  - 2nd line treatments include steroids, vincristine and rapamycin (sirolimus)
- Rapidly involuting congenital hemangioma (RICH; will turn white and involute over 1 year) and non-involuting congenital hemangioma (NICH; does not involute) are present at birth and do not grow after; **p/w ery-**

thematous plaque w/ surrounding pallor and characteristic radiating telangiectatic vessels
- o GLUT-1 (-)

Vascular malformations (port wine stains)

- Unlike infantile hemangiomas, these are **evident at birth**, do not rapidly enlarge (not a true neoplasm), persist into adulthood, do not have gender predilection and GLUT-1 (-)
- p/w flat, pink/light red unilateral patch at birth which over time thickens and develops a rubbery, cobblestoned quality (MC in the head/neck)
- Rx: PDL
- Workup: get ophtho exam and MRI of head if in V1 distribution (Sturge-Weber) and consider MRI of the spine if on lower back (LUMBAR)
    - o PWS is considered low risk for spinal dysraphism but if a/w another low-risk stigmata (e.g., dimple, CALM) or high risk stigmata (midline **hemangioma**, faun tail hypertrichosis, ACC, **lipoma**) then get the spinal MRI (or US if < 4 months old)
- Syndromes with vascular malformations are discussed in section 4.6

Intravascular papillary endothelial hyperplasia (IPEH; Masson's tumor)

- IPEH: Intraluminal (**vein** is MC) Papillary Proliferation of Endothelial cells Entirely contained within a Hyperplastic thrombosed vessel
- p/w PEH: Painful Purple to Erythematous Hard slow growing nodule on the **Head/neck**
- Excision is curative (this represents a Histologic pattern rather than a distinct entity)

Reactive Angio-Endotheliomatosis (RAE)

- The name tells you that it is a reactive hyperplasia of endothelial cells (like IPEH) but it results in luminal obliteration of pre-existing dermal vessels due to vaso-occlusive disorders and systemic infections (Rheumatoid arthritis, Renal failure, IgA monoclonal gammopathies, Antiphospholipid syndrome, Endocarditis)
- p/w RAE: Red Acral (lower legs is MC) nodules or plaques with Ecchymosis or petechia
- Path: proliferation of grouped capillaries in dermal blood vessels (CD31+, vWF+)
- Rx RAE: Revascularization of ischemic limb, Accutane, Evaluate/treat systemic diseases
    - Diffuse Dermal angiomatosis is a variant that occurs on the breasts > legs of women with large pendulous breasts (Double Ds); a/w smoking/ atherosclerosis

Angiokeratoma

- Small, dark (use dermoscopy to rule out melanoma) superficial vascular lesions
- 5 types (all p/w dark red to violaceous nodules)
    - Angiokeratoma Circumscriptum: Children w/ a Collection of lesions forming Confluent plaques unilaterally on a lower extremity (Calf) usually present at birth
    - Angiokeratoma corporis diffusum: child w/ multiple lesions in bathing suit distribution (abdomen, buttocks, thighs) from lysosomal storage diseases (Fabry)
    - Angiokeratoma of Mibelli: lesions located "far from the belly" on the fingers and toes of adolescents and are **a/w chilblains and acrocyanosis** → finger ulceration
    - Angiokeratoma of Fordyce: lesions on scrotum or vulva of older men/women

  - Solitary and multiple angiokeratomas: arise due to chronic trauma in any age
- Path: superficial dilated vessels a/w an acanthotic epidermis ("**bloody SK**")

Targetoid hemosiderotic lymphatic malformation (THLM)

- The old term "Hobnail Hemangioma" is inappropriate as it is a LM, not a hemangioma
- There is a history of Trauma (that is why is it MC on the legs > arms)
- **Targetoid in appearance**: 2 mm red-blue to brown papule which enlarges and is surrounded by a thin pale ring and then a peripheral echymotic ring
- Path: **superficial dilated BVs** w/ endothelial cells that protrude (hobnail) into the lumen in the upper dermis; **lower dermis has thin and slit-like BVs** and there is **hemosiderin**
  - IHC: vessels stain with lymph markers (VEGF-3 and podoplanin/D2-40)

Verrucous venulocapillary malformation (verrucous hemangioma)

- As this is actually a vascular malformation, it presents at birth and does not regress
- Somatic mutations in **MAP3k3** detected in most lesions
- p/w **grouped** or confluent red to purple papules on the distal extremities that darken and **become hyperkeratotic** during childhood → may ulcerate, bleed and scar
- Path: dilated capillaries and venules that stain with CD31 and CD34
- Rx: surgical excision or vascular laser

Pyogenic granuloma (lobular capillary hemangioma)

- Reactive vascular hyperplasia from "events that make you scream" (**Trauma** > **Pregnancy**) and "drugs that make you SCREAM" (Sirolimus, Capecitabine, Retinoids, EGFR inhibitors, Antiretrovirals, MTX)

- p/w a rapidly growing friable red papule that frequently ulcerates (ddx: melanoma)
    - o MC on the **gingiva (esp. in pregnancy)** > fingers > lips > face > tongue
- Path: well-circumscribed, exophytic, capillary proliferation arranged in a lobular pattern
- Rx: shave excision + electrosurgery; application of table salt has also proven effective

Tufted angioma ("tough LUCK")

- p/w with slowly expanding (**Lateral extension**) indurated mottled red patch on trunk
    - o The erythema can be subtle, especially in skin of color
- Utilization of platelets in Congenital cases due to Kasabach-merritt phenomenon (KMP)
- Path: tightly packed Lobules (Ultrastructural studies show Weibel-Palade bodies) of **Capillaries in a "Cannonball" pattern in Clusters** with an empty appearing Crescent surrounding each lobule (Clefting) which represent dilated lymphatic Channels
    - o CD61 confirms platelet trapping in cases of Kasabach-merritt
- Ddx: infantile hemangioma quickly grows outwards (vs slowly grows lateral)
- Rx (LuCK): Lasers (argon, Nd: YAG), Complete surgical excision, Corticosteroids; for Kasabach-merritt you can use vincristine + corticosteroids or use sirolimus
- Workup: MRI (determines extent and to differentiate from other tumors) + coagulation studies to rule out KMP (CBC, PT/PTT, fibrinogen, D-dimer)

Glomeruloid hemangioma ("glome rhymes with POEM")

- Reactive vascular proliferation d/t ↑ **VEGF** seen in POEMS > multicentric Castleman's
    - o POEMS: Polyneuropathy, Organomegaly, Endocrinopathy, Monoclonal gammopathy, Skin lesions (pigmentation, cherry > glomeruloid hemangiomas)
        - Other things that should be in the mnemonic (POEMS): Polycythemia, volume Overload, VEGF, Multicentric castleman's, Sclerotic bone lesions
- Clinically they look like large (1 cm) cherry hemangiomas
- Path: RBCs + capillary loops within dilated vessels (architecture resembles a glomerulus)
- Rx: surgical excision, shave, electrosurgery, and laser

Cherry angioma

- Acquired, slow growing vascular tumor of older adults; a/w pregnancy and POEMS
    - o MC of the acquired cutaneous vascular proliferations
- p/w bright red, dome-shaped polypoid papule on the trunk or extremities of adults
- **Path: dilated capillaries within the papillary dermis**

Microvenular hemangioma

- Acquired, slow growing vascular tumor of young adults; a/w pregnancy and POEMS
- p/w solitary red papulonodule on the forearm > proximal extremities > trunk
- Path: small ("micro") monomorphic flattened blood vessels that fill the dermis

Epithelioid hemangioma (angiolymphoid hyperplasia with Eosinophilia)

- p/w multiple violaceous papulonodules on the head/ neck (esp. around the **Ear**)
- Patients have Enlarged LNs and peripheral Eosinophilia
- Path: Enlarged thickened vessels lined by Enlarged plump Epithelioid Endothelial cells which have intracytoplasmic vacuoles; background of intense **Eosinophilic inflammation**
- Rx: surgical Excision

Congenital Cutaneous Angiomatosis w/ thrombocytopenia ("ABC"; Multifocal lymphangioendotheliomatosis with thrombocytopenia)

- Many Angiomatous Burgundy to red-Brown papules at Birth w/ Central pallor/scar
- p/w **Anemia** in infancy due to similar lesions in the Bowel > lung → **Bleeding**
- Ddx: Blueberry muffin Baby and Blue rubber Bleb nevus syndrome
- Dx: anemia and thrombocytopenia
- Path: thin-walled vessels form intraluminal papillary projections
    - Coexpression of both blood vessel (CD34) and lymphatic (LYVE-1) markers

Sinusoidal hemangioma

- Solitary SQ papulonodule on the arms or trunk (esp. breast) of adult women
- Path: dilated, interconnecting venous channels in a Sieve-like or Sinosoidal pattern
- Ddx: well-differentiated angio-Sarcoma

Spindle cell hemangioma ("spindle MIKE")

- Occurs in Maffucci (some have somatic IDH1 mutations) > Klippel-Trenaunay syndrome

- p/w solitary red-blue nodule seen in Kids on the distal Extremity → become multifocal
- Path (MIKE): Mixture of Cavernous ("Kavernous") spaces and more cellular areas containing spindle cells w/ aggregates of vacuolated Epithelioid cells
    - Resembles "hemorrhagic lung" with alveolar spaces at scanning power
        - "Spindle MIKE vapes all day which gave him a hemorrhagic lung"
- 60% recur following Excision

GlomuS Tumor

- Benign proliferations of perivascular epithelioid cells derived from Suquet-Hoyer canal
- Path: rows of round dark nuclei w little cytoplasm ("String of black pearls") which Surround Subtle vascular Spaces (vs glomangioma which has prominent vessels)
- Compared to glomangiomas (glomulovenous malformation), glomuS Tumors are…
    - Solitary blue nodule on palms or **Subungual** areas w/ Sensitivity to pressure/cold
        - vs multiple painless lesions in glomangiomas
    - Onset is in Teenage years or later (vs infancy in glomangiomas)
    - Three times more common than glomangiomas
    - Treatable with excision (glomangiomas are difficult to treat)

Acroangiodermatitis (pseudo-Kaposi sarcoma)

- Rare angioproliferative entity a/w **venous insufficiency** (MC), AVMs of the leg, dialysis
    - Stewart-Bluefarb: acroangiodermatitis PLUS congenital AVM on the leg
- p/w violaceous nodules/plaques on the B/L lower extremities w/ background of stasis

- Path (stasis-like): proliferation of thick-walled capillaries in a lobular pattern, RBC extravasation, hemosiderin, dermal fibrosis, PV lymphs; plasma cells are also found and may resemble Kaposi's but there is a lack of atypical cells
- Rx: treat underlying conditions (e.g., **compression socks**, embolization of AVM)

Borderline and low-grade malignant vascular neoplasms

Kaposiform hemangioendothelioma

- Thought to represent a deeper version of a tufted angioma
- Like tufted angiomas, they may be congenital or present in early childhood and demonstrate coexpression of blood (CD34) and lymph markers (Prox1, VEGFR-3, LYVE-1)
- More strongly **a/w Kasabach-Merritt Phenomenon** (KMP) than tufted angioma
    - o KMP refers to the consumption of platelets and clotting factors in the tumor
    - o The MCC of death from KMP is thrombocytopenia and direct tumor infiltration
- p/w violaceous plaque w/ ecchymotic edge that becomes massively engorged in KMP
- Path: nodules of spindle cells w/ slit-like lumina containing RBCs (like nodular Kaposi's)
    - o CD61 confirms platelet trapping in cases of Kasabach-merritt
    - o Unlike infantile hemangiomas it is **GLUT-1 negative**
- Rx: sirolimus or vincristine + prednisone (w/ KMP) vs surgery or prednisone (w/o KMP)
    - o Platelet transfusions or FFP given to actively bleeding pts or prior to procedures

- Workup: **MRI**, CBC, coagulation studies, D-dimer, and fibrinogen to detect KMS

Papillary intralymphatic angioendothelioma
- p/w an enlarging dermal or SQ mass on the distal extremity of a child
- Path: papillary intralymphatic growth w/ rosette-like clusters of hobnail endothelial cells

Retiform Hemangioendothelioma
- p/w enlarging exophytic tumor on the distal extremity of a young adult
- Path: arborizing blood vessel pattern reminiscent of Rete testes
- 60% recur after excision

Kaposi Sarcoma (KS; "CATHolics ask for HELP from Christ")
- **HHV-8** is present in all lesions which consist of slow-growing violaceous patches/plaques/nodules with potential visceral involvement (GI, LNs, lungs)
  - **LANA is a product of HHV-8**
- 4 clinical variants ("CATH")
  - CLassic KS: p/w slow growing red-violaceous macules/patches on the **Legs** (Calves) of elderly Ashkenazi Jews, Eastern Europeans or Mediterranean's
    - 1/3rd develop another malignancy (**non-Hodgkin Lymphoma is MC**)
  - African endemic KS: subgroups include nodular (resembles classic KS), florid and infiltrative (biologically aggressive) and lymphadenopathic (affects children, primary tumor is in LNs, course is fulminant and fatal)
  - Transplant-associated KS (due to iatrogenic immunosuppression): like classic KS

        - Only skin limited form (others have lesions in GI, LN, spleen, lung, liver)
    - **HIV-associated KS**: homosexual males with CD4 counts < 500; range from faint oval red macules on the trunk (arranged along lines of cleavage like in Christmas tree pattern;) to purple-black nodules that favor **Head/neck (including mouth)**
        - Purple macules on the nose (ddx lupus pernio), earlobes and behind the ears are very characteristic and can be stigmatizing in this population
- Histology varies depending on stage of the lesion ("HELP")
    - Patch/plaque stage (HELP): subtle or pronounced (in plaque stage) Hemosiderin, **Erythrocyte Extravasation**, infiltration of Lymphatic-like vessels w/ Pale appearing stroma (looks understained), **Plasma cells, Promontory sign**
    - Nodular stage: **nodules composed of fascicles of parallel spindle cells** w/ slit-like lumina containing RBCs; cells are never as atypical as those seen in angiosarcoma
        - IHC (HELP): HHV-8 or latency-associated nuclear antigen (**LANA-1**)
            - Mixed Lymphatic and BV phenotype (LYVE-1, CD34, VEGFR-3)
- **Next step: rule out HIV**
- Rx according to NCCN ("CHRIST")
    - Localized: **IL vinCristine/vinblastine**, Cryo (SE is Hypopigmentation), topical Retinoid (**alitretinoin**) or Imiquimod, Surgical excision, RT or PDT
    - Systemic: Chemo (**liposomal doxorubicin**), **HAART (HIV-associated KS)**, RT, Imatinib, **Sirolimus (Transplant-associated KS),** TSEB, Thalidomide (pts w/ IRIS)

  - Relapsed/refractory: pomalidomide (preferred), lenalidomide, vinorelbine, gemcitabine, bortezomib, imatinib, pembrolizumab (endemic or classic KS)
- Workup: oral exam (oral lesions strongly a/w GI tract involvement), CBC (anemia), FOBT (GI bleeding), CXR (pulmonary lesions), CT (hepatosplenomegaly), endoscopy, HIV test
- Poor prognostic signs: tumor-associated edema or ulceration, extensive oral or GI lesions, KS in organs other than LNs, and CD4 count < 150

High-grade malignant vascular neoplasms

Angiosarcoma

- Aggressive malignant neoplasm of vascular endothelial cell origin
- Presentation variable: may p/w expanding purpuric or echymotic plaque on **scalp** (MC)
- Types ("SARC")
  - Sun-exposed sites: elderly people on sun-damaged sites such as the head/neck
  - Radiation-exposed sites: MC on the breast after radiation of breast cancer
  - Chronic lymphedema sites (lymphangiosarcoma): MC on the arms following axillary LN dissection after breast cancer (Stewart-Treves syndrome)
    - Metastasizes to the lung (MC); 5-year survival is less than 10%
- RFs: lymphedema, radiation, thorotrast (old radiocontrast material) and vinyl chloride
- Path ("SARC"): large, pleomorphic, crowded and protuberant endothelial cells that **Stack on top of each other ("multilayered/piled-on")** and dissect between collagen bundles forming Anastomosing vascular networks + RBC extravasation + Cytoplasmic vacuoles

- IHC ("Angi sarcs and FUCs MY External Genitalia"): FLI-1⁺, Ulex europaeus lectin⁺, **CD31⁺, CD34⁺**, c-MYC amplification (radiation-induced), ERG⁺ (most sens/specific)

- Rx (SARC): Surgery (5 cm margins), Adjunctive propranolol, Radiation, Chemo
- Workup: **CT/MRI** to ascertain extent of bone/soft tissue involvement and asses LNs
- Prognosis: 5-year survival is < 20% (MC spread is to regional LNs > lungs > liver)

Epithelioid hemangioendothelioma

- Malignant but relatively indolent vascular tumor arising in adults
- Clonal endothelial cells w/ **translocations generating a WWTR1-CAMTA1 fusion protein**
- p/w slightly painful mass within deep soft tissue or bone
- 30% will metastasize to regional LNs, lung, liver or bone
- Rx: WLE w/ adjuvant chemotherapy or radiation w/ regional LN evaluation

Chapter 7: Dermatologic Surgery

7.1 Surgical Anatomy

Head and neck anatomy (and other high-yield dermatology locations)

- Arterial system: face receives blood from the External and Internal Carotid A. (ECA/ICA)
    - Branches of the ECA from superior to inferior are "STOMP on his face"
        - Superficial temporal artery: supplies temple, scalp and lateral forehead
        - Transverse facial artery: supplies the parotid gland and lateral face
        - Occipital artery: supplies occipital scalp and posterior neck
        - Maxillary artery ("Max has a high BMI"): branches into Buccal (supplies cheek), Mental (chin) and Infraorbital (midface/nasal dorsum) artery
        - Posterior auricular artery: supplies the scalp behind the auricle
        - Facial artery: branches into inf./sup. labial arteries (supplies lips) before becoming angular artery (arterial injection w/ filler in NL fold may occur)
            - Angular artery anastomoses w/ branches of ICA (**Dorsal Nasal A.**)
                - "DNA is a molecule with many anastomoses"
    - The branch of the ICA that supplies the mid-forehead/midnose is the **ophthalmic artery**

which travels through the optic canal to branch into "SLIDER" → **Supraorbital, Supratrochlear,** Lacrimal, **Infratrochlear** (BUT NOT INFRAORBITAL), Dorsal nasal, External nasal, Ethmoidal (anterior and posterior), Retinal arteries

- Fast pushes of filler if injected into a nasal or glabellar artery can cause retrograde flow of product into the retinal artery → blindness

- Venous system: whereas most veins follow their associated arteries (ex. angular vein → facial vein → internal jugular vein), many veins corresponding to arteries supplied by the ICA (ex. **supratrochlear and infratrochlear veins**) drain directly through the orbit and into the cavernous sinus (infections in this area around the nose can cause cavernous sinus thrombosis, meningitis and brain abscesses)
- Lymphatic system: generally, drains from superior to inferior and medial to lateral
  - o Lymph nodes (LN) from superior to inferior ("PASS that lymph")
    - Posterior cervical LNs: receive lymph from scalp, neck and upper ear
    - Preauricular superficial parotid LNs: cheek, forehead, temple, lateral ear
    - Anterior cervical LNs: oropharynx, tongue, anterior neck, lower ear
    - Submandibular LNs: upper lip/mandibular area
    - Submental LNs: chin, lower lip
- Superficial musculoaponeurotic system (SMAS): fibrous network of lower 2/3rds of face (platysma inferior and zygomatic arch superior) that connects facial muscles to dermis
  - o Allows muscle forces to be evenly distributed and contain infections superficially

- Sensory nerves (CN V) are Superficial and motor nerves (CN 7) are deep to SMAS
- Facial sensory nerves: face supplied entirely by CN V ("LISA IZZ A Bloody Little Mess")
  - V1 (ophthalmic; LISA)
    - Lacrimal nerve: lateral eyelid, conjunctiva, lacrimal gland
    - Infratrochlear nerve: **nasal root/bridge, medial canthus**
    - Supratrochlear n: medial upper eyelid/forehead/frontal scalp/conjunctiva
    - Supraorbital n: lateral upper eyelid/forehead/frontal scalp/conjunctiva
      - Border b/w supratrochlear and supraorbital sensory innervation on forehead skin is an imaginary line drawn up at the medial iris
    - Anterior ethmoidal nerve: inferior central nose (dorsum, tip, columella)
  - V2 (maxillary; IZZ)
    - Infraorbital nerve: nasal sidewall, nasal ala, **upper lip**, medial cheek, **lower eyelid**, upper teeth and maxillary gingiva
    - Zygomaticofacial nerve: malar eminence
    - Zygomaticotemporal nerve: medial temple, supratemporal scalp
  - V3 (mandibular; A Bloody Little Mess)
    - Auriculotemporal nerve: superior anterior ear, auditory canal, tympanic membrane, lateral temple, temporoparietal scalp, TMJ
      - Also has **parasympathetic innervation to parotid**
      - Frequently injured during TMJ surgery or parotidectomy → **Frey syndrome (ear or lateral temple sweats while eating spicy food)**

- Buccal nerve (Boca = mouth in Spanish): angle of mouth, buccal mucosa
- Lingual nerve (Lengua = tongue in Spanish): anterior 2/3rds of tongue
- Mental nerve (mentón = chin in Spanish): chin and lower lip
- **V3 also provides motor innervation to the muscles of mastication**
  - Muscles of mastication arise from 1st branchial arch and are innervated by V3, muscles of facial expression arise from 2nd branchial arch and are innervated by CN7

- Salivary glands: exocrine glands that produce saliva (listed from largest to smallest)
  - Parotid gland: located on the lateral face and commonly encountered during MOHs (path shows triad of **basophilic cells + eosinophilic ducts + adipocytes;** adipocytes predominate in the elderly, obese and those w/ Sjögrens or diabetes)
    - Parasympathetic innervation by auriculotemporal nerve (branch of V3)
    - "Vessels trapped in parotid gland are not FREE" (from superficial to deep)
      - Facial nerve: 2 branches enter the gland and 5 branches exit
      - Retromandibular vein: enters gland as maxillary and superficial temporal vein and exits as facial and posterior auricular vein
      - External carotid artery: exits gland superiorly as the maxillary and the superficial temporal artery
  - Submandibular gland: located deep to the body of the mandible (path shows predominance of clear foamy mucus-rich glands)

        - **Duct crossed laterally by the lingual nerve** (parasympathetic innervation)
        - Gland is supplied by the facial and lingual artery
        - Common site of calculus formation
    - Sublingual gland: located below the floor of the mouth
        - Ducts open onto the floor of the mouth
        - Like submandibular gland, it receives parasympathetic innervation from the lingual nerve (chorda tympani) and is supplied by the facial artery
    - Labial glands: circular (**size of a small pea**) glands located between submucosa and orbicularis oris muscle (labial artery also runs here but is not circular)
        - Labial glands and artery are encountered during MOHs (recognize them!)
- Cervical plexus: come from Erb's point along w/ accessory nerve ("Erb has Great LATS")
    - Great auricular nerve (C2, C3): **angle of jaw, mastoid process**, ear, lateral neck
    - Greater occipital nerve (C2): majority of occipital scalp
    - Lesser occipital nerve (C2): posterior neck, **postauricular scalp**
    - Accessory nerve (CN XI): motor innervation to SCM/trapezius → **damage causes wing scapula, poor shoulder abduction, shoulder/neck pain, trapezius atrophy**
    - Transverse cervical nerve (C2, C3): anterior neck ("where the Thyroid is")
    - Supraclavicular nerve (C3, C4): chest, clavicle, Shoulder ("in-between Shoulders")
- Nose sensory nerves: V2 innervates the B/L nasal dorsum and alae (V1 supplies the rest)

  - Smell is by olfactory nerve (CN1) and the nasal muscles by the facial nerve (CN7)
- Ear sensory nerves: great auricular nerve (C2, C3) innervates entire ear except...
  - **Anterior helix (including crux and tragus) → auriculotemporal nerve (V3)**
  - Conchal bowl → CN7, **CN10 (vagus nerve)** ("I always bowl a 7–10 split")
  - Superior posterior ear: lesser occipital nerve (C2; also supplies scalp behind ear)
  - Posterior portion of external auditory canal: chorda typani (branch of CN7)
- Ring block around ear anesthetizes everything **except conchal bowl** +/- EAM
  - To block the great auricular nerve inject behind inferior aspect of earlobe
  - To block the auriculotemporal nerve inject superior and anterior to tragus
- Hand sensory nerves: Radial, Ulnar and Median nerves ("I drink RUM with my hands")
  - Radial nerve: first 3 and a half digits on **dorsal side** from wrist to PIP joint
    - However, they may show you dorsal side of 2nd/3rd fingertip → median n.
  - Ulnar nerve: **dorsal and ventral** 5th digit and ulnar half of 4th digit
    - Block: inject radial to flexor carpi ulnaris tendon at proximal wrist crease
  - Median nerve: first 3 and half digits on **plantar side** and **dorsal tip of 2nd/3rd digit**
    - Median is Major nerve in hand as it has Most of palm and Most of fingers
    - Block: inject radial to palmaris longis tendon at proximal wrist crease
- Foot sensory nerves (all 5 are branches of sciatic nerve except the saphenous nerve)

- Posterior tibial nerve: heel and **sole of foot** and plantar toes ("Plantar Only")
  - Block: inject Posterior to medial malleolus
- Sural nerve: **lateral** foot, lateral heel and lateral 5th toe
  - Block: inject posterior to lateral malleolus
- Deep peroneal nerve: in-between 1st and 2nd toes
  - Block: lateral to extensor hallucis longus tendon at foot/ankle junction
- Superficial peroneal nerve: dorsal toes and dorsal foot ("per-toe-neal")
  - Block: inject along dorsum of foot from malleolus to malleolus
- Saphenous nerve (branch of the femoral nerve): medial (middle) ankle/foot/calf ("poor sap in the middleclass can't support his femily")
  - Block: inject medial (middle) and superior to medial (middle) malleolus
  - All other foot nerves are branches of the sciatic nerve sciatic nerve block will provide complete anesthesia below the knee w/ the exception of the area innervated by the saphenous nerve (branch of femoral nerve)

- The common peroneal nerve (as it wraps around the head of the fibula) is susceptible to injury in cutaneous surgeries involving the lateral upper leg
- Sensory nerves for digits: to perform digit block inject perpendicular to the digit at Wallace's line at least 1 cm distal to the web space using 1–2 cc on each side (max volume of lidocaine that can be used is 4 mL per digit according to Napier et al.)
  - "If you use > 4 cc of anesthetic in a digit the patient will be left with only 4 digits"
- Tongue nerves
  - Sensory innervation to the anterior 2/3rds of tongue is w/ the lingual nerve of V3

- Taste of anterior 2/3rds of tongue is w/ the chorda tympani branch of CN 7
  - "Taste the Tympani"
- Taste and sensory innervation to posterior 1/3rd of tongue is w/ CN IX
- Motor innervation to tongue is w/ CN 12

- Face motor innervation: **facial nerve** (CN7) emerges from skull base at the stylomastoid foramen, travels in parotid gland, splits into 5 branches ("Ten Zebras Bit Mandy's Cervix")
  - Temporal branch: supplies frontalis (eyebrow elevation; **has no bony attachments**), corrugator supercilia (pulls eyebrows inferiomedially), upper orbicularis occuli (tight closure of eyelids)
    - Injury: can't make shocked face (**can't fully open eyes; no forehead lines**)
    - Botox: frontalis (forehead lines), orbicularis oculi (crow's feet), corrugator supercilli (vertical glabellar lines)
  - Zygomatic branch: supplies alar portion of nasalis (flares nostrils), procerus (horizontal glabellar lines; shortens nose), lower portion of orbicularis occuli (**tight closure of eyelids**), zygomaticus major (elevates upper lip)
    - Injury: **can't make a mean face** ("I call it zygo-mean-icus")
    - Botox: procerus (horizontal glabellar lines), alar nasalis (flared nostrils)
    - CN III (innervates levator palpebrae superioris) opens eyelids ("III looks like three columns keeping eyelids open) whereas CN 7 (innervates orbicularis oculi) closes eyelids ("7 looks like a hook which shuts eyelids")
    - Extensive rami exist so injury to this nerve usually is not permanent

- Buccal branch (boca is mouth in Spanish): supplies Buccinator muscle of mastication (along w/ V3), transverse portion of nasalis (Bunny lines), depressor septi nasi (pulls columella toward lip) and upper lip muscles (orbicularis oris, zygomaticus major/minor, risorius, levator anguli oris, and levator labii superioris)
  - Injury: can't talk (muffled speech), can't kiss (pucker), can't smile (**uneven smile even at rest**), can't eat (food accumulates b/w cheek and teeth)
  - Botox: levator labii superioris (gummy smile), trans. nasalis (bunny lines)
  - Extensive rami exist so injury to this nerve usually is not permanent
  - These muscles converge and are held together by a fibrous tissue known as the modiolus (just superior and lateral to the oral commissure)
- Marginal mandibular branch: supplies lower lip muscles (orbicularis oris, depressor anguli oris, depressor labii inferioris, mentalis, upper platysma)
  - Muscles of facial expression in the lower face have no bony attachments
  - **Most superficial nerve; highest risk of permanent motor deficits**
  - Injury: can't evert lower lip, **uneven smile visible when smiling**
- Cervical branch: supplies platysma (depresses lower jaw and tenses neck skin)
  - Injury: can't depress lower jaw to make a grimace
  - Botox: platysmal bands
- Posterior auricular branch of CN7 (not in mnemonic as it branches before entering the parotid close to the stylomastoid foramen; "Ten Zebras Bit

Mandy's Cervix Auright"): supplies occipitalis muscle and muscles of the ear
  - Facial nerve also provides sensory innervation to the conchal bowl ("bowl 7–10 split"), taste to ant 2/3rds of tongue, parasympathetic innervation to sublingual and submandibular glands, and motor innervation to muscles of mastication
  - CN7 is prone to injury w/ retroauricular surgery in kids (immature mastoid)
- Cutaneous danger zones
  - Labial/angular artery: skin necrosis if injected near the base of ala w/ filler
  - Supratrochlear artery: skin necrosis or blindness if injected in glabella w/ filler
  - Temporal branch of CN7: eyebrow ptosis if severed over zygomatic arch
  - Marginal mandibular branch of CN7: facial asymmetry upon smiling if severed 2–3 cm inferolateral to oral commissure as it passes over the mandible
  - Spinal accessory nerve (CN XI): **shoulder pain** (MC symptom), **inability to abduct arm** (MC sign), **internal rotation of humoral head, winged scapula** and **trapezius atrophy** if severed at Erb's point (6.5 cm below EAM at posterior border of SCM)
  - Parotid duct: sialocele requiring surgery if injured as it courses over masseter

7.2 Instruments and Sterilization

- Scalpel blades (be able to recognize all tools in this section)
  - #10: curved belly that looks like part of a "0" used for cutting thick skin (back)
  - #11: sharp point that looks like a "1" used for I&D or cutting sharp angles

  - #15: shape resembles a portion of a "5" and is the MC blade used in dermatology
  - #15c: variant that is flatter and thinner than the traditional 15 blade
- Scalpel handles that hold the Blade
  - Seigel: round handle used in MOHs surgery (greater maneuverability) that attaches to the same type of blades as the Bard-Parker (rectangular slits)
  - Bard-Parker handle: flat handle (MC handle in dermatology)
  - Beaver handle: round handle but attaches to a blade w/ a small round slit
  - Hair transplant scalpel handle has insertions for multiple blades
- Scissors:
  - Short-handled good for delicate work vs long-handled good for extending reach
  - Curved blades are used for Cysts vs Straight blades for trimming tissue or Sutures
  - Sharp-tipped used for course dissection vs blunt-tipped for delicate undermining
  - Iris scissors: sharp-tipped and short-handled; MC scissor in dermatology
  - Strabismus scissors: looks like iris scissors (short scissors) but w/ blunted end used around the eye ("your eyesight is blunted if you have strabismus")
  - LaGrange scissors: S-shaped body ensures cutting w/ minimal slipping
  - O'brien scissors: off-center angled blade ("Imagine a drunk Irishman off-center")
  - Mayo scissors: 1:1 handle to blade ratio ("Mayo has 1:1 ratio of egg to vinegar")
  - Gradle scissors: blade tapered to a fine point ("Dreidels spin from a fine point")
  - Westcott/castro-viejo scissors: spring loaded instrument used for delicate areas

- Ragnell dissecting scissors: dissecting scissors w/ flat Rounded tips
- Metzenbaum scissors: long handles w/ blunt tips ("Metzen-blunt is a long word")
- Kretzer bandage scissors: Kurved edge adds to pt comfort while **cutting bandage**
- Spencer scissors: curved blade w/ a notch on one blade for **Suture cutting**
- Supercut scissors: one blade has a razor edge; denoted by black handles

- Needle drivers
  - Smaller needle drivers: needle is less damaged but also less secure
  - Larger needle drivers: needle is more damaged but more secure
  - Tungsten carbide may coat the jaws to improve grip, denoted by gold handles
  - Castroviejo needle holder: spring loaded used in delicate areas
  - Webster needle driver: short handle w/ small jaws (good for smaller needles)
  - Crile-wood: longer handle and larger jaws (good for larger needles)
    - "Imagine a small spider web on a much larger piece of wood"
  - Olsen-Hegar needle holder: proximal to the jaws, there is a suture cutting scissor surface, allowing the surgeon to suture and cut suture w/ the same instrument
    - "Dr. Olsen Hegar is a lonely Old Hag" (no MA there to cut sutures)
- Forceps ("Jewish parents teach kids ABC's with A Little Jewish Guilt")
  - Serrated forceps are easier to grab needle but ↑ tissue crush injury

- Toothed forceps are harder to grab needle but handles tissue gently
- Adsons forceps: broad handle that tapers to a narrow tip (MC in dermatology)
- Bishop-Harmon forceps: fine small-tipped; used near eyes; has 3 holes in handles
- Castroviejo forceps: ideal for fine tissue around eye and for nasal cartilage
- **Allis clamps (Allis hemostat)**: clamps used to grasp walls of cysts w/o breaking it
- Littauer cilia forceps: wide jaws w/ fine horizontal serrations
- Jeweler's forceps: very pointy ends used for suture removal
- Graefe forceps: used to Grasp tissue (functions like a hand and looks like a hand)

- Shaw scalpel is a form of electrocautery (heat) used to cut tissue w/ minimal blood loss
  - Commonly used to treat rhinophyma and in parotid gland surgeries
- Skin hooks
  - Two hooks: Joseph (wider apart) vs Freer (narrower)
    - "Joseph is a bigger/wider word than Freer"
  - Single hook: Gillies vs converse
- Hemostats
  - Kelly clamp: has a longer tip than seen in Halsted hemostat
  - Halsted hemostat (mosquito clamp): smaller tip than Kelly clamp

Sterilization (AbCDEFG)

- Autoclave (steam autoclave and Chemiclave)
  - Steam autoclave ("2 is a backwards S"): high pressure, high temperature (2 atm of pressure at **121°C for 20–30 minutes**); **MC to dull Sharp instru-**

ments; must use distilled water (not tap water); **MC method used in office setting**
  - Chemical autoclave ("FAM"): lower humidity than steam; sterilizes via **heated chemicals** (mixture of Formaldehyde, Acetone, Alcohols, Methyl ethyl ketone)
- Cold sterilization: cold solution of **glutaraldehyde/formaldehyde** ("hyde from the cold")
  - Instruments must be used immediately after and Cannot be wrapped for storage
  - Not effective against spores or Hep B so **Cannot use for invasive procedures**
  - Thioureas (neoprene) Cross-reacts w/ **glutaraldehyde** and causes allergic Contact dermatitis in **medical/dental assistant** who sterilize
- Dry heat (oven): **Doesn't Dull sharp instruments**; inexpensive; longer times
  - MC settings (1 hour at 171° C or **6 hours at 121° C**)
- Gas sterilization ("GEOFF has gas") with **Ethylene oxide (MC),** Ortho-pthalaldehyde (new liquid sterilant; stains skin gray) and Formaldehyde gasses
  - Good for large volumes (used in the hospital) but contains toxic/mutagenic gas

7.3 Suture Techniques

- Knots
  - Surgeon's knot: most common; first knot is double thrown to prevent slippage
  - Aberdeen hitch knot: used to tie the end of a running subcuticular suture
    - Advantages: more compact, more secure, uses less suture and less bulky

- Cuticular/epidermal suturing
    - Simple interrupted: used for wounds under moderate to high tension
    - Simple running: used for wounds under minimal tension; ↑ risk of dehiscence
    - Running locked sutures: provides hemostasis but has ↑ risk of strangulation
        - Running locked is best suture to use on the helical rim ("he-lock-al rim")
    - Vertical mattress: gives the most eVersion ("far far near near")
    - Horizontal mattress: gives the most Hemostasis but has **↑ risk of strangulation**
    - Pulley: **approximates wounds under tension** ("far near near far") by promoting mechanical tissue creep prior to placement of dermal sutures
    - Running horizontal mattress: ↓ strangulation risk vs simple horizontal mattress
    - Tip stitch: defined as a **half-buried horizontal mattress suture**
    - Step-off stitch: used to correct uneven dermal sutures by taking a deeper bite on the side that is lower and a more superficial bite on the side that is higher
- Subcuticular/dermal suturing
    - Simple buried suture: the needle enters the deep surface of the wound (SQ fat), passes through the dermis, crosses the wound and enters the opposing dermis, and then exits at the same level of the SQ fat on the opposite side of the wound
        - Advantage: closes dead space
    - Buried vertical mattress: similar to simple buried suture but needle has a heart-shaped path → everts wound edge/better cosmesis/lower risk of spitting sutures

  - Set back suture: most eversion, best cosmesis and lowest risk of spitting sutures
    - Advantage of buried vertical mattress/set back: prevents indented scars
- Running subcuticular: sutures run in superficial dermis/DEJ (**prolene** is best)
    - Advantage: no track marks so best if worried about hypertrophic scar
  - Buried horizontal mattress: suture enters at the papillary dermis and exits on the undersurface of the dermis then on the contralateral side it enters at the undersurface of the dermis and exits at the papillary dermis
    - Advantage: **↓ wound tension**
  - Purse string: used to ↓ wound size and ↓ healing times (vs 2° intention healing)
  - Buried pully suture: series of two or more simple buried sutures which permits wound closure under high tensions but may cause tissue strangulation
  - Figure of 8: used commonly to close punch biopsies or to tie off bleeding vessels
- Suture removal recommendations (largely anecdotal): 1 week on face, 10–14 days on trunk and proximal extremities, and 2 weeks on scalp, ears and distal extremities
- Suspension sutures: anchor overlying tissue to periosteum to remove tension from flap
  - Prevents distortion of a free margin (especially the eyelid)
  - Prevents flap "tenting" across a concavity (**can use to recreate nasolabial fold**)
- Cheese wiring: refers to suture cutting through thin skin in the elderly or those w/ EDS
  - We can place Steri-Strips down and suture over them to prevent this

7.4 Closure Materials

- Absorbable sutures: loses tensile strength within 60 days (used as "deep" sutures)
  - Gut, fast-absorbing gut, chromic gut, polyglactin 910 (vicryl), poliglecaprone-25 (mono), polyglycolic acid (dexon), polyglyconate (maxon), polydioxanone (PDS)
- Nonabsorbable sutures: maintains tensile strength for > 60 days ("superficial" sutures)
  - Names sound like materials in clothes: silk, nylon (ethilon), polypropylene (prolene), polyester, polybutester (novafil)
- Natural fibers (gut and silk): digested by Proteolysis; Rapidly degraded; ↑ risk of inflammatory Reactions (N, P, and R are close in alphabet)
- Synthetic fibers: broken down by hydrolysis; slowly degraded; non-inflammatory
- Monofilament: comprised of a single filament
  - Advantages: slides easily through tissue (because of ↓ COF), harbors less bacteria (because ↓ capillarity), less inflammatory
  - Disadvantages: ↓ knot security (because of ↑ memory and ↓ COF) and poor ease of handling (because of ↓ pliability and ↑ memory)
    - "Monofilament has ↑ Memory"
- Braided (multifilament): "girls w/ braided hair have more SPICE but have bad memories"
  - **↑ knot Security, ↑ tensile Strength, ↑ Pliability, ↑ Infection risk, ↑ Inflammatory potential, ↑ Capillarity, ↑ COF, ↑ Ease of handling, ↓ memory**
  - There are fewer braided sutures so just remember these
    - **Polyester + silk (non-absorbable); vicryl + polyglycolic acid (absorbable)**

- **"Poly and Ester stroke silk as they cry on Poly's acid"**

Key terms

- Plasticity: ability of a suture to maintain a new shape without breaking
    - Stretches for edema but wound may not approximate after edema resolves
- Elasticity: ability of a suture to regain its original shape after being stretched
    - Allows for wounds to stay approximated even after swelling subsides
    - "Think Elastigirl from the movie The Incredibles"
    - Polybutester is known for its elasticity ("poly-butt-ester has great el-ass-ticity")
- Memory: an inherent ability of the suture to maintain its original shape after use
    - Determined by suture size, **plasticity, and elasticity** ("I remember that big ass")
    - **↑memory → ↓knot security and ↓ease of handling ("the more you remember the past, the less secure and at ease you feel in the present")**
- Tissue reactivity: degree of tissue inflammation elicited by the suture
    - The most reactive are natural sutures: **gut** (absorbable) > **silk** (non-absorbable)
    - The least reactive are the ones we use all the time: poliglecaprone 25, aka monocryl (absorbable) and polypropylene, aka prolene (non-absorbable)
- Tensile strength: ability to resist breakage
    - Synthetic sutures are generally stronger but tensile strength is mainly determined by suture size (e.g., 3-0 is stronger than 4-0)
    - Poliglecaprone 25 has highest and gut has lowest initial tensile strength for absorbable sutures while stainless steel (#1) and **polyester** (#2) have

the highest and silk has the lowest initial tensile strength for non-absorbable
  - Polyglyconate (Maxon) and polydioxanone (PDS) have the longest time required to ↓ to 50% of initial tensile strength while fast absorbing gut has the shortest
  - PDS has the longest absorption time while fast absorbing gut has the shortest
    - Beware of trick questions: any non-absorbable suture will last longer than any absorbable suture, even PDS
- Coefficient of friction (COF): degree of friction met while pulling a suture through tissue
  - ↑ COF → ↑ knot security/knot strength and ↑ local tissue damage
  - Polypropylene (prolene) has a low COF → slides easily through tissue so ideal for subcuticular sutures but requires more throws to secure knot
- Knot Security (Strength of the knot): ↑ knot Security is due to ↑ COF and ↓ memory
- Pliability ("playability"): ability to bend
  - ↑pliability → ↑ease of handling ("The more you play the more at ease you are")
- Capillarity: ability of a suture to absorb/transfer fluid
  - ↑ capillarity → ↑ risk of infection
  - Silk is the non-absorbable suture with the highest risk of infection
- Ease of handling: ease with which a suture is used
  - ↑ ease of handling → ↑ pliability and ↓ memory
  - **Silk is gold standard for ease of handling** ("Silk & ease are both 4 letter words")
    - Silk is used in areas where ↓ discomfort is key (mouth, eyelid margin)

Time required for an absorbable suture to decrease to **50% of tensile strength** /absorption time

- Braided absorbable sutures ("2s and 3s")
  - Dexon (polyglycolic acid): **2 weeks** / 3 months
  - **Vicryl (polyglactin 910): 3 weeks** / 2 months
- Guts ("1, 2, 3")
  - Fast-absorbing gut: 1 week / 1 month
  - Plain gut: 2 weeks / 2 months
  - Chromic gut: 3 weeks / 3 months
- Monocryl: 1 week / 3 months
- Maxon (glycolic acid) and PDS have the longest times: 1 month / 6 months

Additional suture information

- Sutures can be coated w/ the antibiotic **triclosan** (denoted by a "+" sign on the package)
- Sutures can be barbed (knot-less suturing method) to hold tissue in place, distribute tension more evenly and offer a faster way to suture wounds
- Tissue adhesives can be used in place of epidermal sutures (↑ risk of dehiscence)
  - Octyl (octyl cyanoacrylate; Dermabond) dry slower and are softer
  - Butyl (butyl cyanoacrylate; Liquiband and GluSeal) dry faster and are more rigid
- Adhesive strips are often used w/ Mastisol after epidermal sutures are removed
- Staples are commonly used on the scalp and are quick/ easy to apply, have ↓ risk of strangulation and ↓ risk of infection compared to epidermal sutures (but have ↑ pain)
- **Photoactivated tissue bonding** (PTB) uses **green light** to crosslink proteins (collagen) between tissue planes and can be used in place of epidermal sutures
  - Blue light for acne and red light for AGA ("Blue is for Blackheads, Red is for bald head, and green

is to attach the epidermis when there is a space between")

7.5 Local Anesthetics and Pain Control

Three major categories of afferent sensory fibers

- Aδ fibers: medium diameter, lightly myelinated fibers; detect sharp pain/temperature
    - 1st to be blocked by local anesthesia ("you shouldn't feel sharp")
- C fibers: small ("Compact") diameter, unmyelinated fibers which detect dull, aching pain
- Aβ fibers: fast-conducting, large diameter (Big), myelinated fibers that transmit vibration
    - Slowest to respond to local anesthesia (in chronological order it is "AD CAB")
        - **Temperature/sharp pain** (Aδ), dull pain (C), light pressure/vibration (Aβ)

Local anesthetics

- Mechanism: reversible inhibition of **sodium** ion influx → blocks nerve conduction
    - Anesthetics prevent action potentials by controlling axonal permeability to Na
- Chemical structure (NOTE: concepts in this section are argued in other review sources)
    - Aromatic end: lipophilic (allows diffusion into cell membranes); **affects potency**
        - "A romantic man loves his wife even if she's fat (lipophilic) and just wants his penis to be potent for her enjoyment"
        - Alternate mnemonic: "that aroma is potent"
        - Potency is proportional to lipid solubility which relates to aromatic end

- Amine end: hydrophilic/lipophobic (determines water solubility which is important for preparation/storage and affects **onset and duration of action**
  - "A mean person would divorce his wife for gaining weight (lipophobic) and just wants sex now (onset) and for it to last long (duration)"
  - Alternate mnemonic: "min" in "amine" for minutes in onset/duration
  - Onset of action is inversely proportional to the pKa (bicarbonate ↑ the pH so it is closer to the pKa resulting in ↓ onset of action) and the duration of action is proportional to the protein binding capacity
- Intermediate chain: mainly determines class (amide vs ester)
  - Amides (lidocaine, mepivacaine, prilocaine, bupivacaine, ropivacaine)
    - Metabolized by **CYP 3A4** in the liver (**CI in end stage liver disease**)
      - Beta blockers/CCBs would ↑ lidocaine toxicity via CYP3A4
    - Allergic reactions rare but occur due to Methyl**paraben** or sodium Metabisulfite (this also ↓pH and makes lido sting) preservative
      - If occurs, switch to preservative-free lidocaine or ropivacaine which has no preservatives
        - "Does Rope have preservatives? Nope"
      - The methylparaben preservative displaces bilirubin from albumin and causes hyperbilirubinemia in infants
  - Esters ("Don't Pester Ester"; Procaine, benzocaine, tetracaine, butacaine)

- Metabolized via Pseudocholinesterase in Plasma; renally excreted
- **Frequent allergic reaction to PABA metabolite**
- Cross-reacts w/ PASTA (PPD, PABA, Para-aminosalicylic acid, Aminophylline, Sulfonamide, Thiazide, ester Anesthetic, and Azo dye)
  - Amide anesthetics do not cross-react w/ ester anesthetics

Testable facts regarding specific anesthetics

- Mepivicaine and Bupivacaine are the only amides not safe in pregnancy (Category C; other amides are category B) as they cause fetal bradycardia ("Miniature Bradycardia")
  - The ester anesthetics are all Category C
  - Lidocaine (**without** epinephrine) is the anesthetic of choice in pregnant women
- Procaine has the **shortest duration** of action (half hour w/o epi and 1 hour w/ epi)
  - "Procaine is the shortest duration of all words, only 8 letters"
- Lidocaine, mepivacaine and prilocaine have a duration of about an hour (30–120 mins)
- Bupivicaine has the longest duration when combined w/ epi (up to 8 hours) but has the highest risk of **cardiac toxicity** ("works great w/ epi but will make your heart Beat Up")
  - Bupivicaine is slow in onset due to its higher pKa of 8.1 (pKa closer to physiologic pH of 7.4 will lead to faster onset of action) and it has a long duration (half-life) because of its high protein binding (nearly 95% of bupivacaine is protein bound)
  - Liposomal bupivacaine (Exparel) is released very slowly and provides safe anesthesia for 72 hours

(can reduce the need for post-operative opioid use)

- Ropivicaine has the longest duration without epi (up to 6 hours; "ropes are long")
- Prilocaine has a risk of methemoglobinemia ("the entire PR Industry does meth")
  - p/w abrupt onset of hypoxia (fatigue, cyanosis, dyspnea, shock, coma, seizures)
  - RFs ("PRI"): G6PD deficiency, Rx meds (e.g., dapsone, HCQ, and sulfa), and Infants (< 1 y/o)
- All anesthetics (**besides cocaine**) vasodilate → lidocaine w/o epi will cause ↑ bleeding

Anesthetic maximum doses

- MC used concentrations: 1% (10 mg/mL), 2% (20 mg/mL), 0.1% tumescent (1 mg/mL)
- Maximum doses of lidocaine allowed is 4.5 mg/kg in adults and 1.5 mg/kg if < 6 months old (without epinephrine) vs 7 mg/kg in adults and 4 mg/kg if < 6 months old (with epi)
  - Epi vasoconstricts and ↓ absorption so you are allowed to use more lidocaine
  - "Just remember **4.5 w/o epi and 7 w/ epi** and subtract 3 from both in pediatrics"
  - Max dose regardless of weight in an adult is **500 mg with epi** and 300 mg w/o epi
- To calculate max cc of lidocaine allowed in adults
  - 4.5 mg/kg (w/o epi) or 7 mg/kg (w/ epi) multiplied by patients' weight in kg (usually 70 kg) and divide this by 10 mg/mL (if 1%) or 20 mg/mL (if 2%)
- Max dose for tumescent anesthesia (0.1% lidocaine w/ **1:1,000,000** epi) is **55 mg/kg**
  - To calculate max cc of lidocaine in tumescent: 55 X kg weight and divide this by 1
    - Always use lidocaine for tumescent anesthesia, bupivacaine is cardiotoxic

- Advantages of tumescent anesthesia: ↓ bleeding, ↑ duration of anesthesia and avoids complications associated with general anesthesia (↓ morbidity/mortality)
- **Caution in end-stage liver disease** (amides are metabolized in the liver)

- Max dose of bupivacaine is 175mg (not based on weight)

Additives to local anesthetics

- Epinephrine (1:200,000 is equally as effective but ↓ toxicity compared to 1:100,000)
  - MOA: vasoconstriction → ↓ anesthetic absorption (stays local)
    - **7–15 minutes to achieve full vasoconstriction**
  - Advantages: ↓ bleeding, ↑ safety and duration of anesthetic
  - Use w/ caution in "the Procaine MATCH": Pregnancy (↓ uterine blood flow; Pregnancy Cat C), **Pheochromocytoma**, Peripheral vascular disease, Propranolol (B-blockers), MAO inhibitors, Acute angle glaucoma, TCAs, **Hyperthyroidism**, uncontrolled Hypertension, severe CV disease
    - The only 2 absolute CIs are hyperthyroidism and pheochromocytoma
- Sodium bicarbonate **8.5% (1 mL per 10 mL of 1% lidocaine)**
  - MOA: raises pH to near physiologic levels (which **↓ pain/Soreness**)
  - Advantages: **↑ Speed of onset because it brings the pH closer to the pKa**
  - Disadvantages: ↓ Shelf-life; ↓ duration of action (↓ protein binding capacity)
  - Notice that it Shorterns all times (onset, duration, shelf-life, and time they're in pain)

- Hyaluronidase ("Thyaluronidase")
  - MOA: digests hyaluronic acid
  - Advantages: ↑ anesthetic diffusion and ↓ Tissue distortion from fluid infiltration
  - Disadvantages: ↓ Time anesthetic works (duration) and ↑ anesthetic Toxicity
    - "Advantages and disadvantages are all the opposite as epinephrine"
  - Contains the contact allergen **Thimerosal**

Presentations of lidocaine overdose

- Mild (< 5 mcg/mL): "Drunk and doing cocaine" → Rx: observe
  - Drunk: euphoria, talkativeness, restlessness, lightheadedness
  - Cocaine: tingling around hands, **circumoral numbness**, metallic taste, **tinnitus**
- Moderate (6 to 10 mcg/mL): "Black out and delirium tremons" → **Rx: check vitals, give oxygen, emergency medical service activation, diazepam, airway maintenance**
  - Black out: nausea, **vomiting**, blurred vision, **slurred speech**, confusion
  - Delirium tremons: psychosis, muscle twitch, tremors
- Severe (> 10 mcg/mL): "About to die of ETOH overdose" → Rx: respiratory support/CPR
  - Life-threatening overdose: seizures, cardiopulmonary depression, and coma

Differential diagnosis of local anesthetic reactions

- Lidocaine/anesthetic toxicity: low blood pressure and low pulse ("like in ETOH toxicity")
  - Rx: discussed below under "Local and Systemic Toxicity" section

- Vasovagal reaction ("patient goes down"): low blood pressure and low pulse
  - o Rx: **Trendelenburg (put their legs up)**, cold compresses, and smelling salts
- Epinephrine reaction ("Epi wakes you up"): high blood pressure and high pulse
  - o Rx: **reassurance/monitor** (usually resolves within minutes)
  - o If patient has history of heart racing, then dilute the epinephrine to 1:400,000
  - o **Any patient with hypertensive emergency must be sent to the ER**
- Anaphylactic reaction: low BP and high pulse (vasodilation w/ reactive tachycardia)
  - o MC to see when using ester anesthetics (PABA allergy)
  - o Rx: epinephrine 1:1000 of 0.3 mL SQ injection, call code/911, support airway

Local And Systemic Toxicity (LAST)

- Local anesthetics inhibit Na channels and cause CNS/CV excitation followed by inhibition
  - o CNS excitation (early; "cocaine"): perioral numbness, tinnitus, and tremors
  - o CNS inhibition (late; "black out"): drowsiness, altered consciousness, and seizures
  - o CV excitation (early; "cocaine"): hypertension and tachycardia
  - o CV inhibition (late, "black out"): hypotension, bradycardia, and cardiac arrest
- If there is a cardiac arrest follow ACLS guidelines; IV lipids improve cardiac conduction and cardiac perfusion by removing liposoluble local anesthetic from cardiac tissue

ACLS review

- If you are alone and see a man down, do this in this order ("look, call, feel")
    - Secure the scene (make sure you and the victim are safe from other hazards)
    - Assess (**look at**) the victim and observe if the victim is breathing or gasping
    - **Call** 911/activate emergency response system
    - Perform CPR (**feel** for a pulse and start CPR if there is none)
- If you are in a medical facility and the patient is at risk of going into cardiopulmonary failure (e.g., anaphylaxis) the first thing you do is "VOMIT on the patient"
    - Vitals, **Oxygen via nasal cannula**, Monitor, IO/IV access, Twelve lead EKG
    - IM Epinephrine (1:1000) would be your next step in cases of anaphylaxis

Management of pre-operative hypertension

- For elevated BP in the hypertensive crisis range (>180/120) it is important to assess for the correct size of the BP cuff and to confirm the BP from the contralateral arm
- **Defer surgery ("STOOOP surg") until PCP eval for BP > 200/100** (Larson et al; Derm Surg)
- For hypertensive Emergency (BP > 180/120 and signs of End organ damage) **send to ER**

Injection techniques to decrease pain

- Most are obvious: pinch surrounding skin at the time of injection ("Gate theory of pain"), use small diameter needle, add bicarbonate to anesthetic, pretreat w/ topical anesthetics or ice-pack to skin, inject slowly, reintroduce needle in previously anesthetized area, and use music or mental distraction to reduce perception of pain

- **Warm anesthetic** to body temperature before injecting
- Use regional blocks (discussed in section 8.1)
    - Risk of blocks include nerve injury, vessel trauma and intravascular infiltration **(pain after block → Rx: stop block, massage, and use plain lidocaine next)**

Topical anesthetics

- EMLA (Eutectic Mixture of Local Anesthesia): 2.5% lidocaine and 2.5% prilocaine
    - "EMLA (Ema) COMBS her hair"
        - Corneal injury (cannot use near eye)
        - Occlusion required
        - **Methemoglobinemia due to prilocaine (CI in infants and in G6PD def)**
        - Broken skin is a CI; Blue color to skin is a SE (causes purpura in children)
        - Basal layer split is seen on path
        - Swelling and vacuolization of upper epidermis is seen on path
- LMX4: lidocaine 4%
- Cocaine: only ester to cause vasoconstriction (all other cause vasodilation)
    - 2nd longest duration of action (2 hours); **dibucaine** has the longest (3–4 hours)
- Benzocaine: topical ester anesthetic used on skin and mucous membranes
    - Shortest onset of action (1 minute)
    - SE: highest risk of ACD and **causes methemoglobinemia in pediatric patients**
- **Tetracaine** and Proparacaine: used for ocular anesthesia ("your eyes are white like TP")
    - Use one of these before placing corneal eye shield
- Benoxinate eye drops contain fluorescein which numbs eye and has a fluorescent color

- True allergies to local anesthetics are rare and usually results from PABA metabolites (like esters) or paraben/ metabisulfide preservatives (like amides)

Anxiety-control measures

- Preoperative anxiolytics (benzodiazepines) → reverse overdose w/ flumazenil

Post-operative pain management

- Pain is at maximal severity on night of surgery and should subside by day 4
  - o Consider infection or hematoma if pain continues beyond this period
- Risk factors include flaps, grafts, high preoperative anxiety, multiple lesions treated at once and surgical sites involving the lip, forehead, scalp, genitalia, nail, chest, and leg
- NSAIDS and acetaminophen alone or in combination are recommended as 1st line
  - o Max dose of tylenol: 4 g/day (< 60 y/o), 3 g/day (> 60 y/o), 2 g/day (liver failure)
  - o Do not prescribe NSAIDS in those with NSAID allergies, pregnancy, peptic ulcers (careful w/ prednisone), renal impairment or cirrhosis (↑ risk of GI bleeding)
- Opioids are 2nd line options for moderate to severe pain (10 tabs of 5mg oxycodone)
  - o MOA: act on the mu receptors in the CNS to produce analgesic effects
  - o Side effects: nausea, constipation, respiratory depression and dependence
- Tramadol has multiple MOA including acting through opioid receptors
  - o ↓ respiratory depression, GI effects and dependance vs traditional opiates

7.6 Antiseptics

General considerations

- Shaving causes abrasions and allows bacteria to enter wound → use clippers instead
- Skin flora is divided into 2 groups
    - Transient bacteria (bad): reside superficially, easily removed w/ hand washing and are responsible for most health care worker transmitted infections
    - Resident bacteria (good): resides deeper, not easily removed, not a/w infections
- Best antiseptics to ↓ bacterial counts: alcohol > chlorhexidine > iodine > triclosan > soap

Antiseptics

- Alcohol (70% is most effective strength)
    - MOA: denatures cell walls ("alcoh-**ol** rhymes w/ wall")
    - **Fastest onset** ("I get drunk fast on alcohol") but offers no residual activity
    - Very broad spectrum but inactive against spores and is not as effective as soap for visibly soiled hands (e.g., dirt, blood, and body fluids)
    - SE: Flammable (caution w/ electrosurgery and lasers); rarely causes cutaneous hemorrhage in neonates
- Chlorhexidine (2%–4%)
    - MOA: **biguanide** which disrupts cells membranes ("only members can dine")
    - Bacteriostatic at low concentrations and bactericidal at high concentrations
    - Rapid onset and has **best residual activity (longest duration)**
        - Does not need to be dry to be effective
    - Very broad spectrum but inactive against spores

  - SE: **ototoxic** and causes **keratitis/corneal ulcers** (never use around eyes or ears)
- Iodine (povidone-iodine)
  - MOA: **halogen** causing oxidation → ↓cell membranes ("only members can dine")
  - Rapid onset but **must wait to dry to be effective** and has poor residual activity
  - **Broadest spectrum** (includes spores) but **inactivated by organic material (blood)**
  - SE: contact dermatitis (must wash it off after), skin irritation, skin discoloration and may cause hypothyroidism in neonates w/ chronic maternal use
- Chloroxylenol (parachlorometaxylenol)
  - MOA: deactivates enzymes/alters cell walls (chloroxylen-**ol** rhymes w/ wall)
  - Slow onset but has good residual activity
  - Broad spectrum but **ineffective against pseudomonas** unless combined w/ EDTA
    - "Chloro = chlorophyl = green = pseudomonal green nail syndrome"
- Hexachlorophene
  - MOA: phenol which inactivates enzymes
  - Slow onset and has only modest residual activity
  - Effective against G(+) but ineffective against G(-), mycobacteria and fungi
  - SE: neurotoxic and teratogenic (pregnancy category X) → not used anymore
    - Can also cause neuropathic symptoms in the fingers of surgeons
- Quaternary ammonium compounds (Benzalkonium)
  - MOA: induces leaks in cytoplasmic Membranes
  - Slow onset but good residual activity
  - Effective against G(+) but ineffective against G(-), mycobacteria and fungi
  - Preservative used in Multi-dose eyedrops

  - Inactivated by organic and some inorganic (cotton gauze) Materials
- Triclosan ("PqRST")
  - MOA: ↓ RNA/Protein Synthesis; binds enoyl-acyl carrier Protein Reductase
  - Rapid onset with good Residual activity
  - Effective against G Positive but ineffective against G(-) and filamentous fungi
  - Used as a coating in Sutures → ↓ Surgical site infections
- Soap and water
  - MOA: detergent; removes dirt, microorganisms and organic substances
  - Very rapid onset but has no residual activity
  - Highly effective against C. difficile and Norwalk viruses and best for soiled hands

7.7 Electrosurgery

- Uses high-frequency **alternating currents** (bi-directional flow) to provide hemostasis
- Cold electrode tip is applied to tissue relaying high frequency alternating current which does not conduct due to the high resistance of human tissue, the electrical energy is converted to thermal energy in skin causing tissue destruction
- Types ("CDEF"): electroCoagulation, electroDesication, electrosEction, electroFulgaration
  - Group the C and E together and remember its characteristics as the early letters; group the D and F together and remember its characteristics as the late letters
- ElectroCoaguation and electrosEction are Biterminal devices and require Grounding pad (Dispersive

Electrode) or biterminal Forceps; Dry waveforms; ↑ **Amperage**; ↓ voltage

- ElectroCoagulation: causes the most Collateral tissue destruction but has the lowest risk to Cardiac defibrillators and pacemakers (besides electroCautery)
- ElectrosEction: **driest** waveform (pure cutting) w/ the **least tissue destruction** of all methods but has **highest current and thus largest risk to ICDs/pacemakers**
  - Immediate hemostasis upon incision by coagulation on both sides of cut

- ElectroDesication/Fulgaration are Monoterminal; Wet (damp) waveform; ↑**Volt**; ↓amp
  - Electro-ful-garation: held at a distance ("full" cm b/w tip and tissue) and causes superficial destruction; **spark** is seen; causes epidermal carbonization ("char")
  - Electrodesication: causes deeper destruction w/ no space b/w tip and tissue
- Alternative mnemonic: "electrosurgery is as easy as ABC'S"
  - ↑ Amperage (↓ voltage); Biterminal → ElectroCoaguation and electroSection

Complications (ABCs)

- If used w/ Aluminum chloride or Alcohol preps while working PeriAnally (methane from bowl gas) it can cause a fire → use chlorhexidine or iodine instead
  - Monopolar devices are the MC source of fires in dermatologic surgery
- Thermoelectric Burns if patient is not properly grounded
- Interference with ICDs (more sensitive) and pacemakers (less sensitive)

- Send for **preoperative Cardiology Consult** or use **Cautery** > electro-Coagulation
- If cautery cannot be used then direct current away from implantable device w/ grounding plate, use short energy bursts (< 5 secs), use low power settings, avoid electrosection (highest risk) and do not use within **5 cm** of an implantable device
- MCC of pacemaker dysfunction from electrosurgery is **oversensing** (when pacer incorrectly senses non-cardiac electrical activity and is inhibited from pacing)
- Use of magnets to pace device at a preset rate is controversial (wrong answer!)
- For noncardiac electrical implantable devices (cochlear implants or deep brain stimulators), **use only bipolar electrodes** no closer to the implant than **1 cm** to avoid device dysfunction (**using monopolar devices on the head/neck is CI**)

Electrocautery

- Portable device with no current (no amperage or voltage) flowing through the patient
- Uses **direct current** to generate heat (calor is hot in Spanish) which provides hemostasis
    - Electrolysis is a hair removal treatment that also uses direct current and is the only form of electrosurgery that uses both low amperage and low voltage
- Maximum tissue destruction of all methods and poses no risk to ICDs and pacemakers
- In contrast to electrosurgery, electrocautery has a hot electrode tip (vs cold), uses **direct current (vs alternating)**, current flows to the device tip (vs to the skin), does not rely on human tissue for energy (vs electrical energy is converted to thermal energy in skin) and has

no risk to implantable devices (vs risk to devices but risk is ↓ w/ biterminal forceps)

- The Shaw scalpel (used for rhinophyma and in parotid surgery) uses electrocautery
  - "Shaw rhymes w/ electro-cau"

7.8 CRYOSURGERY

- Use of a low temperature substance to cause tissue damage
- Mechanism ("CD"): **Cell membrane rupture (via intracellular ice Crystal formation)**, extracellular Dehydration (via extracellular ice Crystal formation), vaso-Constriction (from initial freezing), compensatory vaso-Dilation after thawing (releases free-radicals)
- **Optimal technique: fast freezing + slow thawing (favors intracellular ice crystals)**
- Maximum depth of the ice ball/ice crystals that can form is **1 cm**
- MC cryogen is liquid nitrogen: boiling point is -196° C
- Temperature required for cell death by cell type
  - **Melanocytes (most sensitive): -5° C ("melano-nickels") → SE hypopigmentation**
  - **Benign tumors, keratinocytes and AKs: -25° C ("keratino-quarters")**
  - Dermal fibroblasts: -40° C ("fibro-forty")
  - **Malignant tumors: -50° C**
- Delivery techniques
  - Open technique (MC): liquid nitrogen is released through tips or cannulas
  - Closed technique: uses a probe (pre-cooled metal tip) that Contacts skin
  - Chamber technique: cryogen is released into a chamber and the turbulence within the chamber

allows cryogen to get Colder faster → used for **Cancer**
  - o Intralesional technique: cryogen is injected directly into tissue w/ a needle
- CI on the digit in a pt w/ Raynaud's

7.9 Excisions

- Excisions should be football shaped w/ **apical angle ≤ 30° → length:width ratio ≥ 3:1**
- Variations
  - o Crescent excision: when one side is longer than the other; used in areas such as the Cheek or Chin where relaxed skin tension lines are Curvilinear
  - o M-plasty: used to ↓ length of an excision so it does not abut a free Margin
  - o S-plasty: scar is S-shaped (even though the distance between the two apices stays the same, the total length of the scar is ↑)
    - Redistributes tension along different vectors but tension is ↓ in the center (↓ risk of central Separation/depression and scar contraction)
    - Commonly used on convex surfaces (**Shin, Shoulder, forearm, and cheek**)
  - o Lip wedge excision: repairs up to 1/3rd length of lower lip in a Layered repair:
    - "I saw someone get their lip knocked out in this one epiSODE on ESPN"
      1) **Submucosal layer**: use Soft Sutures like Silk > polyglactin 910
         - o Labial a. lies beneath orbicularis oris and above submucosa

2) **Orbicularis oris (critical step; closed first)**: use Polyglactin 910
    - o Muscle approximation is key to preventing depressed scar
    - o For lip repairs (including mucosal advancement flaps) we undermine in the submucosal plane, deep to minor salivary glands and superficial to orbicularis oris
3) Dermis/SQ: use Polyglactin 910
4) Epidermis: use Nylon w/ hypereversion to prevent depressed scar

- Standing cones ("dog ears") are caused by apical angles ≥ 30°, length:width ratio ≤ 3:1, unequal lengths on each side of wound (longer side will have cones), non-uniform depth of excision, convex surface, inadequate undermining or excess SQ tissue at apical angles
    - o "If you see dog ears, then fix THEM"
        - ▪ Burrows Triangle: triangle of tissue that is excised so that tissue adjacent to the wound w/ the standing cone can be advanced without it buckling
        - ▪ Rule of Halves: standing cone is redistributed along the entire length of an excision by halving it throughout
        - ▪ Extending incision: ↑ length allows for redistribution of excess skin
        - ▪ M-plasty: allows for excision of the standing cone
- Layered closures (e.g., closing SQ space) offers ↓ tension on wound edges (↓ risk of dehiscence) and ↓ dead space (↓ risk of hematoma/seroma) vs simple closures

Undermining planes

- Face: undermining in the SQ plane preserves motor nerves (all deep to SMAS)
    - o Lower forehead: deep SQ plane just above frontalis
    - o Cheek: mid-SQ plane (avoids parotid duct + buccal/zygomatic branches of CN7)
    - o Temple: superficial SQ plane (avoids temporal branch of facial nerve)
    - o Eyebrow: mid SQ deep to hair bulb (minimizes eyebrow hair loss)
    - o Lip and eyelid: above orbicularis oris and oculi, respectively (minimal SQ tissue)
    - o Ear: above perichondrium (minimal SQ tissue here)
    - o Nose: above nasalis (upper 1/3rd of nose) or above perichondrium (lower 2/3rd)
- Lateral neck: superficial SQ (avoids spinal accessory nerve found at Erb's point)
- Scalp: subgaleal space/loose areolar connective tissue (avascular plane)
    - o Scalp layer's ("ED'S GP"): Epidermis, Dermis, SQ, Galea, and Periosteum
- Upper forehead: between deep SMAS and periosteum (V1 sensory nerves initially run deep to forehead muscles as they exit the skull but then superficial to SMAS superiorly)
    - o Forehead layers: skin, SQ, superficial SMAS, frontalis, deep SMAS, periosteum
- Trunk/extremities: mid to deep fat (above fascia for large lesions or melanomas)

Wound/scar strength after closure

- 1 week: 5%
- 2 weeks: 10%
- 3 weeks: 20%
- 4 weeks 40% (notice how in the 1st month, every week it doubles)

- 1 year and beyond: 80% (wound never returns to 100% strength)

Surgical margins w/ WLE (do not do a flap/extensive undermining until clear margins identified)

- Melanoma
  - In-situ: 0.5 cm–1 cm margins and down to deep fat
  - < 1 mm deep: 1 cm margins and down to fascia
  - 1–2 mm deep: 1–2 cm margins and down to fascia
  - > 2 mm deep: 2 cm margins and down to fascia
- BCC: usually 0.4 cm margins; 0.6–1 cm margins if BCC is high risk (see below)
- SCC: usually 0.4–0.6 cm margins; 0.6–1 cm margins if SCC is high risk (see below)
  - Must include peripheral erythema around tumor as part of the cancer
- Others can be remembered with the "SLAM'D Angi Extra" mnemonic
  - SCC and BCC/Sebaceous carcinoma: 0.4–1 cm (melanoma in-Situ is 0.5–1 cm)
  - Leiomyosarcoma/AFX/Merkel cell carcinoma/ Melanoma: 1–2 cm
  - DFSP: 2–5 cm (2 cm → 40% recurrence rate; 3 cm → 15%; 5 cm 5%)
  - Angiosarcoma/Extramammary Paget's disease: 5 cm

High risk factors of NMSC: "HIGH RISK NMSC" (**NCCN high-risk features**)

- **High risk locations (H or M; esp ears/lips for SCC)**; Huge tumor (> 2 cm)
  - > 4 cm wide and > 6 mm deep/invasion beyond fat is very high risk in SCC
    - Any of these would automatically result in SCC being AJCC8 stage T3

- Immunosuppressed patient (transplant/lymphoma/HIV)
- Growth is fast (this feature is specific for SCC)
- **High risk Histology**
    - o BCC: infiltrative, sclerosing, morpheaform, micro-nodular, metatypical
    - o SCC: spindle cell/desmoplastic or adenoid subtype or poorly differentiated tumor
- Radiation previously done at site of cancer; Recurrence
    - o Ill-defined borders; Invasion of nerves > 0.1mm, lymphatics or vessels on path
    - o Scars (Marjolin's ulcers; this feature is specific for SCCs)
    - o Key patient characteristics (genetic syndromes or immunocompromised patients)
    - o Neuro symptoms (SCC only): pain/paresthesia/anesthesia/diplopia (suggests PNI)

High risk (H), Medium risk (M) and low risk (L) areas of body

- H: T-zone of face (near orifices including chin), nipples, hands/feet, and genitals
- M: cheeks, forehead, scalp, neck, jawline, and pretibial surface
- L: trunk and extremities (excluding pretibial surface, nipples, genitals, hands, and feet)

Postsurgical wound care

- Ideal wound dressing helps achieve hemostasis, protects against infection and foreign material, limits tissue movement, provides a moist environment and removes exudate
- Conventional wound dressings can be "layered" with ointments
    - o Petrolatum is better than topical antibiotics (cause antimicrobial resistance/ACD)

- Topical silicone is better than petrolatum as it is nonocclusive, waterproof, gas permeable, is anti-microbial and ↓ inflammation and scar formation

7.10 MOHs Surgery

ABC's of MOHs surgery

- Surgeon cuts tissue at an Acute (30–45°) angle (scalpel is Beveled) so tissue can lie flat (epi is in the same plane as the deep tissue) → allows for horizontal processing and staining of slides using H&E or toluidine Blue w/ complete 360° (Circumferential) margin control (100% of margin is visualized vs 1% in standard bread-loafing technique)
- ↑ Cure rates (↓ recurrences) compared to WLE and to Slow-MOHs (probably because hospital histotechnicians are not as experienced getting 100% of the epidermal margin)
- Conserves healthy (non-cancerous) tissue
- Cost-effective relative to other skin cancer treatments
- Contiguous growth pattern of the tumor is essential
  - Tumors w/ skip lesions may erroneously be read as clear
- CLIA requires that **MOHs slides are preserved for 10 years after date of examination**, paper/EMR notes for 2 years (except path report which is for 10 years), and that tissue remnants are preserved in the cryostat until a diagnosis is made on the specimen
  - Just remember if it relates to path its 10 years, whereas chart notes are 2 years

Steps ("Propper orientation will help you Score In Bed, aka have sex")

1. Orientation/mapping: each specimen should have a distinct hash marks (e.g., 6 o'clock)

2. Scoring/relaxing incisions/prepping to lay flat: relaxation cuts are made 1/3rd the way from outer circumference parallel to the epidermis (30° angle) halfway into specimen
3. Inking/chromacoting: must ink entire edge if no epidermis is present (true margin is when either full epi or full ink is present) and helps w/ orientation
4. Embedding: once specimen is lying flat and inked, it is frozen onto a glass slide using frozen tissue media and transferred to chucks
5. Sectioning: the frozen specimen is sectioned from deep tissue to superficial; the initial sections are discarded (because these usually won't contain 100% of the epi)

Potential pitfalls while reading slides

- Because of the beveling and then flattening of a 3-dimensional structure into a 2-dimesional slide, tumor seen in the deep may really be near the margin and both deep and the epidermal margin should be taken in the next stage
- Scar adjacent to tumor is never a clear margin as scar can lead to discontinuous tumor
    - **If you see scar where you are concerned there may be cancer, get deepers!**
- Inflammation deep to cancer should not be read as clear as this indicates more tumor

MOHs cure rates for cancers that are MOHs appropriate ("BALD and SMEL-E MOHs patients")

- BALD (95%-100% cure): BCC (99%)/SCC (97%), AFX, Apocrine/eccrine carcinoma, Adnexal carcinoma, Adenoid cystic carcinoma, Lentigo maligna, DFSP
    - Only use MOHs for in-situ melanomas on cosmetically sensitive areas (e.g., face)

- SMEL (90–95%): Sebaceous carcinoma, MAC, Erythroplasia of Queyrat, and Leiomyosarcoma
- E (85% cure rate but greatly improved w/ IHC): Extramammary Paget's disease

Indications for MOHs for NMSC: refer to HIGH RISK NMSC mnemonic in section 8.9 and 6.1

- Must know what is MOHs criteria! If it is in the HIGH-RISK NCCN mnemonic, it qualifies
- Important to know High risk (H), Medium risk (M) and low risk (L) areas of body
    - H: facial T-zone (periorificial + temples/chin), nipples, hands/feet/ancles, and genitals
    - M: cheeks, forehead, scalp, neck, jawline, and pretibial surface
    - L: trunk and extremities (excluding pretibial skin, nipples/genitals, and hands/feet)
- Aggressive histology, H-zone area, genetic syndromes, immunocompromised, **recurrent tumors, skin cancer arising in scar or radiation** are particularly heavily weighted factors
- Every skin cancer in the "BALD and SMEL-E" mnemonic is always appropriate for MOHs even w/ primary tumors on low risk (L) area in healthy patients with some exceptions...
    - Non-aggressive SCC (including Bowens) on L area if ≤ 1 cm is inappropriate, and if 1.01–2 cm, it is uncertain (surprisingly, a KA is appropriate on L area if > 1 cm)
        - For SCCs (including Bowens) lesions of any size on M area are appropriate
    - **SCC in situ arising from an AK (AK w/ focal SCC in situ) is NEVER appropriate**
    - **Superficial BCC on L area of any size (even if recurrent) are not appropriate**

        - Genetic syndromes make primary sBCC of any size appropriate on L area
        - Recurrent sBCC on L area are always inappropriate even w/ a syndrome
    - **Superficial BCC on the M area if ≤ 0.5 cm are uncertain** (unless tumor is recurrent or patient is immunocompromised in which case it is appropriate)
    - **Nodular BCC on L area if ≤ 1 cm is inappropriate and if 1.01–2 cm it is uncertain**
        - Any recurrent nodular BCC is appropriate even in the L area
        - Aggressive BCCs ≥ 0.6 cm and nodular BCCs in the immunocompromised ≥ 1 cm are appropriate in the L area
    - Aggressive BCC and SCC subtypes are always appropriate except aggressive BCCs on L area which are uncertain, even if the patient is immunocompromised
- **Merkel cell carcinoma and lentigo Maligna/MIS for MOHs Must be on the M or H area**
    - Uncertain if on L area regardless of size (recurrent lesion makes it appropriate)
- Angiosarcoma is always "uncertain"
- Bowenoid papulosis is always inappropriate
- DTE is not appropriate on L areas and "uncertain" on M or H area

To summarize the highly testable points of MOHs appropriate use criteria for BCCs and SCCs

- Any BCC or SCC is appropriate in H and M zone (except sBCC ≤ 0.5 cm in M zone)
    - And this does not include SCC arising from an AK which is never appropriate
- Any aggressive SCC (e.g., sclerosing) or BCC (infiltrative) is appropriate anywhere

  - Except aggressive BCC ≤ 0.5 cm in the L zone +/- immunocompromise (uncertain)
- Nodular BCCs and non-aggressive SCCs are only appropriate in L zone if ≥ 2 cm
  - Except KA which is not an aggressive SCC but it is appropriate in L zone if ≥ 1 cm
  - Immunocompromise makes these appropriate in L zone if ≥ 1 cm
  - Recurrent non-aggressive BCCs or SCC are always appropriate in L zone
    - Except recurrent SCCIS (uncertain) or sBCC (inappropriate) in the L zone

Stains to be familiar with in MOHs surgery

- BCC: **toluidine blue** (special stain), AE1/AE3 and Ber-EP4 (IHC stains)
- SCC: AE1/AE3 (IHC stain), p63 (IHC stain) can be useful in poorly differentiated SCCs
- Melanoma: **Melan-A/MART-1 (MC)**, Mel-5, SOX10, MITF, and HMB-45 (IHC stains)
- DFSP: CD34 (IHC stain)
- Seb-A-ceous carcinoma: Oil red O (special stain), Adipophilin, EMA, and AE1/AE3 (IHC stains)
- MAC: toluidine blue (special stain) and cytokeratin (IHC stain)
- EMPD: PAS (special stain), **CK7 (most used),** and CEA (IHC stains)
- Merkel cell carcinoma: CK20 (most used), CAM5.2, and AE-1

Interpretation of MOHs surgery slides

- If there is no tumor seen and 100% of the deep/peripheral margin is seen then it is clear
- If there is tumor seen then perform another layer to clear the tumor

- If not 100% of the deep (holes) or epidermal margin is not seen then **ask for a recut**
- If there is an uncertainty in diagnosis or need to appropriately stage tumor then thaw the tissue and send for permanents

7.11 Flaps

- Axial Pattern flaps: flaps based on a named vessel
    - Abbe cross-lip flap (abbe; labial artery)
    - Paramedian forehead flap (supratrochlear artery)
- Random pattern flap: flaps w/ unnamed arteries of the underlying subdermal/dermal vascular plexuses (includes all flaps not listed above)
- "Facial reconstruction is an ART" → Advancement, Rotation, Transposition
    - Advancement: flap is moved linearly onto primary defect producing a tension vector that is opposite the direction of flap movement (**the scar lines are linear**)
        - Only flap which **does not redirect the primary tension vector**
        - **The key stitch** (point of max tension) **is used to close the primary defect**
        - Advantage: burrows triangle can be put far away from a free margin
        - Disadvantage: limited by degree of elasticity of surrounding skin
    - Rotation flap: pivots (rotates) adjacent tissue around an axis to close a defect
        - **Redirects tension vector along on arc** next to the primary defect
        - **They key suture is used to close the primary defect**

        - Advantage: makes use of skin laxity at a distance from the defect
        - Disadvantage: functional Reduction in flap length
    - Transposition: noncontiguous skin is lifting over normal skin into primary defect
        - **Redirects primary tension vector to donor site** (tension vector of the donor site will be the primary tension vector for closure of the defect)
        - **They key suture is used to close the 2° defect (3° defect for bilobed flap)**
            - **Must close 2° defect (3° defect for bilobed flap) first**
        - Advantage: utilizes nearby but nonadjacent tissue reservoir
        - Disadvantage: **Trapdooring/pincushioning** (undermine widely to prevent)
            - Pincushioning occurs in 15% of transposition flaps on the nose
            - Due to insufficient undermining, oversized flap or ↑ SQ fat in flap
            - Rx: **ILK**, CO_2 laser, dermabrasion, debulking, multiple Z-plastys
    - Interpolation: two-stage transpositions that allows for ↑ flap length:width ratio of > 4:1 ("interpolation is long word → long length"); does not cause trapdooring
        - Pedicle is taken down at **3 weeks**
        - MC SE of interpolation flaps is **bleeding**
- Indications: close large defect that cannot be closed by other modalities (linear closure)
- CI: flaps are CI if existing malignancy is not completely cleared (tumor can spread along plane of undermining → ↑ morbidity); smoking is relative CI (advise to stop for surgery)

Notable examples of flaps

- Advancement flaps
  - Unilateral burrows advancement (O → L): displace burrows away from the eyelid
    - Commonly used on the forehead
  - Unilateral crescentic advancement (cheek to nose crescentic): variant of O → L where a crescentic dog ear is removed within the flap body
    - Commonly used for a cheek to nose advancement (lateral nasal defect)
  - Unilateral O → U advancement (helical rim advancement): incisions and Burrows triangle are oriented in the same direction away from the defect
    - Commonly used on Helical rim (Hyper-evert flap to prevent notching)
    - Rintala flap is an O → U that it used for defects on the nasal tip
  - Bilateral O → T advancement: 2 opposing flaps are B/L advanced onto defect
    - Optimal design is flap height (defect + dog ear) is 2X the defect diameter
    - Commonly used on chin and **lower eyelid defects** (no risk of ectropion)
  - Bilateral O → H advancement: essentially a bilateral O → U flap
    - Commonly used on the forehead but forehead numbness is a common SE
  - Island pedicle ("kite flap; V → Y) advancement: unlike other advancements, area under flap body is not undermined (≥ 40% of the pedicle must remain intact) but the periphery is and a V-shaped island w/ underlying pedicle is advanced onto defect (ideal length:width ratio is ≤ 4:1); key stitch is midpoint of leading edge

        - Commonly used next to free margins (nose, eyes, lips)
    - Mucosal advancement: mucosal lip is advanced to cover a vermillion lip defect
        - Undermine deep to minor salivary gland but superficial to orbicularis oris
        - Favored method for restoration of the vermillion (**maintains cupids bow**)
        - SE: lip numbness, drooling and feminization of males
- Rotation flaps
    - Unilateral rotation: curvilinear flap w/ arc length/ width > defect length/width
        - Area of pivotal restraint is widely undermined; back cuts ↑ mobility
        - Commonly used on the scalp, upper cutaneous lip and nose
    - Unilateral rotation Rieger variant (dorsal nasal rotation; Hatchet flap; glabella turn-down): some consider it an axial flap (angular artery) w/ a backcut in the glabella; skin is undermined just above perichondrium
        - Point of maxima pivotal restraint is the **medial canthal tendon**
        - Used for medium to large (up to 2.5 cm) midline nasal tip defects
        - SE: thick glabellar skin is rotated into medial canthus + pig-nose deformity
    - Unilateral rotation Mustarde/Tenzel variant: **lateral cheek/temple skin** is rotated to cover a large (Mustarde) or smaller (Tenzel) lower lid defect
        - Tacking sutures to lateral orbital rim periosteum decreases ectropion risk
    - Bilateral rotation (O → Z): double rotation flap w/ yin-yang shaped used on scalp
- Single staged transposition flaps

- Rhombic flap: classic design is a parallelogram-shaped flap that forms a question mark-shaped scar; 2° defect is closed first (**key stich: midpoint of question mark**)
    - If they ask to which corner a tip of tissue gets flapped onto in a rhombic flap just count 2 corners from the starting point
    - Commonly used on convex surfaces (cheek) but can be used anywhere
    - Webster (narrower pedicle; ↑ ischemia risk) and DuFourmental are variants w/ a shorter arch of rotation → easier to close the 2° defect
- Bilobed flap: multilobed transposition flap that shares tension between all lobes
    - 45° angle from 1° defect to 1° lobe and 45° angle from 2° lobe to 1° lobe
        - Flap has 90° angle in total
        - 1° defect, 1° lobe and 2° lobe should be roughly equal in diameter
    - Undermine above perichondrium (submuscular) as we always do on nose
    - Used for nasal ala defects (little tension on alar rim → no pulling on ala)
    - Variants include Zitelli modification (total transposition arc of 90° to 110°), lateral (modified) bilobed flap (used for defects on nasal tip not ala) and the trilobe flap (uses 3 lobes; total arch of rotation is 120°)
- Banner transposition flap: long skinny (> 3:1 length to width ratio) pedicle gets transposed ≥90° onto 1° defect (prone to necrosis due to narrow pedicle)
    - Used on the upper helical rim, medial canthus and lower eyelid
- Nasolabial (melolabial) transposition flap: skin from medial cheek is transposed onto nasal ala defects using a long skinny pedicle (like the Banner

transposition except the arc of rotation is < 60°); the medial margin of the flap is drawn within the nasolabial fold and the lateral margin is located on the medial cheek

- Used for medium sized defects of the nasal ala
- Flap is supplied from branches of the **angular artery**
- SE: **blunting of alar crease** (and all transposition flaps get pincushioning)
- Place tacking suture from the dermal undersurface of flap to periosteum (in the concavity of the nasofacial sulcus) to ↓ blunting of the alar crease

- Z-plasty: used in revision of "zcars" (lengthen contracted scar or redirect tension)
  - Re-orients scar, but **elongates** central arm of scar (unlike S-plasty which ↑ total scar length but distance between the 2 apices stays the same)
  - ↑ angle used → ↑ length gained and ↑ reorientation of tension
    - **60° angle 75% ↑ in length and 90° tension reorientation**
      - **60 + 15 = 75; 75 + 15 = 90**
    - 45° angle → 50% ↑ in length and 65° tension reorientation
    - 30° angle → 25% ↑ in length and 40° tension reorientation
      - Notice every 15° angle ↓ from baseline (bolded) results in a 25% ↓ in length and a 25° ↓ in tension reorientation
  - The bigger the angle, the ↑ tension b/w the two transposition flaps and the ↑ risk of dog ears; the smaller the angle, the ↑ risk of flap necrosis

    - "I'd rather a big tense dog then a small dead one"
- Interpolation flaps ("Before take down at 3 weeks, interpolation flaps look like a RAMP")
    - Retroauricular flap: Rectangular-shaped Random pattern flap that is Raised in SQ plane from Retroauricular sulcus to the hairline and sutured onto helical defect
    - Abbe' lip switch: Axial flap based on labial artery which transfers orbicularis oris and lip mucosa from lip to cover large defect of opposing lip
    - Melolabial/nasolabial interpolation flap: random pattern flap (perforators of angular artery not angular artery itself) w/ a similar design to melolabial transposition used for large nasal ala defects (but does not blunt alar crease)
    - Paramedian forehead flap: axial flap based on the **supratrochlear artery** where tissue from the forehead is used to repair large defects of the distal nose
        - Supratrochlear artery is found directly under the medial canthal vertical line (1 cm lateral to glabellar midline) and pierces through the corrugator supercilii muscle into the SQ skin 1.5–2.5 cm above the supraorbital rim
        - Pedicles **1 cm** (8–15mm) is adequate for flap mobility and vascular supply
        - Must thin the tip (distal aspect) of the flap (metabolically less demanding)

7.12 Grafts

Graft physiology ("IRS"; notice how the stages are in alphabetical order)

- Imbibition (1 day): "fibrin glue" attaches graft to recipient bed which allows **passive diffusion** of nutrients from fibrin lattice to graft → graft is edematous ("Massive graft")
  - **At 24 hours the graft turns dusky blue** (due to venous congestion); **hyperemia**
- Inosculation (1 day to 1 week): **anastomoses** b/w wound bed and **existing** graft vessels
- Revascularization (1 week to 1 month): vascular proliferation of **new** vessels in graft
- Sensory innervation (1 month to 1 year): reinnervation of new sensory nerves to graft

Types of Grafts ("Sam Bankman Fried is a Crypto Conman")

- Split-thickness skin graft: epidermis and variable amount of dermis ("dermis is split")
  - Specialized instruments are required (e.g., Weck blade, zimmer and mesher)
  - Advantages: covers larger Surface area, ↑ **graft Survival** (thinner grafts have ↓ metabolic demand) and tumor recurrences are more easily Seen
    - Can be used directly over periosteum/perichondrium whereas FTSGs must first allow time for granulation tissue to form at the base of defect
  - Disadvantages: ↑ **contraction (do not use near free margin),** poor cosmesis (adnexal structures not retained), bullae form within graft (↓ anchoring to BMZ)
- Burow's graft: type of FTSG where donor skin is from one of the discarded dog ears of a primary closure that failed to close all the way (thus requiring a graft)

    - Provides excellent tissue match compared w/ grafts harvested from distant sites
- Full-thickness skin graft (FTSG): comprised of epidermis and full thickness dermis
    - **Advantages: ↓ contraction, good cosmesis (retains adnexal structures)**
    - **Disadvantages: poor survival** (thicker graft has ↑ metabolic demand; graft Fails)
        - Poking small fenestrations into the exposed auricular cartilage provides the area w/ access to robust vascular supply from the opposing side of the ear improving graft survival (or granulation if healing by 2° intent)
    - Must oversize graft by Fifteen percent to account for shrinkage after harvesting
        - Consider oversizing 25% on eyelid to ↓ wound contraction (ectropion)
    - De-Fatting of graft is recommended to ↑ graft survival
    - Basting stitch or bolster dressing is recommended to immobilize graft and ↑ graft adherence to wound bed (↑ graft survival)
    - Delayed grafting: wound granulates for 1 to 3 weeks before applying the graft to ↑ graft survival of deep wounds where avascular bone/cartilage is exposed
    - **Dermabrasion may be performed at Five weeks** post-op to ↑ cosmesis
    - Graft necrosis denoted by **black color: do not remove (acts as biologic dressing)**
- Cartilage graft: MC used to prevent nasal valve Collapse in large nasal defects
    - MC source of cartilage grafts are from the antihelix and the Conchal bowl

  - Moderately high metabolic demand (transposition flap after cartilage will ensure the most robust vascular supply and best chance of graft survival)
- Composite graft: most often refers to FTSG + Cartilage (same purpose as cartilage graft)
  - Also useful for full-thickness **alar rim defects** (FTSG may cause alar notching)
  - Thickest graft so has **highest metabolic demand (highest risk of necrosis)**
  - Any graft comprised of cartilage has a higher risk of infection
  - MC source of composite grafts are from Crux of helix and helical rim for nasal ala defects and Concha for nasal sidewall or columella defects

MC FTSG donor sites

- Nasal dorsum/sidewall/tip/ala defects: preauricular sulcus (sun-exposed) donor site
- Lower eyelid defect: upper eyelid or postauricular sulcus (sun-protected) donor site
- Ear defect: pre or postauricular sulcus
- Scalp/forehead defect (SCALP): SupraClavicular region, inner upper Arm, Lateral neck

7.13 Surgical Complications

- "I HID from surgical complications": Ischemia (12 hours), Hematoma/bleeding (2 days), Infection (4 days), Dehiscence (8 days)

Ischemia: due to venous congestion or arterial insufficiency

- Venous congestion (< 4 hours post op): p/w cyanotic skin w/ dark blood on skin-prick
- Arterial insufficiency (12 hours post-op): p/w pallor and no bleeding on skin-prick test

Hematoma/bleeding (highest risk is in the first 48 hours)

- Stable: non-expanding firm to fluctuant red-purple mass w/ **pressure sensation**
    - o If small (5–10 mL), stable and not compromising tissue viability than no surgical intervention is necessary and treat w/ warm compresses (body will reabsorb it)
        - Early (< 2 days) and late (> 10 days) hematomas are fluctuant
            - Rx: can be aspirated w/ large bore needle through suture line
        - Organized hematomas (2–10 days) p/w firm mass (cannot aspirate)
            - Rx: warm compresses (body will reabsorb it)
- Expanding hematoma: enlarging **painful/throbbing** red-purple mass
    - o Any large (> 10 cc) or rapidly expanding (active bleeding) hematoma → **open wound**, cauterize/ **ligate bleeding source and give antibiotics**
    - o Expanding hematoma near Eye (blindness) or neck (asphyxiation) → **send to ER**
- Although **anticoagulation therapy (esp warfarin) and clopidogrel** do put pts at risk for bleeding/hematoma, it is not recommended to stop anticoagulation
    - o It is recommended to hold supplements that ↑ risk of bleeding (e.g., fish oil, vit E, garlic) and aspirin/ ibuprofen taken for pain or preventive measures for 10 days prior to surgery and hold alcohol (causes **vasodilation**) for 3 days after surgery
- Warfarin antagonizes vitamin K and requires monitoring to ensure a pre-op **INR of < 3.5**
- Post-op bleeding is MC w/ non-vitamin K blockers (dabigatran, rivaroxaban, apixaban)

- Reversal agents: warfarin (vitamin K, FFP), ticagrelor (bentracimab), dabigatran (idarucizumab), rivaroxaban and other factor Xa inhibitors (Andexxa)
- Ibrutinib is a chemo agent for B-cell cancers which carries a high risk for severe bleeding

Infection (generally 4 days post-op)

- Defined as any infection that occurs within **30 days** and as a direct result of a procedure
- p/w rubor (redness), dolor (pain), calor (warmth), tumor (swelling) +/- purulence, fevers
- Sterile gloves do not decrease the risk of surgical site infections
- **Diabetes mellites** is the MC risk factor a/w infections (even more than smoking)
- MC site for surgical site infection is genitals followed by lower leg (7%)
    - On leg, infections are MC from flaps then 2° intent (6%) and primary closure (3%)
- **S. aureus** is #1 cause (pseudomonas common after ear surgery; ppx: topical gentamycin)
    - Infection is MC < 6 days after ear surgery; chondritis (Rx NSAIDS) is MC ≥ 6 days
        - Both can be red and painful but purulence points to an infection
- Rx: culture wound, antibiotics (ciprofloxacin x 7 days if by the ear) + I&D any abscesses
- Prevention: use sterile technique, minimize wound tension, perioperative antibiotic ppx
    - Perioperative (1 hour before surgery) antibiotic ppx (Adapted from JAAD 2008)
        - High risk for endocarditis/prosthetic joint infection + breach oral mucosa
        - High risk for endocarditis/prosthetic joint infection + infected skin/wound

- High risk for infective endocarditis: "PUT them on antibiotics"
  - Prosthetic cardiac valve; Prior hx of endocarditis
  - Unrepaired cyanotic congenital heart defect (or repaired w/ residual defects or repaired in last 6 months)
  - Transplanted heart who develops valvopathy
- High risk for prosthetic joint infection: first 2 years after joint replacement, prior prosthetic joint infection, type 1 DM, history of malignancy, immunosuppressed/HIV, malnourishment, hemophilia, connective tissue disease w/ arthropathy (RA, SLE)

- ppx consider in high-risk sites ("She's not a MILF but a Wild GILF")
  - Wedge excisions on lips/ears, Grafts (any site), Groins, extensive Inflammatory skin disease, Lower extremities, Flaps on nose

- Medications: **cephalexin** 2 gm once is the answer unless it is in the oral mucosa (**amoxicillin** 2 gm) or if they are PCN allergic (here the answer is clindamycin 600mg or azithromycin 500mg unless the site is the lower legs or groin and they have a PCN allergy and then you use **levofloxacin** 500mg or TMP-SMX DS)

Dehiscence

- Typically occurs 1–2 weeks post-op
- Major RFs: **smoking**, BMI > 35, DM, age > 65, wound infection, long duration of surgery

Other less tested surgical complications

- Spitting suture: buried suture is extruded from the skin surface before it dissolves and may cause erythema, edema and foreign-body sensation
    - MC w/ polyglactin 910 (Vicryl; "cry and spit")
    - Rx: removed w/ forceps or trim as close as possible to skin surface
- Suture granuloma: granulomatous reaction to suture material; p/w red bumps on scar
    - Can be purulent w/ inflammatory papules and often is mistaken for infection but is in a linear pattern along scar and occurs over a longer timeframe (2 months)
    - Rx: IL Kenalog
- Ectropion: eversion of the lower eyelid margin → inability to fully close eye → dry eye
    - Snap test: delayed retraction after lid pulled from globe indicates high risk
    - Rx: upward massage of eyelid; surgery (wedge tarsectomy or tarsal strip surgery)
- Hypergranulation tissue: p/w beefy red hypertrophic granulation tissue
    - Rx: chemical cautery w/ TCA or silver nitrate sticks; PDL laser
- Graft contamination: if graft falls on the floor, **inform patient of what happened**, **wash the graft in chlorhexidine (or povidone iodine)** and proceed with the procedure
- Needle stick: start post-exposure prophylaxis as soon as possible and until the patient has a negative HIV test (if patient cannot get tested or is positive, continue for 4 weeks)

7.14 Nail Surgery

- Total or partial nail plate avulsion is usually done prior to nail bed or nail matrix biopsy
- Nail avulsion is usually performed with a distal nail avulsion technique (nail elevator is first inserted under the nail plate distally until entire nail plate is separated from nail bed) but if there is distal subungual hyperkeratosis a proximal nail avulsion is performed
- Nail bed biopsy: done to diagnose nail bed pathology
    - Longitudinal excision ("Beds lay longitudinally when you walk in a room")
    - Double punch technique with a 3mm punch biopsy (leaves nail plate intact)
        - Depth of 2nd punch goes to periosteum
        - If punch is less than 3 mm, let it heal by secondary intent; if bigger than 3mm, use an absorbable suture (fast absorbing gut or vicryl)
    - Low risk of nail dystrophy after biopsy of nail bed
- Nail matrix biopsy: done to determine cause of melanonychia or dx tumor of the matrix
    - **Horizontal excision ("Mats lay horizontally when you walk in a house")**
    - Proximal nail fold reflected back with two 5 mm incisions from proximal nail fold
    - ↑ risk of nail dystrophy, nail plate thinning and split nails
        - **Lowest risk of nail deformity with distal nail matrix biopsies**
- Deciding what type of biopsy to do for longitudinal melanonychia
    - Pigment is on the ventral nail plate: distal nail matrix biopsy
    - Pigment is on the dorsal nail plate: proximal nail matrix biopsy

  - For central lesions, horizontal ellipse has best yield, but you can also do...
    - 3 mm punch biopsy if longitudinal melanonychia is < 3 mm
    - Shave biopsy of matrix if longitudinal melanonychia is > 3 mm
  - For lateral lesions, a lateral longitudinal excision has the best yield
- Lateral longitudinal nail biopsy
  - Lateral longitudinal excision used for lesions on lateral nail fold/bed/matrix
  - ↑ risk of spicule/cyst formation due to retention of lateral horn of **nail matrix**
  - Nail width will be permanently narrowed
- A punch biopsy may be done of the bed or matrix
- All biopsies must extend **down to bone/periosteum** (0.8 mm deep); no SQ in nail matrix
- Longest time to leave a tourniquet during a nail procedure is 15–20 minutes
- Matricectomy: removes nail matrix so no new nail plate is formed
  - #1 indication is ingrown nail (onychocryptosis)
  - Done via en-bloc excision (cancer) or chemical matricectomy (onychocryptosis)
  - "I got Post Traumatic Stress from my chemical matricectomy"
    - **Phenol (88%; MC to be used),** TCA (90%), Sodium hydroxide (10%)
  - Complications of nail surgery is "nail RIPPS Off"
    - Reflex sympathetic dystrophy (suspect if pain lasts > 10 days post-op)
    - Infection (new onset pain 48 hours post-op; always use sterile technique)
    - Pain (common in first 24 hours); Pyogenic granuloma

        - Pterygium: occurs if proximal nail fold adheres to open matrix and scars
        - Septic arthritis
        - Osteomyelitis

- Trephination indicated w/ significant **(> 50%)** nail hematomas + painful + < 48 hours old
    - "Make a Hole if Hematoma is greater than Half of nail"
    - X-rays also recommended to rule out fracture of distal pharynx

Chapter 8: Cosmetic dermatology

8.1 Lasers

Speaking the language of lasers

- Laser terminology
  - Energy (Joules): unit of work
  - Fluence (Joule/cm^2): energy per cm (↑ fluence → ↑ energy per unit area)
    - Changing the spot size does not alter fluence
  - Power (Watts = Joule/s): energy as a rate
  - Irradiance (Watts/cm^2): power delivered per cm^2
    - If given irradiance and fluence (dose) and asked how long to keep them in light box, use formula: Fluence (J/cm^2) = Irradiance (J/s cm^2) x Time (s)
      - "People who love UV light are generally more FIT"
  - Pulse width, aka pulse duration (seconds): duration of laser exposure
    - ↑ pulse duration → ↑ energy or heat delivered to tissue
    - Pulse duration should be ≤ TRT to prevent collateral damage to tissue
  - Spot size (mm): diameter of the laser beam hitting skin
    - ↑ **Spot size** → ↓ Scatter → ↑ **Span (depth) of penetration**
  - Wavelength (nm): **longer wavelengths (shorter frequency) penetrate deeper**
    - UV (10–400 nm): excimer laser (308 nm)

        - Visible (400–700): argon (488–514), KTP (532), PDL (585–600), Ruby (694)
        - Infrared (700 nm–1 mm): alexandrite (755), diode (800), Nd: YAG (1064), Erbium: Glass (1540), thulium (1927), Erbium: YAG (2940), CO_2 (10,600)
        - Radiofrequency/microwaves (> 1 mm)
    - Chromophore: absorptive target of laser (e.g., melanin, hemoglobin, and water)
    - Thermal relaxation time (TRT): time for heated tissue to dissipate 50% of its heat
        - TRT (seconds) is proportional to the **square of the target's Radius**
        - Pulse duration should be ≤ TRT ("P is before/less than T or R in alphabet")
        - Since **tattoo** ink and melanosomes are the chromophores with the smallest diameters (0.1 and 0.5 micrometers respectively), they have the smallest TRTs (**10** and 250 **nanoseconds** respectively) and thus require Q-switched lasers with pulse durations in the nanoseconds
        - Standard pulse duration for PDL on **telangiectasias is 10 milliseconds**
            - "Tattoo (ns) and Telangiectasias (ms) are both Ten"
    - Photomechanical effect: sudden heating produces cavitation (Pits/Pockets)
        - **Cavitation causes vessel rupture with PDL** and skin whitening with QS
- Lasers are characterized by the 3 Cs
    - Coherence: light waves travel in phase spatially and temporally
    - Collimation: light waves travel together in a parallel fashion (minimal divergence)

  - Mono-Chromatic: light waves are all same wavelength (which determines color)
- Three different media exist
  - Gas ("You don't gas a check you cash A CHECK"): Argon, CO_2, Helium-neon, Excimer laser (xenon chloride), Copper vapor, and Krypton
  - Liquid ("liquid dye"): pulse dye light (rhodamine dye)
  - Solid: two classes
    - Crystal ("Krystal"): KTP, ruby, Er-YAG, Nd-YAG, alexandrite
    - Semiconductor ("solid semicon-diode"): diode
- Properties of selective photothermolysis of target tissue ("light kills that Pesky Wuhan Flu")
  - **Pulse duration should be ≤ TRT** (thermal relaxation time) minimizes the Propagation of heat and resultant "collateral damage" to tissue
  - **Wavelength** must reach appropriate depth to target the desired chromophore
  - **Fluence** must be high enough to damage target tissue but no higher
- Four types of laser waveforms
  - Continuous: light is emitted continuously; low power (e.g., CO_2, argon)
  - Quasicontinuous: light is emitted in multiple small rapid bursts; low power (e.g., copper vapor, potassium titanyl phosphate (KTP)): "When cops pat you down, they do it in a quasicontinuous way (multiple rapid low power pats)"
  - Pulsed: light is emitted periodically with short pulse durations (milliseconds) and high power (e.g., PDL, ruby, alexandrite, diode, Erbium:glass, Erbium:YAG)
    - These are the lasers from 585 to 2940 nm
  - Quality switched (Q-switched): variant of pulsed lasers with extremely short pulse durations (nano-

seconds); extremely high power (e.g., ruby, alexandrite, Nd:YAG) → laser of choice for pigmented lesions, tattoos and drug deposits

- Treated skin will have one or more of the following four interactions: "STAR light":
  - Scattering: light waves bounce off fibers within dermis/SQ → **limits the Span of penetration** (↑ Spot size → ↓ Scatter → ↑ Span/depth of penetration)
  - Transmission: light waves Transmit Through Tissue without having any effect
  - Absorption (desired effect): light it absorbed by its target tissue
  - Reflection: **4–7% of light it reflected** by skin surface
- Epidermal damage can be minimized by cooling (three methods)
  - Precooling with cryogen (tetraflouroethane) spray; side effect is dyspigmentation (e.g., blue skin); most aggressive and effective method
    - "When you are in preschool (precool) you cry on the flour until you turn blue. Crying is an aggressive but effective way to get what you want."
  - Parallel cooling is done during the laser treatment
  - Postcooling is used to ↓ pain, erythema and edema afterwards (e.g., ice packs)
- The various lasers can be remembered by "Excimer APP ReADY glass TEC"
  - Excimer (308 nm; UVB range): UV light (used for psoriasis and vitiligo)
  - Argon (488–514nm): Blue visible light ("A next to B in alphabet")
  - Potassium titanyl phosphate (KTP; 532 nm): green light ("Green KaTerPillar")
  - PDL (585–600 nm): yellow visible light ("PD-yellow")

- Ruby (694 nm): Red visible light ("69 is a # that makes you blush/turn red")
- Alexandrite (755 nm): infrared light ("Alexander the Great was born in 755 BC")
- Diode (800 nm): infrared light ("I call it Di-ocho because ocho is 8 in Spanish")
- Nd: YAG (1064 nm): infrared light ("YAG lasers are close to 1000 and 3000")
  - **Penetrates deepest, bypassing melanocytes so is safest in skin of color**
- Erbium glass (1540 nm): infrared light ("Glass was discovered in 1540")
- Thulium (1927 nm): infrared light ("Thulium was discovered in 1927")
- Erbium YAG (2940 nm): infrared light ("YAG lasers are close to 1000 and 3000")
- CO_2 (10,600 nm): infrared light

- Nonlaser energy sources are much less selective and less powerful
  - Intense pulsed light (IPL): **xenon flashlamp** emits light that do not follow any of the 3 Cs → noncollimated, noncoherent, polychromatic
    - Broad wavelength (range 500–1200 nm) requires filters to narrow it down
    - **IPL has been shown to Increase expression of p53**
    - **IPL is "No HELP": Non-ablative resurfacing, Hair removal, Erythematotelangiectatic rosacea, Lentigos, Poikiloderma of Civatte**
  - Radiofrequency (RF): alternating electric current **locally heats tissue** ("think Fire")
    - Has specificity for Fat (used to treat cellulitis); potential SE is lipoatrophy
    - Also affective for scars and skin tightening and is **safe in all skin types**

Laser safety

- Lasers are divided into 4 safety classes (1–4) where class 4 is the most hazardous and powerful laser class and also the MC class used in dermatology
- The four main concerns are **ocular damage (blindness)**, inhalation of biohazardous plume (**HPV**), cutaneous burns and fire hazard ("blindly inhaling burning fire")
    - Various ocular complications may arise depending on which laser is used
        - UV laser (excimer) damages the **lens cataracts** ("Lens filter UV")
        - Visible light and near infrared lasers ("APP ReADY"; 400–1400 nm) target **melanin/hemoglobin** → damages pigment containing structures **(retina)**
            - **p/w sudden painless Vision loss** which improves over weeks
                - Painless because the retina does not have pain receptors
            - Near infrared/Q-switched **("ReADY") has highest risk of blindness**
        - Mid and far infrared lasers ("glass TEC"; 1400–100,000 nm) target **water** → damages water containing structures such as the cornea and sclera
            - **CO_2 laser → Corneal ulceration → pain**, tearing and blurry vision
    - Inhalation of biohazardous plume specifically **HPV** particles
        - Concern for oral SCC; prevent w/ smoke evacuator held 1 cm away + N95
    - Cutaneous burns may occur with any laser as a result of operator error
    - Risk of fire hazard is greatest with Erbium:YAG and CO_2 lasers ("TEC") and when oxygen is being

administered (reduce intraoperative O_2 concentration < 40%)

- Other fire hazards ("a fire CAME"): CO_2 lasers, Aluminum chloride (drysol), Alcohol, Malathion, Erbium:YAG lasers

Types of lasers

Vascular lasers (poster child is PDL)

- Utilizes selective Photothermolysis to damage blood vessels
    - Uses: telangiectasias, PWS, superficial hemangiomas, poikiloderma of Civatte, scars, psoriasis, PG, angiofibromas and warts
- Targets hemoglobin: **Oxyhemoglobin** (O next to P in alphabet) > deoxyhemoglobin
    - Absorption peaks are 418, 542 and 577 nm ("I just remember 543 and 567")
- SEs: **Purpura (#1)**, **Pigmentary changes/PIH (#2)** and blisters; **prevent side effects by Precooling, decreasing the fluence and using longer Pulse durations (ms not ns)**
    - In darker skin types: warn patients of transient PIH, increase skin cooling, **lengthen pulse width/duration** and decrease energy/fluence
    - Site of eye damage is retina
- To make vascular lasers more effective you can ↑ fluence or use shorter pulse durations
- Desired treatment endpoint for PDL is Purpura (a result of cavitation and vessel rupture)
    - With pulse durations of 10 ms or more, there is little to no immediate purpura as cavitation and vessel rupture is avoided **(short pulse durations cause purpura)**
    - "Pulse Stacking" w/ PDL changes Shape of RBCs, is more effective and causes less purpura (because

you can ↓ pulse duration) but it causes more Swelling/edema

- Desired treatment endpoint for KTP and Nd:YAG is immediate disappearance of vessels
- PDL is TOC for most vascular lesions except…
  - o Telangiectasia: **KTP** (short wavelength good for superficial lesions), IPL, PDL
  - o Poikiloderma of Civatte: IPL (PDL is next best)
  - o Vascular ectasias on the Lower legs: Long-pulsed Nd:YAG (diode is next best)
    - ▪ Whereas long-pulse Nd:YAG is a vascular/depilatory laser, QS Nd:YAG is a hyperpigmentation/tattoo/nevus of ito laser

Hair reduction lasers and light sources

- Utilizes selective photothermolysis to destroy the **bulge and bulbar stem cells** (ideally)
- Targets melanin (absorption spectra is 300–1000 nm w/ no peaks; linear; "me-line-in")
  - o White hair is impossible to remove because it lacks melanin chromophore
- SEs are PIH (↑ risk in skin of color; **Nd:YAG safest in POC**), leukotrichia, blisters/scars
  - o May see paradoxical hypertrichosis as low fluence induces hair growth (happens in darker skin types because we use lower fluences in these patients)
  - o Site of eye damage is retina
- Can shave before treatment but do not fully remove hair shaft (will lose chromophore)
- Desired treatment endpoint is **transient perifollicular edema**
- Diode is the most efficacious Depilatory laser; Nd: YAG is the safest in skin of color

Resurfacing lasers

- Uses selective photothermolysis to target water (absorption peaks: 1450, 1950, 3000)
    - Uses: skin tightening, wrinkles, age spots, sun damage, **hypertrophic scars**, warts
- May be ablative (vaporization of target tissue) or nonablative (thermal effect on dermis)
    - Ablative lasers (more downtime but requires less treatments)
        - Erbium:YAG (2790 nm) and Erbium:YSGG (2790 nm) have less thermal injury → ↓ coagulation, ↑**bleeding**, ↓ collagen retraction, ↓ down time
        - CO_2 (10,600 nm) has more thermal injury → ↑ Coagulation, ↓ bleeding, ↑ Collagen retraction, ↑ recovery time/PIH/erythema
    - Nonablative lasers (less downtime but requires more treatments)
        - Vascular lasers (PDL), infrared lasers (Nd: YAG, diode, Er:glass), IPL and RF
- May be fractionated (↓ downtime, ↓ erythema but less effective) or nonfractionated
    - Fractionated ablative lasers create columns of thermally damaged skin next to islands of normal skin (these keratinocyte reservoirs lead to more rapid healing)
    - Unlike fully ablative lasers, fractionated lasers can be used on the neck and chest
- SEs are erythema, PIH and infections (↑ risk of HSV in 1st week); consider prophylaxis
    - Site of eye damage is cornea and sclera → corneal ulceration/pain/blurry vision
    - Prophylaxis 1 day before to 10 days after resurfacing laser if history of HSV
    - MC short-term SEs are erythema (100% of patients) and **post-inflammatory hyperpigmentation**

  - (40%); MC long-term SE is **hypopigmentation** (16%)
  - Infrared non-ablative lasers penetrate deeper into the skin (bypass melanocytes) than the ablative lasers and thus cause less PIH in darker skin types
  - Ectropion can occur after periorbital resurfacing (↑ risk if pt had blepharoplasty)
- CI to Ablative lasers: Active infections/inflammation in treatment zone (herpes labialis, impetigo), history of keloid formation, history of AI-CTD (lupus or scleroderma)
- Most sources say to wait between 1 and 6 months after isotretinoin to use fully ablative lasers (and medium/deep peels) but there is no need to wait for other types of lasers such as fractional ablative, non-ablative, PDL and laser hair removal

Hyperpigmentation/tattoo removal lasers

- Targets tattoo pigment: small radius → small TRTs (nanoseconds) → **QS-lasers required**
- For black, blue or brown pigment use ReADY lasers (except diode → hair removal)
  - Alikhan refers to these as the RAN lasers, I call them RAY lasers
  - These QS-RAY lasers are also best for pigmented lesions (lentigines, ephelides, nevus of ota, minocycline pigmentation, post-sclerotherapy hyperpigmentation)
    - QS Ruby 694 ("RAY") works best; **QS-1064 Nd-YAG ("RAY") safest in POC**
- For green pigment use "QS-RA" (QS **ruby 694** is best but QS Alex 755 is safer in POC)
- For turquoise the 755 QS-alexandrite is best
- For Yellow, Red, Violet, White or Orange use the frequency doubled **Nd:YAG (532 nm)**

- "Your Return Visit Will be On May 32" (532 nm frequency doubled Nd:YAG)
- Red tattoos w/ mercuric sulfide (cinnabar) are most likely to cause allergic reactions
- A Granulomatous reaction to red tattoo is a type 4 (Four) delayed hypersensitivity or a Foreign body reaction ("F next to G in alphabet")
- If patient is allergic to tattoo die, laser treatment may cause anaphylaxis
- **Desired endpoint is immediate tattoo whitening (a result of cavitation)**
  - White tattoos may undergo paradoxical darkening 2° to **reduction** of Ti^{4+} Ti^{3+}
    - We can treat this complication w/ further Q-switch laser but it may be permanent (a test spot is recommended to avoid this complication)
  - Flesh toned/light red tattoos (permanent lip liner) may undergo paradoxical darkening 2° to reduction of Ferric oxide (Fe^{3+}) → Ferrous oxide (Fe^{2+})
    - "Think iron in steak which goes from red when rare to black when burnt"
    - Opposite of methemoglobinemia ("ferrous to ferric, will make you sick")
- Tattoo pigment origin: black, blue (cobalt; "blackberry/blueberry cobbler"), brown (ochre; "brown oak tree"), green (chromium; chlorophyll is green), yellow (cadmium; "yellow cab"; cause photoallergic tattoo reactions), white (titanium), **red (mercuric sulfide;** "mercury is the red planet"; **MCC of allergic tattoo reactions**), violet (manganese; "non-ripe mangos are violet")
- Pigment alteration/erythema is the MC SE with Q switch lasers (all lasers really)

- Laser-induced chrysiasis (p/w blue-gray skin) is a SE specific to QS and picosecond lasers that occur in those w/ a history of gold ingestion (old treatment for RA)

8.2 Botulinum Toxin and Fillers

The basics of Botulinum

- Botulinum toxin is a neurotoxin produced by the bacteria Clostridium botulinum
- Botulinum toxin is a **zinc-dependent** protease that cleaves polypeptides for exocytosis
- MOA: inhibits nerve terminal function through presynaptic blockade of SNARE complex which inhibits acetylcholine release resulting in chemical denervation of muscles
  - The heavy chain of botulinum toxin attaches w/ the surface receptor (axon terminals), the **light chain degrades the SNAP receptor** via protease action
    - "Heavy girls get so attached, but SNAP thin/ light girls just degrade you"
    - 3 proteins make up SNARE complex: SNAP-25, synaptobrevin, syntaxin
- Botox is FDA approved for facial rhytids (1st approved for glabella), axillary hyperhidrosis (not palmar), and non-derm indications (Blepharospasm was 1st FDA-approved indication)
- Various subtypes of botulinum toxin inhibit certain regions in the SNARE complex
  - Subtype A blocks SNAP-25 (all botulinum toxin dermatologists use is this type)
    - Onabotulinum toxin A: only one **w/o a sugar** moiety (best in diabetes)

    - Incobotulinum toxin A: only product **without complexing proteins** and which does not require refrigeration before reconstitution
    - PurTox (if approved) will lack complexing proteins also
    - Abobotulinum toxin A: should be avoided if patient has **cow milk Allergy**
    - Prabotulinum toxin A-xvfs is the newest toxin approved in 2019
    - Dilution: Ona (Botox) to inco (Xeomin) to prabo (Jeuveau) to abo (Dysport) has a 1:1:1:3 ratio (dilute 100 botox units in 2.5 mL of NaCl)
  - Subtype B blocks synaptoBrevin/VAMP (Vesicle Associated Membrane Protein)
    - Faster onset and duration of action than subtype A ("more Brief")
  - Subtypes A-H exist; vowels (A/E) block SNAP, consonants block synaptobrevin
    - Except subtype C which blocks syntaxin ("C-ntaxin")
  - Can add **benzoyl alcohol** preservative during reconstitution to ↓ **injection pain** and to ↑ shelf-life ("Ben'z alcohol helps to numb the pain of botox")
  - Manufacture can add Albumin to prevent Adhesion to the walls of the glass vial
- Before injecting botox, think about your ABCs
  - Active infection at injection site and neuromuscular disorders due to ↓ Acetylcholine from nerve terminal (ALS, myasthenia gravis) are CI
  - Allergy to any constituents (e.g., cow's milk allergy w/ Abobotulinum toxin) is a CI
  - Aminoglycosides (e.g., tobramycin) **increase** neurotoxin effect
  - Acetylcholinesterase inhibitors (donepezil) **diminish** neurotoxin effect

  - Breastfeeding/pregnancy and patients w/ Body dysmorphic disorder are CI
  - Cyclosporine and CCBs (e.g., verapamil) **increase** neurotoxin effect
- SEs: headaches and ptosis are the two MC
  - Rx ptosis w/ α-agonist to stimulate Mullers muscle ("ptosis is a PAIN so give Oxy")
    - Phenylephrine, Apraclonidine, **Iopidine,** Naphazoline, and Oxymetazoline
  - **↑ incidence of eyelid ptosis in Asian subjects after Botox**
  - Antibodies against botulinum toxin A is from hemagglutinin protein complex

High yield muscles we commonly inject neurotoxin into

- Nasalis: treats "bunny lines"
- Frontalis: treats and paralyzes horizontal forehead lines
- Orbicularis oris: treat perioral rhytides ("crow's feet")
- Levator labii superioris alaeque nasi: treats gummy smile
- Depressor anguli oris: treats downturned oral commissures
  - Diffusion medial into the depressor labii inferioris p/w asymmetric smile at rest

Fillers

- Non-HA fillers of importance
  - Autologous Fat
    - Liposuction from donor area (buttocks, abdomen) is used to extract fat
    - **Can be Frozen and used several months later**
    - 50% of the fat survives but the fat that remains lasts **Forever** (permanent)
  - Polymethacrylate (Artefill)

        - **Permanent filler** which contains polymethacrylate and bovine collagen
            - "Pol rhymes with Col"
            - **Skin testing required** (due to collagen) to prevent anaphylaxis
    - Calcium Hydroxyapatite (Radiesse)
        - Semi-permanent filler commonly used in HIV lipoatrophy and to fill Hands
        - Radio-opaque (seen on imaging) due to calcium
        - Hyper-dilute Radiesse is used for skin tightening
    - Poly-L-lactic acid (Sculptra)
        - Semi-permanent filler used in HIV lipoatrophy and for skin tightening
        - Stimulates fibroblasts resulting in collagen formation over several months
            - Considered a stimulatory filler
        - Must inject deep or else nodules may form
        - Must massage (5 times a day for 5 minutes for 5 days total)
        - Delayed reactions (cellulitis-like nodule) 2° to **idiopathic immunologic rxn**
            - "The acid makes me think of HIV positive hippies doing acid which stimulates different parts of the brain (stimulates fibroblasts), and makes the hippies think deep (must inject deep) and give each other massages. A side effect of acid is a delayed trip (flashback)"
- HA fillers (Juvaderm, Restylane, Prevelle, Hydrelle, Belotero)
    - Restylane/Juvederm HA fillers are derived from the bacteria streptococcus equi
    - Restylane and Juvederm Ultra/Ultra plus are used for facial wrinkles and folds

  - Restylane silk and Juvederm Volbella are used for lips and perioral rhytides
  - Restylane lift and Voluma are for age related volume loss in the midface
  - Degree of cross linking: ↑ cross-linking (e.g., Vollure) → ↑ **durability/longevity** of HA fillers → filler lasts longer but is more resistant to hyaluronidase
  - G′: **↑G′ → ↑ resistance to movement (elasticity)**, ↑ spread, ↑ volume support
    - "I imagine a G (a guy who women love) who is grounded, is not affected by external forces and who supports his woman"
    - Juvaderm Ultra has lowest and Resylane Lift has the highest G′
    - Important property for mid-facial volume restoration
- Complications (B's and 3's)
  - Bruising
  - Bleeding (avoid aspirin or vitamin E before treatment)
  - Burning (usually transient)
  - Beading/nodules (can be Blue if injected superficially due to the Tyndall effect)
    - Non-inflammatory: p/w painless nodule from too much product injected
      - Rx: observe, massage, needle aspiration, hyaluronidase
    - Inflammatory: p/w tender nodule due to infection
      - Rx: culture and treat w/ macrolide or tetracycline x 2–6 weeks
    - Delayed non-inflammatory (> 30 days post-procedure): p/w granuloma
      - Rx: oral/IL steroids, hyaluronidase, IL 5-FU, surgery is TOC

    - Delayed inflammatory (> 30 days post-procedure): p/w infectious Biofilm
      - Rx: clarithromycin + moxifloxacin, ciprofloxacin, or minocycline
  - Blanching is the first sign of arterial occlusion → cutaneous necrosis
    - Rx: warm compress, nitropaste, massage, **hyaluronidase** (may even help in non-HA fillers by dissolving native hyaluronan), hyperbaric oxygen, ASA
      - Pts w/ hx of anaphylaxis to **Bee stings** should be sent to allergist before dissolving filler w/ hyaluronidase due to cross-reaction)
      - > 3 days post-procedure all you can do is wound care (petrolatum)
  - Blindness is possible when injecting nose (now the MC location) and glabella
  - Anaphylaxis (rare) is a risk with Bovine collagen → 2 skin tests before treatment

8.3 Sclerotherapy

- Venous anatomy
  - A deep and a superficial venous compartment connected by perforating veins
  - Most important veins of the Superficial venous system = small and great Saphenous veins (typically the most cosmetically disturbing)
    - The lateral venous system, a third superficial system, is the most common source of telangiectasias
    - Superficial varicosities on medial thigh = greater saphenous insufficiency

    - Most important veins of the deep venous system = femoral and popliteal veins
- Etiology of varicose veins: ↑ superficial venous pressure, valvular incompetence, hormones, gender, age, pregnancy, body mass index and family history
- Sclerotherapy: sclerosing agent causes thrombosis and eventual collapse of the vein
    - **Postprocedural compression required** (20 mmHg x 3 days)
    - **Sclerotherapy is TOC for telangiectasias and reticular veins of the legs**
        - Long pulsed Nd-YAG (1064 nm) is the laser of choice
    - Foaming (ratio of **1:4** liquid to air) may allow treatment for larger varicose veins but are CI in patients w/ symptomatic Foramen ovale → TIA
- **Detergents**: sodium morrhuate, STS, polidocanol and ethanolamine oleate produce endothelial damage by Denaturing cell surface proteins; pain virtually absent
    - Sodium morrhuate and ethanolamine oleate can produce **severe necrosis** with extravasation and harbor a risk for **allergic reactions** and are thus rarely used
        - Sodium morrhuate is the "most hot" (huate) → **anaphylaxis**/arrythmias
        - Ethanolamine oleate is the 2nd most hot → **urticaria** but it also causes acute renal failure and hemolytic reactions ("mine, ren and hem rhyme")
    - Sodium tetradecyl sulfate (STS) has a high risk of **Serum Sickness reaction**, Skin Sloughing/necrosis/ulceration and **hyperpigmentation** ("Skin Too Shady")
    - Polidocanol has lowest risk of pain and anaphylaxis among detergents but can get **disulfiram-like reactions** and **venous thrombotic events (DVTs)**

- **Hyperosmotic agents**: **Hypertonic saline** with and without dextrose cause **dehydration** of endothelial cells through osmosis resulting in endothelial/RBC dehydration
    - Little to no allergenicity
    - SEs: **pain/muscle cramps**, **necrosis of skin** (if extravasated) and is the sclerosant most likely to cause **Hyperpigmentation** (which is MC SE of sclerotherapy; 30%)
- **Chemical irritants**: polyiodide iodine and chromated glycerin work as corrosives by poisoning cell surface and disrupting chemical bonds; too weak to use for large veins
    - Polyiodide iodine can cause anaphylaxis and iodine hypersensitivity reactions
    - Chromated glycerin can cause pain and hematuria; **lowest risk for hyperpigmentation, telangiectatic matting and anaphylaxis**
        - RFs for telangiectatic matting (distal angioplasia): obesity, OCPs
- MC site for inadvertent arterial injection after sclerotherapy is the medial malleolus (posterior tibial artery) causing cutaneous necrosis of the foot/ankle region → next step after arterial injection is apply ice, attempt to flush and hospitalize w/ IV anticoagulation

8.4 Liposuction and Fat Reduction

- Fat reduction techniques
    - Tumescent liposuction: allows liposuction to be performed under local anesthesia → ↓ risk of major SEs (bleeding and bowel perforation)
        - SEs: temporary breast enlargement, abdominal distention, bruising and **compartment syndrome (occurs after liposuction in arms**

and legs due to post-op edema causing capillary ischemia)
- Post-op compression socks help bruising/compartment syndrome

- With tumescent method, lidocaine limit is **55 mg/kg**
    - 10-fold dilution of standard 1% lidocaine w/ 1:100,000 epinephrine → 0.1% lidocaine w/ **1:1,000,000 epinephrine**
- Max volume that can be safely withdrawn in a liposuction session is **5 L**
    - "Saying tumes-cinco helps me remember 55 mg/kg and 5 L"

- Cryolipolysis (CoolSculpting): Cold-induced apoptosis of adipose cells
    - SEs: numbness, bruising and paradoxical adipocyte hyperplasia (0.005%)
    - CI: Complex regional pain syndrome, Cryoglobulinemia, Chilblains
- Deoxycholic acid injections: chemical Degradation of adipocytes
    - SEs: numbness, bruising, edema, pain
    - FDA approved for submental fat contouring ("Double chin")
- Radiofrequency devices: heat-induced apoptosis of adipose cells
    - SEs: erythema, edema and may induce focal atrophy
- Mesotherapy: involves injecting microscopic quantities of a variety of pharmaceutical agents, extracts from plants, homeopathic agents and vitamins into the mesoderm in order to degrade adipose cells (not FDA regulated)
    - SEs: infections, panniculitis and scarring

- These procedures should **NOT be used as a form of weight loss in obese people**

8.5 Hair Transplantation

- Performed under local anesthesia
- More favorable candidates have more years of life (> 25 years old), more thickness to hair follicles (> 70 microns), more hair at donor site (> 80 follicular units/cm^2; 40 is minimum needed), a more anterior baldness (effecting frontal scalp) and more hair colors ("salt and pepper", red or blond hair; Black hair only is Bad for hair transplants)
- Best candidates have stable alopecias (triangular temporal or stable scarring alopecia)
- Active hair loss (e.g., perifollicular erythema in FFA) is a CI
- Donor dominance: transplanted hair retains characteristic of where hair was taken from
    - Harvest graft from "safe zone" in occipital scalp (will never be affected by AGA)
    - Harvest from axilla or pubic area for the eyebrows
- Two methods to harvest grafts
    - Strip (elliptical) excision: cannot exceed 30 cm^2
        - Typically, 65–85 follicular units/cm^2 in occipital scalp donor strip
        - Leaves linear Scar in occipital scalp
    - Follicular unit extraction (FUT)
        - Removal of individual follicular units using manual or robot devices
        - Punches used in FUE vary between 0.8 to 1 mm in diameter
        - Punch depth of 3–3.5 mm should be maintained to minimize transection
        - Posterior scalp is trimmed to **1 mm in length** to allow harvesting of graft
            - This mandatory trimming of hair is not ideal for female patients

    - Given the minimal scars left by FUE, body hair can also be used as donor sites (beard hair in submandibular area is best)
- Eyebrow transplants are micrografts (grafts composed of a single follicular unit)
- Post-transplant telogen effluvium occurs 2–3 weeks post-op (self-resolves)
- New hair growth seen at 3 to 4.5 months post-op (6–9 months for full effect)
- SEs: lidocaine toxicity, cobblestoning, pruritis, post-operative edema, folliculitis, hypoesthesia, hypertrophic scar at donor site, and violaceous discoloration at recipient site

8.6 Chemical Peels

Superficial peels: depth is to papillary dermis and used for melasma, hyperpigmentation, acne, photo-aging, fine lines ("The Jessner and Sali Glines Twins at age 10–25 were so superficial")

- Jessner's peel ("Don't let Jessner think LESR of you"): composed of Lactic acid, Ethanol, **Salicylic acid** (SE: **tinnitus**), **Resorsinol** (SE: ochronosis, **syncope and hypothyroidism)**
    - o Jessner's peel + 35% TCA peel become medium depth peel good for AKs
- Salicylic acid (20%–30%; β-hydroxy acid): "Sali is SALTI"
    - o **Safe to use in Fitzpatrick V and VI skin up to 30%**
    - o Works well for **Acne** due to its **Lipophilic**, keratolytic and comedolytic properties
    - o SEs: **Tinnitus** and Immediate white frosting due to precipitation of salicylic acid crystals ("looks like their face is salty")
- Glycolic acid (35%–70%): require post-peel **neutralization** w/ sodium bicarb, emollient or saline; safe to

use in POC in concentrations up to 50% and safe in pregnancy

- o **α-hydroxy acid ("Alpha males give Good TLC Man"): Glycolic acid, Tartaric acid, Lactic acid, Citric acid, and Mandelic acid**
- o β-hydroxy acid ("Beta males Salty b/c the alphas get the girls"): Salicylic acid

- TCA (10–25%): best for melasma; frosting occurs in concentrations **> 20%** and occur from precipitation of denatured proteins (less safe in POC than salicylic or glycolic acid)
- The only peels that do not show frosting are Jessner's and Glycolic acid
  - o "Jessica Glynne (famous singer) ain't no frosty bitch"

Medium depth peels: depth is in the papillary to upper reticular dermis (0.45 mm)

- TCA (35–50%): used for AKS, SKs, dyspigmentation, and medium-sized wrinkles
  - o Frosting occurs within 2 minutes and lasts for 20 minutes
    - ▪ Do not reapply another layer until you wait the full 2 minutes
  - o Post-peel erythema lasts for about 20 days (**persistent erythema after medium or deep peel is a/w potential for scarring**)
  - o Like resurfacing lasers, HSV ppx is recommended for medium to deep peels in those w/ a history of herpes labialis (valacyclovir 1g BID x 7 days is common)

Deep peels: depth is in mid-reticular dermis and is mainly used for Deeper wrinkles; main cutaneous side effect is Depigmentation/ scarring

- TCA (> 50%): focal use only; causes more frosting than 35–50%; SE is depigmentation
- Baker-Gordon ("Silly Cardiotoxic Deep Peel"): Sepsitol liquid soap (8 drops), Croton oil (3 drops), Distilled water (2 mL) and Phenol 88% (3 mL)
    - Efficacy and side effects of peel is most strongly related to **croton oil** which increases depth of penetration by dissolving keratin
    - Use mineral oil to flush eyes if contact occurs
        - Remember like dissolves like → mineral oil dissolves the croton oil
    - SEs (depigmentation/scars/milia) include arrythmias (cardiac monitoring required), renal toxicity (IV hydration recommended), hepatotoxicity, post-peel erythema lasting 3 months, laryngeal edema, and skin atrophy

8.7 Cosmeceuticals

- Arnica, vitamin K and Bromelein (derived from pineapples) all ↓ bruising/purpura
    - "Artistically Kills Bruising"
- Vitamin C: primary antioxidant in the skin that interacts w/ copper to inhibit tyrosinase, assists in collagen formation (hydroxylation) and prevention of UVB-induced erythema
    - L-Ascorbic acid: most biologically active form but is easily oxidized (e.g., air, light)
        - Reducing pH (addition of ferulic acid) aids in stabilization
    - Tetrahexyldecyl ascorbate: analog of L-Ascorbic acid that is more stable

- Cysteamine: lightening agent that lightens melanin in s. corneum via antioxidant effects
    - Double enzyme inhibition of tyrosinase and peroxidase
- Tranexamic acid: hemostatic and lightening agent which ↓ melanogenesis by inhibition of plasminogen to plasmin (blocks interaction between melanocytes and keratinocytes)
- Soy, Niacinamide and Licochalcone (licorice extract) treat acne and rosacea
    - "Saturday Night Live actors never have acne or rosacea"
    - Soy/niacinamide also treat melasma by ↓ melanosome transfer to keratinocytes
- Kojic acid and azelaic acid: treat melasma/hyperpigmentation by decreasing melanin production in melanocytes via **tyrosinase inhibition**
    - Phenylalanine, Hydroquinone, Azelaic acid, Retinoids, Cysteamine, vitamin C and Kojic acid inhibit tyrosinase ("PHARCCK I inhibited tyrosinase")
- Retinoids treat hyperpigmentation by inhibiting tyrosinase, ↓ melanin synthesis, ↓ transfer of melanocytes to keratinocytes, ↑ exfoliation (eliminates pigment) and can help other agents (e.g., hydroquinone) work better by ↑ penetration

8.8 Dermabrasion and Microneedling

Dermabrasion/dermasanding

- Resurfacing procedure that uses a rapidly rotating device to sand the outer layers of skin
- Manual dermabrasion

  - Better control over depth, lower cost, less risk of aerosolizing infectious particles and lower incidence of post-inflammatory hypopigmentation
- Motorized dermabrasion ("Motor-boat her BREAST")
  - Better for Benign neoplasms (e.g., syringomas), Rhynophyma, Extensive Epidermal lesions, **Acne scars**, Surgical/traumatic scars, Tattoos unresponsive to lasers

Microdermabrasion

- Aluminum oxide crystals are used
- Compared to dermabrasion, microdermabrasion has no bleeding and has less downtime

Microneedling

- Creates tiny controlled epidermal and dermal wounds
- Used for rhytides, scars and striae
- Safe in skin of color (minimal risk of dyspigmentation)
- Avoid topical application of any product **during** the procedure (risk of granuloma)
  - Topicals w/ growth factors, hyaluronic acid, and vitamin C are used after

8.9 Cosmetic Considerations in Skin of Color

- Neuromodulators tend to have more side effects (eyelid ptosis and headache) and show a lower response rate in patients w/ darker skin tones
- SEs of fillers specific to POC include hyperpigmentation (11%; MC), hypopigmentation, hemosiderin deposition, and keloid scar formation
- Stick to superficial peels in POC as deeper peels can result in dyspigmentation

- Long-pulsed 1064-nm Nd:YAG is the preferred depilatory laser in POC
    - o Before treatment: avoid sun and shave 1 week before (plucking is discouraged)
    - o After treatment: **proper cooling**, avoid sun and can apply hydroquinone
- Keloids are common in POC and history of keloids should be elicited before procedures
- Peels safe in POC (all exert effects at or above basal layer): 35–70% glycolic acid, 20–30% salicylic acid, 40% mandelic acid, Jessner solution, 88% lactic acid, phytic acid, < 15% TCA

Chapter 9: Dermatopathology

9.1 Essential Concepts in Dermatopathology

Normal skin anatomy

- Scalp skin: numerous **terminal hair follicles that extend deep into the SQ fat**
- Facial skin: thin epidermis w/ basket weave stratum corneum, numerous hair follicles and sebaceous glands that extend down into the dermis, demodex mites common
    - Nose: abundant sebaceous glands
    - Eyelid: numerous vellus hair follicles and skeletal ("sk-eye-letal") muscle
    - Ear: numerous vellus hair follicles and cartilage
    - Dry vermillion lip: keratinized (stratum corneum) w/ skeletal muscle
    - Wet mucosal lip: non-keratinizing (lacks corneal and granular layer), lacks hair follicles (glabrous) and has pale, glycogen-rich keratinocytes
- Mouth: gingiva, hard palate, and dorsal tongue are keratinizing (contains a s. corneum)
    - The other oral areas are non-keratinizing (basal and spinus layers only)
    - Tongue: keratinized (dorsal side only) stratified squamous epithelium w/ underlying skeletal muscle (nuclei is off to the periphery)
- Trunk skin: Thick dermis (esp from the back) w/ scattered hair follicles
- Areolar skin: abundant smooth muscle ("feel good skin") + mammary ducts

- Anogenital skin: abundant smooth muscle ("feel good skin") + papillomatous epidermis
  - o Hypodermis virtually absent in eyelid, scrotum, penis and dorsal hand
- **Axilla: abundant apocrine glands + terminal hairs** + papillomatous epidermis
- Volar skin: massively thickened stratum corneum, compact orthohyperkeratosis, Meissner's corpuscles in dermal papillae, and no hair follicles (glabrous)
  - o Digit: thick orthokeratosis w/ haphazard nerve bundles
- Nail bed: orthokeratosis w/ no underlying granular layer; dermis sits directly over the periosteum of the distal phalanx (no SQ), no melanocytes (only in nail matrix)

High-yield dermatopathology bodies (know what these look like)

- Asteroid bodies: star-shaped intracytoplasmic inclusions seen in Sarcoid ("Star-coid")
- Banana bodies: yellow dermal bodies seen in ochronosis (alkaptonuria vs hydroquinone)
- Caterpillar bodies: eosinophilic BMZ material (Collagen IV+/PAS+) in blister roof in PCT
- Cigar bodies: oval yeasts (PAS+ and GMS+) seen in sporotrichosis
- Civatte/colloid/cytoid bodies: apoptotic keratinocytes seen in lichen planus
- Comma-shaped bodies: seen in benign Cephalic histiocytosis on electron microscopy
- Cowdry A and B bodies: **intranuclear** inclusions seen in Herpes and Polio, respectively
  - o "Her Polio made her turn into a dry cow and stay inside her cozy nook (nucleus)"

- Donovan bodies: intracytoplasmic safety pin-shaped bacteria within macrophages seen in granuloma inguinale
- Dutcher bodies: pseudo-intranuclear pink mass of immunoglobins within plasma cells seen in malignant B-cell processes such as B-cell lymphoma and multiple myeloma
    - Dutcher = Dead (vs Russel bodies: "happy pregnant plasmas" in benign diseases)
- Gamma-Favre bodies: intracytoplasmic basophilic inclusions within endothelial cells seen in lymphogranuloma venereum (LGV)
- Guarnieri bodies: eosinophilic cytoplasmic inclusions seen in smallpox
- Henderson-Paterson bodies: pink intracytoplasmic inclusions seen in molluscum
- Kamino bodies: eosinophilic BMZ material (Collagen IV+/PAS+) in epidermis in Spitz nevi
- Medlar bodies: brown round yeasts forms ("Copper pennies") seen in **Chromomycosis**
- Michaelis-Gutmann bodies: calcified laminated bacterial remnants seen in **Malakoplakia**
- Odland (lamellar) bodies: oval granules seen on EM (major role in barrier function) in the upper spinous/granular layer which are **↓ in Harlequin fetus and Flegel's disease**
- Papillary mesenchymal bodies: condensed clusters of fibroblasts which recapitulates the normal hair bulb seen in desmoplastic/classic trichoepithelioma or trichoblastoma
- Psammoma bodies: concentric, calcified laminated spheres seen in Papillary thyroid cancer, Meningioma, Mesothelioma, and Ovarian cancer
- Pustulo-ovoid bodies of Millan: round eosinophilic cytoplasmic inclusions comprised of lysosomes (PAS+ and diastase-resistant) seen in granular cell tumor

- Rocha-Lima bodies: intracytoplasmic inclusions in endothelial cells seen in Oroya fever/verruga peruana
- Russel bodies: collections of immunoglobins in the cytoplasm of plasma cells seen in benign conditions such as **Rhinoscleroma** or granuloma inguinale
- Schaumann bodies: calcified laminated collections seen in Sarcoid
- Verocay bodies: rows of long palisaded nuclei surrounding amorphous pink material seen in the hypercellular (Antoni A) areas of **schwannoma's**
- Weibel-Palade bodies: cytoplasmic organelle of endothelial cells which contains vWF and **P-selectin** and seen in blood vessel tumors (e.g., glomus tumor, tufted angioma)

High-yield dermatopathology cells/entities (know what these look like)

- Antoni A: cellular areas of schwannomas which contain abundant Verocay bodies
- Antoni B: hypocellular areas of schwannomas
- Bean bag cells: histiocytes that have engulfed WBCs, RBCs and nuclear debri (cytophagocytosis) seen MC in cytophagic histiocytic panniculitis
- Cholesterol clefts: needle-shaped clear spaces filled w/ cholesterol
    - Seen within adipocytes in SQ fat necrosis of the newborn, sclerema neonatorum and poststeroid panniculitis
    - Seen within the dermis in **NXG** > NLD, plane xanthoma, and eruptive xanthoma
    - Seen within arterioles in cholesterol embolism
- Clover leaf (flower cells): atypical T-cells with a cloverleaf or flower-like nucleus seen in the peripheral blood of HTLV-induced adult T-cell lymphoma

- Corps ronds/grains: two special types of dyskeratotic keratinocytes seen in "DAWG" → Darier's, Acantholytic dyskeratotic acanthoma, Warty dyskeratoma, Grover's
    - Ronds: Red Round cells w/ perinuclear halo found in the spinous layer
    - Grains: smaller, flattened cells found in the Granular or corneal layer
- Flame figure: major basic protein which is deposited on collagen seen in Wells syndrome
- Ghost cells: blue calcium outlines in necrotic lipocytes seen in pancreatic panniculitis
- **Globi: encapsulated collections of mycobacterium seen in lepromatous leprosy**
- Hallmark (horseshoe) cells: large atypical T-cells w/ a horseshoe-shaped nucleus seen in anaplastic large cell lymphoma
- **Miescher's radial granuloma: giant cell located in the fat septae of erythema nodusum**
- Mikulicz cells: foamy histiocytes containing gram-negative rods of Klebsiella rhinoscleromatis seen in rhinoscleroma ("Mike licks his nose"); also see Russel bodies
- Mulberry cells: large pink fat cells w/ central nucleus (vs peripheral in normal fat cells) and a multivacuolated, granular cytoplasm seen in hibernoma (tumor of brown fat)
- Morula: GMS/PAS$^+$ organism w/ internal septations ("soccer ball") seen in protothecosis
- Reed-Sternberg cells: large atypical B-cells (Both CD30$^+$ and CD15$^+$) w/ Bilobed nucleus w/ central nucleolus within each nucleus ("Owl eyes") seen in Hodgkin's lymphoma
- Reed-Sternberg-Like cells: appear similar to Reed-Sternberg cells but are T-cells (CD30$^+$ and CD15$^-$) and are seen in Lymphomatoid papulosis
- Sézary cells: atypical lymphocytes w/ cerebriform nuclei seen in Sézary syndrome

- Signet ring cells: cells w/ large amounts of intracytoplasmic mucin which pushes nucleus to the periphery seen in metastatic adenocarcinoma (MC is gastric)
- Sunburn cells: dyskeratotic keratinocytes in the epidermis seen in phototoxic drug rash
- Virchow cells: histiocytes containing acid fast bacilli seen in lepromatous leprosy
- von Hansemann cells: histiocytes containing Michaelis-Gutmann bodies (calcified bacterial remnants) seen in Malakoplakia

High-yield giant cells seen in dermatology ("giants have LOFTy goals")

- **Langhans giant cells**: nuclei in a horseshoe pattern ("hands and shoes") seen in Syphilis, Leprosy, Invasive fungal infections, TB and Sarcoidosis ("horseshoes have SLITS")
- Osteoclast-like giant cells: have central nuclei seen in giant cell tumor of tendon sheath
- Floret cells: multinucleated giant cells w/ peripheral overlapping nuclei (resembles flowers) seen in pleomorphic lipoma
- Foreign-body type giant cells: haphazard pattern of nuclei seen in foreign body reaction
- Touton giant cells: giant cells w/ wreath-like arrangement of nuclei seen in JXG/xanthomas and contain hemosiderin in DF (never seen in DFSP)

Transport media

- Routine H&E: 10% buffered formalin
- Electron microscopy: 2.5% glutaraldehyde solution
- Flow cytometry: fresh specimen on saline soaked gauze or RPMI medium
- Immunofluorescence: Michel's medium (**ammonium sulfate**)

- If Michel's is not available, phosphate buffer saline can be used to hold tissue

Common issues with the biopsy

- Lost specimen → inform the patient (take new biopsy)
- Wrong label → verify photography
- There is improved diagnostic accuracy (esp w/ melanocytic lesions) w/ second dermpath opinion so do not be afraid to speak to your dermpath and request a second opinion
- If anything seems suspicious (e.g., young child w/ melanoma), **just call your dermpath!**

9.2 Stains

Special stains

Special mucin stains ("PACT with mucin")

- Periodic acid Schiff (PAS): stains neutral MPS (BMZ), fungi and glycogen Pink-red
  - Does not stain acid MPS (hyaluronic acid and other mucins)
- Alcian blue: stains sulfated acid MPS (dermatan or chondroitin sulfate) blue at low (0.5) and high (2.5) pH **but only stains non-sulfated MPS (hyaluronic acid) at high pH (2.5)**
- Colloidal iron: stains sulfated and non-sulfated acid MPS blue on a pink background
  - Hyaluronidase can be added to distinguish b/w hyaluronic acid and other mucins
- Toluidine blue: stains acid MPS (and mast cells) purple on a blue background
  - Metachromatic stain: stain is blue but mast cells/ acid MPS is highlighted purple

- Mucicarmine: stains epithelial mucin (Paget's, crypto) pink-red on a yellow background

Mast cell stains: "Master (mast cells) KIT Led them on a Trip to the Tall blue Gems"

- KIT (CD117): immunostain (not dependent on the presence of mast cell granules)
- Leder stain: stains mast cell granules red (not dependent on mast cell granules either)
- Tryptase: immunostain
- Toludine blue: stains mast cell granules purple (metachromatic)
- Giemsa: stains mast cell granules purple (metachromatic)
    - o 1st two in mnemonic (KIT/Leder stains) function even after recent degranulation
    - o Last 2 in mnemonic (toluidine blue/giemsa) are the metachromatic stains

Other special stains

- Verhoeff-van Gieson (VVG): stains **elastin** (black) and collagen (red)
- Orcein: stains elastin (black-brown) and collagen (red-pink); also stains Hep B
- Masson trichrome: stains **Collagen (Blue or Green)** and **Smooth muscle (Red)**
    - o "C is close to B and G, while S is close to R in the alphabet"
- Movat's pentachrome: stains elastin (black), collagen (yellow) and smooth muscle (red)
- Phosphotungistic acid hematoxylin (PTAH): stains smooth muscle (purple), collagen (red)
- Oil-red-O, Sudan black B and Scarlet red all stain lipids (the color in their name)
    - o All lipid stains must be performed on frozen tissue only

- Perls (Prussian blue): stains iron/hemosiderin blue on a pink-red background ("opposite as the Fite stain and Ziel-Neelson colors")
- Fontana-Masson: a silver stain that stains melanin black on a pink-red background
- **Von Kossa stains calcium black** on a pink-red background and Alizarin red stains calcium red on a yellow background
    - "von Cossa and Alizarin red are Calcium stains"
- Congo red: stains amyloid pink-red (apple green birefringence when polarized)
- **Thioflavin T: stains amyloid yellow-green on a black background** (looks like a DIF and requires fluorescence microscopy like a DIF)
- PAS: stains **fungi**, Glycogen and Neutral MPS (basement membrane) Pink
    - "Fun Guys stay Neutral and pass (PAS) on politically charged conversations"
    - Glycogen is sensitive to diastase so it will no longer stain after adding diastase (clear-cell acanthoma, trichilemmoma) but fungi and neutral MPS are resistant
- Grocott's methenamine silver (GMS): **stains fungal walls black**
- Gram stain (Brown-Hopps): stains G- bacteria red and G+ bacteria blue
- **Fite stain ("Fight for your LANd"): stains Leprosy, Atypical mycobacteria, Nocardia red on blue-green background** ("looks like a fite in the ocean with red blood in a blue sea")
- Ziehl-Neelson: stains acid-fast bacteria (TB) red on a blue-green background (like Fite)
- Auramine-rhodamine: stains acid-fast bacteria yellow-green on black background (requires fluorescent microscopy so looks like a DIF/thioflavin T stain)

- Warthin-Starry stain: stains Spirochetes (syphilis, borrelia) and bacteria in bacillary angiomatosis, granuloma inguinale, rhinoscleroma black on a golden yellow background
    - "A starry sky is golden yellow stars in a black background, this stain is opposite"
- Steiner stain: like Warthin-Starry it stains Spirochetes black on a gold yellow background
- Giemsa ("Rick gave Lisa Chlamydia and His Massive purple-blue gem"): stains Rickettsia, Leishmania, Chlamydia, Histoplasma and Mast cells purple-blue

Immunohistochemical stains

- IHC stains can supplement normal H&E slides using the same paraffin-embedded tissue
- Antibodies directed towards the antigen of interest are conjugated to **peroxidases**

Epithelial markers

- AE1/AE3: cocktail of low (AE1) and high (AE3) molecular weight keratin antibodies
    - (+) in epithelial tumors (SCC/adnexal) except sarcomatoid (spindle cell) SCC
- CK polyclonal keratin (pankeratin) and MNF116: greater sensitivity than AE1/AE3
- CK5/6: high molecular weight keratin immunostain
    - (+) in primary cutaneous SCC and adnexal carcinomas, negative in metastasis
- p63: positive in normal epidermis and adnexa
    - (+) in primary cutaneous **SCC** and adnexal carcinomas, negative in metastasis
    - p63 expression is associated w/ a worse prognosis in Merkel cell carcinoma

- p40: p63 isoform; nuclear marker positive in SCC of any site (e.g., skin, lung, urothelium), BCC and skin adnexal tumors (e.g., hidradenoma)
- CAM5.2: low molecular weight keratin immunostain against CK8 (glandular epithelium)
  - (+) in Paget's, EMPD and eccrine glands/tumors
- CK7: stains benign and malignant adnexal ("adnexal has 7 letters") neoplasms and used w/ CK20 to discover origin of adenocarcinoma; (+) in Pagets and non-GI adenocarcinoma
  - CK7+/CK20- ("the Kids LOST By 7"): mets from Kidney (papillary RCC), **Lung,** non-mucinous Ovarian carcinoma, **Salivary glands, Thyroid and Breast**
  - CK7-/CK20+: Merkel and mets from **large intestine (large intestine = larger #)**
  - CK7+/CK20+ ("U R POSitive"): mets from Urinary tract/bladder, Rectum, Pancreaticobiliary, Ovarian (mucinous carcinoma), Stomach
  - CK7-/CK20- ("ALL clear"): Adrenals, Liver (HCC), Clear cell RCC, prostate also
- **CK20: stains Merkel cell carcinoma in a perinuclear dot pattern, marker of large intestinal adenocarcinoma and stains benign follicular tumors (trichoepithelioma)**
- CDX2: marker for intestinal adenocarcinoma (positive in GI metastases)
- Thyroid transcription factor (TTF-1): marker for metastatic small cell lung carcinoma
  - Commonly performed w/ CK20 as small cell lung cancer looks like MCC on path
- EMA (epithelial membrane antigen): stains sebaceous and sweat glands
  - (+) in Paget's, EMPD, sebaceous carcinoma, SCC and epithelioid sarcoma
- CEA: stains sebaceous and sweat glands

  - (+) in Paget's, EMPD, sweat gland neoplasms and most adenocarcinomas
- Gross cystic disease fluid protein (GCDFP-15): apocrine marker
  - (+) in EMPD but not of EMPD stemming from internal cancer
- Ber-EP4: marks most epithelial cells but not those undergoing squamous differentiation
  - (+) in BCC and (-) in SCC

Mesenchymal markers

- Desmin: (+) in skeletal muscle and most smooth muscle but not vascular smooth muscle
  - DESMIN: "Doesn't Emphasize Smooth Muscle that is INtravenous"
- Smooth muscle actin (SMA): (+) in skeletal muscle and smooth muscle
  - Diffuse staining in leiomyoma/leiomysarcoma
  - Tram-track staining in myofibroblastic tumors like AFX and dermatomyofibroma
- Vimentin (fibroblast intermediate filament): marker for **sarcomas**; stains endothelial cells, fibroblasts, melanocytes, lymphocytes, macrophages but **not keratinocytes**
- Factor13a: marker for type 1 dermal dendrocytes (which reside in the papillary dermis)
  - (+) in DF and fibrous papule of the face (angiofibroma); (-) in DFSP
- CD34: marker for vascular endothelium and T2 dermal dendrocytes (in reticular dermis)
  - (+) in "THINK DFSP" → Trichilemmoma, epithelioid Hemangioendothelioma, Ischemic fasciitis, NSF, Kaposi's, DFSP, Fibrofolliculoma, Spindle cell lipoma, Solitary fibrous tumor, Sclerotic fibroma, Pleomorphic fibroma

  - Does not stain DFs; decreased staining in morphea/ scleroderma
- CD31: more specific vascular marker than CD34; (+) in angiosarcoma (angiosarc stains…)
  - "Angi sarcs and FUC's MY External Genitalia": FLI-1, UEA, CD31, CD34, MYC, ERG
  - FLI-1: nuclear stain; improvement over CD31 and CD34 but not as good as ERG
  - UEA-1 (Ulex europaeus agglutinin): binds vascular endothelium; (+) in angiosarc
  - MYC: marker for radiation and chronic lymphedema-associated angiosarcoma
  - **ERG: most sensitive and specific marker for angiosarcoma**
- GLUT-1 (glucose transporter): expressed in endothelial cells
  - (+) in infantile hemangiomas (not congenital hemangiomas) and perineurial cells
  - (-) in vascular malformations
- D2-40 (podoplanin): lymphatic marker; can be used to detect lymphovascular invasion

Neuroectodermal markers (melanocytes; "Some Pretty Huge Melanocyte Stains")

- S100: cytoplasm and nuclear stain; marker for neural crest cells and mesenchymal lines
  - (+) in melanocytes, Langerhans cells, Sweat glands, nerves, Schwann cells myoepithelial cells, fat, muscle and chondrocytes
    - Examples: melanoma, LHC, granular cell tumor, Rosai-Dorfman disease
      - Most sensitive IHC stain for melanoma
- S100A6 (calcyclin): member of the S100 superfamily
  - (+) in cellular neurothekeoma (S100 is negative) and in diffuse staining in Spitz nevus (spitzoid melanomas have weak or patchy staining)

- p16: positive in Spitz but often lost in spitzoid melanomas; (+) in SCC
    - Notice how **p16 and S100A6 stain spitz** but are lost in spitzoid melanoma
        - "Six rhymes w/ Spitz much better than it rhymes w/ spitzoid mel"
    - **p16 also stains HPV-associated anogenital lesions and Bowens/SCC**
- PRAME (Preferentially expressed Antigen in Melanoma): diffusely positive in the nuclei of melanoma but negative in benign nevi
- p75 (nerve growth factor): sensitive marker in spindle and desmoplastic melanoma
- HMB-45 (**gp100**; "Good Premelanosome stain"): cytoplasmic **premelanosome** marker
    - Loss of staining of melanocytes w/ descent into the dermis is a manifestation of loss of premelanosomes and serves as marker for normal maturation
    - Uniform staining in blue nevi and melanoma (but not desmoplastic melanoma)
- Melan-A (MART-1): cytoplasmic stain that recognizes a protein in melanosomes
    - Does not stain desmoplastic melanoma reliably
- MITF (microphthalmia-associated transcription factor): **nuclear** melanocytic marker
    - Does not stain desmoplastic melanoma reliably
- Sox-10: **nuclear** marker of Schwann cells and melanocytes
    - Sensitive melanoma marker including Spindled/Sarcomatoid/desmoplastic types

Neuroendocrine stains ("CNS"; all stain for Merkel cell carcinoma)

- Chromogranin, Neuron-specific enolase, and Synaptophysin

- Besides Merkel, other neuroendocrine tumors include small cell lung cancer, carcinoid tumors, islet cell tumors, medullary thyroid cancer, and pheochromocytomas

Hematopoietic markers

- CD45 (Leucocyte Common Antigen): marker for all hematopoietic cells except RBCs
    - o CD45Ra: naïve T-cells
    - o CD45Ro: memory T-cells
- CD3 (Three): pan-T-cell marker (sensitive and specific T-cell marker)
    - o CD5 and CD7 are less sensitive because are commonly lost in T-cell lymphoma
- CD4: marker for helper T-cells
- CD8: marker for cytotoxic T-cells
- CD30 (Ki-1, BERH2; "30 y/o MALE"): positive in activated lymphocytes of tumor stage MF, Anaplastic large cell lymphoma, LyP, Exaggerated bug-bite including scabies nodule
- CD10: marker for B-cell differentiation and expressed in AFX and clear cell neoplasms (clear cell RCC, clear cell hidradenoma, balloon cell nevi, sebaceous tumors)
    - o Also stains the stroma of trichoblastomas and epithelial cells of BCC
    - o To differentiate metastatic RCC and clear cell hidradenoma do p63 or p40
- Kappa/lamda: normally expressed in a ratio of 2/3rd kappa to 1/3rd lambda (deviation from this ratio suggests a clonal B-cell proliferation)
    - o "K comes right before L in alphabet so there is more Kappa"
- CD79a: marker for plasma cells and B-cells
- CD138 (syndecan-1): marker for plasma cells
- CD86: dendritic cells → remember, for costimulatory signal to occur CD28 on T-cells binds B7-1 or B7-2

(CD80 or CD86) on APCs ("8 looks like B") such as dendritic or B cells

- CD123: marker for plasmacytoid dendritic cells
    - ↑ in 1st, 2nd, 3rd letter of LGBtq: Lupus (but not DM), GA, Blood cancers (AML)
- CD163: marker for monocytes and macrophages (along w/ CD 68, lysozyme, α-1 antitrypsin, HAM-56, CD11b, CD14b, factor 13a, MAC-387 and vimentin)
- CD117 (c-KIT): marker for mast cells and melanocytes
- CD207 (langerin): marker for Langerhans cells (along w/ CD1a, S100, peanut agglutinin)
- CD56: marker for NK cells (along w/ CD57, granzyme A/B, TIA-1)
- MPO (myeloperoxidase): marker for granules of neutrophils; (+) in AML/leukemia cutis
- ALK-1: (+) in systemic anaplastic large cell lymphoma (ALCL) and epithelioid cell histiocytoma; (-) in primary ALCL
- MUM-1: (+) in primary cutaneous diffuse large B-cell lymphoma ("your MUM is large")
- BCL2: (+) in BCC (diffuse staining), trichoepithelioma (only stains outermost epithelial layer), primary cutaneous and systemic marginal zone lymphoma and mantel cell lymphoma; **BCL-2 inhibits apoptosis**
- BCL6: (+) in follicle center lymphomas and pseudolymphoma (reactive germinal centers)

Proliferation markers

- **Mib-1** (Ki-67): nuclear proliferation marker that stains cells in all phases of the cell cycle
    - **Diffuse and deep staining in melanoma**
- pHH3: mitotic marker that only stains cells in the M phase of the cell cycle

Other mnemonics related to stains

- Sweat glands stains ("ECCrine Gland Stains"): EMA, CEA, Cytokeratin, GCDFP-15, S100
- Sebaceous gland stains ("Seb-A-ceous"): Adipophilin, AR > EMA
- Nerves: axons (Neuron specific enolase$^+$ and neurofilament$^+$), Schwann cells (S100$^+$), perineurim (EMA$^+$; "EMA is a groupie because she always surrounds the nerves")

9.3 Dermpath Differentials

Neutrophils

Neutrophils in the horn/corneum ("SPASTIC")

- Seb derm: psoriasiform spongiotic dermatitis w/ perifollicular neutrophilic scale/crust
- Psoriasis: discussed later under reaction patterns section
- Amicrobial pustulosis of the folds
- Syphilis: long Sexy Skinny rete, Swelling of vessel lumen, plasma cells
- Tinea: neuts and horizontal hyphae in stratum corneum which is commonly basket-weave w/ a narrow zone of compact corneum just above the granular layer
- Impetigo: neutrophils and **clusters of gram-positive cocci** in the stratum corneum
- Candida: neutrophils and pseudohyphae (often vertically oriented) in stratum corneum
    - "Tinea swims and candida dives (candi-dives)"

Subcorneal neutrophilic pustule ("A CAT PISS")

- IgA pemphigus: intrepidermal neutrophilic infiltrate with minimal acantholysis (IEN type) or subcorneal pustule (subcorneal pustular dermatosis type); both have **(+) DIF**

  - DIF: intercellular IgA in upper epidermis (IEN) or lower/entire epidermis (SPD)
- AGEP: in contrast to IgA pemphigus and Sneddon-Wilkinson, AGEP has **eosinophils** in the dermal infiltrate, papillary dermal edema and necrotic keratinocytes
- Candida: neutrophils and pseudohyphae (often vertically oriented) in stratum corneum
- Acropustulosis of infancy: intraepidermal neutrophils and eos → subcorneal pustule
- Transient neonatal pustular melanosis: subcorneal (superficial) pustule w/ (-) gram stain
- Tinea: may show a subcorneal pustule but would see hyphae on GMS or PAS
- Pustular psoriasis: subcorneal pustule w/ other psoriasis features (hypogranulosis, etc.)
- Impetigo: neutrophils and clusters of gram-positive cocci in the stratum corneum
- SSSS: subcorneal split w/ neuts but no bacterial colonies (vs bullous impetigo)
- Sneddon-Wilkinson (subcorneal pustular dermatosis): subcorneal pustule w/ **(-) DIF**

If there are many neuts in the dermis, next question to ask yourself is if there's a vasculitis

- Vasculitides: pink fibrinoid degeneration of vessel wall w/ neutrophils extravasating the vessels walls and karyorrhexis/leukocystoclasia/nuclear dust ("ant particles")

Medium vessel vasculitis (polyarteritis nodosa)

- LCV with necrotizing arteritis of medium sized arteries in the superficial SQ

Mix of small and medium vessel leukocytoclastic vasculitis ("Big 5 pattern of vasculitis")

- Involves both small vessels (post-capillary venules) and large ones in the reticular dermis
- Endothelium is frequently necrotic with fibrin deposition → RBCs extravasation
- Karyorrhexis (neutrophilic debris) w/ RBC extravasation
- MARS: Mixed cryoglobulinemia, ANCA vasculitis, Rheumatoid vasculitis, Septic vasculitis
    - Granulomatosis w/ polyangiitis (Wegener's granulomatosis): LCV evolves into stellate abscesses (palisaded granuloma w/ central neutrophils) and giant cells
        - "Blue granuloma"
    - Churg-Strauss: LCV evolves into stellate abscesses (palisaded granuloma w/ central eosinophils); granuloma composed of epithelioid cells w/o giant cells
        - "Red granuloma"
    - Microscopic polyangiitis: no granuloma so only non-distinct ANCA+ vasculitis
    - ANCA-positive vasculitis secondary to drug (eosinophils) or levamisole (thrombi)
    - Septic vasculitis: CSSV + thrombi + dense dermal inflammation

Small vessel leukocytoclastic vasculitis ("Little 5 pattern")

- Involves only small vessels (post-capillary venules)
- Endothelial necrosis is rare but will still see fibrin deposition within the vessel wall
- Karyorrhexis (neutrophilic debris) w/ RBC extravasation
- "Small vessel vasculitis is A HUGE Sickness": Acute hemorrhagic edema of infancy, **Henoch-Schönlein purpura**, Urticarial vasculitis, Granuloma faciale, EED, Serum Sickness, Secondary CSVV (ABCD; Autoimmune, Bug, Cancer, Drug)

  - o Granuloma faciale: Grenze zone w/ mixed infiltrate; facial skin (no granuloma)
  - o EED: LCV early w/ onion skin fibrosis in later lesions; not on facial skin

Stellate abscesses (palisaded granuloma w/ central neutrophils): "No CLAST"

- Nocardia: stellate abscess w/ acid fast and gram-positive filaments present
- Cat scratch: stellate abscess that stains w/ Warthin-Starry or B. henslae IHC
- Lymphogranuloma venereum: stellate abscess w/ plasma cell infiltration and sinus tracts
- Atypical mycobacteria: stellate abscess w/ acid fast-positive organisms within histiocytes
- Sporotrichosis: stellate abscesses +/- cigar-shaped yeasts
- Tularemia: stellate abscess
- Other conditions that show stellate abscesses include Churg-Straus and GPA (would also show vasculitis) and mycetomas (would also show Splendore-Hoeppli phenomenon)

Neutrophils in the dermis but no obvious vasculitis or stellate abscess ("NEUTS")

- Neutrophilic dermatosis of the dorsal hand: diffuse neutrophilic dermal infiltrate
- Erythema marginatum: superficial perivascular neutrophilic infiltrate
- Urticaria: superficial dermal vessels filled w/ neutrophils (early) → perivascular and interstitial neutrophilic infiltrate and superficial dermal vessels filled w/ neutrophils
- TRAPS and other autoinflammatory periodic fever syndromes: neutrophilic infiltrate

- Sweet's syndrome: diffuse infiltrate of neutrophils w/ marked papillary dermal edema
- PG, Behçet's and Bowel-Bypass syndrome can all look like Sweets

Lymphocytes

Perivascular lymphoid infiltrate ("LGBT Plus PRIDe" where PRIDe represents a true lymphocytic vasculitis → damage/edema to vessel walls w/ lymphocytes extravasating vessel walls)

- Lupus: **vacuolar interface** w/ dermal **mucin**, **dense PV/PA lymphocytes**, BMZ thickening
- Gyrate erythema: dense "coat-sleeve" perivascular lymphoid infiltrate
  - Includes erythema marginatum (neuts and lymphs), erythema migrans, EGR, EAC
- Bullous lupus: subepidermal blisters w/ neuts, dermal PV/PA lymph infiltrate, ↑ mucin
- Tumid lupus: PV/perieccrine lymphocytic infiltrate, ↑ mucin, minimal vacuolar interface
- PMLE: **superficial** > deep **PV lymph infiltrate w/ papillary dermal edema; not acral skin**
- PPD (capillaritis): purely lymphoid inflammation which surrounds capillaries (above level of the post-capillary venule), RBC extravasation and hemosiderin deposits over time
- Pityriasis lichenoides (PLEVA): **compact hyperkeratosis w/ Parakeratosis** (+/- neuts in the horn), Lichenoid to vacuolar infiltrate but w/ lymph in every whole, Extravasated RBCs, V (wedge)-shaped dermal lymph infiltrate w/ neuts but never any eosinophils, Apoptotic/dyskeratotic keratinocytes in a spongiotic epidermis w/ exocytosis of lymphs
- Perniosis: **superficial and deep PV lymphoid infiltrate w/ papillary dermal edema**, edema around ves-

sels and expansion of vessel walls without fibrin deposition; **acral skin**

- Rickettsial disease: lymphohistiocytic perivascular infiltrate w/ RBC extravasation edema, vacuolar interface +/- fibrin thrombi, capillary wall necrosis and karyorrhexis
- Insect bites: **dense wedge (V)-shaped perivascular lymphoid infiltrate w/ eosinophils and papillary dermal edema** +/- focal LCV
- Degos disease: V-shaped (superficial and deep) PV lymphoid infiltrate w/ vessel damage (chronic lesions display a central epidermal depression w/ necrosis of dermal structures)

Lupus ddx (dense nodular Lymphiod infiltrate in the dermis)

- Lupus: vacuolar interface w/ mucin and **PV/PA lymphocytes** and BMZ thickening
- Light (PMLE): papillary dermal edema and a dense **perivascular lymphocytic** infiltrate
- Lymphoma: lymphocytes are diffuse and atypical
- Lymphocytoma cutis: nodular lymphocyte-predominant infiltrate in the dermis
- **Lichen striatus: LP-like interface at the DEJ and peri-eccrine lymphocytic inflammation**
- Lues (syphilis): psoriasiform hyperplasia with long "sexy" rete ridges, lichenoid interface, abundant lymphocytes and plasma cells and endothelial cell swelling

Eosinophils

Eosinophilic spongiosis ("HAAPIED")

- Herpes gestationis: histologically indistinguishable from BP (subcorneal split w/ eos)
- Arthropod bite: moderately dense superficial and deep infiltrate of lymphs and eos

- Allergic contact dermatitis: spongiotic dermatitis w/ many eosinophils
- Pemphigus (early stage): prior to an intrepidermal split you see eosinophilic spongiosis
- Pemphigoid (early urticarial stage): perivascular and interstitial infiltrate of lymphocytes and many eosinophils that tend to line up at the DEJ
- Incontinentia pigmenti (early vesicular stage): eosinophilic spongiosis w/ **dyskeratosis**
  - Verrucous stage: hyperkeratosis w/ papillomatosis w/ whorls of dyskeratosis
  - Pigmented stage: pigment incontinence
  - Hypopigmented stage: decreased melanocytes
  - Erythema toxicum neonatorum: spongiosis adjacent to follicle + eosinophils
- Drug reaction: variable but commonly includes interface dermatitis w/ necrotic keratinocytes, spongiosis and superficial and deep mixed infiltrate w/ eosinophils
  - This pattern is not distinct and can be seen in viral exanthems also

Perivascular lymphocytic infiltrate with eosinophils ("BAD eos hang around blood vessels")

- BP (urticarial phase): **superficial** eos going into the epidermis or lining up at the DEJ
- Arthropod/Well's: infiltrate is **deeper** (even down into the SQ) and more dense
  - May also see papillary dermal edema (discussed below in "PASTE" mnemonic)
- Drug: this is favored if the eos are not superficial (epi → BP) or deep (near fat → bug)
  - Path is variable but commonly see a vacuolar interface and a polymorphous infiltrate w/ eosinophils which is less exuberant than in arthropod assault

Plasma cells: "KRLASMA"

- Kaposi's, Rhinoscleroma, **Rosai-Dorfman**, Leishmaniasis, Lymphomas, nodular Amyloid, Syphilis, Scleroderma, SCC, SPAP, Melanoma, Morphea, AK
- So if you are ruling out one of these conditions, try not to take a biopsy from an area of the body that also commonly recruits PLASMA Cells (Posterior neck, face esp near the Lips, Anogenital area, Shins, **Mouth**, Axilla, Chest/breasts)

Granulomas

- All CD68+ and HAM56+ except Langerhan cell histiocytosis
- Always perform special stains on all these to rule out fungal and mycobacterial infections and examine under polarized light to exclude foreign material
  - Fungal infections are discussed below
  - Cutaneous tuberculosis (e.g., lupus vulgaris): lymphocytic and suppurative (neuts) granuloma w/ epithelioid histiocytes and Langhan (horse-shoe shaped) giant cells palisading around **central caseous necrosis**

"GRANulomas R XL": GRAN are palisading and R XL are a sea of histiocytes in dermis

- Granuloma annulare (palisade around **mucin/degenerated collagen**): eosinophils in 40%
  - Interstitial pattern (MC): interstitial histiocytes + lymphs (busy dermis) + mucin
    - Ddx: breast cancer/leukemia cutis (look for nuclear atypia)
  - **Palisading pattern: histiocytes surround altered dermal collagen and mucin**

        - Ddx: NLD (deeper, more fibrosis, layered cake pattern), actinic granuloma (on actinically damaged skin, elastophagocytosis, less mucin)
    - Deep (SQ): histiocytes palisading around degenerated collagen in deep dermis
        - Ddx: looks similar to rheumatoid nodule but color is not as bright pink
- Gout: feathery crystals of uric acid w/ surrounding granulomatous inflammation (looks amorphous from low power but it actually has a feathery/needle-shaped appearance)
    - Ddx: similar to IL ken which shows palisade around amorphous bubbly material
- Rheumatoid nodule: large palisading granuloma surrounding **pink fibrin (no mucin)**
- Actinic granuloma (annular elastolytic giant cell granuloma): looks like palisading GA except it **lacks mucin and there is solar elastosis**; VVG shows loss of elastic tissue
- Acne agminata (lupus miliaris disseminates faciei): palisaded granuloma w/ central light pink caseous necrosis
    - Ddx: TB (e.g., miliary TB/lupus vulgaris) also has a palisading around caseous necrosis (lighter pink than the fibrin in rheumatoid nodule) but TB should have horseshoe-shaped Langhan Giant cells and would stain for acid-fast bacilli
- Necrobiosis lipoidica: palisade of histiocytes w/ pale degenerated collagen in a sclerotic dermis forms a **"layered cake"** appearance; square punch biopsy w/ plasma cells
- Necrobiotic xanthogranuloma (NXG): neutrophils, histiocytes and **large Touton giant cells palisading around large X-shaped pink zones of necrosis** w/ **cholesterol clefts**

- Reticulohistiocytoma: "sea" of mononuclear histiocytes in the dermis w/ a two-toned (one lighter and one darker area) cytoplasm ("reticulohistiocy-two-ma")
- Rosai-Dorfman disease: sheets of **lymphocytes** (dark-staining), **plasma cells** and histiocytes (light-staining) w/ emperiopolesis (lymphocytes passing through histiocytes)
    - IHC: CD68+ and **S100+**
- Xanthogranuloma: sea of histiocytes w/ **many Touton giant cells** (no hemosiderin vs DF)
- Langerhans cell histiocytosis (LCH): superficial sea of histiocytes w/ reniform nuclei that commonly shows epidermotropism (Langerhan cells are meant to be in the epidermis)
    - IHC: S100+, CD1a+, peanut agglutinin+, langerin (**CD207**)+; CD68-
    - Ddx: mastocytoma looks similar on low power but mast cells are "fried egg" or "polka dot" in appearance and do not cross the DEJ into the epidermis

Sarcoidal ("naked") granulomas: "Get naked and talc about Milking Sir Crohns tattooed cactus and Sarcing Ross' silly berries" (look for $CD68^+$ foreign body giant cells in foreign body ones)

- Talc granulomas: sarcoidal granulomas w/ white birefringent crystals on polarized light
- Milkersson-Rosenthal: granulomatous (especially sarcoidal) inflammation of lip stroma
- Zirconium: non-polarizable foreign material
- Cutaneous Crohn's: sarcoidal granulomas and crypt irregularities
- Tattoo granuloma: **black** material in the dermis (melanin and hemosiderin are brown)
- Cactus granuloma: sarcoidal or foreign body granulomas w/ PAS+ spines
- Sarcoidosis: epithelioid histiocytes forming naked granulomas (no lymphs); **no necrosis**

- Granulomatous rosacea (lupus miliarius disseminates facei is a variant): folliculocentric sarcoidal granulomas **(caseating necrosis in LMDF); dilated blood vessels**
- Silica granuloma: sarcoidal granulomas w/ polarizable birefringent crystalline particles
- Beryllium granuloma: non-polarizable foreign material
- Tuberculoid leprosy: sarcoidal granulomas that track horizontally along nerves

Foreign body granulomas: "foreign languages don't STICK AZ well as A-B-Z"

- Silica (Silicon dioxide): Sarcoidal granulomas containing birefringent crystalline particles
- Starch: foreign body granulomas w/ ovoid basophilic **PAS+** starch granules
- Splinters (wood): PAS+ birefringent material made of regularly sized cells
- Spines of Jellyfish/coral/sea urchin: lichenoid dermatitis w/ birefringent calcite crystals
- Suture: foreign body granulomas w/ birefringent suture material within a scar
- Tattoo ink: black material in the dermis (melanin and hemosiderin are brown)
- Talc (hydrous magnesium silicate): sarcoidal granulomas w/ white birefringent crystals on polarized light ("Don't talc to white cops")
- IL steroids: foreign body granulomas w/ central pale bluish material (resembles mucin)
- Cactus (Opuntia): sarcoidal or foreign body granulomas w/ PAS+ spines
- Keratin: foreign body granulomas w/ birefringent keratin flakes on polarized light
- Arthropod parts: PAS+ birefringent material on polarized light
- Zinc: dense neutrophilic infiltrate w/ birefringent **rhomboidal** crystals on polarized light

- Aluminum: granulomas w/ no polarizable particles seen
- Beryllium: caseating granulomas w/ no polarizable particles seen
- Zirconium: sarcoidal granulomas; no (Zero) polarizable particles seen
    - A-B-Z (words also end in "ium") are the ones that are non-birefringent
    - Arthropod parts, Aluminum, Starch, cactus Spines and wood Splinters are PAS+

Foreign body reactions to filler material

- Hyaluronic acid: amorphous basophilic material that stains w/ mucin stains
- Paraffin: **cystic spaces of varying sizes (Swiss-cheese)** which stain with Oil red O
- Silicone: **cystic spaces of varying sizes (Swiss-cheese)** which do not stain with Oil red O
- PMMA w/ bovine collagen (Artefil): round non-birefringent bodies in cystic spaces
- PMMA w/ hyaluronic acid (DermaLive): irregular polygonal, pink, non-birefringent particles that resemble broken glass in cystic spaces
- Poly-L-lactic acid (Sculptra): irregular fusiform, oval and Spikey ("Sculptra and Spikey sound alike") birefringent particles in cystic spaces that resemble suture material
- Calcium hydroxylapatite (Radiesse): blue-gray round or oval microspheres
    - "Looks kind of like the saponified calcium seen in pancreatic panniculitis"

Xanthomas ("Plane VET")

- Planar xanthomas (DIXX): **foam cells** (lipidized histiocytes) located **superficially**
    - Diffuse plane xanthoma: a/w IgG paraproteinemia but no lipid abnormalities

  - Intertriginous xanthoma: a/w type 2 hyperlipoproteinemia (2 antecubital fossae)
  - Xanthoma striatum palmaris: a/w type 3 hyperlipoproteinemia (3 palmar lines)
  - Xanthelasma: lipid levels are normal in around half of patients
    - Path also shows many vellus follicles and **striated muscle** (eyelid skin)
- **Verruciform xanthoma**: papillomatosis and parakeratosis ("wart on fire") w/ foam cells in dermal papillae; a/w CHILD but not a/w lipid abnormalities; MC in mouth (esp tongue)
- Eruptive xanthoma: foam cells + extracellular lipid (looks like mucin → confused w/ GA)
- **Tuberous xanthoma**/Tendinous xanthoma: foam cells + fibrotic nodule

Reaction patterns

Lichenoid: sawtooth rete, band-like lymphoid infiltrate, Civatte bodies and hyperkeratosis

- Lichen planus: only one that never has parakeratosis or eosinophils
- Benign lichenoid keratosis: usually can see a solar lentigo or SK towards the periphery
- Lichenoid drug: lichenoid interface dermatitis often w/ **eosinophils** +/- parakeratosis
  - Civatte bodies can be seen up higher in the epidermis than in LP
- Lichenoid GVHD: lichenoid interface that may have parakeratosis but rarely has eos
- Lichenoid regression of a melanoma: lichenoid interface on heavily sun-damaged skin
- Hypertrophic lupus: lichenoid interface (rarely has parakeratosis or eos) w/ superficial and deep infiltrate that

is often peri-adnexal (↑ CD123^{+} plasmacytoid dendritic cells)

- Syphilis can also have a lichenoid interface but do not have the other features of LP
    - o "Looks like LP and psoriasis had a messy baby"; **plasma cells are your main clue**

Vacuolar interface w/ a lymph in every hole ("Most Bangable Player puts it in every hole")

- Mycosis fungoides: large angular hyperchromatic lymphocytes in the epidermis (sometimes in Pautrier's microabscesses) and at the DEJ w/ papillary dermal fibrosis
- Benign lichenoid keratosis (early): vacuolar interface > lichenoid interface
- PLEVA: **compact hyperkeratosis w/ Parakeratosis** (+/- neuts in the horn), Lichenoid to vacuolar infiltrate but w/ lymph in every whole, **Extravasated RBCs**, V (wedge)-shaped dermal lymph infiltrate w/ neuts but never eos or plasma cells, Apoptotic/dyskeratotic keratinocytes in a spongiotic epidermis w/ exocytosis of lymphs
    - o PLC is a variant with less pronounced histologic features (less interface, less inflammation, less RBCs, less apoptotic keratinocytes)
    - o Ddx: syphilis is the great imitator and can look similar (look for plasma cells!)

Vacuolar interface ("when you see holes at the DEJ, you DELVe G")

- DM: similar to lupus but generally has more dermal Mucin and epidermal atrophy
- Drug including fixed drug eruption: many eosinophils (w/ pigment incontinence in FDE)
- EM: basket weave stratum corneum, vacuolar interface w/ spongiosis and dyskeratosis

- Lupus: vacuolar interface w/ thin epidermis, PV/PA lymph infiltrate and BM thickening
  - o From ACLE to SCLE to DLE, the vacuolar interface becomes more obvious, lymphoid infiltrate becomes deeper, epidermis becomes thinner w/ more follicular plugging
  - o Tumid lupus is not in this ddx because while it has ↑ dermal mucin and PV/PA lymph infiltrate, it lacks epidermal changes (vacuolar interface, BM thickening)
  - o DIF: continuous **granular** band of IgG/A/M and C3 (full house) at the BMZ
- Viral exanthem: mild vacuolar interface w/ perivascular lymphocytes (non-specific)
- GVHD: discussed below

Vacuolar interface with Dyskeratotic cells in the epidermis (abcDEFG)

- EM: **more dyskeratosis** (can be full thickness in areas) than the others, basket weave stratum corneum, superficial PV lymphocytic infiltrate +/- eosinophils
  - o Early (macules/papules): mild lymph vacuolar interface, dyskeratosis, pap dermal edema, spongiosis (intercellular edema) and ballooning (intracellular edema)
  - o Fully developed (vesicles): more lymph vacuolar interface which progresses to subepidermal vesicle, confluent necrotic keratinocytes, more papillary dermal edema and more spongiosis/ballooning (intraepidermal vesicle)
- FDE: mixed infiltrate that extends Deeper into the dermis than the others with **Eosinophils**, **pigment incontinence** and dermal fibrosis
- acute GVHD
  - o Vacuolar interface w/ lymphs next to apoptotic cells (satellite cell necrosis)

  - o **Hair follicles** are also affected w/ dead keratinocytes and interface change
  - o Dysmaturation of epidermis (resembles Bowenoid AK)
- Paraneoplastic pemphigus and PLEVA can also be in this differential

Psoriasis

- Neutrophils alternating w/ confluent parakeratosis (sandwich sign) in stratum corneum
- Collections of neutrophils in stratum corneum (Munro microabscesses)
- Collections of neutrophils in spinous layer (spongiform pustules of Kogoj)
- Regular acanthosis w/ skinny, club-shaped rete that are "test-tube like" (vs irregular and thick rete in LSC) w/ thin suprapapillary plates (vs thick in PRP), hypogranulosis (vs hypergranulosis in LSC) and dilated capillaries in dermal papillae

Psoriasisiform ddx ("My BIG Necrolytic PSoRIATIC Plaque")

- Mycosis Fungoides: large angular hyperchromatic lymphocytes in the epidermis (no neutrophils) and at the DEJ w/ papillary dermal fibrosis
- Bowen's disease: atypical keratinocytes at all levels of the epidermis
- ILVEN: **horizontally alternating ortho and parakeratosis** with ↓ granular layer under areas of parakeratosis (which is typical when we see parakeratosis)
- Granular parakeratosis: stratum corneum w/ granules and parakeratosis w/ a preserved granular layer (whereas the granular layer is usually ↓ under areas of parakeratosis)
- Necrolytic acral erythema: psoriasiform hyperplasia **w/ necrotic keratinocytes**

- PRP: no neuts in the stratum corneum, Parakeratosis (but no neuts) and **acantholysis** at follicular ostia, horizontally and vertically alternating **"checkerboard" ortho- and parakeratosis** and acanthosis w/ **thick** suprapapillary plates
- Seb derm: Spongiosis w/ Superficial PV/PF lymph infiltrate; neuts next to follicular ostia
- Syphilis: Sexy Skinny rete, Swelling of vessel lumen and plasma cells (looks like LP and psoriasis had a messy baby; PLEVA is also in the ddx but this does not have plasma cells)
- Reiter's disease: looks identical to psoriasis
- ILVEN: see above description
- Acrodermatitis enteropathica (and other nutritional deficiencies like pellagra or necrolytic acral erythema): psoriasiform hyperplasia w/ **pallor** of the upper epidermis
- Geographic Tongue: looks like psoriasis but in mouth (no granular or corneal layer)
- ILVEN: see above description
- **Clear cell acanthoma**: sharp demarcation of clear (glycogenated) psoriasiform epidermis
- **Porokeratosis**: look for **cornoid lamella** (angled column of parakeratosis w/ dyskeratotic cells below); zone between cornoid lamella may appear lichenoid or psoriasiform

Mounds (patchy/non-confluence) of parakeratosis ("PEGS")

- PR: mounded Parakeratosis, RBC extravasation, PV lymph infiltrate, mild spongiosis
- EAC: mounds of parakeratosis, **dense "Coat sleave"** PV lymph infiltrate, mild spongiosis
- Guttate psoriasis: **neuts above mounded para**, RBC extravasation, mild spongiosis
- Small plaque parapsoriasis (antiquated term): mounds of parakeratosis, mild spongiosis

Spongiotic dermatitis (edema between keratinocytes:): "SAND PITZ"

- Stasis dermatitis: cannonball-like angioplasia in the superficial dermis with hemosiderin
    - **Acroangiodermatitis (pseudo-kaposi) is clinically like Kaposi but on path can show features of both stasis and Kaposi's sarcoma**
- Seb derm: psoriasiform spongiotic dermatitis w/ perifollicular neutrophilic scale/crust
- Allergic contact dermatitis: eosinophilic spongiosis (HAPPIED mnemonic below)
- Nummular dermatitis: spongiosis of the epidermis
- Dyshidrotic dermatitis: spongiosis of the epidermis
- Pityriasis Rosea: spongiosis w/ Parakeratotis focally, RBC extravasation
- ID reaction: spongiosis of the epidermis
- Tinea: hyphae in a stratum corneum with a basket weave layer above a compact layer
- **Zoon's balanitis: pale flattened, diamond-shaped keratinocytes in a thin epidermis, w/ dilated dermal capillaries and a dermal infiltrate composed entirely of plasma cells**
- Candida: neutrophils and vertically oriented pseudohyphae in the stratum corneum

Stages of spongiotic dermatitis

- Early (papules): spong w/ superficial perivascular infiltrate and basket-weave corneum
- Early (vesicles): spongiotic microvesiculation, parakeratosis/scale-crust, psoriasiform hyperplasia and superficial perivascular infiltrate
- Late (psoriasiform plaques): LSC changes (compact orthokeratosis, hypergranulosis w/ stratum lucidum, psoriasiform hyperplasia and course collagen fibers in vertical streaks in the papillary dermis) with no spongiosis

  - Only time you will see a stratum lucidum on hair bearing skin ("hairy palm" sign)

Blisters

- Get a DIF

Subcorneal split (all attack desmoglein 1 except friction blister; "I have to take a Frickin' PISS")

- Friction blisters: superficial split just below the granular layer **w/ epidermal necrosis**
- Pemphigus foliaceus: subcorneal acantholysis w/ scattered **eosinophils**; **DIF (+)**
  - DIF: netlike pattern of IgG (upper epidermis > lower epidermis)
    - Pemphigus erythematosus is a variant which also has linear MBZ staining
- bullous Impetigo: **neutrophils** within the subcorneal bullae +/- **staph colonies**; DIF (-)
- SSSS: clean subcorneal split w/ no inflammation or staph colonies; DIF (-)

Intra-epidermal acantholysis ("Pem-PHHAAA-gus")

- Pemphigus vulgaris: **acantholysis above basal layer ("tombstoning")** that **tracks down hair follicles**; + **eosinophils**
  - DIF: net-like deposition of IgG and C3 (lower epidermis > upper epidermis)
- IgA Pemphigus (IEN type): intraepidermal **neutrophilic** infiltrate w/ minimal acantholysis
  - DIF: intercellular IgA in upper epidermis (SPD type) or lower/entire epi (IEN type)
- Paraneoplastic pemphigus: **lichenoid or vacuolar infiltrate** w/ necrotic keratinocytes

    - DIF: net-like IgG and C3 (like PV) **but also linear deposition at the DEJ** (this DIF pattern is most reminiscent of pemphigus erythematosus)
- Hailey-Hailey: **acantholysis at all levels of an acanthotic epidermis (resembles a dilapidated brick wall)** but **does not track down follicle**; minimal dyskeratosis; DIF (-)
- **HSV 1-3 (M)**: intraepidermal blister w/ solitary keratinocytes w/ nucleic changes of viral infection→ Multinucleated keratinocytes, **Margination of chromatin**, nuclear Molding
- Acantholytic acanthoma: acantholysis of acanthotic epidermis like in Hailey-Hailey but does not have any dyskeratosis
- **Acantholytic AK/SCC**: large atypical acantholytic keratinocytes (usually a/w hair follicle)
- Bullous Arthropod assault: intraepidermal acantholysis w/ dense superficial PV lymphocytic infiltrate w/ numerous eosinophils

Intra-epidermal acantholysis w/ prominent dyskeratosis (corps ronds and grains; "DAWG")

- Dariers (keratosis follicularis): intraepidermal acantholysis can be seen at all levels of the epidermis w/ numerous dyskeratotic cells including corps Ronds (cells w/ pyknotic nucleus, clear perinuclear halo and brightly Red/eosinophilic cytoplasm) and corps grains (oval cells w/ elongated cigar-shaped nuclei and abundant keratohyalin granules mostly seen in the stratum corneum); orthokeratosis; lymphs (but no eos) in the dermis
- Acantholytic dyskeratoma: solitary lesion w/ acantholytic dyskeratosis
- Warty D: cup shaped/**endophytic** solitary lesion w/ acantholytic dyskeratosis

- Grovers: smaller involved foci than in Darier's +/- **eosinophils** (absent in Darier's)
    - In reality, these are not able to be differentiated from each other on H&E

Subepidermal autoimmune (positive DIF) blistering diseases: "ABCDE"

- linear IgA bullous dermatosis: sup-epidermal split w/ **neutrophils** lined up at the DEJ
    - DIF: linear IgA at DEJ
- Bullous lupus: sub-epidermal blister w/ **neutrophils**
    - DIF: full house (IgG, C3, IgA, IgM) in a granular pattern along the DEJ
- BP: sub-epidermal split with **eosinophils** and neutrophils in vessel cavity ("BAD eos": BP, Arthropod and bullous Drug can all do this so you will need DIF to differentiate)
    - DIF SSS: stains roof of blister cavity (vs stains floor in EBA)
    - DIF: linear C3 and IgG along DEJ in an n-serrated pattern ("bullous pen-phigoid")
- Cicatricial pemphigoid: subepi split w/ lymphs > plasma cells and eos; **dermal fibrosis**
    - DIF: linear IgA, IgG and C3 along the DEJ and along appendageal structures
- DH: sup-epidermal split w/ **neutrophilic micro-abscesses in tips of dermal papillae**
    - DIF: granular IgA within dermal papillae
- EBA: noninflammatory subepi split (mechanobullous) vs BP-like (inflammatory form)
    - DIF SSS: stains floor of blister cavity (vs stains roof in BP)
    - DIF: linear IgG > C3 at DEJ in u-serrated pattern ("epidermoysis bulossa aquisita")

Non-autoimmune subepidermal blisters (all are pauci-inflammatory except bullous CSVV)

- **PCT**: subepidermal split on acral skin w/ minimal inflammation, protuberance of rigid dermal papillae into blister cavity ("festooning"), amphophilic BMZ (type 4 collagen) material in overlying epidermis above blister cavity ("caterpillar bodies") and thickened hyalinized PAS+ material around BVs under blister cavity w/ surrounding solar elastosis
    - o DIF (typically negative): **IgG, IgM and C3 in vessels** >> linear at DEJ
- SJS/TEN: subepidermal bulla w/ **eosinophils** and **full-thickness epidermal necrosis**
- Bullous dermatitis artifacta (self-inflicted): subepidermal blister w/ epidermal necrosis
- Bullous CSVV: LCV with massive subepidermal edema and epidermal necrosis
- Coma blisters: cell poor subepidermal blister with **necrosis of eccrine glands**
- Edema blisters: marked epidermal spongiosis w/ dilated dermal BVs and mild infiltrate
- Bullous drug eruption: variable presentations but tend to show a blister w/ eosinophils
- Bullous diabeticorum, delayed postburn/postgraft blisters, fracture blisters and suckling blisters also fit into the category of pauci-inflammatory subepidermal split

Neoplastic

Squamous eddies ("Eddy is Tricky IF Very Irritated")

- Trichilemmoma: smooth lobules of glycogenated cells hanging down from the epidermis w/ a peripheral palisade and outlined by a thick eosinophilic basement membrane

  - IHC: $CD34^{+}$; PAS^{+} (becomes negative if diastase is added due to ↑ glycogen)
- IFK (inverted follicular keratosis): endophytic lesion resembling an expanded hair follicle
- Verruca vulgaris: exophytic, papillomatosis, rounded parakeratosis, coarse hypergranulosis, koilocytes (vacuolated cells w/ hyperchromatic shriveled nuclei)
  - Myrmecia (palmoplantar wart; HPV-1): endophytic w/ **red** cytoplasmic inclusions
  - Verruca plana (flat wart): bird's eye cells (like koilocytes but lack shriveled nuclei)
  - Epidermodysplasia verruciformis: widespread flat warts w/ **blue cytoplasm**
  - Condyloma acuminata: SK-like (horn cysts/squamous eddies) but in genitals
- Irritated SK: type of SK (loose keratin, acanthosis, horn cysts) but w/ squamous eddies
  - Other types of SKs include pigmented (pigmented keratinocytes), hyperkeratotic (papillomatosis), inflamed (lymphocytes), **clonal (islands of small keratinocytes)**, Dowling-Degos disease (SK coming off hair follicles); refer to 6.1 for more on SKs

Clonal ("Clone Chriss BoSH")

- Clonal Bowens: clonal islands of atypical keratinocytes w/ pagetoid scatter
- Clonal SK: clonal islands of small keratinocytes w/ bland uniform nuclei
  - Regular SKs are too easy so this is the type of SK most likely to be tested
  - Hidroacanthoma simplex (intraepidermal poroma): clonal islands of small eosinophilic acrosyringial keratinocytes but w/ small ducts in the center

Malignant tumors in the epidermis/Pagetoid spread ("Bowens SPITS")

- Bowens: atypical keratinocytes w/ clear cytoplasm which crush basal layer ("eye-liner sign"); abnormal keratinocyte maturation ("wind-blown appearance"); **parakeratosis**
  - AK only has atypical keratinocytes in the lower epidermis (not full thickness)
  - Keratin stains (p63, HMWK)
- SebAceous carcinoma (ocular type): malignant epidermal sebaceous-appearing cells w/ scalloped nuclei and clear cytoplasm containing microvesicles; no parakeratosis
  - Adipophilin, Androgen receptor, EMA
- Paget's/EMPD: **large cells (some are signet ring) w/ ample bluish mucinous cytoplasm (glandular differentiation apparent)** spitting into the epidermis and crushing basal layer
  - Clue: apocrine glands, dilated dermal blood vessels (gives the red "strawberry and cream" color clinically); no parakeratosis or solar elastosis (vs Bowens)
  - IHC: EMA, PAS (diastase resistant), CEA, CK7, gross cystic protein (GCDFP-15)
    - "EMA passed by and resisted a sea of 7 cocks, gross"
    - Disease extending from internal cancer is **CK20**$^{+}$, CK7^{-}, and **GCDFP-15**$^{-}$
      - "But internally EMA wanted 20 cocks and did not find them gross"
- Spitz nevus: well-circumscribed lesion w/ large junctional nests that "rain down" and exhibit clefting +/- Kamino bodies (pink clumps of collagen 4) in the

epidermis; Pagetoid spread of melanocytes and superficial mitoses can be seen
  - IHC: p16$^+$, Melan-A$^+$, S100$^+$, S100A6$^+$ ("when a girl PMS'S she spitz at you")
    - p16 is positive in Spitz but lost in atypical Spitz/spitzoid melanomas
- Intraepidermal porocarcinoma: like poroma but w/ cytologic atypia and atypical mitoses
  - IHC: CEA, EMA, and PAS highlight ducts and intracytoplasmic lumina
- Thin melanomas (in-situ): **basal layer involved (so it is not crushed)**; look for pigment and **nests of atypical melanocytes** at all levels of epi (usually spits into the s. corneum)
  - Lentigo maligna: confluence of atypical melanocytes at the DEJ (less pagetoid)
  - IHC: melan-A, S100, SOX10

Stages of Paget's/extramammary Paget's (EMPD)

- Neoplastic cells in Paget's migrate to the epidermis from **lactiferous ducts** whereas in **EMPD they begin in the epi ("adenocarcinoma in situ")** and migrate down into adnexa
  - EMPD due to mets from GI/GU/cervix adenocarcinoma makes up < 20% of cases
- Early lesions (patch): single Paget cells in epidermis, especially lower half
- Fully developed (plaque): Paget cells nested in aggregates throughout entire epidermis
- Late lesions of EMPD due to GI/GU/cervix adenocarcinoma: aggregates of Paget cells in epidermis, dermis, superficial SQ and within vascular spaces

BCC look-a-likes ("Bacon Lettuce Tomato")

- BCC: blue islands w/ peripheral palisade and retraction artifact in a fibromyxoid stroma
  - Variants: superficial (blue buds come off epidermis), nodular (large round blue islands), micronodular (small round blue islands), infiltrative (spikey blue islands), morpheaform (thin infiltrative strands of BCC in sclerotic stroma), infundibulocystic (pink strands, blue buds, horn cysts), fibroepithelioma of pinkus (pink strands, blue buds, eccrine ducts), adenoid (clear spaces in islands)
  - IHC: **Ber-EP4; strong diffuse BCL-2 staining and androgen receptor**
- Lymphadenoma (adamantanoid trichoblastoma): tumor islands w/ 1–2 layers of basaloid cells peripherally and clear cells centrally
  - IHC: same as trichoblastoma
- Trichoblastoma: large blue islands in the dermis but there is no peripheral palisade, retraction is seen between collagen in stroma not between tumor and stroma, stroma is fibroblast-rich and papillary mesenchymal bodies may be seen in stroma
  - Trichoepithelioma is a variant which is smaller (trichoblastoma is bigger) and has cribriform (Swiss-cheese) basaloid nodules
  - IHC: CD10, CK20, CD34 (stroma), BCL-2 (stains periphery of islands)

SCC-like

- SCC: atypical keratinocytes invading the dermis w/ a jagged border
- KA: invasive proliferation of glassy red keratinocytes w/ keratin-filled crater, neutrophilic microabscesses and trapping of elastic fibers peripherally
- **Verrucous carcinoma**: well-differentiated glassy eosinophilic keratinocytes w/ blunt/rounded border

that push into the underlying tissue in a bull-dozing fashion
    - Seen in anogenital region (Buschke-Lowenstein tumor), mouth (oral florid papillomatosis) and foot (epithelioma caniculatum); HPV-6, 11
- **Lymphoepithelioma-like carcinoma**: at scan it looks like a germinal center but on closer look there are keratin-positive atypical epithelial cells surrounded by inflammation

Papillomatosis ("An Erratic Church Spire Pattern): undulation of epi in a "church spire" pattern

- Acanthosis nigricans, Axillae/groin skin, Acroverruciformis of Hopf, Epidermal nevi, CARP, Stucco keratoses, Papillomatous/hyperkeratotic SK
- Differentiation between entities in this mnemonic based on pathology is not possible

Malignant spindle cells SLAM against the epidermis

- Spindled (sarcomatoid) SCC: biphasic tumor w/ thin epithelial elements surrounded by spindled cells; may have epidermal component
    - HMWK, CK5/6, p63, and p40 (newest and most specific)
- Leiomyosarcoma: no epidermal component; tumor is very pink; cells are cigar-shaped w/ perinuclear vacuoles ("glycogen-snack" for these muscle cells)
    - SMA, desmin
- Atypical fibroxanthoma: no epidermal component; cells are very pleomorphic, multinucleate and bizarre
    - Can be (+) for S100A6, **CD10** and SMA
- **Melanoma (desmoplastic)**: can have epidermal component (usually lentigo maligna pattern); **lymphoid aggregates is a great clue;** may or may not see melanin
    - **S100, Sox-10, p75**

Cysts: "A DUMB Cystic VEST"

- Apocrine/eccrine hydrocystoma: flat cuboidal epithelium w/ large empty cystic space
- Apocrine cystadenoma: has been used interchangeably w/ apocrine hydrocystoma but inside the cyst there are papillary projections ("mix between HPAP and hydrocystoma")
    - o Ddx: tubular apocrine adenoma has many small cyst-like spaces w/ these papilla
- Auricular pseudocyst: cystic space in cartilage w/ no epithelial lining or chondritis
- Dermoid cyst: stratified squamous epithelium (SSE) w/ granular layer and adnexal structures (sebaceous/ eccrine/apocrine glands and **hair follicles**); may contain red shark-tooth lining like steatocystomas; lamellar keratin is inside cyst cavity
- Digital mucus cyst/ganglion cyst: mucin inside pseudocyst (no epithelial lining)
- Urachal cyst: ectopic bladder epithelium (cuboidal or flat, atrophic epithelia)
    - o Ddx: omphalomesenteric duct remnant (GI mucosa w/ goblet cells on path) vs umbilical granuloma (vascular proliferation on path)
- Median raphe cyst: dirty debris ("penis' are dirty") in cyst; genital skin features
- Mucocele: mucin inside pseudocyst (no epithelial lining) +/- adjacent salivary glands
- Branchial cleft: variable lining w/ surrounding **Lymphoid Aggregates (germinal centers)**
- Bronchogenic cyst: ciliated columnar epithelium; cartilage, smooth muscle, goblet cells
- Cutaneous Ciliated Cyst (lower legs) and Ciliated Cysts of vulva: Columnar Ciliated epithelium +/- dirty debris in cyst ("vulvas are dirty")

- Cutaneous endometriosis ("GIRL"): cyst-like Glandular spaces, Iron, RBCs, Loose concentric fibromyxoid stroma
- Verrucous cyst: looks like a pilar cyst but w/ papillomatosis, hypergranulosis, koilocytes
- Vellus hair cyst: looks like epidermoid cyst but w/ multiple vellus hairs in cyst cavity
- Ear pits: lined by stratified squamous epithelium (SSE) w/ a granular layer
- Epidermoid cyst: cystic cavity filled w/ **laminated keratin** lined by SSE w/ granular layer
- Steatocystoma: lined by SSE w/ no granular layer and thin bright pink corrugated ("Shark-tooth") cuticle w/ Sebaceous glands in wall (no hair follicles in cyst wall or lamellar keratin in cyst cavity like in dermoid cysts)
- Trichilemmal: SSE w/ no granular layer and dense pink homogenized keratin +/- calcium
- Thyroglossal duct cyst: variable lining w/ bright pink thyroid follicles in the wall

Melanocytic neoplasms

- Ephelides/CALMs: ↑ basilar keratinocyte hyperpigmentation w/o ↑ melanocyte density
- Solar lentigo: long rete ridges w/ basilar keratinocyte hyperpigmentation ("dirty socks")
- Lentigo simplex: ↑ basilar keratinocyte hyperpigmentation; mild ↑ melanocyte density
- Mucosal melanotic macule: acanthosis with mild basilar hyperpigmentation and mild ↑ in melanocyte density
- Becker's nevus: ↑ basal melanocytes w/ a smooth muscle hamartoma in the dermis
- Dermal melanocytosis: dendritic melanocytes oriented east to west in lower dermis

- Nevus of Ito/Ota: dendritic melanocytes oriented east to west scattered between collagen bundles in the upper 1/3rd of the dermis; no sclerotic stroma
- Common blue nevus: small: wedge-shaped lesion in upper 2/3rd of dermis composed entirely of long dendritic melanocytes embedded in a sclerotic stroma
- Cellular blue nevus: proliferation of both epithelioid (plump) and dendritic melanocytes in a sclerotic stroma that bulges into the SQ ("big black ball in the fat")
- Epithelioid blue nevus: proliferation composed entirely of epithelioid (plump) melanocytes but no sclerotic stroma
- Deep penetrating nevus (DPN): very similar to cellular blue nevus (both have epithelioid melanocytes diving deep into SQ) but DPN'S Dive Down (more wedge-shape; classically tracking down adnexa/nerves), more Pigmented, more Nested and are more Spitzoid (cells have more abundant cytoplasm) compared to a cellular blue nevus
- Spitz nevus ("shpitz"): symmetric and circumscribed lesion w/ large junctional nests of epithelioid melanocytes Hanging down from a Hyperplastic epidermis; overlying Hyperkeratosis and Hypergranulation; **kamino bodies** within epidermis
- Pigmented spindle cell nevus of Reed: like spitz but more superficial (superficial dermis), more pigmented (more melanophages) and melanocytes are spindled (vs epithelioid)
- BAP-1 inactivated nevus: combined nevi composed of conventional nevus (w/ preserved BAP-1 expression) and zone of large spitzoid cells w/ amphophilic cytoplasm (BAP loss)
- Recurrent melanocytic nevus: atypical junctional melanocytic proliferation (resembling MIS) located above a

dermal scar; benign dermal nevus seen below/next to dermal scar

- Balloon cell nevus: > 50% dermal melanocytes are "balloon cells" (large pale melanocytes w/ vacuolated cytoplasm); always can find conventional nevus somewhere
- Halo nevus: bland nevus w/ lymphocytes intertwined w/ melanocytes ("cocktail party")
- Congenital melanocytic nevus: symmetrical broad proliferation of melanocytes in the dermis w/ maturation, splaying between collagen bundles and permeation of erector pilli muscles, blood vessels, adnexal structures, and nerves (this is not worrisome)
- Acquired melanocytic nevus: symmetrical and circumscribed junctional, compound or intradermal proliferations of nested epithelioid nevoid cells which show maturation w/ depth (cells are more spindled/neuroid and singly spaced in the deep dermis)
- Dysplastic (Clark's) nevus: asymmetry, atypical nests at the junction extend > 2 rete ridges beyond dermal component, "bridging" of junctional nests, papillary dermal fibrosis, and cytologic atypia (graded based on degree of architectural and cytologic atypia)
- Melanoma: asymmetry, poor circumscription, irregular nests w/ discohesion, confluent melanocytes along DEJ, pagetoid growth, epidermal consumption w/ extension down adnexa, lack of maturation of dermal component (large nests at base), and cytologic atypia

Melanoma variants

- Melanoma in situ (MIS): broad lesion, nests vary in size and shape and are found at all levels of the epidermis and extend down adnexa
- Lentigo maligna: form of MIS on sun-damaged skin; confluence of atypical melanocytes at the DEJ (junctional growth w/o Pagetoid spread)

- Lentigo maligna melanoma: lentigo maligna w/ a vertical growth phase
- Superficial spreading melanoma: broad lesion w/ buckshot scatter of atypical melanocytes in the epidermis, nests are not confined to tips and sides of rete (vs dysplastic nevus) and are not evenly spaced
- Nodular melanoma: may be symmetrical, no in situ component, dermal component consists of a cohesive nodule of tumor cells with pushing border, deep mitoses and necrosis; plasma cells common in center and lymphs common at base ("riot police")
- Regressing melanoma: effaced rete pattern, dermal fibrosis and lichenoid inflammation w/ abundant melanophages
- Desmoplastic melanoma: elongated spindle cells (long fascicles of parallel nuclei) and abundant fibrous stroma; foci of **lymphoid aggregates** is a useful clue
    - Tumors w/ ↑ cellularity and ↓ stroma best classified as spindle cell melanoma

Benign adnexal neoplasms

- Eccrine poromas: endophytic proliferation of epidermal poroid cells (small red cuboidal cells) w/ variably spaced sweat ducts in the epidermis and a highly vascularized stroma
    - Poroma variants
        - Hidroacanthoma simplex: nests of small poroid cells only in the epidermis
        - Dermal duct tumor: dermal nodules of poroid cells; no connection to epi
        - Hidradenoma ("SPoCK, aka eyebrows are high"): Squamoid cells + Poroid cells + Clear cells (any of these 3 cell types may dominate) + Cystic degeneration + Keloidal collagen
- Syringoma: tadpole or comma-shaped sweat ducts (amorphous sweat within lumen) in a sclerotic stroma

confined to the upper half of dermis (benign superficial tumor)

- Mixed tumor (chondroid syringoma): circumscribed tumor made of glandular structures in a Myxoid stroma; branching (apocrine) and small tubular (eccrine) types exist
- Spiradenoma: large "blue ball" in the dermis w/ cystically dilated ducts and PAS+ hyaline droplets (3 types of cells on high power: large pale + small blue + lymphocytes)
- Cylindroma: jigsaw pattern of tumor lobules encircled by thick hyalinized BMZ material
- Syringocystadenoma papilliferum: papillary glandular proliferation w/ decapitation secretions which opens to Skin Surface ("looks like you can Slide in"); many plasma cells
- Hidradenoma papilliferum: papillary proliferation w/ decapitation secretions "hiding" in the dermis (lacks epidermal connection) w/ a maze-like architecture ("hide in the maze")
    - o Ddx: nipple adenoma (looks like an HPAP but it is on the nipple), apocrine cystadenoma (mix b/w hidrocystoma and HPAP w/ papillary fronds budding into the lumen of the cyst), tubular apocrine adenoma ("small cystic mazes") and aggressive digital papillary adenocarcinoma (consider if HPAP-like lesion on digit)
- Papillary eccrine adenoma (PEA) and tubular apocrine adenoma (TAA): proliferation of small round sweat ducts w/ Papillary projections in lumen
    - o "Whereas HPAP is one huge maze, PEA/TAA looks like many tiny mazes"
- Syringofibroadenoma: long strands of sweat-duct epithelium that hang down from epi
- Hidrocystoma: cyst lined by cuboidal or columnar cells +/- decapitation secretions

Aggressive and Malignant adnexal neoplasms

- Aggressive digital papillary adenocarcinoma: looks like SPAP/HPAP due to numerous papillary projections but it is deeply infiltrative w/ ↑ mitoses and atypia
- Adenoid cystic (S sound) carcinoma: cribriform ("Swiss-cheese") appearance of basaloid tumor nodules with mucin in the cribriform lumens extending deep into the SQ fat; **PNI**
- Mucinous carcinoma: blue tumor cells in sea of mucin ("blue islands in a sea of snot")
- Microcystic adnexal carcinoma (MAC): deeply infiltrative basaloid proliferation w/ Multi-lineage differentiation (horn cysts and sweat ducts), PNI and lymphoid aggregates

Follicular neoplasms ("There is hair on my Filthy Toilet Paper")

- Fibrofolliculoma: central follicle w/ numerous thin strands of immature (**no mature follicle/hair shafts**) follicular epithelium radiating from it; loose fibromyxoid stroma
- Trichofolliculoma: dilated central follicle w/ smaller but still **fully formed vellus follicles radiating from it** ("mother and her babies")
- Trichoepithelioma: well-Circumscribed tumor of basaloid Cribriform nodules, numerous horn Cysts, Calcification and papillary mesenchymal bodies in a pink Collagenous stroma
    - Desmoplastic TE: Cords of blue cells in Collagenous stroma, Calcium, horn Cysts
- Trichilemmoma: circumscribed proliferation of clear outer root sheath cells (contains glycogen) that hangs down from the epidermis (broad connection to epi) and has a peripheral palisade w/ hyalinized BMZ and a warty surface
    - Desmoplastic trichilemmoma: **often mistaken for invasive SCC** due to pseudo-infiltrative epithe-

lial strands but you see a classic trichilemmoma embedded in a sclerotic stroma off to the periphery

- Trichoadenoma: dermal proliferation of keratinizing milia-like cysts in a sclerotic stroma (cysts are often in pairs resembling eyeglasses)
- Tumor of the follicular infundibulum: downward epidermal proliferation of clear cells that run parallel to the epidermis (clinically and histologically may mimic superficial BCC)
- Pilar sheath acanthoma: similar to trichofolliculoma but babies radiating from central dilated pore are acanthotic ("fat fingers radiating from dilated pore")
- Pilomatricoma: cystic architecture w/ "rolls and scrolls", blue matrical cells which have an abrupt transition to anucleate shadow cells
- Proliferating pilar tumor: same "rolls and scrolls" architecture as pilomatricoma but has dense keratin instead of shadow cells and lacks basaloid matrical cells

Sebaceous neoplasms

- Nevus sebaceous of Jadassohn: "broad, bald (no terminal hairs), bumpy (papillomatous) and bubbly (↑ sebaceous and apocrine glands)"
- Sebaceous hyperplasia: enlarged sebaceous glands w/ normal architecture (central mature white sebocytes w/ thin peripheral rim of immature blue seboblasts)
- Sebaceous adenoma: **superficial** proliferation w/ central mature sebocytes w/ thicker rim of blue seboblasts ("but still more white than blue")
    - "In sebaceous adenoma we just add some blue seboblasts to the periphery"
- Sebaceous epithelioma (sebaceoma; "sa-blue-ce-oma"): purely intradermal mass comprised of **more blue seboblasts than white sebocytes ("more blue than white")**
- Sebaceous carcinoma

- Ocular: intraepithelial spread of malignant cells in a pagetoid pattern w/ minimal sebaceous differentiation (need stains to identify)
  - IHC (Seb-A-ceous): EMA, AR, Adipophilin, Factor XIIIa (AC-1A1)
- Extraocular: infiltrative sebaceous basaloid proliferation ("may have more white than blue or more blue than white") w/ atypia, mitoses and tumor necrosis

Paisley tie: all show tadpole shaped islands in a red sclerotic stroma (**Tied** up think BDSM)

- BCC (morpheaform): clefts Between epithelium and stroma; no sweat ducts
  - IHC: (+) for BCL2 diffusely and Ber-EP4
- DTE (think Cs): Clefts within stroma, **Central dell (umbilication), horn Cysts (follicular differentiation)**, Calcifications on Cheek of Child (young female); **no sweat ducts**
  - IHC: (+) for CK20, CD10 in stroma, CD34, PHLDA, BCL-2 only stains periphery
- Syringoma: Small benign tumor (never deep) of eccrine gland w/ Sweat in ducts
- MAC: deep infiltrative pattern w/ horn cysts, **perineural extension and lymphoid aggregates w/ bi-linear differentiation** (follicular horn cysts + sweat ducts; "MAC is bi")

Downward epidermal proliferations ("Peanut Butter STICKS")

- Poroma: epidermal proliferation of small monotonous keratinocytes w/ ducts
- BCC (superficial, fibroepithelioma of Pinkus and infundibulocystic)
- Seborrheic keratosis: broad sheets of small polygonal keratinocytes w/ intervening horn cysts; loose lamellar "shredded wheat" keratin

- Tumor of the follicular infundibulum: acanthoma composed of pale pink cells forming anastomosing narrow strands that run parallel (just underneath) to the epidermis
- Inverted follicular keratosis: endophytic lesion w/ squamous eddies
- Clear cell acanthoma: distinct transition between normal epidermis and acanthoma made of clear glycogenated (PAS+ diastase sensitive) cells w/ overlying parakeratosis
- Syringofibroadenoma of Mascaro: Slender downward ductal proliferation

Deep dermal tumors: "SANS SANG with a deep voice

- Spiradenoma: big blue ball in dermis composed of dark cells, light cells, lymphocytes, hyaline droplets and widely ectatic blood vessels
- Angiolipoma: proliferation of capillary sized blood vessels and lipocytes
- Nodular hidradenoma ("SPoCK"): Squamoid cells + Poroid cells + Clear cells (any of these 3 cell types may dominate) + Cystic degeneration + Keloidal collagen
    - Clear cell hidradenoma mimics metastatic RCC but in **hidradenoma you see ductal structures** and in metastatic **RCC you see RBCs and vascular spaces**
- Spindle cell lipoma: "I call it a ropey myxoid spindle cell lipoma to remind me that you see ropey collagen in a myxoid stroma with surrounding spindle cells and lipocytes"
    - Pleomorphic lipoma looks like a Spindle cell lipoma but it has floret giant cells
- Schwannoma: deep encapsulated tumor w/ hypercellular Antoni A areas containing Verocay bodies (looks like leaves raked into piles) and hypocellular Antoni B areas

- Angioleiomyoma: deep nodule of smooth muscle with round slit-like vascular spaces
- NoduLAR fasciitis: Loose myxoid stroma, Large pleomorphic fibroblasts, Aggregates of inflammatory cells, RBC extravasation and Red thick collagen bundles in older lesions
- Giant cell tumor of the tendon sheath: deep tumor composed of foamy macrophages, plump fibroblasts, hemosiderin in a fibrous pseudo-capsule; osteoclast-like giant cells

Fibrohistiocytic neoplasms: "JACK F***ING DIES and the Police Department is PAGED Fast"

- Benign (JACK F***ING DIES)
    - Juvenile hyaline fibromatosis: pink amorphous hyaline material in dermis
    - Angiofibroma: dermal proliferation of stellate factor 13a+ fibroblasts w/ concentric perivascular fibrosis and ectatic thin-walled vessels
    - Multinucleate cell Angiohistiocytoma: looks like an angiofibroma but contains **bizarre, angulated Multinucleated giant cells**
    - Adult myofibroma: fibrovascular proliferation w/ myofibroblasts, staghorn vessels and large nodules w/ a blue hue ("adult myofi-blue-ma")
    - Acquired digital fibrokeratoma: compact hyperkeratosis and acanthosis w/ vertical collagen bundles in the dermis; no nerves (vs supernumerary digit)
    - Calcifying aponeurotic fibroma: plump epithelioid fibroblasts palisading around foci of **cartilage or calcification** +/- osteoclast-like giant cells
    - Keloid/scar: discussed elsewhere
    - Fibromatosis: proliferation of long fascicles of corkscrew-shaped myofibroblasts
    - Fibrous hamartoma of infancy: Fat cells (S100+), Fibroblast cells consisting of plump spindle cells

in Fascicles (Actin+), Myxoid Mesenchymal cells (Vimentin+)

- Pleomorphic Fibroma: skin tag w/ hyperchromatic, bizarre, multinucleated cells
- Infantile myofibromatosis: same path as in fibromatosis (above)
- Nodular fasciitis: described above in deep dermal tumor mnemonic
- Giant cell tumor of the tendon sheath: above in deep dermal tumor mnemonic
- Dermatofibroma ("DF'S"): Dermal spindle cell proliferation w/ collagen trapping, thickened epidermis w/ Folliculo-sebaceous induction; when present, ringed lipidized Siderophages are pathognomonic
  - IHC (DF'S): D2-40, Factor 13a ("13A you're A OK"), Stromelysin-3
- Dermatomyofibroma: spindle cells w/ east-west orientation that respect adnexa
- Infantile digital fibroma entire ("intire") dermis is filled w/ intersecting fascicles of plump spindle cells which contain pink-red inclusion bodies
- Elastofibroma dorsi: large fibrous tumor w/ beaded elastic fibers visible on VVG
- Epithelioid cell histiocytoma: well-circumscribed dermal proliferation of epithelioid cells (spitz nevus-like) w/ epidermal collarette and dermal sclerosis
- Sclerotic fibroma: acellular collagen bundles w/ van Gogh's Starry night pattern

- Borderline (Police Department)
  - Plexiform fibrohistiocytic tumor: Poorly demarcated dermal or SQ mass w/ multinodular Plexiform fascicles of fibrohistiocytic spindle cells +/- giant cells
  - Desmoid tumor (aggressive fibromatosis; "ABCDEFG"): Aggressive fibromatosis, Bland wavy

nuclei on path, β-Catenin mutation, Desmoid tumor, Deep infiltration, Fibroblastic proliferation, a/w Gardner's syndrome

- Malignant (PAGED Fast)
    - Pleomorphic undifferentiated sarcoma: similar to AFX but more deeply located
    - Pleomorphic dermal sarcoma: similar to AFX but more deeply located
    - AFX: fairly well-circumscribed but overtly malignant dermal proliferation of anaplastic, pleomorphic cells w/ high mitotic rate and wildly atypical mitoses which fills the dermis but does not invade into the fat (if it does then call it a PDS or superficial UPS/PUS); composed of 4 cell types ("call it atypical fibro-histiocytic xanthoma") → bizarre atypical multinucleated giant cells, spindle cells, histiocyte-like cells, xanthomatous cells
        - IHC (non-specific): **CD10**, CD68
    - Giant cell fibroblastoma: multinucleated giant cells lining pseudovascular spaces
    - Epithelioid sarcoma: transition from epithelioid to plump pleomorphic spindle cells **w/ central necrosis** and a surrounding lymphohistiocytic infiltrate
        - "Looks like a palisaded granuloma"
    - DFSP: Densely hypercellular Dermal proliferation infiltrating **Fat (creates a "honeycomb" pattern)** consisting of Spindled cells w/ a **Storiform Pattern**
        - IHC: **CD34+** (D2-40, Factor 13a and Stromelysin-3 negative)
        - 15% of DFSP's may undergo fibrosarcomatous degeneration → ↑ atypia, ↑ cellularity, ↑ mitoses w/ **"herringbone" pattern**, loss of CD34 staining
    - Fibrosarcoma: densely hypercellular tumor w/ herringbone ("Fir tree") pattern

Vascular neoplasms

- Infantile hemangioma: lobular proliferations of GLUT-1 (+) dermal capillaries lined by plump endothelium (transiently positive for LYVE-1 but lacks other lymphatic markers)
- Intravascular papillary endothelial hyperplasia (IPEH): Intraluminal Papillary Proliferation of Endothelial cells Entirely contained within a Hyperplastic thrombosed vessel (e.g., vein)
- Reactive Angioendotheliomatosis: proliferation of grouped capillaries in dermal BVs
- Angiokeratoma: superficial dilated vessels a/w an acanthotic epidermis ("**bloody SK**")
- Targetoid hemosiderotic lymphatic malformation: **superficial dilated BVs** with endothelial cells that protrude (hobnail) into the lumen in the upper dermis; the **lower dermis has hemosiderin and BVs get thin and slit-like**; vessels stain w/ lymph markers
- Verrucous venulocapillary malformation (verrucous hemangioma): dilated capillaries and venules that stain with CD31 and CD34
- Pyogenic granuloma: circumscribed, exophytic capillary proliferation in a lobular pattern
- Tufted angioma ("tough LUCK"): tightly packed Lobules (Ultrastructural studies show Weibel-Palade bodies) of **Capillaries in a "Cannonball" pattern in Clusters** with an empty appearing Crescent surrounding each lobule (Clefting) which represent dilated lymphatic Channels; CD61 confirms platelet trapping in cases of Kasabach-merritt
- Glomeruloid hemangioma: RBCs + capillaries in dilated vessels (resembles glomerulus)
- Cherry angioma: dilated capillaries within the papillary dermis
- Microvenular hemangioma: small flat monomorphic blood vessels that fill the dermis

- Epithelioid hemangioma: Enlarged thickened vessels lined by Enlarged plump Epithelioid Endothelial cells which have intracytoplasmic vacuoles; **Eosinophilic inflammation**
- Congenital Cutaneous Angiomatosis w/ thrombocytopenia: thin-walled vessels form intraluminal papillary projections; Coexpresses BV (CD34) and lymph (LYVE-1) markers
- Sinusoidal hemangioma: dilated intersecting channels in a Sieve-like/Sinosoidal pattern
- Spindle cell hemangioma: mixture of cavernous spaces and more cellular areas containing spindle cells w/ aggregates of vacuolated epithelioid cells
    - o Resembles "hemorrhagic lung" with alveolar spaces at scanning power
- Glomus tumor: rows of round dark nuclei w/ little cytoplasm ("String of black pearls") which Surround Subtle vascular Spaces (vs glomangioma which has prominent vessels)
- Acroangiodermatitis (pseudo-Kaposi sarcoma): proliferation of thick-walled capillaries in a lobular pattern, RBC extravasation, hemosiderin, dermal fibrosis, and PV lymphs; plasma cells are also found and may resemble Kaposi's, but there is a lack of atypical cells
- Kaposiform hemangioendothelioma: nodules of spindle cells w/ slit-like lumina containing RBCs (like nodular Kaposi's)
    - o CD61 confirms platelet trapping in cases of Kasabach-merritt
    - o Unlike infantile hemangiomas it is **GLUT-1 negative**
- Kaposi Sarcoma
    - o Patch/plaque stage (HELP): subtle or pronounced (in plaque stage) Hemosiderin, **Erythrocyte Extravasation**, infiltration of Lymphatic-like

vessels w/ Pale appearing stroma (looks under-stained), **Plasma cells, Promontory sign**

- Nodular stage: **nodules composed of fascicles of parallel spindle cells** w/ slit-like lumina containing RBCs; cells are never as atypical as those seen in angiosarcoma
  - IHC (HELP): HHV-8 or latency-associated nuclear antigen (**LANA-1**)
    - Mixed Lymphatic and BV phenotype (LYVE-1, CD34, VEGFR-3)

- Angiosarcoma ("SARC"): large, pleomorphic, crowded endothelial cells that **Stack on top of each other ("multilayered/piled-on")** and dissect between collagen bundles forming Anastomosing vascular networks w/ RBC extravasation and Cytoplasmic vacuoles
  - IHC ("Angi sarcs and FUCs MY External Genitalia"): FLI-1^{+}, Ulex europaeus lectin^{+}, CD31^{+}, CD34^{+}, c-MYC amplification (radiation-induced), ERG^{+} (most sens/specific)

Neural neoplasms (M-T)

- **Merkel cell carcinoma**: tightly packed and atypical small blue cells w/ ↑ N:C ratio which exhibit nuclear molding, numerous mitoses and speckled salt and pepper chromatin
  - **IHC: perinuclear dot pattern w/ CK20**
- MPNST: densely cellular (hypercellularity is more characteristic than atypia) proliferation of atypical intersecting spindle cells ("herringbone pattern") w/ large areas of necrosis; low power shows marbling due to alternating hypo- and hypercellular areas
- Neuroblastoma: small blue cells which form a dermal/SQ nodule
- Neurofibroma: loose arrangement of haphazard small wavy (S-shaped) spindle cells in pale myxoid stroma; numerous mast cells

- Neurothekeoma: multiple (plexiform) myxoid lobules containing bland spindle cells
- Cellular Neurothekeoma: multiple nests/lobules of epithelioid or spindled cells
- Nasal glioma: astrocytes w/ round vesicular nuclei in a loose neurofibrillary stroma
- Perineuroma: circumscribed tumor of spindle cells w/ onion skin-like whorls
- PEN: **superficial** dermal tumor w/ a **thin delicate capsule surrounding fascicles of spindle cells separated by clefts** (recapitulates normal nerve; Schwann cells:axons = 1:1)
    - May see **adjacent sebaceous glands and vellus hair follicles** typical of facial skin
- "Qutaneous" ganglioneuroma: localized collection of wavy Schwann cells admixed w/ large polygonal ganglion cells (big cells hanging on in the superficial dermis in "gangs")
- gRanular cell tumor: sheets of large polygonal cells w/ granular cytoplasm due to pink cytoplasmic inclusions (**Pustulo-Ovoid bodies)** w/ pseudoepitheliomatous hyperplasia
- Schwannoma (neurilemmoma): deep encapsulated proliferation of plump wavy Schwann cells w/ hypercellular (Antoni A) areas containing Verocay bodies (palisaded nuclei around acellular pink material) and hypocellular (Antoni B) myxoid areas
- Supernumerary digit: acral (thick stratum corneum) papule w/ nerve bundles
- Traumatic neuroma: like PEN, there is a haphazard proliferation of small nerve fascicles (resembles normal nerve in that Schwann cells and axons are in 1:1 ratio) separated by clefts however traumatic neuroma also has a background of scar and is not on the face

Neoplasms of fat ("fatty FLAPS")

- Fibrolipoma: large collagen bundles ("fibro") + mature fat ("lipoma")
- Lipoma: well-circumscribed tumor of mature lipocytes
- Angiolipoma: thrombosed capillary sized blood vessels ("angio") + mature fat ("lipoma")
- Angiomyolipoma: smooth muscle coming off vessel walls ("Angiomyo") + fat ("lipoma")
- Pleomorphic lipoma: **multinucleate floret cells** (overlapping nuclei arranged at the periphery like petals of a flower) + myxoid areas + ropey collagen bundles + mature fat
- Spindle cell lipoma (like pleomorphic lipoma w/o the floret cells): myxoid areas + ropey collagen bundles + mature fat ("I call it a ropey myxoid spindle cell lipoma to remind me of the ropey collagen in a myxoid stroma with surrounding spindle cells and lipocytes")

Smooth muscle neoplasms

- Pilar leiomyoma (piloleiomyoma): circumscribed but non-encapsulated (ill-defined) dermal nodule of intersecting bundles of smooth muscle cells (spindle cells w/ bright Pink cytoplasm and cigar-shaped nuclei w/ Perinuclear vacuole containing glycogen)
- Genital leiomyoma: similar to pilar leiomyoma but often larger and less circumscribed
- Angioleiomyoma: deep SQ nodule of smooth muscle containing slit-like vascular spaces
- Leiomyosarcoma: like leiomyoma but ↑ cellularity, atypia, pleomorphism and mitoses
- Smooth muscle hamartoma: numerous haphazard bundles of smooth muscle in the dermis (bundles are fewer and more discrete than those seen in leiomyoma)

CTCLs w/o a cytotoxic phenotype

- Mycosis fungoides: lichenoid band w/ epidermotropism of lymphs which may be in clusters (Pautrier's microabscesses) and lined up at the DEJ
- Lyp: discussed below
- Primary cutaneous anaplastic large cell lymphoma (ALCL): diffuse sheets of large, atypical $CD4^{+}$ > $CD30^{+}$ cells in the dermis +/- Hallmark (horseshoe) cells

Cytotoxic CTCLs: "EGS are fatty (located in fat) and toxic (cytotoxic: granzyme B+, TIA-1+)"

- Extranodal NK/T-cell lymphoma, nasal type: dense lymphoid infiltrate in SQ and dermis with angiodestruction; EBV+, CD2+, CD3epsilon+, and CD56+
- Gamma-delta T-cell lymphoma: **infiltrate in SQ, dermis and epidermis**; CD3+, CD56+
- Subcutaneous panniculitis-like T-cell lymphoma: **infiltrate is in SQ in a lace-like pattern with rimming of adipocytes (no dermis/epi involvement)**; CD8+
- Primary cutaneous aggressive epidermotropic CD8+ cytotoxic T-cell lymphoma has a cytotoxic phenotype but is superficial and epidermotropic (looks like MF)

Lymphomatoid papulosis subtypes ("My Ana is aggressive and a little Extra")

- Type A (typical LyP): wedge-shaped dermal infiltrate w/ lymphocytes, neutrophils, **eosinophils** and large $CD30^{+}$ (Ki-1) Reed-Sternberg-like cells
    - Resembles PLEVA but PLEVA never has large $CD30^{+}$ cells or eosinophils
- Type B (Mycosis fungoides-like): epidermotropic infiltrate of CD30 negative cells
- Type C (Anaplastic large cell lymphoma-like): diffuse sheets of large cells in the dermis

- Type D (primary cutaneous aggressive epidermotropic CD8⁺ cytotoxic T-cell lymphoma-like): markedly epidermotropic CD8⁺/CD30⁺/TIA-1⁺/granzyme B⁺ cells
- Type E (extranodal NK/T-cell lymphoma-like): angioinvasive CD30⁺/β F-1⁺ cells

Primary cutaneous B-cell neoplasms ("Full MIL")

- As the mnemonic progresses, the entities go from more common to less common, the MC location goes from superior to inferior and the prognosis gets worse
- Follicle center cell lymphoma: irregular neoplastic follicles which lack follicle polarity, lacks a well-defined mantle zone, lacks tingible body macrophages and lacks t(14;18) translocation (vs systemic follicular lymphoma); **BCL-6**⁺/BCL-2⁻
- Marginal zone lymphoma: "inverse" pattern of central darker benign reactive lymphocytes w/ surrounding neoplastic Monocytoid B-cells (marginal zone cells) and numerous plasma cells, some w/ Dutcher bodies; BCL-6⁻/**BCL-2**⁺
- Intravascular B-cell lymphoma: large, atypical B-cells within vessels; CD20⁺, CD79a⁺
- Diffuse Large B-cell lymphoma: dense infiltrate of Large atypical cells; **MUM**⁺/BCL2⁺/BCL6⁺/FOXP1⁺ ("Your MUM is quite large")

Connective tissue and depositional diseases

Occlusive/thrombotic vascular disease ("SCLE")

- Stasis change: **cannonball tufting of vessels in the superficial dermis**, RBC extravasation, dermal hemosiderin +/- thrombi of small vessels
- Coagulopathy (APLS, factor V Leiden, purpura fulminans, etc.): thrombi in vessels
- Cryoglobulinemia (type 1): **pink jelly** material **occluding vessel lumen**, RBC extravasation

- Livedoid vasculopathy (atrophie blanche): **hyalinized vessel walls ("pink crayon")** w/ thrombi and stasis change (cannonball tufting of superficial vessels, hemosiderin, RBCs)
- **Cholesterol Embolization: arteriole containing cholesterol clefts**

Square punch/dermal sclerosis ("Nice Sclerotic Cutis Can Make Good Square Biopsies")

- Necrobiosis lipoidica: horizontal acellular, pale degenerated collagen alternating w/ horizontal layers of granuloma ("layered cake"); plasma cells +/- cholesterol clefts
- Nephrogenic systemic fibrosis (NSF): ↑ CD34+ dermal fibroblasts, ↑ dermal mucin
    - Can be indistinguishable from scleromyxedema but in NSF the process is **deeper**, denser, more cellular, and less mucinous than in scleromyxedema
        - May extend into adipose, fascia and muscle (need deep incisional biopsy)
        - May see osseous metaplasia ("lollipop bodies")
- Scleromyxedema: ↑ CD34+ dermal fibroblasts ("sclero"), ↑ mucin ("myxedema")
- Scleredema: thickened dermis w/ widened spaces between collagen bundles (more evident in the deep dermis) filled w/ mucin (can be subtle and mimics normal back skin)
- Stiff skin syndrome: Sclerosis of the fascia but unlike deep morphea, there is no inflammation at the dermal/SQ junction, and it does not trap adnexal structures
- Connective tissue nevus: thick dermis due to excessive collagen and/or elastic tissue
- Chronic radiation dermatitis: papillary dermal pallor **w/o vacuolar change or a lymphoid band (vs LS&A)**, large stellate fibroblasts, loss of adnexa and superficial dilated vessels

- Morphea/scleroderma: **thick, closely packed (hyalinized) collagen bundles**, loss of adventitial fat resulting in **"trapped" eccrine glands**, ↓ CD34+ fibroblasts in the dermis, **lymphoplasmacytic infiltrate at dermal-SQ junction (can mimic panniculitis)**
- GVHD (sclerodermoid): dermis is thickened and sclerotic w/ no adnexal structures
- Scar: fibroblasts w/ east-west orientation and blood vessels w/ north-south orientation
    - Hypertrophic scar: nodules or whorls of thickened collagen and fibroblasts
    - Keloid: hyalinized "bubble gum" collagen in a background of hypertrophic scar
- Back skin: thick dermis (extends deeper than other sites); **no mucin (vs scleredema)**

Other sclerotic conditions not in the square punch mnemonic

- Lichen sclerosis ("red, white, blue"): compact stratum corneum w/ follicular plugging ("red"), papillary dermal pallor ("white") overlying a deeper lymphoid band ("blue")
    - **Process is too superficial to cause a square punch biopsy**
    - LS&A can also occur after radiation and look like radiation dermatitis on path but **LS&A has a lymphoid band, subtle vacuolar changes and lacks large fibroblasts**
- Eosinophilic fasciitis: thick eosinophilic fascia due to fibrosis and hyalinized collagen
    - Process is too deep to make a square punch (it's more dumbbell shaped)

Perforating disorders ("Emergency Room PA")

- Elastosis perforans serpiginosa: tortuous (serpiginous) channel through an acanthotic epidermis w/ extrusion of pink (Eosinophilic) elastic fibers
  - Penicillamine-induced EPS shows "bramble bush" elastic fibers (lateral buds)
- Reactive perforating collagenosis: broad (cup-shaped) vertical channel through an acanthotic epidermis w/ extrusion of basophilic collagen bundles
- Perforating calcific elastosis: keratotic plug w/ calcified elastic fibers (like PXE)
- Acquired perforating dermatoses (Kyrle's disease): most resembles RPC

Huge superficial mucin deposits ("Myxoid DFSP")

- Myxoid DFSP: like DFSP (bland spindled cells w/ storiform pattern) in a myxoid stroma
- Myxoid neurothekeoma (dermal nerve sheath myxoma): multinodular growth pattern w/ fibrous bands separating the nodules; nodules composed of cords of S100, GFAP and CD57-positive spindled or stellate cells in a background of abundant myxoid matrix
- Mucocele: pseudocystic space containing mucin +/- adjacent salivary gland
- DM/tumid lupus: abundant mucin in the dermis w/ PV/PA lymphs; mild interface change
- Digital mucoid cyst: **dome-shaped papule containing a pool of mucin on acral skin**
- Focal cutaneous mucinosis: **resembles digital mucoid cyst but is not on acral skin**
- Spindle cell lipoma/pleomorphic lipoma: **bland CD34+ spindle cells**, mature **adipocytes**, **wiry/ropy collagen** in a myxoid stroma (pleomorphic lipoma has floret cells)

- Pretibial myxedema: **large amounts of mucin throughout the entire dermis (deep too) w/ attenuation of collagen fibers (reduced to thin wisps)**
- Scleredema is not listed since the mucin (between collagen bundles) is deep and subtle

Calcification

- Calciphlaxis: **calcified small vessels in the SQ fat** w/ overlying epidermal necrosis
- Subepidermal calcified nodule: **pseudoepitheliomatous hyperplasia** w/ calcium deposits
- Scrotal calcinosis: **calcium masses; smooth muscle and rugated epidermis** (genital skin)

Deposition of fissured amorphous pale pink dermal material ("The MALE is pale")

- Colloid Milium: **very fragmented/fissured**, pale pink material in the superficial dermis; atrophic epidermis and surrounding solar elastosis
  - o Stains w/ amyloid stains (crystal violet, congo red, thioflavin t) except pagoda red
- Amyloid (nodular): large fissured pale pink nodules in the dermis; **many plasma cells**
  - o Primary systemic amyloid: amorphous eosinophilic fissured material
  - o Macular/lichen amyloid: small superficial dermal deposits (invisible dermatosis)
- Lipoid proteinosis: pale pink hyaline deposits which tend to be arranged perpendicular to the epidermis and around blood vessels, adnexal structures and eccrine glands
  - o Alcian blue+; PAS+ diastase resistant; usually negative for Amyloid stains
- Erythropoietic protoporphyria (EPP): PAS+ hyaline cuff (reduplicated basement membrane) **around superficial blood vessels** (post-capillary venules)

- There will be no solar elastosis (vs colloid milium) because patients avoid the sun
- PCT has much smaller hyaline cuffs of BMZ material around superficial vessels

Disorders of skin appendages and panniculitides

Non-scarring alopecia (all have ↑ % of catagen/telogen hairs; "All tricky tracts tell the pattern")

- "All tricky tracts": huge ↑ (> 50%) of hairs in catagen/telogen phase
  - Alopecia areata: **peri-bulbar lymphs ("swarm of bees")**, lymphs/eos/melanin within fibrous tract remnants, follicular miniaturization (resembles vellus hairs)
    - Syphilitic alopecia may be identical to alopecia areata but w/ plasma cells
  - Trichotillomania: **trichomalacia + melanin in hair canal (pigment casts)**
  - Traction alopecia: resembles trichotillomania on path
- "Tell the pattern": mild ↑ (25–50%) of hairs in catagen/telogen phase
  - Telogen effluvium: normal hair density w/ mild ↑ of catagen/telogen hairs
  - Pattern (androgenetic) alopecia: **miniature** anagen **follicles** w/ variable diameter (**anisotrichosis**), normal hair density and ↑ sebaceous glands (↑ androgens)
    - The scalp biopsy looks like facial skin (↑ sebaceous glands w/ vellus hairs)

Scarring/cicatricial alopecia (differentiate based on predominant cell type)

- Lymphocytes
  - CCCA: **Concentric lamellar fibrosis** + perifollicular lymphs (less dense than LPP)
    - Many dermatopathologists believe LPP and CCCA are on a spectrum
  - LPP (including FFA variant): **dense lichenoid interface at level of infundibulum**
    - Late stage: wedge-shaped scar (like wedge-shaped hypergranulosis in LP)
    - DIF: shaggy linear fibrin and cytoid bodies
  - Discoid lupus: dense lymphoid infiltrate (vacuolar or lichenoid) at level of isthmus (**deeper**), follicular hyperkeratosis, BMZ thickening, melanin pigment incontinence under DEJ, vertical columns of lymhs, PV/PA/PE lymphs, and mucin
    - Late stage: scar throughout entire dermis
    - DIF: continuous granular band of IgG/A/M and C3 at the follicular BMZ
- Neutrophils (2nd letter is an "e")
  - Dissecting cellulitis: neutrophilic abscesses, sinus tracts and granulation tissue
    - Hidradenitis suppurativa looks like this but on axillary/genital skin
  - Folliculitis decalvans: dense neutrophilic infiltrate at level of infundibulum
- Mixed (lymphoplasmacytic and neutrophilic) infiltrate
  - Acne keloidalis nuchae: perifollicular inflammation, plasma cells (posterior neck location), hypertrophic scar (not keloid) w/ concentric lamellar fibrosis
- Epithelioid histiocytes
  - Acute Langerhans cell histiocytosis: perifollicular epithelioid histiocytes w/ kidney-shaped nuclei at the level of the infundibulum

Septal panniculitis (erythema nodosum)

- Septal panniculitis: thickened and inflamed septa w/ lipocytes similar in size and shape ("looks like Cheerios") vs "oil-in-water" appearance of fat cells in lobular panniculitides
    - Septa: neuts in acute phase; granulomas (Miescher granuloma) in chronic phase

Lobular panniculitis (just like scarring alopecia, differentiate based on cell type)

- Lymphocytes
    - Lupus panniculitis (lupus profundus): **hyalinized septae**, **nodular lymphoid aggregates** w/ plasma cells, overlying interface dermatitis and dermal mucin
        - Ddx: SQ panniculitis-like Lymphoma (both entities display a lobular lymph infiltrate w/ lymphs rimming fat cells, but lupus panniculitis is more likely to show epidermal atrophy, interface changes w/ thickened BM, mucin, follicular plugging, hyaline lipomembraneous change, B-cell follicles and a mixed infiltrate of plasma cells, and plasmacytoid dendritic cell aggregates
- Granulomatous (giant cells + histiocytes)
    - SQ fat necrosis of the newborn/post-steroid panniculitis/sclerema neonatorum: **fat crystallization** (radial crystals in fat)
    - Cytophagic histiocytic panniculitis: beanbag cells (giant cells engulf RBCs/WBCs)
- Eosinophils
    - Eosinophilic panniculitis: eosinophils in the fat lobules and septae
- Neutrophils ("I'M A neutrophilic lobular panniculitis")
    - Infectious: mixed inflammation and necrosis of fat lobules (rule out with stains)

  - Myelodysplastic syndrome
  - Alpha$_1$-antitrypsin deficiency: neuts + liquefactive necrosis of septum and dermis
- Neutrophils w/ vasculitis
  - Nodular vasculitis/erythema induratum: LCV of all vessel sizes (in dermis and fat)
- Others
  - Pancreatic panniculitis: calcium soap outlining necrotic lipocytes (saponification)
  - Lipodermatosclerosis (stasis panniculitis): **lipomembraneous change ("frost on a window") w/ overlying stasis change** (nodular angioplasia and hemosiderin)
  - Cold panniculitis (deep perniosis): lobular fat necrosis w/ mixed infiltrate (lymphs, histiocytes, neuts) and overlying perniosis (papillary dermal edema)

Infectious

Bacterial rods or cocci in the stratum corneum ("PIE")

- Pitted keratolysis: pit in stratum corneum w/ G+ rods and cocci at base of dell; acral skin
- Impetigo: **clusters of G+ cocci and neutrophilic crust in stratum corneum**
- Erythrasma: G+ rods forming vertical filaments in stratum corneum (normal skin ddx)
- Ecthyma ("ulcerated impetigo"): **G+ cocci (staph colonies) at the base of an ulcer**
  - Don's confuse w/ ecthyma gangrenosum: G- bacteria around vessels (light blue haze) + lack of inflammation (no dark blue lymphs) + pink necrosis of vessels

PEH w/ neutrophilic intraepidermal pustule ("Here Come Big Green Leafy Veggies")

- Halogenoderma: pseudoepitheliomatous hyperplasia (PEH) + pus but **no organisms**
- Chromomycosis: **round copper-colored Medlar bodies ("Copper pennies")**
- Blastomycosis: organisms have an asymmetric refractile wall w/ dark Blue nucleus; if Budding is present it is Broad-Based ("looks like a snowman")
- Granuloma inguinale: organisms within histiocytes (Donovan bodies)
- Leishmaniasis: parasitized organisms at periphery of histiocytes (marquee sign)
- Pemphigus vegetans: PEH w/ **eosinophilic pustules;** no organisms

Parasitized histiocytes/organisms within histiocytes ("pH GIRL")

- Penicillium marneffei: looks like histoplasmosis on path but patient is from SE Asia
- Histoplasmosis: small uniform dots evenly spaces within histiocytes; no kinetoplasts
    - African histoplasmosis: large clear yeast evenly spaced within histiocytes
- Granuloma inguinale: organisms in histiocytes (Donovan bodies)
- Rhinoscleroma: **sheets of plasma cells**, Russell bodies (plasma cells filled with bright pink immunoglobin), Mikulicz cells (histiocytes with large round collections of bacilli)
- Leishmania: organisms at periphery of histiocytes (marquee sign) +/- kinetoplasts
- **Lepromatous leprosy: sheets of histiocytes containing globi (amphophilic collections of mycobacteria which stain w/ Fite stain); grenz zone**

- o Tuberculoid leprosy: epithelioid granulomas ("sausages") running east-west in dermis (tracks along nerves) and lacks globi (so Fite stain is negative)

Deep fungal infections not in PEH + pus or pH GIRL mnemonics

- Coccidioidomycosis: **large spherules** (much larger than surrounding cells) w/ gray lacy and granular cytoplasm; uniform size and shape; refractile wall +/- PEH + pus
- Cryptococcus: **yeast w/ clear gelatinous capsule** (around same size as surrounding cells)
  - o Capsule stains red w/ mucicarmine; organisms stain w/ Fontana-Masson
  - o Ddx: round yeast are same size and shape to blastomycosis but blasto has PEH + pus and yeast in crypto have a clear gelatinous capsule
- Paracoccidioides (South-American Blasto): **Mariner's wheel pattern** of budding yeast
- Lobomycosis: **organisms in chains** ("resembling pop-beads")
- Sporotrichosis: palisaded neutrophilic abscess +/- **cigar-shaped yeasts** (not usually seen)
- Zygomycosis (Rhizopus): **Red 90° (Right-angle) non-septate hyphae** ("Red Ribbon")
- Hyalohyphomycosis (Aspergillosis/fusariosis): non-pigmented **septate** hyphae that **invade vessels, branch at a 45° angle (Acute)**; surrounded by bright pink immunoglobin (Splendore-Hoeppli phenomenon but not in BEAN mnemonic as it does not coat grains)
- Protothecosis: non-pigmented algae which demonstrate **soccer ball-like Murula**
- Rhinosporidiosis: huge sporangia (larger than coccidioidomycosis) w/ many endospores

Splendore-Hoeppli phenomenon (deposition of pink immunoglobin at the edge of grain/BEAN)

- Botryomycosis: grains composed of huge staph colonies; neuts/sinus tracts
- Eumycetoma: grains composed of fungal hyphae (may be pigmented); neuts/sinus tracts
    - Pigmented eumycetoma ("My Lousy Greasy Jeans are black"): Madurella mycetomatis, Leptosphaeria spp, M. grisea, Exophiala jeanselmei)
    - The MC eumycetoma is the non-pigmented P. boydii ("white boy")
- Actinomycetoma: grains composed of filamentous bacteria; neuts/sinus tracts
    - Nocardia brasiliensis (white grains; "white note cards"), Actinomyces israelii (yellow), Actinomadura pelletieri (red), Actinomadura madurae (pink/cream)
- Nocardia: MC type of actinomycetoma

Pigmented fungi ("the dark art of CPT code manipulation")

- Chromoblastomycosis: PEH + pus; round pigmented medlar bodies in the dermis
- Phaeohyphomycosis: long thin **pigmented hyphae in the dermis**
    - Pheaeomycotic cysts have these hyphae in cyst walls (MC organism is Exophiala jeanselmei and unlike phaeohyphomycosis, occurs in immunocompetent people)
- Tinea nigra: **pigmented hyphae in thickened (acral skin) stratum corneum**

HPV infections

- Verruca vulgaris: papillomatous exophytic lesion w/ hypergranulosis and koilocytes (keratinocytes w/ clear cytoplasm and shrunken "raisin-like" nuclei)

- Myrmecia: endophytic lesion w/ course red cytoplasmic inclusions
- Verruca plana: flatter lesion w/ rounded koilocytes ("bird-eyes") w/o shriveled nuclei
- Epidermodysplasia verruciformis (β HPV types): verruca plana w/ **βlue cytoplasm**
    - The truncal tinea versicolor-like macules also look like this
- Condyloma acuminatum (CA): **path looks like SK in genitals** w/ vacuolated keratinocytes, round parakeratosis and course hypergranulosis
- **Bowenoid papulosis: can look like CA but w/ Bowenoid full thickness atypia**
- Verrucous cyst: cyst with wart-like lining
- Heck's disease: rounded parakeratosis (red) atop epithelial pallor (white)

HSV infections

- HSV 1–3: **Multinucleated keratinocytes w/ nuclear Molding and Margination of chromatin to the periphery** (looks like a cluster of grapes or egg-shells)
- HSV5 (CMV): large swollen endothelial cells w/ intranuclear inclusions ("owl's eye")

Poxvirus

- Smallpox: epidermal necrosis w/ reticular degeneration and eosinophilic inclusions
- Monkeypox: like smallpox but w/ Multinucleated keratinocytes
- Molluscum contagiosum: cup-shaped lesion w/ Henderson-Paterson bodies
- Parapox (Orf and Milker's nodules): → **"ENBREL"**
    - Epidermal Necrosis (late lesions)
    - Bodies (eosinophilic cytoplasmic viral inclusion bodies in keratinocytes)
    - Reticular degeneration (intraepidermal vesiculation)

- o Eosinophilic viral inclusions are characteristic of parapox virus infection
- o Long slender epidermal acanthosis

Other viruses

- Coxsackievirus (hand-foot-mouth): **reticular or ballooning degeneration and necrotic keratinocytes** affecting the upper half of the epidermis ("cox-half-ie"); often acral skin
- Gianotti-Crosti syndrome: non-specific but shows papillary dermal edema, spongiosis and a superficial perivascular lymphoid infiltrate

Parasites ("My there are LOTS of parasites")

- Myiasis: fly larva w/ thick undulating chitinous wall w/ pigmented setae
    - o "My undulating chitinous wall"
- Larva currens: larval nematode within the dermis
- Cutaneous Larva migrans: may see worm in the epidermis
- Onchocerciasis: microfilaria within lymphatics
- Tungiasis: chitinous gravid flea w/ striated muscle and guts ("looks Trippy") on acral skin
- Tick: organism w/ chitinous wall, striated muscle and blood-filled guts attached to skin
- Sparganosis: Subcutaneous cestode w/ Smooth muscle and calcareous bodies
- Scabies: chitinous pigtails within the Stratum corneum

Miscellaneous dermpath differentials

Papillary dermal edema ("PASTE"): differentiate these based on cells type

- PMLE: superficial **lymphocytic** infiltrate; **not on acral skin** +/- dyskeratotic keratinocytes

- Perniosis: superficial and deep **lymphocytic** infiltrate with damaged vessels; **acral skin**
    - o The deep lymphocytes are primarily around eccrine glands (vs follicles in lupus)
- Arthropod assault/Well's syndrome: superficial and deep **eosinophilic** infiltrate
- Sweet's syndrome: diffuse **neutrophilic** infiltrate
- Tinea (bullous): variable infiltrate w/ PAS+ hyphae in the epidermis
- Erythema multiforme: vacuolar infiltrate w/ keratinocyte death; mostly lymphocytes
- Early EED: looks like Sweets (later lesions show onion skin fibrosis)

Invisible dermatosis: "TRUMPS ALIVE but we can't see him because he's invisible (cancelled)"

- TMEP: **subtle increase in perivascular spindle-shaped mast cells in the upper dermis**
- Tinea: non-pigmented hyphae in stratum corneum that is compact just above granular layer and normal basket weave on the very top (may see parakeratosis or neutrophils)
- Tinea versicolor: short curved hyphae and round spores (ziti and meatballs) in corneum
- Regressing melanoma: may see a subtle lichenoid inflammation w/ melanophages
- Urticaria: intravascular and perivascular neutrophilic infiltrate
- Ulerythema ophryogenes (and all KP variants): plugging of hair follicles + hyperkeratosis
- Macular amyloid: subtle pink material in the papillary dermis outlined by melanophages
- PXE: **curly calcified elastic fibers ("twigs on the bramble bush")** in the dermis
- Psoriasis (guttate): mounds of parakeratosis w/ neutrophils and mild spongiosis

- Scleredema: **mucin separating collagen in the deep dermis** (looks like normal back skin)
- Argyria: **tiny gray/black granules concentrated around eccrine glands**
- Atrophoderma (superficial morphea): dermis is less thick and individual collagen bundles are smaller (H&E changes subtle unless compared against normal adjacent skin)
- Anetoderma: elastic fibers are absent in the superficial and mid-dermis (normal H&E)
    - Mid-dermal elastolysis: absent elastic fibers in the mid-dermis only
    - Cutis laxa: absent elastic fibers at all levels of the dermis
- Lichen amyloid: same as macular amyloid but with overlying acanthosis + hyperkeratosis
- Ichthyosis vulgaris: **compact hyper-orthokeratosis with a paradoxically diminished granular layer** (pityriasis rotunda looks identical on path)
- Vitiligo: absence of melanocytes in basal layer
- Erythrasma: very small/thin G+ rods forming vertical filaments in the stratum corneum

Note, the mnemonic above are things that resemble normal skin at scan, **nevus anemicus** however is histologically and ultrastructurally identical to normal skin

Busy dermis ("Busy Dermis Can Kill Grandmas Sweet Niece")

- Blue nevus: pigmented dendritic melanocytes in a sclerotic dermis; pigment extends to the base but there are no deep mitoses or necrosis
- Desmoplastic melanoma: busy dermis w/ spindled cell proliferation in a sclerotic dermis that looks scar-like but cells are more hyperchromatic; **lymph aggregates** is a good clue

- Dermal spitz: enlarged epithelioid cells intersecting through collagen bundles; pigment
- Dermatofibroma: interstitial spindle cell proliferation, collagen trapping towards the periphery, overlying plate-like acanthosis w/ follicular induction
- Cutaneous metastasis: varies based on type for example breast carcinoma, carcinoma en cuirasse and leukemia cutis have large atypical cells lining up single file (Indian filing); RCC shows tubules of clear cells w/ prominent blood vessels and RBC extravasation
- Kaposi's (patch/plaque stage): dermal vessels give a busy appearance; **promontory sign**
- Granuloma annulare (interstitial): patchy interstitial histiocytes, lymphocytes and **mucin**
- Scleromyxedema: ↑ dermal fibroblasts, fine collagen fibers and interstitial mucin
- Neurofibroma: comma-shaped spindle cells in a pale mucinous stroma w/ mast cells

Index

A

B

C

D

E

F

G

H

M

N

Q

R

S

T

U

V

W

X

Y

Z

About the Author

Dr. Jeffrey Morris is a dual board-certified dermatologist and Mohs surgeon. He was born and raised in Fort Lauderdale, Florida, and graduated with honors from Rollins College in Winter Park, Florida. There he was inducted into the college's hall of fame in men's tennis.

Afterwards, he went to medical school at Nova Southeastern University in Fort Lauderdale, where he was selected into the highly coveted Nova Southeastern University Research Fellowship program, which gave him a full academic scholarship and allowed him to pursue his research interests.

During the fellowship, he published numerous peer-reviewed articles on the subject of skin cancer and dermoscopy.

After medical school, he completed his internship in Miami at Larkin Community Hospital and then completed his dermatology residency in Detroit at Beaumont, where he was chief resident.

Currently, he practices in The Villages, Florida, where he does a mix of Mohs surgery, general dermatology, and cosmetics.

Mnemonics has always helped him remember medical jargon, and over the years in his medical training, he has become quite adept at creating helpful mnemonics that allows him to remember the facts necessary to go into his various in-service and board exams with confidence. After acing the updated dermatology board exam, he wanted to share these mnemonics with his future colleagues. He hopes they help you as much as they helped him.

www.ingramcontent.com/pod-product-compliance
Lightning Source LLC
LaVergne TN
LVHW052202200926
848481LV00001B/11

* 9 7 9 8 8 9 3 0 8 4 4 8 1 *